THE WASHINGTON MANUAL™
OF CRITICAL CARE

THE WASHINGTON MANUAL™ OF CRITICAL CARE

2nd Edition

Marin H. Kollef, MD

Professor of Medicine
Virginia E. and Sam J. Golman Chair in Respiratory Intensive Care Medicine
Director, Respiratory Care Services
Director, Critical Care Research
Division of Pulmonary and Critical Care Medicine
Washington University School of Medicine
Barnes-Jewish Hospital
St. Louis, Missouri

Warren Isakow, MD

Assistant Professor of Medicine
Director, Medical Intensive Care Unit
Division of Pulmonary and Critical Care Medicine
Washington University School of Medicine
Barnes-Jewish Hospital
St. Louis, Missouri

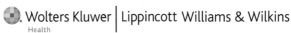
. Wolters Kluwer | Lippincott Williams & Wilkins
Health

Philadelphia · Baltimore · New York · London
Buenos Aires · Hong Kong · Sydney · Tokyo

Acquisitions Editor: Brian Brown
Product Manager: Nicole Dernoski
Production Manager: Bridgett Dougherty
Senior Manufacturing Manager: Benjamin Rivera
Design Coordinator: Holly McLaughlin
Production Service: Aptara, Inc.

Library of Congress Cataloging-in-Publication Data
The Washington manual of critical care / [edited by] Marin H. Kollef, Warren Isakow.
   p. ; cm.
   Manual of critical care
   Includes bibliographical references and index.
   ISBN 978-1-4511-1022-7
   I. Kollef, Marin H.   II. Isakow, Warren.   III. Title: Manual of critical care.
   [DNLM: 1. Critical Care–methods–Handbooks.   2. Critical Illness–therapy–
Handbooks. WX 39]
   LC classification not assigned
   616.02'8–dc23   2011031694

Care has been taken to confirm the accuracy of the information presented and to describe generally accepted
practices. However, the authors, editors, and publisher are not responsible for errors or omissions or for any
consequences from application of the information in this book and make no warranty, expressed or implied,
with respect to the currency, completeness, or accuracy of the contents of the publication. Application of the
information in a particular situation remains the professional responsibility of the practitioner.

   The authors, editors, and publisher have exerted every effort to ensure that drug selection and dosage
set forth in this text are in accordance with current recommendations and practice at the time of publication.
However, in view of ongoing research, changes in government regulations, and the constant flow of
information relating to drug therapy and drug reactions, the reader is urged to check the package insert for
each drug for any change in indications and dosage and for added warnings and precautions. This is
particularly important when the recommended agent is a new or infrequently employed drug.

   Some drugs and medical devices presented in the publication have Food and Drug Administration
(FDA) clearance for limited use in restricted research settings. It is the responsibility of the health care
providers to ascertain the FDA status of each drug or device planned for use in their clinical practice.

To purchase additional copies of this book, call our customer service department at (800) 638-3030 or fax
orders to (301) 223-2320. International customers should call (301) 223-2300.

Visit Lippincott Williams & Wilkins on the Internet: at LWW.com. Lippincott Williams & Wilkins
customer service representatives are available from 8:30 am to 6 pm, EST.

10 9 8 7 6 5 4 3 2 1

We dedicate this manual to all health care providers involved in the care of critically ill patients and their families. We acknowledge their efforts and sacrifices and hope that this manual can assist them in some meaningful manner.
To our families for their support and to the critical care and academic communities of Washington University and Barnes-Jewish Hospital for their commitment to the education and well-being of medical students and house staff physicians.

Contributors

Anupam Aditi, MD
Resident
Department of Medicine
Washington University School of Medicine
Barnes-Jewish Hospital
St. Louis, Missouri

Jennifer Alexander-Brett, MD, PhD
Fellow
Division of Pulmonary and Critical Care Medicine
Washington University School of Medicine
Barnes-Jewish Hospital
St. Louis, Missouri

Richard G. Bach, MD
Associate Professor of Medicine
Cardiovascular Division
Director, Cardiac Intensive Care Unit
Washington University School of Medicine
Barnes-Jewish Hospital
St. Louis, Missouri

Timothy Bedient, MD
Fellow
Division of Pulmonary and Critical Care Medicine
University of Colorado Denver
Aurora, Colorado

Morey A. Blinder, MD
Associate Professor of Medicine, Pathology and Immunology
Division of Hematology
Washington University School of Medicine
Barnes-Jewish Hospital
St. Louis, Missouri

Linda Bobo, MD, PhD
Fellow
Division of Infectious Diseases
Washington University School of Medicine
Barnes-Jewish Hospital
St. Louis, Missouri

Alan C. Braverman, MD
Alumni Endowed Professor in Cardiovascular Disease
Professor of Medicine
Cardiovascular Division
Chief of Service, Inpatient Cardiology Firm
Director, Marfan Syndrome Clinic
Washington University School of Medicine
Barnes-Jewish Hospital
St. Louis, Missouri

Stephen R. Broderick, MD
Fellow
Division of Cardiothoracic Surgery
Washington University School of Medicine
Barnes-Jewish Hospital
St. Louis, Missouri

Steven L. Brody, MD
Associate Professor of Medicine
Division of Pulmonary and Critical Care Medicine
Washington University School of Medicine
Barnes-Jewish Hospital
St. Louis, Missouri

Derek E. Byers, MD, PhD
Assistant Professor of Medicine
Division of Pulmonary and Critical Care
  Medicine
Washington University School of Medicine
Barnes-Jewish Hospital
St. Louis, Missouri

Bernard C. Camins, MD, MSCR
Assistant Professor of Medicine
Division of Infectious Diseases
Associate Hospital Epidemiologist
Washington University School of
  Medicine
Barnes-Jewish Hospital
St. Louis, Missouri

Jeanine F. Carbone, MD
Fellow
Department of Obstetrics and Gynecology
Washington University School of Medicine
Barnes-Jewish Hospital
St. Louis, Missouri

Mario Castro, MD, MPH
Professor of Medicine and Pediatrics
Division of Pulmonary and Critical Care
  Medicine
Washington University School of Medicine
Barnes-Jewish Hospital
St. Louis, Missouri

Murali M. Chakinala, MD
Associate Professor of Medicine
Division of Pulmonary and Critical Care
  Medicine
Washington University School of Medicine
Barnes-Jewish Hospital
St. Louis, Missouri

Alexander Chen, MD
Assistant Professor of Medicine and
  Surgery
Director of Interventional Pulmonology
Division of Pulmonary and Critical Care
  Medicine
Washington University School of Medicine
Barnes-Jewish Hospital
St. Louis, Missouri

Steven C. Cheng, MD
Assistant Professor of Medicine
Renal Division
Washington University School of
  Medicine
Barnes-Jewish Hospital
St. Louis, Missouri

William E. Clutter, MD
Associate Professor of Medicine
Division of Endocrinology, Metabolism,
  and Lipid Research
Washington University School of
  Medicine
Barnes-Jewish Hospital
St. Louis, Missouri

Daniel H. Cooper, MD
Assistant Professor of Medicine
Cardiovascular Division
Washington University School of Medicine
Barnes-Jewish Hospital
St. Louis, Missouri

Jeffrey S. Crippin, MD
Marilyn Bornefeld Chair in
  Gastrointestinal Research and Treatment
Division of Gastroenterology
Medical Director, Liver Transplantation
Washington University School of
  Medicine
Barnes-Jewish Hospital
St. Louis, Missouri

Alex E. Denes, MD
Associate Professor
Division of Oncology
Director, Inpatient Oncology
Washington University School of
  Medicine
Barnes-Jewish Hospital
St. Louis, Missouri

Jeremiah Depta, MD
Fellow
Cardiovascular Division
Washington University School of
  Medicine
Barnes-Jewish Hospital
St. Louis, Missouri

Rajat Dhar, MD, FRCPC
Assistant Professor of Neurology
Department of Neurology
Washington University School of Medicine
Barnes-Jewish Hospital
St. Louis, Missouri

Erik R. Dubberke, MD, MSPH
Assistant Professor
Associate Hospital Epidemiologist
Division of Infectious Diseases
Washington University School of Medicine
Barnes-Jewish Hospital
St. Louis, Missouri

Michael J. Durkin, MD
Instructor in Medicine
Department of Medicine
Washington University School of
    Medicine
Barnes-Jewish Hospital
St. Louis, Missouri

Gregory A. Ewald, MD
Associate Professor
Cardiovascular Division
Medical Director, Cardiac Transplant
    Program
Washington University School of
    Medicine
Barnes-Jewish Hospital
St. Louis, Missouri

Derrick R. Fansler, MD
Fellow
Cardiovascular Division
Washington University School of
    Medicine
Barnes-Jewish Hospital
St. Louis, Missouri

Saad Ghafoor, MD
Fellow
Department of Pediatrics
Washington University School of
    Medicine
St. Louis Children's Hospital
St. Louis, Missouri

Jennifer L. Gnerlich, MD
Resident
Division of General Surgery
Washington University School of
    Medicine
Barnes-Jewish Hospital
St. Louis, Missouri

Seth Goldberg, MD
Assistant Professor of Medicine
Renal Division
Washington University School of
    Medicine
Barnes-Jewish Hospital
St. Louis, Missouri

Jonathan M. Green, MD
Associate Professor of Medicine, Pathology
    and Immunobiology
Associate Dean for Human Studies
Executive Chair of the Institutional
    Review Board (IRB)
Division of Pulmonary and Critical Care
    Medicine
Washington University School of
    Medicine
Barnes-Jewish Hospital
St. Louis, Missouri

Brenda J. Grossman, MD, MPH
Associate Professor of Pathology and
    Immunology
Medical Director, Transfusion Medicine
    Services
Department of Laboratory and Genomic
    Medicine
Washington University School of
    Medicine
Barnes-Jewish Hospital
St. Louis, Missouri

**Chandra Prakash Gyawali, MD,
MRCP**
Professor of Medicine
Division of Gastroenterology
Washington University School of
    Medicine
Barnes-Jewish Hospital
St. Louis, Missouri

Ahmed Hassan, MD
Assistant Professor of Neurology
Department of Neurology
Washington University School of
  Medicine
Barnes-Jewish Hospital
St. Louis, Missouri

Hitoshi Honda, MD
Fellow
Division of Infectious Diseases
Washington University School of Medicine
Barnes-Jewish Hospital
St. Louis, Missouri

Molly Houser, MD
Fellow
Department of Obstetrics and Gynecology
Washington University School of Medicine
Barnes-Jewish Hospital
St. Louis, Missouri

Yen-Michael S. Hsu, MD, PhD
Resident
Department of Pathology and
  Immunology
Washington University School of
  Medicine
Barnes-Jewish Hospital
St. Louis, Missouri

Howard J. Huang, MD
Instructor in Medicine
Division of Pulmonary and Critical Care
  Medicine
Washington University School of
  Medicine
Barnes-Jewish Hospital
St. Louis, Missouri

Warren Isakow, MD
Assistant Professor of Medicine
Director, Medical Intensive Care Unit
Division of Pulmonary and Critical Care
  Medicine
Washington University School of Medicine
Barnes-Jewish Hospital
St. Louis, Missouri

Peter Juran, MD
Postdoctoral Fellow
Renal Division
Washington University School of
  Medicine
Barnes-Jewish Hospital
St. Louis, Missouri

Andrew M. Kates, MD
Associate Professor of Medicine
Director, Cardiovascular Fellowship
  Program
Cardiovascular Division
Washington University School of
  Medicine
Barnes-Jewish Hospital
St. Louis, Missouri

Jeremy Kilburn, MD
Fellow
Division of Pulmonary and Critical Care
  Medicine
Washington University School of
  Medicine
Barnes-Jewish Hospital
St. Louis, Missouri

John P. Kirby, MD
Associate Professor of Surgery
Division of General Surgery
Director, Wound Healing Program
Washington University School of
  Medicine
Barnes-Jewish Hospital
St. Louis, Missouri

Marin H. Kollef, MD
Professor of Medicine
Virginia E. and Sam J. Golman Chair in
  Respiratory and Intensive Care Medicine
Director, Respiratory Care Services
Director, Critical Care Research
Division of Pulmonary and Critical Care
  Medicine
Washington University School of
  Medicine
Barnes-Jewish Hospital
St. Louis, Missouri

Kevin M. Korenblat, MD
Associate Professor of Medicine
Division of Gastroenterology
Washington University School of Medicine
Barnes-Jewish Hospital
St. Louis, Missouri

Mrudula V. Kumar, MD
Fellow
Division of Gastroenterology
Washington University School of Medicine
Barnes-Jewish Hospital
St. Louis, Missouri

Andrew Labelle, MD
Fellow
Division of Pulmonary and Critical Care
   Medicine
Washington University School of Medicine
Barnes-Jewish Hospital
St. Louis, Missouri

Shane J. LaRue, MD
Fellow
Cardiovascular Division
Washington University School of Medicine
Barnes-Jewish Hospital
St. Louis, Missouri

Steven J. Lawrence, MD
Assistant Professor of Medicine
Division of Infectious Diseases
Washington University School of Medicine
Barnes-Jewish Hospital
St. Louis, Missouri

Tinting Li, MD
Assistant Professor of Medicine
Renal Division
Washington University School of Medicine
Barnes-Jewish Hospital
St. Louis, Missouri

Stephen Y. Liang, MD
Fellow
Division of Infectious Diseases
Washington University School of Medicine
Barnes-Jewish Hospital
St. Louis, Missouri

Michael Lippmann, MD
Professor of Medicine
Division of Pulmonary and Critical Care
   Medicine
Washington University School of Medicine
St. Louis Veterans Affairs Medical Center
St. Louis, Missouri

John E. Mazuski, MD, PhD
Professor of Surgery
Division of General Surgery
Washington University School of Medicine
Barnes-Jewish Hospital
St. Louis, Missouri

Kevin W. McConnell, MD
Assistant Professor of Surgery
Department of Acute and Critical
   Care Surgery
Emory University
Atlanta, Georgia

Scott T. Micek, PharmD
Clinical Pharmacist
Department of Pharmacy
Washington University School of Medicine
Barnes-Jewish Hospital
St. Louis, Missouri

Nicholas M. Mohr, MD
Assistant Professor of Medicine
Department of Anesthesiology
Department of Emergency Medicine
Washington University School of Medicine
Barnes-Jewish Hospital
St. Louis, Missouri

James C. Mosley III, MD
Attending Physician
Department of Hematology
Southeast Hospital
Cape Girardeau, Missouri

Daniel K. Mullady, MD
Assistant Professor of Medicine
Division of Gastroenterology
Washington University School of Medicine
Barnes-Jewish Hospital
St. Louis, Missouri

Hannah Otepka, MD
Resident
Department of Medicine
Washington University School of Medicine
Barnes-Jewish Hospital
St. Louis, Missouri

Laura A. Parks, MD
Assistant Professor
Department of Obstetrics and Gynecology
Washington University School of Medicine
Barnes-Jewish Hospital
St. Louis, Missouri

Varun Puri, MD
Assistant Professor of Surgery
Division of General Thoracic Surgery
Washington University School of Medicine
Barnes-Jewish Hospital
St. Louis, Missouri

Amy M. Richmond, RN, MHS, CIC
Department of Medicine
Washington University School of
Medicine
Barnes-Jewish Hospital
St. Louis, Missouri

David Rometo, MD
Fellow
Division of Endocrinology, Metabolism,
and Lipid Research
Washington University School of Medicine
Barnes-Jewish Hospital
St. Louis, Missouri

Ryan P. Roop, MD
Fellow
Divisions of Hematology and Oncology
Washington University School of Medicine
Barnes-Jewish Hospital
St. Louis, Missouri

Jamie M. Rosini, PharmD
Clinical Pharmacist
Department of Pharmacy
Washington University School of Medicine
Barnes-Jewish Hospital
St. Louis, Missouri

Michael A. Rubin, MD
Assistant Professor of Neurology
Department of Neurology
Washington University School of
Medicine
Barnes-Jewish Hospital
St. Louis, Missouri

Tonya D. Russell, MD
Associate Professor of Medicine
Director, Pulmonary & Critical Care
Medicine Fellowship
Division of Pulmonary and Critical Care
Medicine
Washington University School of
Medicine
Barnes-Jewish Hospital
St. Louis, Missouri

Douglas J.E. Schuerer, MD
Associate Professor of Surgery
Director of Trauma
Director of Surgical Critical
Care Fellowship
Division of General Surgery
Washington University School of
Medicine
Barnes-Jewish Hospital
St. Louis, Missouri

Jennifer Shaffer, MD
Fellow
Division of Pulmonary and Critical Care
Medicine
Washington University School of
Medicine
Barnes-Jewish Hospital
St. Louis, Missouri

Jay Shah, MD
Fellow
Cardiovascular Division
Washington University School of
Medicine
Barnes-Jewish Hospital
St. Louis, Missouri

Devin P. Sherman, MD
Fellow
Division of Pulmonary and Critical Care
Medicine
Washington University School of
Medicine
Barnes-Jewish Hospital
St. Louis, Missouri

Lee P. Skrupky, PharmD
Clinical Pharmacist
Department of Pharmacy
Washington University School of
Medicine
Barnes-Jewish Hospital
St. Louis, Missouri

Robert Southard, MD
Assistant Professor of Surgery
Division of General Surgery
Washington University School of
Medicine
Barnes-Jewish Hospital
St. Louis, Missouri

Molly J. Stout, MD
Fellow
Department of Obstetrics and Gynecology
Washington University School of
Medicine
Barnes-Jewish Hospital
St. Louis, Missouri

Toshibumi Taniguchi, MD
Fellow
Division of Infectious Diseases
Washington University School of
Medicine
Barnes-Jewish Hospital
St. Louis, Missouri

**Beth E. Taylor, MS, RD, CNSD,
FCCM**
Clinical Dietician
Department of Food and Nutrition
Washington University School of
Medicine
Barnes-Jewish Hospital
St. Louis, Missouri

Garry S. Tobin, MD
Associate Professor of Medicine
Division of Endocrinology
Director, Diabetes Center
Washington University School of Medicine
Barnes-Jewish Hospital
St. Louis, Missouri

Ahsan Usman, MD
Clinical Fellow
Renal Division
Washington University School of
Medicine
Barnes-Jewish Hospital
St. Louis, Missouri

Anitha Vijayan, MD
Associate Professor of Medicine
Renal Division
Medical Director, Acute Dialysis Unit
Washington University School of Medicine
Barnes-Jewish Hospital
St. Louis, Missouri

Sundeep Viswanathan, MD
Instructor in Medicine
Department of Medicine
Washington University School of
Medicine
Barnes-Jewish Hospital
St. Louis, Missouri

David K. Warren, MD, MPH
Associate Professor of Medicine
Division of Infectious Diseases
Hospital Epidemiologist
Washington University School of
Medicine
Barnes-Jewish Hospital
St. Louis, Missouri

Chad A. Witt, MD
Fellow
Division of Pulmonary and Critical Care
Medicine
Washington University School of
Medicine
Barnes-Jewish Hospital
St. Louis, Missouri

Keith F. Woeltje, MD, PhD
Professor of Medicine
Division of Infectious Diseases
Director, Clinical Advisory Group
  and Healthcare Informatics
Washington University School of
  Medicine
Barnes-Jewish Hospital
St. Louis, Missouri

Roger D. Yusen, MD, MPH, FCCP
Associate Professor of Medicine
Medical Director, Lung Volume Reduction
  Surgery
Division of Pulmonary and Critical Care
  Medicine
Washington University School of Medicine
Barnes-Jewish Hospital
St. Louis, Missouri

Preface

This is the second edition of *The Washington Manual™ of Critical Care*, building upon the first edition and adding to the long tradition of medical education promoted by *The Washington Manual™ of Medical Therapeutics* and the associated medical and surgical subspecialty manuals published from Washington University. Our continued goal in publishing this manuscript is to provide experienced clinicians and trainees a resource containing comprehensive and current treatment algorithms for the bedside diagnosis and management of the most frequently encountered illnesses and problems in the intensive care unit (ICU). In this edition, we continue to focus on the delivery of concise algorithms in order to expedite bedside decision-making. The chapters include annotated bibliographies of select references to guide more in-depth reading when time permits. We again include sections on common ICU procedures, equations, nutrition, and pharmacology. All chapters were written by Washington University faculty physicians and experts in their respective fields, often with the assistance of subspecialty fellows and residents.

We recognize that the field of critical care is constantly changing with the availability of new study results. Therefore, this manual is meant to be a starting place for the initial care and stabilization of critically ill patients. The tables and figures that accompany each chapter are meant as guides and may not be applicable for all patients. We strongly encourage further reading of the literature and consultation with more expert clinicians to optimize the outcomes of critically ill patients.

We again especially give our sincerest thanks to Becky Light for her devoted efforts in preparing chapters and for acting as the liaison between the chapters' authors and Lippincott Williams & Wilkins. We also thank the entire production staff at Lippincott Williams & Wilkins and Wolters Kluwer for their efforts in the production of this manual.

M.H.K. would like to thank his loving family for all their support and encouragement. W.I. would like to thank his wife for her support and understanding.

Acknowledgments

The editors thank Becky Light who expertly coordinated all of the chapter communications, preparation, and revisions.

Contents

1

Introduction to Shock

Marin H. Kollef

Shock is a common problem in the intensive care unit, requiring immediate diagnosis and treatment. It is usually defined by a combination of hemodynamic parameters (mean blood pressure <60 mm Hg, systolic blood pressure <90 mm Hg), clinical findings (altered mentation, decreased urine output), and abnormal laboratory values (elevated serum lactate, metabolic acidosis). The first step is to identify the cause of shock, as each condition will require different interventions. The overall goal of therapy is to reverse tissue hypoperfusion as quickly as possible in order to preserve organ function. Table 1.1 and Algorithms 1.1 and 1.2 offer an approach for determining the main cause of shock. Specific management of the various shock states is presented in the following chapters. Early evaluation with echocardiography, intraesophageal aortic waveform assessment, or right heart catheterization will allow determination of the cause of shock and will assist in management.

TABLE 1.1	Hemodynamic Patterns Associated with Specific Shock States[a]							
Type of Shock	CI	SVR	PVR	SvO$_2$	RAP	RVP	PAP	PAOP
Cardiogenic (e.g., myocardial infarction or cardiac tamponade)	↓	↑	N	↓	↑	↑	↑	↑
Hypovolemic (e.g., hemorrhage and intravascular volume depletion)	↓	↑	N	↓	↓	↓	↓	↓
Distributive shock (e.g., septic and anaphylaxis)	N-↑	↓	N	N-↑	N-↓	N-↓	N-↓	N-↓
Obstructive (e.g., pulmonary embolism)	↓	N-↑	↑	N-↓	↑	↑	↑	N-↓

[a]Equalization of RAP, PAOP, diastolic PAP, and diastolic RVP indicates cardiac tamponade. CI, cardiac index; SVR, systemic vascular resistance; PVR, pulmonary vascular resistance; SvO$_2$, mixed venous oxygen saturation; RAP, right arterial pressure; RVP, right ventricular pressure; PAP, pulmonary artery pressure; PAOP, pulmonary artery occlusion pressure; ↑, increased; ↓, decreased; N, normal.

ALGORITHM 1.1 Main Causes of Shock

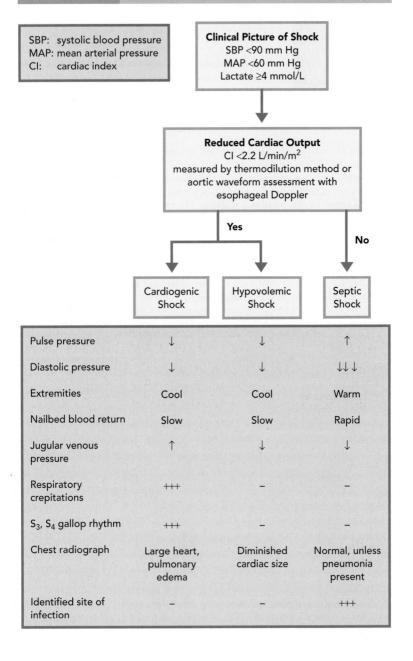

SBP: systolic blood pressure
MAP: mean arterial pressure
CI: cardiac index

Clinical Picture of Shock
SBP <90 mm Hg
MAP <60 mm Hg
Lactate ≥4 mmol/L

Reduced Cardiac Output
CI <2.2 L/min/m²
measured by thermodilution method or
aortic waveform assessment with
esophageal Doppler

Yes

No

	Cardiogenic Shock	Hypovolemic Shock	Septic Shock
Pulse pressure	↓	↓	↑
Diastolic pressure	↓	↓	↓↓↓
Extremities	Cool	Cool	Warm
Nailbed blood return	Slow	Slow	Rapid
Jugular venous pressure	↑	↓	↓
Respiratory crepitations	+++	–	–
S₃, S₄ gallop rhythm	+++	–	–
Chest radiograph	Large heart, pulmonary edema	Diminished cardiac size	Normal, unless pneumonia present
Identified site of infection	–	–	+++

ALGORITHM 1.2 Miscellaneous Causes of Shock

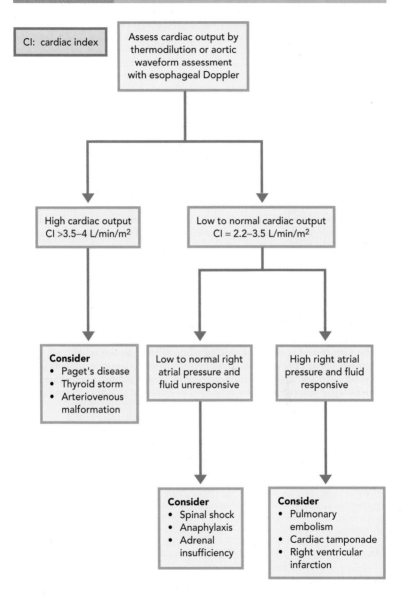

CI: cardiac index

Assess cardiac output by thermodilution or aortic waveform assessment with esophageal Doppler

High cardiac output
CI >3.5–4 L/min/m^2

Low to normal cardiac output
CI = 2.2–3.5 L/min/m^2

Consider
- Paget's disease
- Thyroid storm
- Arteriovenous malformation

Low to normal right atrial pressure and fluid unresponsive

High right atrial pressure and fluid responsive

Consider
- Spinal shock
- Anaphylaxis
- Adrenal insufficiency

Consider
- Pulmonary embolism
- Cardiac tamponade
- Right ventricular infarction

2 Hypovolemic Shock

Marin H. Kollef

Hypovolemic shock occurs as a result of decreased circulating blood volume, most commonly from acute hemorrhage. It may also result from heat-related intravascular volume depletion or fluid sequestration within the abdomen. Table 2.1 provides a classification of hypovolemic shock based on the amount of whole blood volume lost. In general, the greater the loss of whole blood, the greater the resultant risk of mortality. However, it is important to note that other factors can influence the outcome of hypovolemic shock including age, underlying comorbidities (e.g., cardiovascular disease), and the rapidity and adequacy of the fluid resuscitation.

Lactic acidosis occurs during hypovolemic shock because of inadequate tissue perfusion. The magnitude of the serum lactate elevation is correlated with mortality in hypovolemic shock and may be an early indicator of tissue hypoperfusion, despite near-normal–appearing vital signs. The treatment of lactic acidosis depends on reversing organ hypoperfusion. This is reflected in the equation for tissue oxygen delivery shown here. Optimizing oxygen delivery to tissues requires a sufficient hemoglobin concentration to carry oxygen to tissues. In addition, ventricular preload is an important determinant of cardiac output. Providing adequate intravascular volume will ensure that stroke volume and cardiac output are optimized to meet tissue demands for oxygen and other nutrients. If, despite adequate preload, cardiac output is not sufficient for the demands of tissues, then dobutamine can be employed to further increase cardiac output and oxygen delivery.

TABLE 2.1	Classification of Hypovolemic Shock	
Category	Whole Blood Volume Loss (%)	Pathophysiology
Mild (compensated)	<20	Peripheral vasoconstriction to preserve blood flow to critical organs (brain and heart)
Moderate	20–40	Decreased perfusion of organs such as the kidneys, intestine, and pancreas
Severe (uncompensated)	>40	Decreased perfusion to brain and heart

ALGORITHM 2.1   Management of Hypovolemic Shock

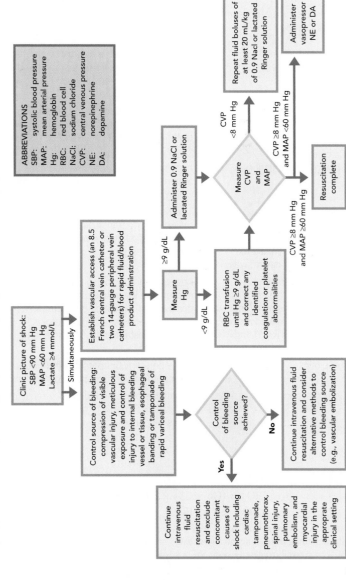

ABBREVIATIONS
SBP: systolic blood pressure
MAP: mean arterial pressure
Hg: hemoglobin
RBC: red blood cell
NaCl: sodium chloride
CVP: central venous pressure
NE: norepinephrine
DA: dopamine

Clinic picture of shock:
SBP <90 mm Hg
MAP <60 mm Hg
Lactate ≥4 mmol/L

Simultaneously

Establish vascular access (an 8.5 French central vein catheter or two 14-gauge peripheral vein catheters) for rapid fluid/blood product adminstration

Control source of bleeding: compression of visible vascular injury, meticulous exposure and control of injury to internal bleeding vessel or tissue, esophageal banding or tamponade of rapid variceal bleeding

Measure Hg

≥9 g/dL

<9 g/dL

Administer 0.9 NaCl or lactated Ringer solution

RBC transfusion until Hg ≥9 g/dL and correct any identified coagulation or platelet abnormalities

Measure CVP and MAP

CVP <8 mm Hg

Repeat fluid boluses of at least 20 mL/kg of 0.9 NacI or lactated Ringer solution

CVP ≥8 mm Hg and MAP <60 mm Hg

Administer vasopressor NE or DA

CVP ≥8 mm Hg and MAP ≥60 mm Hg

Resuscitation complete

Control of bleeding source achieved?

Yes

No

Continue intravenous fluid resuscitation and exclude concomitant causes of shock including cardiac tamponade, pneumothorax, spinal injury, pulmonary embolism, and myocardial injury in the approprate clinical setting

Continue intravenous fluid resuscitation and consider alternative methods to control bleeding source (e.g., vascular embolization)

TABLE 2.2	Adjunctive Therapies for Hypovolemic Shock
Therapy	Rationale
Airway control	To provide appropriate gas exchange in the lungs and to prevent aspiration
Cardiac/hemodynamic monitoring	To identify dysrhythmias and inadequate fluid resuscitation (Algorithm 2.1)
Platelet/fresh-frozen plasma administration	Required because of dilutional effects of crystalloid and blood administration as well as consumption from ongoing bleeding. The prothrombin time and partial thromboplastin time should be corrected and the platelet count should be kept >50,000/mm^3 with ongoing bleeding
Activated Factor VII	Should be considered in the presence of diffuse or nonoperative ongoing hemorrhage when clotting abnormalities have been corrected
Calcium chloride, magnesium chloride	To reverse ionized hypocalcemia and hypomagnesemia resulting from the administration of citrate with transfused blood, which binds ionized calcium and magnesium
Rewarming techniques (e.g., warm fluids, blankets, radiant lamps, head covers, warmed humidified air, heated body cavity lavage)	Hypothermia is a common consequence of massive blood transfusion that can contribute to cardiac dysfunction and coagulation abnormalities
Monitor and treat for transfusion-related complications including transfusion-related acute lung injury (TRALI) and transfusion reactions	These are immunologically mediated, requiring appropriate use of mechanical ventilation with positive end-expiratory pressure for TRALI and bronchodilators and corticosteroids for severe bronchoconstriction, subglottic edema, and anaphylaxis
Antibiotics	When open dirty or contaminated wounds are present to prevent and treat bacterial infections
Corticosteroids	For patients presumed to have adrenal injury and patients unable to mount an appropriate stress response

$$\dot{D}O_2 = CaO_2 \times CO$$
$$CaO_2 = (Hb \times 1.34 \times SaO_2) + 0.0031\, PaO_2$$
$$CO = SV \times HR$$

where $\dot{D}O_2$ = oxygen delivery, CaO_2 = arterial oxygen content, CO = cardiac output, Hb = hemoglobin concentration, SaO_2 = arterial hemoglobin oxygen saturation, PaO_2 = arterial oxygen tension, SV = stroke volume, and HR = heart rate.

The treatment goals in hypovolemic shock are to control the source of hemorrhage and to administer adequate intravascular volume replacement. Control of the source of hemorrhage may be as simple as placing a pressure dressing on an open bleeding wound, or it may require urgent operative exploration to identify and control the bleeding source from an intra-abdominal or intrathoracic injury. Angiographic embolization of a bleeding vessel may also be helpful for bleeding injuries that are not amenable to surgical intervention (e.g., multiple pelvic fractures with ongoing hemorrhage). Therefore, most episodes of hypovolemic shock are managed by trauma specialists, usually in the emergency department setting. However, all clinicians caring for critically ill patients should be able to recognize the early clinical manifestations of hypovolemic shock and to initiate appropriate fluid management.

An algorithm for the fluid management of hypovolemic shock is provided in Algorithm 2.1. At least two large-bore (14 to 16 gauge or larger) peripheral vein catheters and/or an 8.5 French central vein catheter should be placed to allow rapid blood product and crystalloid administration. A mechanical rapid transfusion device should also be used to decrease the time required for each unit of blood or liter of crystalloid to be infused. In a patient with ongoing hemorrhage, initial administration of 2 to 4 L of crystalloid (0.9 NaCl or lactated Ringer solution) and group O blood should be given. Most hospitals will employ four units of Rh-positive O blood for men and women who are not in childbearing age and Rh-negative O blood for women who are in childbearing age. Type-specific blood is usually administered after the first four units of nontyped blood are given. The goal of blood transfusion therapy during ongoing hemorrhage is to maintain the hemoglobin value above 8 g/dL.

In addition to the initial administration of crystalloid and red blood cells, other therapies will be required in patients with hypovolemic shock. These are summarized in Table 2.2 and are especially important for patients requiring massive transfusions or those with ongoing blood loss.

SUGGESTED READINGS

Bilkovski RN, Rivers EP, Horst HM. Targeted resuscitation strategies after injury. *Curr Opin Crit Care.* 2004;10:529–538.
> *Provides end points for the management of hypovolemic shock in patients with blunt or penetrating injury.*

Kelley DM. Hypovolemic shock: an overview. *Crit Care Nurs Q.* 2005;28:2–19.
> *A concise review of hypovolemic shock including initial evaluation and management.*

Nunez TC, Cotton BA. Transfusion therapy in hemorrhagic shock. *Curr Opin Crit Care.* 2009;15:536–541.
> *Current review on strategies aimed to optimize resuscitation and the bleeding diathesis in bleeding patients.*

Stein DM, Dutton RP. Use of recombinant factor VIIa in trauma. *Curr Opin Crit Care.* 2004;10:520–528.
> *Summarizes potential uses of recombinant factor VIIa in patients with trauma and ongoing hemorrhage.*

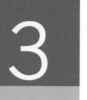

3

Severe Sepsis and Septic Shock

Marin H. Kollef and Scott T. Micek

Severe sepsis is an infection-induced syndrome resulting in a systemic inflammatory response that is complicated by dysfunction of at least one organ system. In the United States, approximately 750,000 cases of sepsis occur each year. The mortality associated with severe sepsis ranges from 30% to 50%, with mortality increasing with advancing age. Although complex, the pathophysiology of sepsis involves a series of interacting pathways involving immune stimulation, immune suppression, hypercoagulation, and hypofibrinolysis. Cardiovascular management plays an important role in the treatment of septic shock. Hypotension occurs because of failure of vasoconstriction by vascular smooth muscle resulting in peripheral vasodilation. Goal-directed cardiovascular resuscitation has been demonstrated to be an important determinant of survival in patients with septic shock. In addition to cardiovascular management, appropriate initial antimicrobial treatment of patients with severe sepsis also appears to be an important determinant of patient outcome.

The unscrambling of the complex pathophysiology associated with severe sepsis and septic shock has made much progress, and current understanding of this process is no longer rudimentary. Novel drug entities and new therapeutic strategies targeting these pathways have demonstrated efficacy in reducing patient mortality (Table 3.1). The challenge for clinicians is the integration of these pharmacotherapies to confer the recognized survival benefit into critical care practice. The Surviving Sepsis Campaign has teamed with the Institute for Healthcare Improvement to create the Severe Sepsis Bundles, which are designed in an effort to optimize the timing, sequence, and goals of the individual elements of care as delineated in the Surviving Sepsis Guidelines. The benefits associated with the use of comprehensive treatment protocols integrating goal-directed hemodynamic stabilization, early appropriate antimicrobial therapy, and associated adjunctive severe sepsis therapies initiated in the emergency department and continued in the intensive care unit have been reported in several prospective trials (Algorithms 3.1–3.3). However, several ongoing trials evaluating the individual elements of goal-directed therapy and drotrecogin alfa (activated) in shock will likely lead to modification of these recommendations.

The significance of early, aggressive, volume resuscitation and hemodynamic stabilization was demonstrated in a randomized, controlled, single-center trial in patients who presented to the emergency department with signs of the systemic inflammatory response syndrome and hypotension, as published by Rivers et al. Administration of crystalloids, red blood cell transfusions, vasopressors, and inotropes based on aggressive monitoring of intravascular volume and a tissue oxygen marker within 6 hours of

TABLE 3.1	Medications Commonly Used in Septic Shock			
I. Vasopressors		**CO**	**MAP**	**SVR**
Norepinephrine	0.05–0.5 μg/kg/min	–/+	++	+++
Dopamine	5–20 μg/kg/min	++	+	++
Epinephrine	0.05–2 μg/kg/min	++	++	+++
Phenylephrine	2–10 μg/kg/min	0	++	+++
Vasopressin	0.04 units/min	0	+++	+++
II. Inotrope				
Dobutamine	2.5–10 μg/kg/min	+++	–/+	–/0
III. Drotrecogin alfa (activated)	24 μg/kg/hr for 96 hr			
IV. Corticosteroids				
Hydrocortisone (+/– fludrocortisone 50 μg daily)	50 mg every 6 hr			
V. Antibiotic management				
(see Algorithm 3.3)				

CO, cardiac output; MAP, mean arterial blood pressure; SVR, systemic vascular resistance.

presentation to the emergency department resulted in a 16% decrease in absolute 28-day mortality. The major differences in treatment between the intervention and control groups were in the volume of intravenous fluids received, the number of patients transfused packed red blood, the use of dobutamine, and the presence of a dedicated study team for the first 6 hours of care.

The implementation of treatment pathways mimicking the interventions of the well-scripted, carefully performed procedures employed by Rivers et al. has been put into practice in the clinical setting. Micek et al. employed standardized order sets that focused on intravenous fluid administration and the appropriateness of initial antimicrobial therapy for severe sepsis and septic shock. Patients managed in this manner were more likely to receive intravenous fluids >20 mL/kg of body weight prior to vasopressor administration, and consequently were less likely to require vasopressor administration at the time of transfer to the intensive care unit. Patients managed with this approach were also more likely to be treated with an appropriate initial antimicrobial regimen. As a result of the aggressive management initiated in the emergency department and continued in the intensive care unit, patients managed via the severe sepsis order sets had statistically shorter hospital lengths of stay and a lower risk for 28-day mortality. Similar results have recently been reported from a multicenter study coordinated by the Surviving Sepsis Campaign Group.

In summary, the initial management of patients with septic shock appears to be critical in terms of determining outcome. Institution of standardized physician order sets, or some other systematic approach, for the management of patients with severe infections appears to consistently improve the delivery of recommended therapies and, as a result, may improve patient outcomes. Given that evidence-based treatment pathways typically have no additional risks and are associated with little to no acquisition

ALGORITHM 3.1   Fluid Management of Septic Shock

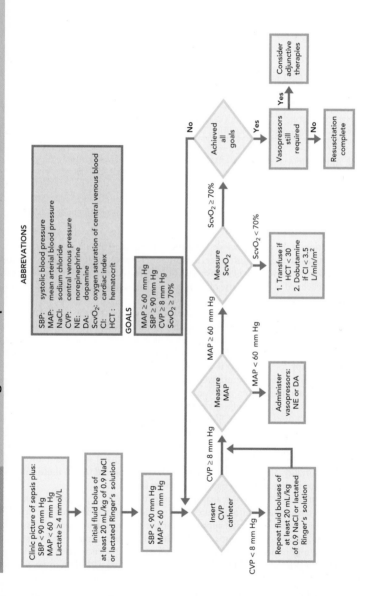

ABBREVIATIONS

SBP: systolic blood pressure
MAP: mean arterial blood pressure
NaCl: sodium chloride
CVP: central venous pressure
NE: norepinephrine
DA: dopamine
ScvO₂: oxygen saturation of central venous blood
CI: cardiac index
HCT : hematocrit

GOALS

MAP ≥ 60 mm Hg
SBP ≥ 90 mm Hg
CVP ≥ 8 mm Hg
ScvO₂ ≥ 70%

Clinic picture of sepsis plus:
SBP < 90 mm Hg
MAP < 60 mm Hg
Lactate ≥ 4 mmol/L

Initial fluid bolus of
at least 20 mL/kg of 0.9 NaCl
or lactated Ringer's solution

SBP < 90 mm Hg
MAP < 60 mm Hg

Insert CVP catheter

CVP < 8 mm Hg

Repeat fluid boluses of
at least 20 mL/kg
of 0.9 NaCl or lactated
Ringer's solution

CVP ≥ 8 mm Hg

Measure MAP

MAP < 60 mm Hg

Administer vasopressors:
NE or DA

MAP ≥ 60 mm Hg

Measure ScvO₂

ScvO₂ < 70%

1. Transfuse if HCT < 30
2. Dobutamine if CI < 3.5 L/min/m²

ScvO₂ ≥ 70%

Achieved all goals

No

Yes

Vasopressors still required

Yes

Consider adjunctive therapies

No

Resuscitation complete

ALGORITHM 3.2   Adjunctive Therapies for Septic Shock

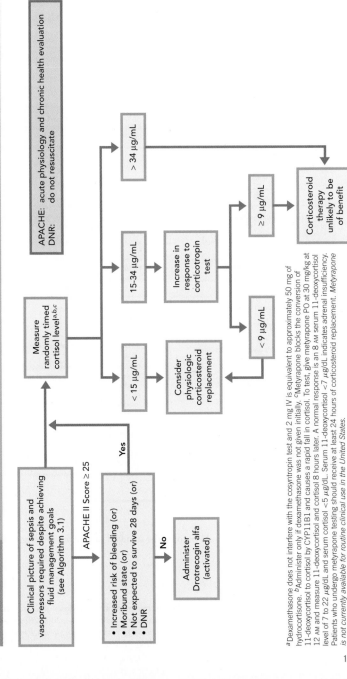

APACHE: acute physiology and chronic health evaluation
DNR: do not resuscitate

Clinical picture of sepsis and vasopressors required despite achieving fluid management goals (see Algorithm 3.1)

APACHE II Score ≥ 25

- Increased risk of bleeding (or)
- Moribund state (or)
- Not expected to survive 28 days (or)
- DNR

No → Administer Drotrecogin alfa (activated)

Yes → Measure randomly timed cortisol level[a,b,c]

- < 15 μg/mL → Consider physiologic corticosteroid replacement
- 15-34 μg/mL → Increase in response to corticotropin test
  - < 9 μg/mL → Consider physiologic corticosteroid replacement
  - ≥ 9 μg/mL → Corticosteroid therapy unlikely to be of benefit
- > 34 μg/mL → Corticosteroid therapy unlikely to be of benefit

[a]Dexamethasone does not interfere with the cosyntropin test and 2 mg IV is equivalent to approximately 50 mg of hydrocortisone. [b]Administer only if dexamethasone was not given initially. [c]Metyrapone blocks the conversion of 11-deoxycortisol to cortisol by CYP11B1 and causes a rapid fall in cortisol. To test, give metyrapone PO at 30 mg/kg at 12 AM and measure 11-deoxycortisol and cortisol 8 hours later. A normal response is an 8 AM serum 11-deoxycortisol level of 7 to 22 μg/dL and serum cortisol <5 μg/dL. Serum 11-deoxycortisol <7 μg/dL indicates adrenal insufficiency. Patients who undergo metyrapone testing should receive at least 24 hours of corticosteroid replacement. *Metyrapone is not currently available for routine clinical use in the United States.*

11

ALGORITHM 3.3 Antibiotic Management of Severe Sepsis and Septic Shock

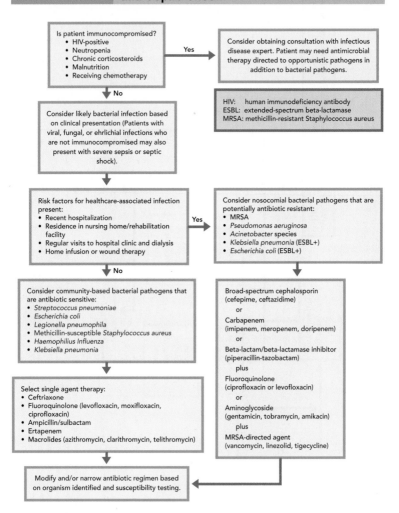

Is patient immunocompromised?
• HIV-positive
• Neutropenia
• Chronic corticosteroids
• Malnutrition
• Receiving chemotherapy

Yes → Consider obtaining consultation with infectious disease expert. Patient may need antimicrobial therapy directed to opportunistic pathogens in addition to bacterial pathogens.

No ↓

HIV: human immunodeficiency antibody
ESBL: extended-spectrum beta-lactamase
MRSA: methicillin-resistant Staphylococcus aureus

Consider likely bacterial infection based on clinical presentation (Patients with viral, fungal, or ehrlichial infections who are not immunocompromised may also present with severe sepsis or septic shock).

Risk factors for healthcare-associated infection present:
• Recent hospitalization
• Residence in nursing home/rehabilitation facility
• Regular visits to hospital clinic and dialysis
• Home infusion or wound therapy

Yes → Consider nosocomial bacterial pathogens that are potentially antibiotic resistant:
• MRSA
• *Pseudomonas aeruginosa*
• *Acinetobacter* species
• *Klebsiella pneumonia* (ESBL+)
• *Escherichia coli* (ESBL+)

No ↓

Consider community-based bacterial pathogens that are antibiotic sensitive:
• *Streptococcus pneumoniae*
• *Escherichia coli*
• *Legionella pneumophila*
• Methicillin-susceptible *Staphylococcus aureus*
• *Haemophilius Influenza*
• *Klebsiella pneumonia*

Broad-spectrum cephalosporin (cefepime, ceftazidime)
or
Carbapenem (imipenem, meropenem, doripenem)
or
Beta-lactam/beta-lactamase inhibitor (piperacillin-tazobactam)
plus
Fluoroquinolone (ciprofloxacin or levofloxacin)
or
Aminoglycoside (gentamicin, tobramycin, amikacin)
plus
MRSA-directed agent (vancomycin, linezolid, tigecycline)

Select single agent therapy:
• Ceftriaxone
• Fluoroquinolone (levofloxacin, moxifloxacin, ciprofloxacin)
• Ampicillin/sulbactam
• Ertapenem
• Macrolides (azithromycin, clarithromycin, telithromycin)

Modify and/or narrow antibiotic regimen based on organism identified and susceptibility testing.

costs, their implementation should become the standard of care for the management of septic shock.

SUGGESTED READINGS

Annane D, Sebille V, Charpentier C, et al. Effect of treatment with low doses of hydrocortisone and fludrocortisone on mortality in patients with septic shock. *JAMA.* 2002;288:862–871. *Randomized trial demonstrating survival benefit amongst patients with septic shock not responding appropriately to administration of corticotropin.*

Bernard GR, Vincent JL, Laterre PF, et al. Efficacy and safety of recombinant human activated protein C for severe sepsis. *N Engl J Med.* 2001;344:699–709.

A randomized blinded trial demonstrating the mortality advantage of patients receiving activated protein C for severe sepsis and high acuity of illness.

Dellinger RP, Levy MM, Carlet JM, et al. Surviving Sepsis Campaign: international guidelines for management of severe sepsis and septic shock: 2008. *Crit Care Med.* 2008;36:296–327.

Evidence-based recommendations for the initial resuscitation and treatment of patients with septic shock and severe sepsis.

Kortgen A, Niederprum P, Bauer M. Implementation of an evidence-based "standard operating procedure" and outcome in septic shock. *Crit Care Med.* 2006;34:943–949.

Evaluation of an algorithm defining resuscitation according to early goal-directed therapy, glycemic control, administration of stress doses of hydrocortisone, and use of recombinant human activated protein C demonstrating improved clinical outcomes.

Levy MM, Dellinger RP, Townsend SR, et al. The Surviving Sepsis Campaign: results of an international guideline-based performance improvement program targeting severe sepsis. *Intensive Care Med.* 2010;36:222–231.

A multicenter experience instituting an algorithm to improve the outcomes of patients with sepsis.

Micek ST, Roubinian N, Heuring T, et al. A before-after study of a standardized hospital order set for the management of septic shock. *Crit Care Med.* 2006;34:2707–2713.

A before-after study demonstrating improvements in 28-day mortality and length of stay for patients with septic shock managed with a standardized order set in the emergency department.

Micek ST, Welch EC, Khan J, et al. Empiric combination antibiotic therapy is associated with improved outcome against sepsis due to Gram-negative bacteria: a retrospective analysis. *Antimicrob Agents Chemother.* 2010;54:1742–1748.

Discusses importance of combination antibiotic therapy to appropriately treat resistant pathogens.

Rivers E, Nguyen B, Havstad S, et al. Early goal-directed therapy in the treatment of severe sepsis and septic shock. *N Engl J Med.* 2001;345:1368–1377.

Randomized trial demonstrating the survival benefit of a goal-directed approach to the initial resuscitation of patients with severe sepsis and septic shock.

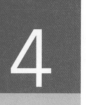

Cardiogenic Shock
Sundeep Viswanathan and Richard G. Bach

Cardiogenic shock refers to a condition in which there is inadequate circulation and compromised organ perfusion primarily due to cardiac dysfunction. This failure of pump function results in an inability to maintain circulation to vital organs that, without treatment, will lead to multisystem failure and death. Cardiogenic shock is characterized by prolonged hypotension (systolic blood pressure <90 mm Hg) in the setting of decreased cardiac output (typically <1.8 L/min/m² without support and <2.2 L/min/m² with support) despite adequate intravascular volume (left ventricular end-diastolic pressure >18 mm Hg and/or pulmonary artery occlusion pressure >15 mm Hg). Clinically, this is suggested when there are signs of systemic hypoperfusion manifested by cool mottled extremities, altered mentation, and/or oliguria. However, these classic signs may not always be present. Despite recent advances in management, cardiogenic shock from pump failure remains associated with a very high mortality. Among patients hospitalized with an acute myocardial infarction (AMI) that is complicated by cardiogenic shock, the rate of death within the first 30 days is in the range of 40% to 50%, although this rate has been on the decline in parallel with increasing rates of early reperfusion by primary percutaneous coronary intervention (PCI) for AMI.

ETIOLOGY

Cardiogenic shock has multiple possible causes (Table 4.1), although the most common cause is acute myocardial dysfunction in the setting of AMI. Shock occurs in approximately 5% to 10% of patients with AMI. It may develop as a consequence of either left or right ventricular infarction, although hemodynamically significant right ventricular infarction occurs most commonly in combination with inferior wall, left ventricular infarction. The severity of shock from left ventricular infarction is generally related to the quantitative loss of functional myocardium, although other factors also play a role. Complications of AMI, such as arrhythmias, ventricular septal defects, papillary muscle dysfunction, or myocardial rupture causing pericardial tamponade, may also trigger the onset of shock. Less frequently, cardiogenic shock may be caused by severe cardiomyopathy (dilated, hypertrophic, or stress induced), acute myocarditis, or severe valvular disease.

PATHOPHYSIOLOGY

Cardiogenic shock generally occurs when myocardial dysfunction exceeds a critical threshold from a single large myocardial infarction (MI) (typically considered to

TABLE 4.1	Causes of Cardiogenic Shock

Acute myocardial infarction
  Left ventricular pump failure
    Large infarction
    Smaller infarction with preexisting LV dysfunction
  Mechanical complications
    Free wall rupture/tamponade
    Papillary muscle dysfunction/rupture
    Right ventricular infarction
    Ventricular septal defect
    Aortic dissection

Severe cardiomyopathy/congestive heart failure
  Dilated cardiomyopathy
  Stress-induced or Tako-tsubo cardiomyopathy

Acute myocarditis (infectious, toxin/drug, transplant rejection)

Myocardial contusion

Calcium channel or beta blocker overdose

Acute/severe valvular insufficiency
  Acute mitral regurgitation (e.g., chordal rupture)
  Acute aortic insufficiency

Obstruction to left ventricular outflow
  Hypertrophic obstructive cardiomyopathy
  Aortic stenosis

Obstruction to ventricular filling
  Pericardial effusion/tamponade
  Mitral stenosis
  Left atrial myxoma

involve >40% of the myocardium), a cumulative amount of damage from multiple infarctions, or from diffuse myocardial injury from other inciting factors. With shock there is increasing myocardial oxygen demand due to elevated end-diastolic ventricular pressure along with decreasing oxygen supply from hypotension and falling cardiac output. This results in a self-perpetuating spiral of progressive ischemia and cardiac dysfunction, ultimately culminating in death (Algorithm 4.1). Treatments of cardiogenic shock have sought to interrupt this spiral at various steps. The situation is further complicated by the fact that the majority of patients with cardiogenic shock secondary to AMI have significant multivessel coronary artery disease (CAD) that can limit any compensatory increase in contractility of noninfarct territories. Recent observations of the inflammatory cascade have modified traditional thinking on this syndrome. First, the average left ventricular ejection fraction among patients with AMI and cardiogenic shock is 30%, not lower as might be expected, and yet many patients with an ejection fraction significantly <30% still do not develop cardiogenic shock. In addition, the systemic vascular resistance in patients with cardiogenic shock is often not elevated and may be unexpectedly low. This may be the result of a systemic inflammatory

ALGORITHM 4.1 Pathophysiology of Cardiogenic Shock

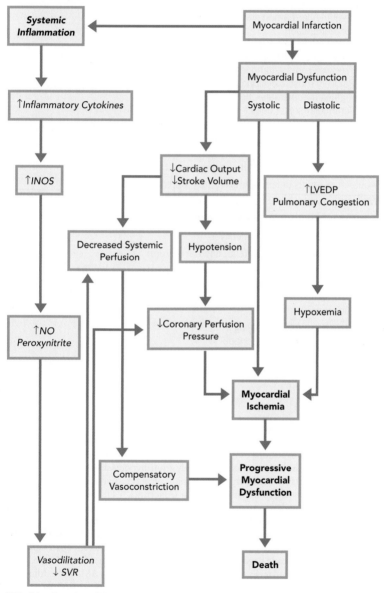

INOS, nitric oxide synthase; NO, nitric oxide; LVEDP, left ventricular end-diastolic pressure; SVR, systemic vascular resistance.

response syndrome not unlike septic shock and putatively related to high levels of cytokines and systemic/vascular nitric oxide, which have both negative inotropic and vasodilatory effects.

PATIENT CHARACTERISTICS

Shock is more likely to develop in the setting of AMI among patients who are older, female, and who have significantly more comorbid conditions (diabetes, prior known CAD, history of cerebrovascular disease, and history of renal insufficiency). Cardiogenic shock can complicate ST elevation MI or non-ST elevation MI; it is more common in patients with anterior location of MI. By angiography, the left anterior descending artery is most commonly the culprit vessel, but patients with cardiogenic shock are also likely to have multivessel CAD. Signs and symptoms of cardiogenic shock usually develop after hospital admission (median, 6.2 hours after initial MI symptoms), and the majority of patients develop shock within the first 24 hours. A significant minority (~25%) of patients may develop cardiogenic shock after 24 hours, possibly due to recurrent ischemia. Note should be made of a select subset of cardiogenic shock patients who present with poor cardiac output and evidence of systemic hypoperfusion but without frank hypotension. These so-called normotensive cardiogenic shock patients have a lower mortality than their hypotensive counterparts (43% vs. 66%, respectively), but their risk of death is still much higher than AMI patients without hypoperfusion.

EVALUATION

Prompt recognition of cardiogenic shock is essential for management, as timely and appropriate treatment can significantly reduce mortality. Patients with low blood pressure (<90 mm Hg) should be quickly assessed for the presence of pulsus paradoxus (potentially indicating cardiac tamponade), signs of congestive heart failure (elevated jugular venous pressure, pulmonary edema, S3 gallop), and evidence of end-organ hypoperfusion (cool, mottled extremities; weak pulses; clouded mental status; reduced urine output). A careful cardiac examination should be performed to assess for the presence of valvular disease or uncommon mechanical causes, although in the setting of AMI or low cardiac output, the murmurs of mitral regurgitation or critical aortic stenosis or insufficiency may be diminished or virtually inaudible. An electrocardiogram should be obtained without delay to look for evidence of acute ischemia or infarction and to assist in triage for emergency reperfusion when indicated. Serum cardiac biomarkers should be measured at presentation and serially to diagnose acute myocardial injury even when the electrocardiogram is nondiagnostic. A bedside echocardiogram is usually indicated as soon as possible at initial evaluation to assess left and right ventricular function, valvular function, and to exclude cardiac tamponade. When detected, certain mechanical causes of circulatory failure, such as acute mitral regurgitation or ventricular rupture, warrant emergency surgical intervention. When the etiology remains unclear, bedside pulmonary artery catheterization can be helpful in differentiating cardiogenic from other forms of shock, although in cases of shock due to suspected acute myocardial ischemia or infarction, such studies should not delay definitive evaluation by left heart catheterization and coronary angiography. In addition to assisting with diagnosis, pulmonary artery catheter monitoring can help to guide therapy with vasopressor and inotropic medications and gauge hemodynamic improvement versus deterioration prior to any clinically evident signs.

TREATMENT

Initial Medical Management

Patients with cardiogenic shock require immediate attention to the stabilization of adverse hemodynamics in order to interrupt the viscous cycle of tissue hypoperfusion and the potential for rapid development of irreversible organ damage (Algorithm 4.2). Such patients typically need central venous access, continuous monitoring of arterial pressure and urine output, and mechanical ventilation in a hospital environment where advanced management options are readily available such as PCI, circulatory assist devices, and cardiac surgery. The cause must be considered when choosing therapeutic interventions because the application of certain therapies commonly used in other forms of shock can be deleterious to the acutely dysfunctional heart, especially in the setting of AMI. Regarding antiplatelet therapy, like any patient with an acute coronary syndrome, patients with cardiogenic shock where acute ischemia or infarction is a likely etiology should receive full dose aspirin and early consideration of an adenosine diphosphate receptor blocker, unless contraindicated. Given their potential for increased perioperative bleeding, thienopyridines may be withheld until coronary anatomy is defined and the possible need for emergent surgical intervention has been determined, but should be administered as early as possible before PCI if indicated. It is important to avoid early beta blockade and angiotensin-converting inhibitors initially until hemodynamic stability is reached. In the absence of overt pulmonary congestion, fluid resuscitation may help reverse hypotension but must be monitored carefully to avoid pulmonary edema and respiratory failure. Systemic hypotension may initially require treatment with vasopressor therapy, although it should be remembered that peripheral vasoconstrictors typically further increase afterload and oxygen demand for the failing myocardium. For this reason, the lowest dose of pressor empirically effective in achieving an adequate blood pressure response should be employed. While the evidence defining first-line pressor selection in cardiogenic shock is limited, both norepinephrine (starting dose, 1 to 40 μg/min) and dopamine (starting dose, 5 to 20 μg/kg/min) can be used and titrated to hemodynamic effect. Dopamine has combined inotropic and vasopressor effects and theoretical preservation of renal perfusion by mesenteric vasodilation at low doses, although its use may be associated with a higher rate of arrhythmias. Of note, in a recent analysis assessing outcome among a subgroup of 280 patients with cardiogenic shock out of 1679 total patients with various etiologies of shock randomly assigned to receive dopamine versus norepinephrine, there was a significantly higher rate of adverse events and of 28-day mortality associated with dopamine compared with norepinephrine. If hypotension remains refractory, combinations of pressors may be necessary.

In patients with relatively stable blood pressure (systolic blood pressure >90 mm Hg) but low cardiac output and evidence of hypoperfusion, dobutamine (2.5 to 10 μg/min) may provide additional benefit due to its inotropic effect. Because of its potential for peripheral vasodilation, dobutamine should be avoided or used with caution in patients with hypotension. Milrinone (0.375 to 0.75 μg/kg/min, with or without a loading dose of 50 μg/kg), another potent inotrope, typically causes significant vasodilation and should be used with great caution in the patient with low blood pressure and avoided in patients with renal insufficiency. Because of the potential adverse effects of pressor agents and the favorable effects of intra-aortic balloon pump (IABP) counterpulsation or mechanical ventricular assist devices, patients with shock due to primary pump failure should always be considered for IABP or another form of mechanical support early in the course of shock. If, however, the rare circumstance

ALGORITHM 4.2   Management of Suspected Cardiogenic Shock

Suspected CS
- SBP <90 mm Hg
- Signs of Low Cardiac Output
(Oliguria, Poor MS, Pulmonary Edema)

↓

Initial Evaluation & Rapid Stabilization
Immediate ECG
*Look for Evidence of AMI
(ST Elevation, LBBB (new), Suspected Posterior MI)
Supplemental 02 / Mech Ventilation (for Hypoxia)
BP Support
SBP <90 mm Hg
Dopamine (5–15 µg/kg/min)
SBP <80 mm Hg (w Dopa)
Norepinephrine (1–20 µg/min)
Goal MAP >65 mm Hg
*All Patients on Vasopressors should have Intra-arterial
Pressure Monitoring

If ECG(+) ↓   If ECG(−) ↓

Immediate Reperfusion Therapy

Emergent Echocardiogram
Evaluate LV/RV function
r/o Mechanical Complications Resulting in CS
- Acute MR/Papillary Muscle Rupture, VSD,
Free Wall Rupture, RV Infarction
PA Catheter Monitoring
Confirm Cardiac Etiology
CI <2.2 L/min/m²
PCWP >15 mm Hg

Thrombolysis/IABP
*Only if Cath Lab not
Immediately Available*

Then Transfer for ↓

Cardiac Catheterization
- <36 hr from Onset of AMI
- <12–18 hr from Onset of Shock
*No other Contraindication to
Anticoagulation*
IABP Support

No Revascularization Possible
Continued Medical Support
if BP Stable Consider
Inotropic Support
Dobutamine (2.5–10 µg/min)
Milrinone (0.375–0.75 µg/kg/min)
Avoid In Hypotension, Renal Failure(Milrinone)

Suitable for Revascularization
PCI (Infarct artery only)
Rec. Use Of Stents And Abciximab
or Emergent CABG
(3V dz, L Main dz, or PCI not possible)

Refractory Shock
*Consider LVAD, Transplant
Evaluation*

CS, cardiogenic shock; SBP, systolic blood pressure; MS, mental status; ECG, electrocardiogram; AMI, acute myocardial infarction; ECG, electrocardiogram; AMI, acute myocardial infarction; BP, blood pressure; MAP, mean arterial pressure; LV/RV, left ventricular/right ventricular; IABP, intra-aortic balloon counterpulsation; MR, mitral regurgitation; VSD, ventricular septal defect; PA, pulmonary artery; PCI, percutaneous coronary intervention; CABG, coronary artery bypass surgery; LVAD, left ventricular assist device.

of hypertrophic cardiomyopathy and shock due to outflow tract obstruction is suspected, drugs with positively inotropic effects and intra-aortic balloon pumping should be avoided and the peripheral vasoconstrictor phenylephrine considered as the pressor of choice.

Reperfusion Therapy: Thrombolytic Therapy and Primary Percutaneous Coronary Intervention

A fundamental concept of current treatment of cardiogenic shock in patients with ischemic heart disease is the recognition that rapid reperfusion of AMI and early revascularization for patients with obstructive CAD are key interventions that have been proven in clinical trials to reduce mortality. Because randomized trials of reperfusion for ST elevation MI have suggested that the presence of cardiogenic shock is associated with reduced efficacy of pharmacologic reperfusion by thrombolytic therapy and superior outcomes after successful PCI, timely primary PCI is strongly preferred as the method of reperfusion when available for patients with cardiogenic shock complicating AMI. There is a significant increase in mortality for such patients even with delays to reperfusion as short as minutes to hours. However, for patients who cannot undergo timely coronary angiography or more invasive therapy, there is limited data that thrombolysis combined with intra-aortic balloon counterpulsation may have benefited as a temporizing measure to be followed by mechanical revascularization when feasible.

Coronary Revascularization

Patients with evidence of an acute coronary syndrome and cardiogenic shock should be referred for urgent left heart catheterization and revascularization if coronary anatomy is suitable. Results from the randomized SHOCK trial comparing early revascularization with conservative management showed that patients (age <75 years) with AMI and cardiogenic shock had significant mortality benefit from early PCI or coronary artery bypass surgery. Current guidelines recommend early revascularization, when feasible, for patients who are within 36 hours of the onset of AMI. Of note, reflecting the complex and extensive CAD in these high-risk patients, 36% of the patients in the SHOCK trial who underwent revascularization received coronary artery bypass surgery. Nonrandomized data show that there may also be a benefit from early revascularization in those patients older than 75 years. Current guidelines recommend that such patients should be considered for early revascularization on an individual basis.

Circulatory Assist Devices

Intra-aortic Balloon Counterpulsation

An intra-aortic balloon catheter is a device inserted via an accessible artery, usually the femoral artery, into the descending aorta where balloon counterpulsation is implemented to provide hemodynamic support for patients in shock. By rapid balloon inflation using helium gas that is timed just after aortic valve closure and deflation just prior to the next ventricular systole, balloon pump counterpulsation is the only means to augment central aortic pressure and vital organ perfusion (including coronary blood flow) while simultaneously reducing afterload and myocardial oxygen demand. Early IABP support can be beneficial as a bridge to revascularization, to recovery following transient myocardial stunning, or en route to more advanced support devices or cardiac transplantation. It should be considered as an early intervention for most patients with cardiogenic shock in whom there are no contraindications (severe aortic insufficiency, severe peripheral vascular disease, aortic dissection, bleeding diathesis, or sepsis). Data on optimal timing of IABP support is still under debate, but many experts recommend insertion before or immediately after primary PCI.

Percutaneous and Surgical Ventricular Assist Devices

When medical therapy and IABP support are inadequate to stabilize vital organ perfusion, more advanced forms of support may be necessary and should be considered before irreversible end-organ damage occurs. Left ventricular assist devices (LVADs) that are inserted surgically or, more recently, percutaneously can provide significant improvements in cardiac output, blood pressure, pulmonary artery wedge pressure, and end-organ perfusion that can be lifesaving. In a suitable patient with cardiogenic shock, an LVAD is most commonly used as a means of temporary support or as a "bridge" to definitive treatment such as orthotopic heart transplantation. LVADs are also now approved for longer-term management of cardiogenic shock in select patients with end-stage cardiac dysfunction. The percutaneous transvalvular LVADs (Impella™ 2.5 and 5.0; Abiomed, Inc.) and percutaneous left atrial-to-femoral artery ventricular assist device (TandemHeart™; CardiacAssist, Inc.) may be better tolerated in patients deemed poor candidates for surgically implanted devices. The Impella™ works on the principle of an Archimedes screw. A large bore pigtail catheter with a miniature impeller pump is percutaneously inserted in the femoral artery and advanced across the aortic valve. The inlet at the distal catheter is positioned in the left ventricle and the device can continuously pump up to 2.5 to 5.0 L/min of blood (depending on model catheter size) into the ascending aorta. The TandemHeart™ System involves a large bore venous catheter inserted into the left atrium via transseptal puncture for withdrawal of oxygenated blood and an arterial catheter placed in the femoral artery for blood return, with an intervening extracorporeal centrifugal pump that can provide up to 5.0 L/min of flow.

Although experience with LVADs is growing, the evidence regarding their effect on outcome for patients with cardiogenic shock remains limited. In a small randomized comparison involving only 26 patients, a percutaneously inserted Impella 2.5 compared favorably with an IABP with respect to improved hemodynamic indices while there was no difference in the high rate of 30-day mortality. Although theoretically appealing, further outcome data using these devices in cardiogenic shock are needed. Contraindications to LVAD insertion include aortic regurgitation, aortic dissection/aneurysm, severe peripheral vascular disease, bleeding diathesis, and sepsis. Device-related complications, including bleeding, vascular compromise, thromboembolic events, and infections, pose continued challenges to management in this critically ill patient population.

CARDIAC TAMPONADE

Cardiac tamponade represents a unique cause of shock in which external compression of the heart significantly restricts filling and limits output. Because it represents a not uncommon and rapidly reversible form of shock, prompt recognition is essential. Cardiac tamponade remains a clinical diagnosis. Important clinical signs on examination include the presence of exaggerated pulsus paradoxus, where the inspiratory fall in systolic blood pressure exceeds ~10 mm Hg; distended jugular veins; and muffled heart sounds. The most common cause is a significant pericardial effusion, although more unusual causes of impaired filling—such as a localized thrombus compressing the left atrium of a patient following cardiac surgery—are possible. Echocardiography may demonstrate the classic findings of a significant pericardial effusion with evidence of diastolic compression of the right side of the heart and exaggerated respiratory variation in Doppler-measured mitral inflow velocities. When hypotension is present, rapid infusion of intravenous fluids may help maintain blood pressure, but removal of the offending pericardial fluid by percutaneous pericardiocentesis or surgical drainage may be needed without delay. If the diagnosis is in question, pulmonary artery catheterization may be useful to confirm hemodynamic evidence of tamponade, suggested by equalization of elevated right atrial, right ventricular diastolic, pulmonary artery diastolic, and pulmonary artery wedge pressures.

CONCLUSION

Cardiogenic shock is a condition associated with profound cardiac dysfunction from several potential causes, but it is seen most commonly in the setting of AMI. It is associated with a high rate of death, although with increasing application of early primary PCI for AMI the incidence and mortality appear to be decreasing. Optimal management requires early recognition and aggressive medical and mechanical intervention. When anatomically feasible for patients with acute coronary syndromes and shock, early revascularization has been shown to be effective for improving both short- and long-term survival.

SUGGESTED READINGS

Cheng JM, den Uil CA, Hoeks SE, et al. Percutaneous left ventricular assist devices vs. intra-aortic balloon counterpulsation for treatment of cardiogenic shock: a meta-analysis of controlled trials. *Eur Heart J.* 2009;10:1093

De Backer D, Biston P, Devriendt J, et al. Comparison of dopamine and norepinephrine in the treatment of shock. *N Engl J Med.* 2010;362:779–789.
    Results of the randomized SOAP II trial showing higher adverse event rates and 28-day mortality associated with dopamine use among the subgroup of patients with cardiogenic shock.

Hochman JS. Early revascularization in acute myocardial infarction complicated by cardiogenic shock. *N Engl J Med.* 1999;341:625–634.
    Published results of the landmark SHOCK trial showing reduced mortality for patients (less than age 75) randomized to a strategy of early revascularization vs. conservative management.

Hochman JS. Cardiogenic shock complicating acute myocardial infarction: expanding the paradigm. *Circulation.* 2003;107:2998–3002.
    A review of cardiogenic shock including newer information regarding pathophysiology and management.

Hochman JS. Cardiogenic shock: current concepts and improving outcomes. *Circulation.* 2008; 117:686–697.

Hollenberg SM, Kavinsky CJ, Parrillo JE, et al. Cardiogenic shock. *Ann Intern Med.* 1999;131: 47–59.
    A general review of cardiogenic shock and evidence-based management.

Seyfarth M, Sibbing D, Bauer I, et al. A randomized clinical trial to evaluate the safety and efficacy of a percutaneous left ventricular assist device versus intra-aortic balloon pumping for treatment of cardiogenic shock caused by myocardial infarction. *J Am Coll Cardiol.* 2008;52:1584–1588.
    Two articles regarding use of percutaneous left ventricular assist devices compared with IABP counterpulsation in the management of cardiogenic shock.

Menon V, White H, Hochman J. The clinical profile of patients with suspected cardiogenic shock due to predominant left ventricular failure: a report from the SHOCK Trial Registry. *J Am Coll Cardiol.* 2000;36(3, Suppl 1):1071–1076.
    JACC supplement with several publications on clinically relevant sub-studies from the SHOCK trial and Registry.

5 Anaphylactic Shock
Timothy J. Bedient and Marin H. Kollef

Anaphylaxis refers to the characteristic and often life-threatening clinical manifestations of the immunoglobulin E (IgE)-mediated immediate hypersensitivity reaction, involving mast cell and basophil degranulation with release of histamine, tryptase, prostaglandins, and leukotrienes, that occurs following exposure to various substances. Anaphylactoid reactions are clinically indistinguishable from anaphylaxis, but are not IgE-mediated. They are thought to result from direct mast cell degranulation independent of IgE, or from alterations in arachidonic acid metabolism. The substances that trigger anaphylaxis and anaphylactoid reactions differ, and are outlined in Table 5.1.

Reactions can develop within minutes, but usually <1 hour, after exposure to a triggering substance. More rapid reactions occur with parenteral exposure. Initial symptoms include flushing, pruritis, and a sense of doom. Characteristic clinical manifestations of varying severity develop involving the skin, eyes, respiratory and gastrointestinal tracts, and cardiovascular and central nervous systems, as listed in Table 5.2. Cardiovascular collapse (shock) occurs in approximately 30% of cases and results from (a) hypovolemia induced by increased vascular permeability and loss of intravascular volume, (b) hypotension from peripheral vasodilation, (c) myocardial depression, and (d) bradycardia. Up to 50% of patients describe respiratory symptoms, which can progress to respiratory failure from severe upper airway edema, bronchospasm, and cardiogenic and noncardiogenic pulmonary edema. Biphasic reactions occur in up to 20% of patients, characterized by a second round of symptoms 1 to 8 hours after the initial reaction (although up to 72 hours has been reported).

Diagnosis is clinical and involves a broad differential diagnosis including urticaria, status asthmaticus, "red man" syndrome (vancomycin), scromboidosis (histamine-like compound in spoiled fish such as tuna, mackerel, mahi-mahi, and blue fish), carcinoid, pheochromocytoma, mastocytosis, monosodium glutamate ingestion, and panic attacks. Serum levels of tryptase (especially the beta subtype) and histamine, when elevated, support the diagnosis. Tryptase levels are elevated for 1 to 6 hours after the event, but serum histamine levels fall within 30 to 60 minutes. A 24-hour urine N-methyl histamine level compared to a later baseline can be a helpful alternative. Patients should be questioned about exposure to potential triggers, but no substance is identified in up to 60% of cases.

Treatment is outlined in Algorithm 5.1 and is based on the joint recommendations of the American Academy of Allergy, Asthma, and Immunology and the American College of Allergy, Asthma, and Immunology. Pharmacologic therapy involves epinephrine to reverse the respiratory and cardiovascular effects, and blocking the effects of histamine with histamine 1 and 2 receptor blockers. There are no contraindications to the use of epinephrine, and numerous studies have shown that it

TABLE 5.1	Causes of Anaphylaxis and Anaphylactoid Reactions (Substances are Paired with the Most Common Associated Mechanism)

Anaphylaxis (IgE-mediated)
   Foods (especially nuts, eggs, fish, shellfish, and cow's milk)
   Antibiotics (especially penicillin; 4% positive by allergy testing also test positive to cephalosporins)
   Vaccines
   Anesthetics
   Insulin and other hormones
   Antitoxins
   Blood and blood products
   Insect stings and bites (bee, wasp, and ant)
   Snake bites
   Latex
   Allergy immunotherapy

Anaphylactoid reactions (direct mast cell degranulation, altered AA metabolism)
   Nonsteroidal anti-inflammatory drugs (especially aspirin)
   Opiates
   Sulfites
   Radiocontrast media
   Neuromuscular blocking agents (curoniums and succinylcholine)
   Gamma globulin
   Antisera
   Exercise

IgE, immunoglobulin E; AA, arachidonic acid.

TABLE 5.2	Clinical Manifestations of Anaphylaxis and Anaphylactoid Reactions

Eyes
   Pruritus
   Lacrimation
   Conjunctival erythema
   Periorbital edema

Cardiovascular
   Hypotension
   Tachycardia (bradycardia when severe)
   Arrhythmias
   Cardiac arrest

Gastrointestinal
   Nausea/vomiting
   Diarrhea
   Abdominal pain

Skin
   Pruritus
   Flushing
   Urticaria
   Angioedema

Respiratory
   Dyspnea
   Stridor/wheezing/hoarseness
   Difficulty swallowing
   Pulmonary edema

Neurologic
   Anxiety and "sense of doom"
   Presyncope and syncope
   Seizures

ALGORITHM 5.1 Acute Treatment of Patients with Anaphylaxis and Anaphylactoid Reactions

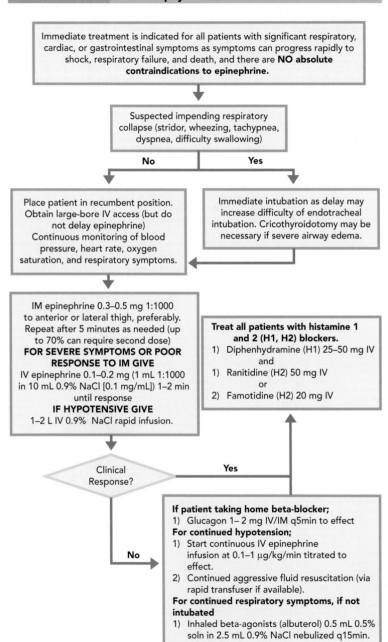

Immediate treatment is indicated for all patients with significant respiratory, cardiac, or gastrointestinal symptoms as symptoms can progress rapidly to shock, respiratory failure, and death, and there are **NO absolute contraindications to epinephrine.**

Suspected impending respiratory collapse (stridor, wheezing, tachypnea, dyspnea, difficulty swallowing)

No   **Yes**

Place patient in recumbent position. Obtain large-bore IV access (but do not delay epinephrine) Continuous monitoring of blood pressure, heart rate, oxygen saturation, and respiratory symptoms.

Immediate intubation as delay may increase difficulty of endotracheal intubation. Cricothyroidotomy may be necessary if severe airway edema.

IM epinephrine 0.3–0.5 mg 1:1000 to anterior or lateral thigh, preferably. Repeat after 5 minutes as needed (up to 70% can require second dose) **FOR SEVERE SYMPTOMS OR POOR RESPONSE TO IM GIVE** IV epinephrine 0.1–0.2 mg (1 mL 1:1000 in 10 mL 0.9% NaCl [0.1 mg/mL]) 1–2 min until response **IF HYPOTENSIVE GIVE** 1–2 L IV 0.9% NaCl rapid infusion.

Treat all patients with histamine 1 and 2 (H1, H2) blockers.
1) Diphenhydramine (H1) 25–50 mg IV and
1) Ranitidine (H2) 50 mg IV or
2) Famotidine (H2) 20 mg IV

Clinical Response?   **Yes**

No

If patient taking home beta-blocker;
1) Glucagon 1– 2 mg IV/IM q5min to effect
For continued hypotension;
1) Start continuous IV epinephrine infusion at 0.1–1 μg/kg/min titrated to effect.
2) Continued aggressive fluid resuscitation (via rapid transfuser if available).
For continued respiratory symptoms, if not intubated
1) Inhaled beta-agonists (albuterol) 0.5 mL 0.5% soln in 2.5 mL 0.9% NaCl nebulized q15min.

IV, intravenous; IM, intramuscular.

is underused in emergency treatment, with delay resulting in shock and respiratory failure. In a study by Korenblat et al., 70% of patients with severe symptoms required at least two epinephrine injections. Intravenous steroids have no role in the acute treatment of anaphylaxis but may prevent phase 2 reactions that can occur up to 72 hours after initial presentation. Steroids are given as an initial dose of 1 to 2 mg/kg of intravenous methylprednisolone, or equivalent, and continued for up to 4 days (intravenously or orally). On discharge, patients should be referred to an allergist for testing and monitoring, and provided with home epinephrine self-injectors (EpiPen).

SUGGESTED READINGS

Joint Task Force on Practice Parameters; American Academy of Allergy, Asthma and Immunology; American College of Allergy, Asthma and Immunology; Joint Council of Allergy, Asthma and Immunology. The diagnosis and management of anaphylaxis: an updated practice parameters. *J Allergy Clin Immunol.* 2005;115:S483–S523.
> *Joint recommendations on the definition, causes, manifestations, diagnosis, and treatment for patients with anaphylaxis and anaphylactoid reactions.*

Korenblat P, Lundie MJ, Dankner RE, et al. A retrospective study of epinephrine administration for anaphylaxis: how many doses are needed? *Allergy Asthma Proc.* 1999;20:383–386.
> *Retrospective review of 105 anaphylactic episodes to determine the level of severity and corresponding number of epinephrine injections required for symptom reversal.*

Sheikh A, Shehata YA, Brown SG, et al. Adrenaline for the treatment of anaphylaxis: cochrane systematic review. *Allergy.* 2009;64:204–212.
> *A systematic evidence-based review on the use of epinephrine for the treatment of anaphylaxis.*

6

Mechanical Causes of Shock

Howard J. Huang

Mechanical shock can be precipitated by an array of syndromes that produce an acute loss of pulmonary vascular cross-sectional area, either by direct obstruction of pulmonary vasculature or through vasoconstriction driven by vasoactive mediators. The end result is an acute rise in pulmonary vascular resistance (PVR), which leads to right ventricular (RV) strain, RV failure, and shock. *Mechanical shock* is also called *obstructive shock;* these terms are used interchangeably in the literature. Cardiac tamponade, discussed in Chapter 4, can also be considered a mechanical cause of shock. However, its pathophysiology is distinct from the other forms of shock discussed here. Although the various etiologies of shock are discussed in isolation in this manual, it is important to recognize that several forms of shock may be present at the same time.

This discussion will focus on four major etiologies of mechanical shock: (1) massive pulmonary embolism, (2) air embolism, (3) fat embolism, and (4) amniotic fluid embolism. The degree of hemodynamic compromise caused by any of these causes of mechanical shock is determined by (1) the magnitude of pulmonary arterial vascular obstruction and/or vasoconstriction, (2) RV performance and reserve, and (3) preexisting cardiopulmonary disease (CPD). For example, a segmental pulmonary embolus normally survivable in an otherwise healthy postpartum patient may produce mechanical shock in a patient with preexisting pulmonary arterial hypertension and marginal RV function.

The pulmonary circulation is normally a high-capacitance, low-resistance circuit. In general, a right ventricle cannot acutely compensate for a mean pulmonary arterial pressure (mPAP) >40 mm Hg. Therefore, the finding of mPAP values >40 mm Hg without clinical signs of RV failure suggests a subacute or chronic cause of pulmonary arterial hypertension. In the absence of preexisting CPD, the increase in RV afterload and mPAP is directly proportional to the magnitude of pulmonary vascular obstruction and/or vasoconstriction. Echocardiographic findings of acute RV dysfunction may be evident following a 25% to 30% reduction in pulmonary vascular cross-sectional area. However, the degree of obstruction necessary to cause hemodynamic compromise and shock may be much lower in a patient with preexisting CPD.

Without aggressive intervention, an acute elevation in PRV beyond the capacity of RV compensation precipitates a deleterious chain of events that ends in refractory shock, circulatory collapse, and death. Algorithm 6.1 illustrates the interdependent nature of the multiple factors that contribute to obstructive shock. Successful management of mechanical shock syndromes requires early recognition and rapid initiation

ALGORITHM 6.1 Pathophysiology of Mechanical Shock

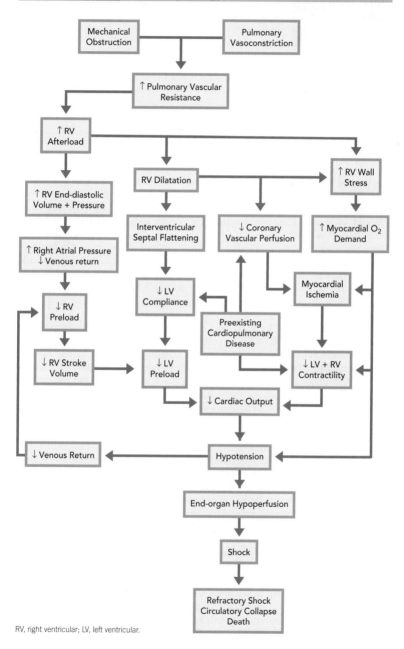

RV, right ventricular; LV, left ventricular.

of supportive measures to restore hemodynamic stability and prevent end-organ dysfunction.

Common clinical findings in mechanical shock states include tachycardia, hypotension, and signs of end-organ hypoperfusion (i.e., decreased urine output, cool and mottled extremities, and altered mental status). Physical examination should reveal signs of decompensated RV failure, including jugular venous distention, tricuspid regurgitation murmur, accentuated P2, hepatojugular reflux, and Kussmaul's sign. Dysregulation of ventilation–perfusion matching results in hypoxemia and tachypnea. In catastrophic cases, ventricular fibrillation, pulseless electrical activity, or asystole may be the initial presentation.

Diagnostically, sinus tachycardia is frequently seen on electrocardiogram (EKG), with or without changes suggestive of RV strain and myocardial ischemia. Echocardiographic signs of RV dysfunction, including RV dilatation, hypokinesis, tricuspid regurgitation, and flattening of the interventricular septum, may also be present. Common laboratory findings include hyponatremia, elevated serum brain natriuretic peptide (BNP), and markers of myocardial injury (troponin T or I).

The following sections discuss the unique features, pathophysiology, and management of four common mechanical shock syndromes. Table 6.1 contains a list of risk factors and presenting signs and symptoms for each syndrome.

PULMONARY EMBOLISM

Venous thromboembolism (VTE) is a common complication in critically ill medical and surgical patients. Most intensive care unit (ICU) patients have multiple major risk factors for VTE, including trauma, prolonged immobilization, malignancy, and indwelling vascular access devices. Clinical studies in medical ICUs have shown that up to one-third of patients not receiving deep venous thrombosis prophylaxis will eventually develop VTE at some point during their hospital course. Approximately 5% to 10% of patients with VTE develop pulmonary embolism (PE), with approximately 10% of these cases causing hemodynamically significant or massive PE. The presence of shock in the setting of PE is associated with a five- to sevenfold increase in mortality. Patients presenting with cardiopulmonary arrest have mortality rates exceeding 65%.

Bedside 2-D echocardiography is a useful diagnostic tool for evaluating hemodynamic status in patients with suspected massive PE. Alternative diagnoses, such as cardiomyopathy, valvular disease, cardiac tamponade, and aortic dissection, can be quickly excluded from the differential diagnosis. McConnell's sign, a classic echocardiographic sign of massive PE, is characterized by global RV hypokinesis with relative sparing of the apical segments.

Initiation of therapy should not be delayed for confirmatory diagnostic testing. Treatment should be focused on (1) restoring hemodynamic stability, (2) maintaining adequate oxygenation, and (3) reducing clot burden and preventing recurrent embolus. A management algorithm for massive PE is shown in Algorithm 6.2.

Multiple randomized controlled trials have addressed the role of thrombolytic (fibrinolytic) therapy versus anticoagulation with unfractionated or low-molecular-weight heparin as initial treatment for PE. Yet, no trial to date has demonstrated a clear mortality benefit for thrombolytic therapy over anticoagulant therapy. However, a meta-analysis of 11 randomized controlled trials showed that early thrombolytic therapy reduced the risk of recurrent embolus and death in hemodynamically unstable patients. Moreover, thrombolytic therapy has been associated with faster recovery of

TABLE 6.1	Risk Factors and Common Manifestations of Mechanical Shock States	
State	Risk factors	Common signs and symptoms
Massive pulmonary embolism	• Immobilization • Surgery within last 3 months • Prior history of VTE • Malignancy • Chronic CPD • Trauma • Obesity • Central venous catheters • Hypercoagulable state	• Pleuritic chest pain • Respiratory distress • Cough • Wheezing • Hemoptysis • Hypoxemia • Cyanosis • Fever
Air embolism syndrome	• Open surgical site above RA (craniotomy, cesarean section) • Use of medical gases in laparoscopic or endoscopic procedures • Volume depletion • Barotrauma • Pulmonary vasodilators • Biopsy of airway or lung parenchyma • Venous access devices • Contrast injection • Trauma	• Anxiety • Sense of impending doom • Chest pain • Respiratory distress • Wheezing • Cyanosis • Hypoxemia • Gasp reflex • Mill-wheel murmur • Agitation, delirium, seizure activity (arterial gas embolization)
Fat embolism syndrome	• Blunt-force trauma resulting in long-bone and pelvic fractures • Orthopedic procedures • Extensive rib fractures • Burn injury • Acute pancreatitis • Diabetes mellitus • Sickle cell anemia • Liposuction • Parenteral lipid infusion	• Agitation • Delirium • Seizure activity • Fevers and chills • Chest pain • Respiratory distress • Wheezing • Cyanosis • Hypoxemia • Petechial rash involving axilla and upper trunk
Amniotic fluid embolism syndrome	• Pregnancy • Peripartum • Postpartum (up to 48 hours) • Difficult labor • Use of labor induction agents • Amniocentesis • First or second trimester abortion • Trauma	• Agitation and delirium • Seizure activity • Fevers and chills • Nausea and vomiting • Respiratory distress • Wheezing • Chest pain • Cyanosis • Hypoxemia • Profuse hemorrhage with no obvious structural cause • Fetal bradycardia or late decelerations

VTE, venous thromboembolism; CPD, cardiopulmonary disease; RA, right atrium.

ALGORITHM 6.2 Management Algorithm for Massive Pulmonary Embolism

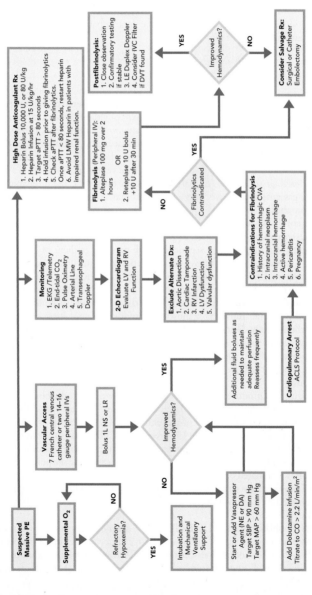

PE, pulmonary embolism; IVs, intravenous catheters; EKG, electrocardiogram; aPTT, activated partial thromboplastin time; LMW, low-molecular-weight; NS, normal saline; LR, lactated ringers; LV, left ventricular; RV, right ventricular; DVT, deep venous thrombosis; IVC, inferior vena cava; NE, norepinephrine; DA, dopamine; SBP, systolic blood pressure; MAP, mean arterial pressure; ACLS, advanced cardiac life support; CVA, cerebral vascular accident; LE.

RV function and improvement in hemodynamic status. Accordingly, in hemodynamically unstable patients without absolute contraindications to thrombolysis, the early use of thrombolytics should be considered. For patients with major contraindications to thrombolytic therapy or unresponsive to pharmacologic thrombolysis, catheter thrombectomy or open surgical embolectomy may be attempted as salvage therapy.

Once hemodynamic stability is restored, definitive diagnosis can be established by computed tomographic angiography or pulmonary angiography. An evaluation for deep venous thrombosis by duplex Doppler ultrasound should be performed with consideration of inferior vena cava filter placement in patients with marginal cardiac function and high clot burden.

AIR EMBOLISM

Air embolism syndrome (AES) occurs when gas enters the arterial or venous circulation driven by a pressure gradient favoring entrainment of gas, or through direct injection. Arterial gas embolization may occur through anatomic shunts (e.g., patent foramen ovale, vascular malformations), pulmonary vasodilator administration, or if the filtration capacity of the pulmonary circulation is overwhelmed by a large volume of gas entering the venous circulation. Indeed, each case of venous air embolism is a potential case of arterial air embolism. Arterial AES typically does not cause mechanical shock. However, gas entering the coronary circulation may cause myocardial ischemia and cardiogenic shock.

Gas enters the venous circulation when there is a negative intrathoracic pressure in the presence of an open central or peripheral vein, or if the open vein is elevated above the right atrium. Even a seemingly small pressure gradient of -5 cm H_2O is sufficient to allow gas to enter the venous circulation at up to 100 mL/sec through a 14-gauge peripheral IV. In the setting of volume depletion and decreased central venous pressure, or if the extravascular environment is under positive pressure (e.g., CO_2 insufflation during laparoscopic surgery), the risk of venous gas embolism increases significantly. Animal studies have shown that sudden, large-volume gas embolism is lethal. Although slow, continuous small-volume gas embolism is survivable, even if the cumulative volume of gas is large. In humans, the estimated lethal dose in venous AES is approximately 200 to 300 mL, and up to 500 mL if gas is entrained slowly. However, acute embolism of as little as 50 mL of gas may be sufficient to cause hemodynamic compromise.

Venous AES produces mechanical shock mainly through the obstruction of the RV outflow tract. The severity of hemodynamic and gas exchange abnormalities depends on (1) the total volume of gas entrained, (2) the rate at which gas enters the pulmonary arterial circulation, (3) preexisting CPD, and (4) the severity of the inflammatory response triggered by gas deposited in the pulmonary circulation. Unlike embolism of solid materials such as thrombus or fat, gas entering the pulmonary arterial circulation is eliminated continuously by diffusion across alveolar capillaries. Thus, if the portal of gas entry is eliminated, and if RV performance is capable of compensating for the elevated PVR, AES-induced mechanical shock should resolve as the embolized gas is cleared.

AES should be considered in the differential diagnosis for patients presenting with acute hemodynamic instability and gas-exchange abnormalities in the proper clinical setting. Table 6.1 lists common risk factors for AES. Mechanical shock induced by AES may be difficult to distinguish from other etiologies of shock. If arterial air embolism occurs and air enters the coronary arterial circulation, cardiogenic shock is added to the picture. Early assessment of hemodynamic function using 2-D echocardiography, transesophageal Doppler, or pulmonary arterial (PA) catheter can determine the predominant cause of shock. Therapy for AES is supportive and should focus on (1) eliminating the portal of gas entry, (2) restoring hemodynamic stability, and (3) promoting clearance of the entrained gas. A management algorithm for AES is shown in Algorithm 6.3.

Although there is no randomized clinical trial data, air aspiration from the RV through a central venous catheter has been reported to remove up to 50% of the embolized gas, producing rapid hemodynamic improvement. The patient is placed in the left lateral decubitus position, elevating the RV above its outflow tract and promoting migration of entrained air back into the RV. A central venous catheter is then placed with the tip approximately 2 cm below the superior vena cava/right atrial junction, and air is aspirated through the distal port. In the setting of refractory cardiopulmonary arrest, emergency thoracotomy, cardiac massage, and direct aspiration of air through the right ventricle may be attempted as a last resort.

Emphasis should be placed on prevention of gas embolization during surgical and medical procedures through adequate hydration, proper patient positioning, avoidance of barotrauma, and observing proper procedures for vascular access insertion and removal. Patients at high risk for AES should be closely monitored via capnography or precordial Doppler ultrasound to detect gas embolization during surgical procedures. Early detection and prompt supportive treatment of AES can dramatically improve outcomes.

FAT EMBOLISM

Fat embolism syndrome (FES) occurs when fat from necrotic bone marrow or adipocytes is released into the venous circulation following trauma or tissue injury, causing mechanical obstruction of the pulmonary vascular bed and triggering a systemic inflammatory response. Approximately 90% of cases of FES occur following blunt trauma resulting in pelvic and long-bone fractures. The risk of developing FES rises with the severity of the injury and the number of large marrow-containing bones involved.

The pathobiology of FES remains incompletely understood. Studies have shown circulating fat in blood specimens collected from patients undergoing orthopedic surgery. This observation suggests that the presence of fat in the circulation is necessary but not sufficient to precipitate FES. The severity of FES-induced mechanical shock probably depends on multiple factors, including (1) the total volume and rate of fat embolization, (2) the immunogenicity of the embolized material, (3) the intensity of the host inflammatory response, and (4) preexisting CPD.

Shock in the early phase of FES is mainly caused by mechanical obstruction of the pulmonary vasculature causing RV failure. Within 24 to 72 hours of the initial insult, toxic free fatty acid metabolites cause systemic inflammation, acute lung injury, and end-organ dysfunction with hemodynamic derangements similar to those found in septic shock. A classic triad of clinical findings consisting of hypoxemia, neurologic dysfunction, and petechial rash involving the upper trunk and axilla may be found in some patients.

No specific diagnostic test is available for FES. Treatment is supportive and should be focused on (1) restoring hemodynamic stability and (2) maintaining adequate

ALGORITHM 6.3   Management Algorithm for Air Embolism Syndrome

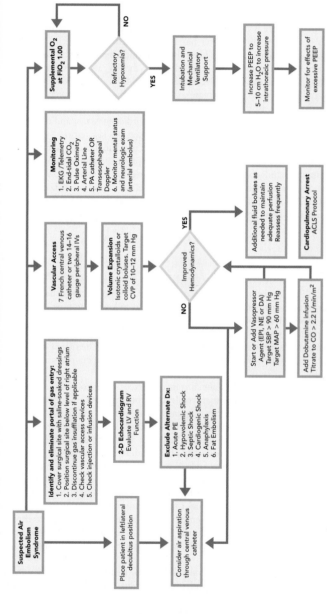

LV, left ventricular; RV, right ventricular; CVP, central venous pressure; PE, pulmonary embolism; EPI, epinephrine; NE, norepinephrine; DA, dopamine; SBP, systolic blood pressure; MAP, mean arterial pressure; IVs, intravenous catheters; EKG, electrocardiogram; PA, pulmonary arterial; PEEP, positive end-expiratory pressure; ACLS, advanced cardiac life support.

ALGORITHM 6.4 Management Algorithm for Fat Embolism Syndrome

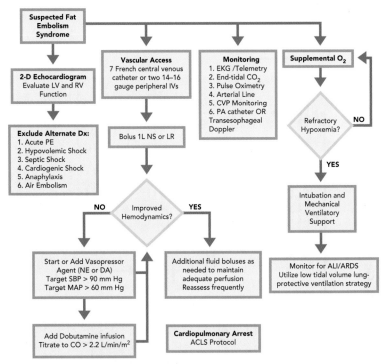

LV, left ventricular; RV, right ventricular; PE, pulmonary embolism; IVs, intravenous catheters; NS, normal saline; LR, lactated ringers; NE, norepinephrine; DA, dopamine; SBP, systolic blood pressure; MAP, mean arterial pressure; EKG, electrocardiogram; CVP, central venous pressure; PA, pulmonary arterial; ARDS, acute respiratory distress syndrome; ACLS, advanced cardiac life support; ACI.

oxygenation to avoid end-organ dysfunction. There is some evidence for prophylactic administration of corticosteroids in patients at high risk for FES. However, there is no evidence to support corticosteroid use after the FES has occurred. A management algorithm for FES is shown in Algorithm 6.4. A high clinical index of suspicion and early institution of supportive care is necessary to improve outcomes for patients with FES.

AMNIOTIC FLUID EMBOLISM

Amniotic fluid embolism syndrome (AFES) occurs when amniotic fluid (AF) enters the maternal circulation during labor and delivery or in the postpartum period due to cervical, uterine wall, or placental membrane disruption. Classic findings include the acute onset of shock, hypoxemia, encephalopathy, coagulopathy, and disseminated intravascular coagulation. A fulminant presentation of AES can lead to circulatory

ALGORITHM 6.5   Management Algorithm for Amniotic Fluid Embolism Syndrome

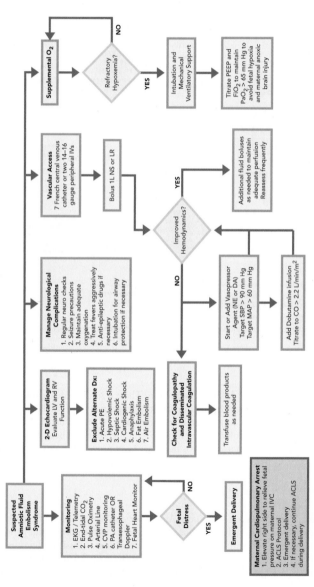

EKG, electrocardiogram; CVP, central venous pressure; PA, pulmonary arterial; RV, right ventricular; LV, left ventricular; PE, pulmonary embolism; IVs, intravenous catheters; NS, normal saline; LR, lactated ringers; NE, norepinephrine; DA, dopamine; MAP, mean arterial pressure; IVC, inferior vena cava; ACLS, advanced cardiac life support; PEEP, positive end-expiratory pressure.

collapse and death within a matter of hours. Survivors of this devastating syndrome are frequently left with severe neurologic impairment.

The pathogenesis of AFES remains incompletely understood. AF contains a heterogeneous mixture of water, electrolytes, hormones, and fetal components. AF components are routinely found in blood specimens from asymptomatic pregnant women, suggesting that entry of AF components into the maternal circulation is necessary but not sufficient to cause AFES. The development of AFES is likely determined by multiple factors, including (1) the absolute volume of AF and its rate of entry into the maternal circulation, (2) AF composition that affects its immunogenicity and vasoactive properties, (3) maternal immune response, and (4) preexisting maternal CPD.

The etiology of AFES-induced shock is often multifactorial and temporally heterogeneous. The early phase of AFES is dominated by severe acute left ventricular (LV) systolic dysfunction and cardiogenic shock. This may be accompanied by arrhythmias including bradycardia, ventricular fibrillation, pulseless electrical activity, or even asystole. Deposition of AF in the pulmonary circulation triggers intense pulmonary vasoconstriction, RV failure, and precipitates mechanical shock. The late phase of AFES, typically occurring 1 to 2 hours later, is frequently complicated by distributive shock caused by the severe systemic inflammatory response triggered by immunogenic AF components. Cardiogenic and obstructive shock may persist into the late phase of AFES, but usually improve over time. Disseminated intravascular coagulation and coagulopathy may add hemorrhagic shock to the picture.

The acute onset of agitation, altered mental status, dyspnea, and hemodynamic instability in a pregnant or peripartum woman should raise clinical suspicion for AFES. No specific test is available for diagnosing AFES. Management of AFES is supportive and consists of the following goals: (1) restoring and maintaining maternal hemodynamic stability, (2) maintaining adequate oxygenation to prevent maternal and fetal hypoxia, (3) correcting anemia and coagulopathy, (4) treating neurologic manifestations, and (5) expediting delivery of the fetus. A management algorithm for AFES is shown in Algorithm 6.5.

Bedside 2-D echocardiography is a useful modality for rapidly assessing LV and RV function. As multiple etiologies of shock are commonly encountered during the course of AFES, a transesophageal Doppler or PA catheter is useful for monitoring changing hemodynamic status and for guiding fluid resuscitation and titration of vasopressors and inotropes. Successful management of AFES requires early recognition, prompt initiation of supportive measures, and close coordination between the intensivist, obstetrician, and anesthesiologist.

SUGGESTED READINGS

Agnelli G, Becattini C. Current concepts: acute pulmonary embolism. *N Engl J Med.* 2010;363:266–274.
  Review of diagnostic strategy and management of acute PE, including risk stratification for hemodynamically stable patients with PE.
Goldhaber SZ. Echocardiography in the management of pulmonary embolism. *Ann Intern Med.* 2002;136:691–700.
  Review of common echocardiographic findings in pulmonary embolism.
Jorens PG, Van Marck E, Snoeckx A, et al. Nonthrombotic pulmonary embolism. *Eur Respir J.* 2009;34:452–474.
  Review of various nonthrombotic etiologies that can produce mechanical shock.

Marek MA, Lele AV, Fitzsimmons L, et al. Diagnosis and treatment of vascular air embolism. *Anesthesiology.* 2007;106:164–177.

Mellor A, Soni N. Fat embolism. *Anaesthesia.* 2001;56(2):145–154.
  A review of etiology, diagnosis, and treatment of fat embolism syndrome.

Moore J, Baldisseri MR. Amniotic fluid embolism. *Crit Care Med.* 2005;33(Suppl):S279–S285.
  Thorough discussion of pathogenesis, diagnosis, and treatment of the amniotic fluid embolism syndrome.

Piazza G, Goldhaber SZ. The acutely decompensated right ventricle: pathways for diagnosis and management. *Chest.* 2005;128:1836–1852.
  Overview of the signs and symptoms and general management strategy for acute right ventricular decompensation.

Wood KE. Major pulmonary embolism: review of a pathophysiologic approach to the golden hour of hemodynamically significant pulmonary embolism. *Chest.* 2002;121:877–905.
  Comprehensive review of the pathogenesis, diagnosis, and management of hemodynamically significant pulmonary embolism.

7 An Approach to Respiratory Failure

Warren Isakow

Respiratory failure is a common reason for intensive care unit admission and is the final pathway for a number of diseases of differing pathophysiology. A mechanism-based approach enables the clinician to identify the most likely cause for the respiratory failure and to treat appropriately. In general, patients with respiratory failure may be classified into two groups, depending on the component of the respiratory system that is involved.

- Hypercapnic respiratory failure is a consequence of ventilatory failure and is recognized by an elevated $PaCO_2$ above normal (>45 mm Hg at sea level). This denotes failure of the respiratory pump and can occur with normal lungs.
- Hypoxemic respiratory failure is a consequence of gas exchange failure and is recognized by hypoxemia (PaO_2 <60 mm Hg) with or without widening of the alveolar-arterial O_2 gradient.

HYPERCAPNIC RESPIRATORY FAILURE

The hallmark of hypercapnic respiratory failure is an elevated $PaCO_2$ above 45 mm Hg.

$$PaCO_2 = K \times \frac{VcO_2}{(1 - Vd/Vt) \times VA}$$

where $PaCO_2$ = the partial pressure of carbon dioxide in the blood, K = constant, VcO_2 = carbon dioxide production, Vd/Vt = dead-space ratio of each tidal volume breath, and VA = minute ventilation.

Analysis of the previous equation shows that hypercapnia can occur from three processes: (a) an increase in CO_2 production, (b) a decrease in minute ventilation, and (c) an increase in dead-space ventilation. Understanding of the "respiratory pump" enables the clinician to systematically consider the cause of hypercapnic respiratory failure in different patients, as depicted in Algorithm 7.1.

The acuity of onset of the hypercapnia is also an important determinant of management. An acute change in $PaCO_2$ of 10 mm Hg will change the blood pH by 0.08 in the opposite direction. In patients with chronic hypercapnia, renal compensation occurs by bicarbonate retention and tends to correct the pH toward normal. In these cases, a change in $PaCO_2$ of 10 mm Hg is reflected by a change of 0.03 in the blood

ALGORITHM 7.1 Causes of Hypercapnic Respiratory Failure Based on Components of the Respiratory Pump

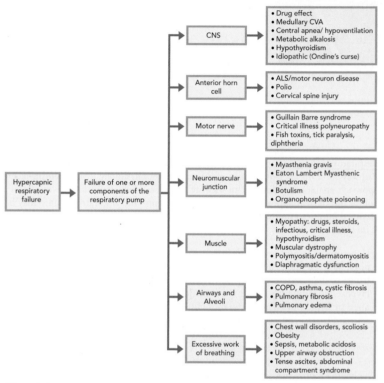

CVA, cerebrovascular accident; ALS, amyotrophic lateral sclerosis; COPD, chronic obstructive pulmonary disease; CNS, central nervous system.

pH in the opposite direction. Recognition of acute hypercapnia or acute on chronic hypercapnia is vitally important as it is a harbinger of an imminent respiratory arrest and potential development of severe hypoxemia.

Important principles in managing patients with hypercapnia are as follows:

- Never sedate a patient with hypercapnia or a patient who has neuromuscular weakness.
- Cautious use of supplemental oxygen is necessary as oxygen can worsen hypercapnia by a number of mechanisms: worsening of V/Q matching, the Haldane effect, and suppression of central hypoxemic drive. Enough oxygen should be given to keep the hemoglobin molecules >90% saturated with oxygen.
- Rapidly institute adequate ventilation: in carefully selected patients, noninvasive ventilation can be tried prior to intubation and mechanical ventilation.

HYPOXEMIC RESPIRATORY FAILURE

Hypoxemic respiratory failure occurs because of impaired gas exchange or hypoventilation and is defined by a PaO_2 of <60 mm Hg. The first step in ascertaining a cause is looking for concomitant hypercapnia as would occur with hypoventilation or severe intrinsic lung disease with increased dead-space ventilation, and calculating the alveolar-arterial oxygen gradient by using the alveolar gas equation. The approach to hypoxemic respiratory failure is summarized in Algorithm 7.2.

The alveolar gas equation follows:

$$PAO_2 = FiO_2(PB - PH_2O) - \frac{PaCO_2}{R}$$

where PAO_2 = alveolar partial pressure of oxygen, FiO_2 = fraction of inspired oxygen, PB = barometric pressure (760 mm Hg at sea level), PH_2O = water vapor pressure (47 mm Hg), $PaCO_2$ = partial pressure of carbon dioxide in the blood, and R = respiratory quotient, assumed to be 0.8.

The alveolar–arterial oxygen gradient = PAO_2–PaO_2. The normal value is between 10 and 15 mm Hg and is influenced by age, increasing by 3 mm Hg every decade after the age of 30 years. For an FiO_2 = 21%, it should be 5 to 25 mm Hg and for an FiO_2 = 100%, it should be <150 mm Hg. Hypoxemic respiratory failure with a widened alveolar–arterial oxygen gradient is caused by V/Q mismatching or shunt pathophysiology. These two processes can be differentiated by improvement in the hypoxemia with supplemental oxygen, in the case of V/Q mismatch, and no improvement in cases with shunt. Diseases that cause airspace flooding, atelectasis, airway disease, or pulmonary vascular problems are common causes of hypoxemic respiratory failure.

Management principles for patients with hypoxemic respiratory failure include the following:

- Rapid restoration of an adequate arterial saturation, which often requires intubation and mechanical ventilation. Patients with hypoxemia as a group respond less well to noninvasive ventilation.
- Use of adequate amounts of positive end-expiratory pressure to reduce FiO_2 to nontoxic levels (FiO_2 <60%).
- A low tidal volume strategy with permissive hypercapnia in patients with acute lung injury/acute respiratory distress syndrome.
- General supportive care in the intensive care unit while the patient's pulmonary process resolves.

It is worthwhile to note that hypoxia refers to an oxygen deficit at a tissue level and depends on oxygen delivery. Therefore, hypoxia can be a result of any process that affects oxygen delivery to the tissues, and includes the following:

- Hypoxic hypoxia (low arterial oxygen saturation and a low PAO_2)
- Anemic hypoxia (low circulating hemoglobin with impaired oxygen delivery)
- Circulatory hypoxia (low cardiac output states)
- Histotoxic hypoxia (poisoning with cyanide where oxygen is delivered to the tissues but cannot be used).

Oxygen delivery = Cardiac Output × Arterial Oxygen Content

$$DO_2 = CO \times CaO_2$$
$$DO_2 = CO \times (1.39 \times [Hb(g/dL)] \times SaO_2) + 0.003 \times PaO_2$$

ALGORITHM 7.2 General Approach to Hypoxemic Respiratory Failure

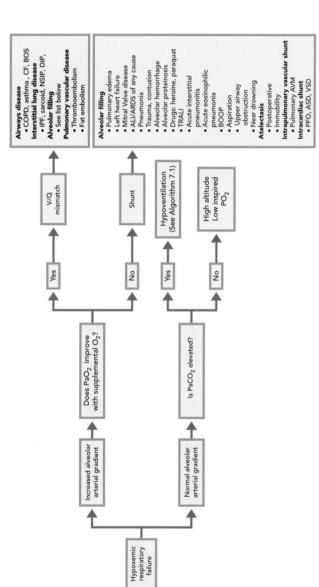

COPD, chronic obstructive pulmonary disease; CF, cystic fibrosis; BOS, bronchiolitis obliterans syndrome; IPF, interstitial pulmonary fibrosis; NSIP, nonspecific interstitial pneumonitis; DIP, desquamative interstitial pneumonia; ALI/ARDS, acute lung injury/acute respiratory distress syndrome; TRALI, transfusion-related acute lung injury; BOOP, bronchiolitis obliterans-organizing pneumonia; AVM, arteriovenous malformation; PFO, patent foramen ovale; ASD, atrial septal defect; VSD, ventricular septal defect.

SUGGESTED READINGS

Lanken PN. Approach to acute respiratory failure. In: Lanken PN, ed. The intensive care unit manual. Philadelphia, PA: Saunders, 2001:1–12.

A superb concise chapter focusing on developing a pathophysiological approach to all patients with respiratory failure.

Wood LDH. The pathophysiology and differential diagnosis of acute respiratory failure. In: Hall JB, Schmidt GA, Wood LDH, eds. Principles of critical care. New York: McGraw-Hill, 2005:417–426.

Another superb textbook chapter focusing on pathophysiology.

8 Initial Ventilator Setup

Warren Isakow

The initiation of mechanical ventilation is a critical period during the course of a patient's stay in the intensive care unit. The clinician is encouraged to monitor the patient closely during initiation of mechanical ventilation as this period often provides important answers regarding a patient's underlying pathophysiologic abnormality. This simple bedside process allows for verification of the underlying cause of the decompensation requiring ventilatory support, assessment of severity of the disease process, the likely response to standard therapies, and it helps with planning of care during the next few days to weeks.

Table 8.1 provides a general guideline to the initial ventilator settings in different clinical circumstances. The table is simply a guide, and the reader should understand that every patient is unique and should have the ventilator adjusted according to the individual's clinical status.

Algorithm 8.1 is a management algorithm for troubleshooting the situation of a patient with persistent high peak airway pressures, a common ventilator-related problem in the intensive care unit. Table 8.2 provides potential causes for an alarm resulting from a low exhaled tidal volume/low minute ventilation.

TABLE 8.1 Guidelines for Initial Ventilator Settings in Different Clinical Scenarios

Indication for mechanical ventilation	Mode of choice	Respiratory rate (breaths/min)	Tidal volume (mL/kg)	FiO_2	PEEP	Additional ventilator issues	Adjunctive therapies	Additional comments
Airway protection, spontaneously breathing patient (e.g., hepatic encephalopathy, upper airway obstruction)	AC (volume) SIMV PSV	10–14	8–10	100%, obtain ABG and wean for sats >92% to goal FiO_2 of 40%	5	Peak flow 60 L/min Trigger sensitivity –2 cm H_2O	DVT GI	Maintain on MV until upper airway issues resolved Patients with hepatic encephalopathy are prone to develop a respiratory alkalosis, so TV may need to be reduced
Asthma exacerbation	AC (volume)	Set rate low, 8–12	6–8	100%, obtain ABG and wean for sats >92% to goal FiO_2 of 40%	0–5	Set peak flows high, allow adequate expiratory time Consider square wave ventilation. Use flow-by for easier triggering	BD ST AB SDN DVT GI	Tolerate hypercarbia, higher peak airway pressures Monitor for auto-PEEP and barotrauma Do not ventilate for a "normal" ABG Apply external PEEP to overcome intrinsic PEEP when triggering Often need heavy sedation initially Once bronchospasm and acute issues adequately resolved do not do prolonged weaning trials, consider trial of extubation

(continued)

45

TABLE 8.1 Guidelines for Initial Ventilator Settings in Different Clinical Scenarios *(Continued)*

Indication for mechanical ventilation	Mode of choice	Respiratory rate (breaths/min)	Tidal volume (mL/kg)	FiO₂	PEEP	Additional ventilator issues	Adjunctive therapies	Additional comments
COPD exacerbation	AC (volume)	Set rate low, 8–12	6–8	100%, obtain ABG and wean for sats >92% to goal FiO₂ of 40%	0–5	Set peak flows high, allow adequate E time Use flow by for easier triggering	BD ST AB DVT GI NUTR	Monitor for auto-PEEP Avoid posthypercapnic alkalosis Tolerate hypercarbia; do not ventilate for a "normal" ABG Monitor for barotrauma Apply external PEEP to overcome intrinsic PEEP when triggering Consider extubation to NIPPV
Hypoxemic respiratory failure with pneumonia or pulmonary edema	AC (volume)	Often need high rates, 16–24 because of high V_E requirements	6–8	100%, obtain ABG and wean for sats >92% to goal FiO₂ of 40%	5–10	Often have high V_E requirements	BD AB DVT GI NUTR	Secretion management is important In septic patients, allow full MVS to divert CO from the respiratory muscles to other vital organs Follow improvement clinically as improved pulmonary compliance

Condition	Mode	Rate	FiO₂	PEEP	Comments	Complications	Notes
ALI/ARDS	AC (volume) PCV, high-frequency oscillator, APRV	Often need high rates, up to 30, because of high V_E requirements	100%, obtain ABG and wean for sats >92% to "safe" FiO₂ of <60%	5–15	May need I:E of 1:1 or 1.5:1 (IRV) Need higher mean airway pressures Allow permissive hypercarbia to pH of 7.20	BD DVT GI NUTR SDN	Consider nebulized prostacyclin, nitric oxide, or oscillator Monitor for barotrauma Often require heavy sedation Try to avoid neuromuscular blockade if possible Consider adjunctive steroids Monitor for septic complications
Postoperative respiratory failure	AC (volume)	Set rate at 10–16	100%, wean rapidly for sats >92% to goal FiO₂ of 30%	5	Verify placement of all lines, tubes placed in OR Peak flow 60 L/min	DVT GI	Await sedatives, paralytics to be cleared and perform weaning rapidly Prone to hypoventilation after extubation Prone to atelectasis and splinting due to pain that can cause hypoxemia
Hypoventilation from CNS depression, neuromuscular weakness	AC (volume)	Set rate at 10–16	100%, obtain ABG and wean rapidly for sats of <92% to goal FiO₂ of 30%	5	Peak flow 60 L/min	GI DVT NUTR	Avoid sedatives Prone to atelectasis Follow NIF in patients with weakness

PEEP, positive end-expiratory pressure; AC, assist control; SIMV, synchronized intermittent mandatory ventilation; PSV, pressure support ventilation; ABG, arterial blood gas; sats, hemoglobin oxygen saturation; DVT, deep venous thrombosis; GI, gastrointestinal; MV, mechanical ventilation; TV, tidal volume; BD, bronchodilator; ST, steroids; AB, antibiotics; SDN, sedation; COPD, chronic obstructive pulmonary disease; NIPPV, noninvasive positive pressure ventilation; V_E, minute ventilation; MVS, mechanical ventilator support; CO, cardiac output; PCV, pressure control ventilation; I:E, expiratory time ratio; IRV, inverse ratio ventilation; NUTR, nutritional support; OR, operating room; NIF, negative inspiratory force; APRV, airway pressure release ventilation.

ALGORITHM 8.1 Management Algorithm for High Peak Airway Pressures

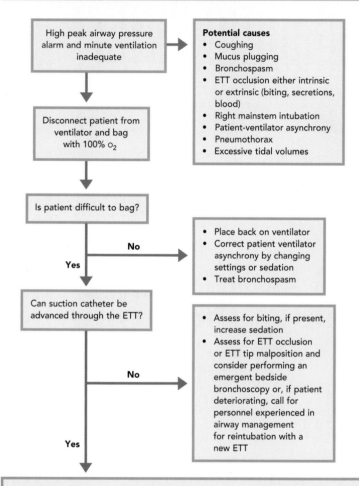

ETT, endotracheal tube; ICS, intercostal space.

TABLE 8.2	**Potential Causes for a Low Exhaled Tidal Volume/Low Minute Ventilation Alarm**

Leak in the circuit
- Tracheal cuff leak
- Patient inadvertently extubated or endotracheal tube tip high, causing a leak
- Ventilator circuit disconnected at any point from the patient to the ventilator
- Large bronchopleural fistula with leak through a chest tube

In patients on pressure support ventilation
- Worsening respiratory system compliance
- Decreased patient effort
- Decreased patient respiratory rate
- Inadequate pressure support being provided

In patients on pressure control ventilation
- Worsening respiratory system compliance

SUGGESTED READING

Reily DJ, Lanken PN. Ventilator alarm situations. In: Lanken PN, ed. The intensive care unit manual. Philadelphia, PA: Saunders, 2001:553–561.
   A practical chapter with clinical information on how to deal with common ventilator alarms.

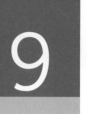

9 Upper Airway Obstruction

Warren Isakow

Upper airway obstruction is a medical emergency that requires rapid evaluation of the patient with simultaneous therapy to ensure adequate oxygenation and ventilation of the patient. Prompt recognition of premonitory symptoms and signs may enable the physician to buy precious time for evaluation and planning patient care. The common causes of upper airway obstruction are presented in Table 9.1, and an algorithm for the rapid assessment and management of the patient is presented in Algorithm 9.1. It is important to note that with most patients, upper airway obstruction is a clinical diagnosis that does not allow for laboratory testing, arterial blood gas analysis, or even imaging in the acute setting, and all resources should be directed to preventing cardiorespiratory arrest and securing the airway. Figures 9.1–9.5 review the anatomy of the upper airway, intubation technique, and illustrate practical aspects of performing emergent airway access.

Some common etiologies and their management are briefly reviewed in the following text.

INFECTIOUS EPIGLOTTITIS AND LARYNGITIS

Routine pediatric vaccination against *Haemophilus influenzae* has now made epiglottitis more common in adults than in children. The potential pathogens include *Haemophilus influenzae* and *Haemophilus parainfluenzae, Streptococcus pneumoniae, Streptococcus pyogenes, Staphylococcus aureus,* and occasionally anaerobes, while laryngitis is often caused by viruses and rarely *Corynebacterium diphtheriae,* which is more common in unvaccinated individuals.

The classic presentation is of an adult who is drooling, appears toxic, and is sitting upright in the tripod position. These patients have a high potential for complete occlusion of the airway and should be treated with empiric intravenous (IV) antibiotics (ceftriaxone, 2 g IV every 24 hours, or TMP-SMX, 10 mg/kg per day divided every 6 hours if allergic to penicillin). Personnel with experience in handling difficult airways should be called in to evaluate the patient, and a tracheostomy set should be brought into the examining room. If an examination is to be performed fiberoptically, preferentially this should be done in the operating room with a tracheostomy set available. The examination needs to be performed cautiously so as not to precipitate further narrowing of the airway.

In cases of epiglottitis, the epiglottis appears swollen and beefy. Diphtheria is characterized by a gray membrane. Blood cultures may occasionally be positive for

TABLE 9.1	Etiology and Specific Therapy of Upper Airway Obstruction by Site	
Site of obstruction	**Etiology**	**Specific therapy**
Nasopharynx	• Nasal polyps • Nasal tumors, lymphoma • Adenoidal hypertrophy • Trauma • Nasal packing	• Nasal steroids, surgery • Radiation, surgery, chemotherapy • Adenoidectomy • Fracture reduction, incise hematomas • Prophylactic antibiotics for sinusitis, humidified oxygen
Oropharynx	• Ludwig's angina • Odontogenic abscess • Retropharyngeal abscess • Peritonsillar abscess • Tonsillar enlargement • Macroglossia • Angioedema • Stevens–Johnson syndrome • Burkitt lymphoma • Salivary tumors • LeFort fractures 2 and 3 • Obstructive sleep apnea	• Antibiotics, drainage, may need tracheotomy • Antibiotics and drainage • Antibiotics and drainage • Tonsillectomy • Supportive, tracheotomy • Antihistamines, steroids, epinephrine (see text) • Supportive care, tracheotomy • Chemoradiation • Resection • Tracheotomy, fixation • CPAP, UPPP, tracheotomy
Laryngopharynx	• Epiglottitis • Acute bacterial laryngotracheitis (diphtheria) • Neoplasms: SCC, papillomatosis • Angioedema • Rheumatoid arthritis • Relapsing polychondritis • ANCA positive vasculitis • Midline granuloma • ETT injury: subglottic stenosis • Trauma, burns, inhalation injury • Hemangiomas • Foreign body aspiration, dislodged tooth • Iatrogenic: laryngospasm, epistaxis	• Antibiotics • Antibiotics • Resection, laser removal • Antihistamines, steroids, epinephrine (see text) • Corticosteroids, tracheotomy • Corticosteroids, tracheotomy • Corticosteroids, cyclophosphamide, tracheotomy • Radiation • Resection, dilation, cryotherapy • Tracheotomy • Laser, intralesional steroids, tracheotomy • Endoscopy • Supportive

CPAP, continuous positive airway pressure; UPPP, uvulopalatopharyngoplasty; SCC, squamous cell carcinoma; ETT, endotracheal tube.

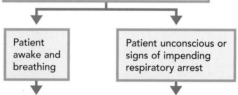

Airway obstruction suspected by history and physical examination:
- Inspiratory stridor: lesion at or above glottis
- Biphasic stridor and wheeze: subglottic lesion or below the glottis
- Impaired phonation
- Poor air entry
- Suprasternal retractions
- Universal choking sign
- Respiratory distress
- Tachycardia
- Agitation
- Angioedema
- Wheezing
- Neck swelling

Patient awake and breathing

Patient unconscious or signs of impending respiratory arrest

- Attempt to localize cause by history and examination
- Assemble help with personnel experienced in difficult airways (anesthesia, ENT)
- Assemble intubation equipment and a tracheostomy tray
- Consider transfer to the operating room to optimize available equipment and personnel
- Careful performance of indirect laryngoscopy or fiberoptic nasopharyngolaryngoscopy

- Call for help to assemble personnel experienced in difficult airways (anesthesia and/or ENT)
- Head tilt-chin lift
- Jaw thrust (if C-spine unstable)
- Insert an oral or nasal airway
- Ventilate with a bag-valvemask
- Attempt direct laryngoscopy and endotracheal intubation
- Surgical airway (bedside tracheostomy)
- Cricothyroidotomy or needle cricothyrotomy if personnel not available to perform a bedside surgical airway

- Management based on diagnosis
- Can use heliox or BiPAP if etiology not progressive
- Close monitoring

- Additional management based on etiology

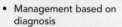

ENT, ear, nose, and throat specialist.

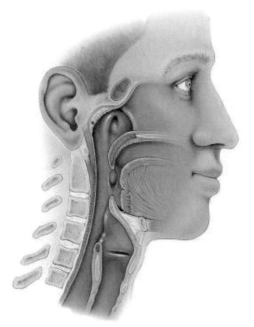

Figure 9.1 Anatomy of the pharynx and larynx—sagittal section. (Adapted from ACC Systems and Structures Chart Images, Anatomical Chart Company, with permission.)

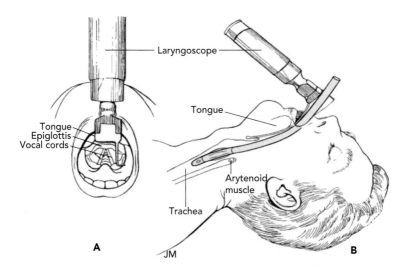

Figure 9.2. Endotracheal intubation in a patient without a cervical spine injury. **A:** The primary glottic landmarks for tracheal intubation as visualized with proper placement of the laryngoscope. **B:** Positioning the endotracheal tube. (Adapted from Smeltzer SC, Bare BG. Textbook of medical-surgical nursing. 9th ed. Philadelphia, PA: Lippincott Williams & Wilkins, 2000.)

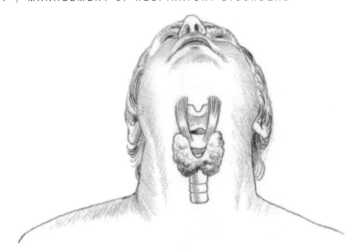

Figure 9.3. Landmarks for performing a cricothyrotomy. (Adapted from Nursing procedures. 4th ed. Philadelphia, PA: Lippincott Williams & Wilkins, 2004.)

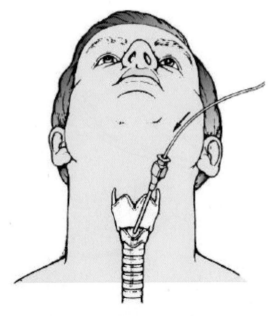

Figure 9.4 Needle cricothyrotomy with a 12- or 14-gauge needle. The catheter should be attached to high-flow oxygen from a wall source (15 L/min). (Adapted from Nettina SM. The Lippincott manual of nursing practice. 7th ed. Philadelphia, PA: Lippincott, Williams & Wilkins, 2001.)

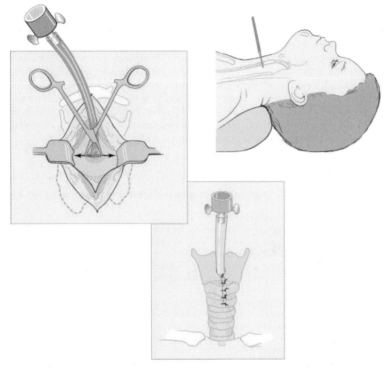

Figure 9.5. Cricothyrotomy. Illustrations showing scalpel in position to perform horizontal incision through cricothyroid membrane; hemostats maintain opening for insertion of tracheal tube, and tracheal tube is secured in place. (Adapted from LifeART Image. Philadelphia, PA: Lippincott Williams & Wilkins. All rights reserved.)

bacteria, and a lateral radiograph of the neck may show the swollen epiglottis. The patient should not be sent out of the intensive care unit for any studies and should not be left alone. Most patients improve rapidly with antibiotics; patients with diphtheria should also receive equine antitoxin and a macrolide antibiotic.

ANGIOEDEMA

Angioedema can occur through a variety of mechanisms and results in painless swelling of the soft tissues of the face. The common precipitants are angiotensin-converting enzyme inhibitors, immunoglobulin E-mediated allergic reactions to foods or medications, and complement activation through an inherited or acquired C1 esterase inhibitor deficiency/impairment.

Patients are treated with antihistamines, steroids, and epinephrine, with airway management as noted in the algorithm. Patients with hereditary deficiency of C1 esterase inhibitor respond to therapy with purified C1 inhibitor concentrate, fresh frozen plasma, or ecallantide (a kallikrein inhibitor).

POSTEXTUBATION STRIDOR

Stridor occurs in up to 15% of patients after extubation, and most cases are caused by laryngeal edema. Laryngospasm and secretions in the airway are less common causes of stridor in this situation. Immediate management should consist of nebulized racemic epinephrine, which will cause local vasoconstriction and reduce edema. Most physicians also use short courses of IV corticosteroids; however, there are no randomized data to support this treatment. These patients need to be monitored in the ICU with all airway precautions fulfilled, as noted in the algorithm. Prevention of this problem by doing a cuff-leak test prior to all extubations is controversial because failing a cuff-leak test is not an accurate predictor of postextubation stridor.

SUGGESTED READINGS

Aboussouan LS, Stoller JK. Diagnosis and management of upper airway obstruction. *Clin Chest Med.* 1994;15(1):35–53.
  An excellent review article on the topic.
Gehlbach B, Kress JP. Upper airway obstruction. In: Hall JB, Schmidt GA, Wood LDH, eds. Principles of critical care. 3rd ed. New York: McGraw-Hill, 2005:455–464.
  An excellent review article on the topic.
Goodenberger D. Medical emergencies. In: Carey CF, Lee HH, Woeltje KF, eds. The Washington manual of medical therapeutics. 29th ed. Philadelphia, PA: Lippincott, Williams & Wilkins, 1998:494–526.
  An excellent concise chapter on the management of common emergencies in the ICU.
Jaber S, Chanques G, Matecki S, et al. Post extubation stridor in intensive care unit patients: risk factors, evaluation and importance of the cuff leak test. *Intensive Care Med.* 2003;29:69–74.
  Risks for stridor include increased severity of illness, medical cause for intubation, traumatic and difficult intubations, a history of self extubation, overdistended endotracheal tube cuffs, and a prolonged period of intubation.
Khosh MM, Lebovics RS. Upper airway obstruction. In: Parillo JE, Dellinger RP, eds. Critical care medicine. 2nd ed. St Louis: Mosby, 2001:808–825.
  A thorough textbook chapter which divides etiologies into anatomic location.
Nzeako UC, Frigas E, Tremaine WJ. Hereditary angioedema. A broad review for clinicians. *Arch Intern Med.* 2001;161:2417–2429.
  Reviews the genetic forms of the disease, the clinical presentation, diagnosis and therapeutic options as well as options for prophylaxis.
Zuraw BL. Hereditary angioedema. *N Engl J Med.* 2008;359:1027–1036.
  Case vignette followed by review of treatment strategies and formal guidelines.

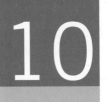

10 Acute Lung Injury and the Acute Respiratory Distress Syndrome

Timothy J. Bedient and Marin H. Kollef

Acute lung injury (ALI) and the acute respiratory distress syndrome (ARDS) are life-threatening examples of acute pulmonary edema. Although a distinction between ALI and ARDS was originally conceived as representing a spectrum of severity (ALI less severe than ARDS), overlap between the two entities is sufficiently great that most experts no longer believe the distinction is clinically important.

The incidence of ALI/ARDS in the United States is estimated to be 200,000 cases per year, with a mortality rate of 35% to 40%, which has significantly decreased from a rate of 65% to 70% in the early 1980s. While the major physiologic consequence of ALI/ARDS is hypoxia, most patients ultimately die from the underlying cause (e.g., sepsis) or associated complications (e.g., multiorgan failure) rather than from refractory hypoxemia *per se*. Current therapy for ALI/ARDS centers around treatment of the underlying cause, a pressure-targeted strategy of low tidal volume ventilation aimed at preventing further lung injury and appropriate fluid management.

In 1994, the American-European Consensus Conference on ARDS convened to develop a set of diagnostic criteria for ALI and ARDS. With these criteria, in conjunction with the more recent view that there is little importance in the distinction between ALI and ARDS, along with evolving changes in the use of hemodynamic monitoring (see later discussion), the diagnosis of ALI/ARDS should be considered whenever the following criteria are met (Algorithm 10.1): (a) an appropriate clinical setting (i.e., a likely underlying cause), (b) the development of bilateral alveolar and/or interstitial infiltrates of acute onset (<72 hours) on frontal chest radiograph, (c) a ratio of the pulmonary arterial oxygen pressure in millimeters of mercury (PaO_2) divided by the fraction of inspired oxygen (FiO_2) of <300, and (d) no clinical evidence that left ventricular failure or intravascular volume overload is the principal cause for the acute radiographic pulmonary infiltrates.

ALI/ARDS can arise from direct injury to the lung parenchyma or from indirect systemic insults transmitted to the lung by the pulmonary circulation (Table 10.1). Direct causes of ALI/ARDS include pneumonia, gastric aspiration, blunt chest trauma, near drowning, and toxic inhalations. Common indirect causes include sepsis, large-volume blood transfusions (typically >15 units), massive tissue trauma, lung transplantation, reperfusion after cardiopulmonary bypass, drug overdoses, and pancreatitis. Although more than 60 conditions have been associated with ARDS, the most frequent cause is sepsis, followed by pneumonia and aspiration.

ALGORITHM 10.1 Ventilator Management in Acute Lung Injury/Acute Respiratory Distress Syndrome

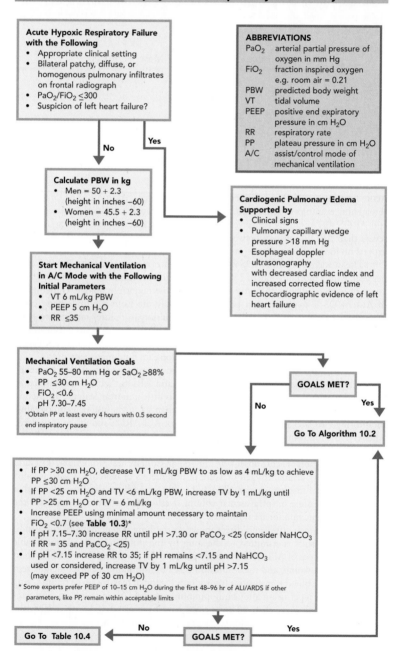

Acute Hypoxic Respiratory Failure with the Following
- Appropriate clinical setting
- Bilateral patchy, diffuse, or homogenous pulmonary infiltrates on frontal radiograph
- $PaO_2/FiO_2 \leq 300$
- Suspicion of left heart failure?

ABBREVIATIONS
PaO_2 — arterial partial pressure of oxygen in mm Hg
FiO_2 — fraction inspired oxygen e.g. room air = 0.21
PBW — predicted body weight
VT — tidal volume
PEEP — positive end expiratory pressure in cm H_2O
RR — respiratory rate
PP — plateau pressure in cm H_2O
A/C — assist/control mode of mechanical ventilation

No / Yes

Calculate PBW in kg
- Men = 50 + 2.3 (height in inches −60)
- Women = 45.5 + 2.3 (height in inches −60)

Cardiogenic Pulmonary Edema Supported by
- Clinical signs
- Pulmonary capillary wedge pressure >18 mm Hg
- Esophageal doppler ultrasonography with decreased cardiac index and increased corrected flow time
- Echocardiographic evidence of left heart failure

Start Mechanical Ventilation in A/C Mode with the Following Initial Parameters
- VT 6 mL/kg PBW
- PEEP 5 cm H_2O
- RR ≤35

Mechanical Ventilation Goals
- PaO_2 55–80 mm Hg or SaO_2 ≥88%
- PP ≤30 cm H_2O
- FiO_2 <0.6
- pH 7.30–7.45

*Obtain PP at least every 4 hours with 0.5 second end inspiratory pause

GOALS MET?

No / Yes

Go To Algorithm 10.2

- If PP >30 cm H_2O, decrease VT 1 mL/kg PBW to as low as 4 mL/kg to achieve PP ≤30 cm H_2O
- If PP <25 cm H_2O and TV <6 mL/kg PBW, increase TV by 1 mL/kg until PP >25 cm H_2O or TV = 6 mL/kg
- Increase PEEP using minimal amount necessary to maintain FiO_2 <0.7 (see **Table 10.3**)*
- If pH 7.15–7.30 increase RR until pH >7.30 or $PaCO_2$ <25 (consider $NaHCO_3$ if RR = 35 and $PaCO_2$ <25)
- If pH <7.15 increase RR to 35; if pH remains <7.15 and $NaHCO_3$ used or considered, increase TV by 1 mL/kg until pH >7.15 (may exceed PP of 30 cm H_2O)

* Some experts prefer PEEP of 10–15 cm H_2O during the first 48–96 hr of ALI/ARDS if other parameters, like PP, remain within acceptable limits

Go To Table 10.4 ← No — **GOALS MET?** — Yes

TABLE 10.1	Common Causes of Acute Lung Injury and Acute Respiratory Distress Syndrome	
Direct causes	**Indirect causes**	
Pneumonia	Sepsis	
Aspiration	Severe traumatic shock	
Inhalation injuries	Large-volume blood transfusions (>15 units)	
Blunt pulmonary trauma	Pancreatitis	
Near drowning	Reperfusion after cardiopulmonary bypass	

The pathogenesis of ARDS starts with a pulmonary or systemic insult that triggers an inflammatory response within the lungs. The resulting "noncardiogenic, increased permeability" form of pulmonary edema follows a predictable clinical and pathologic course that has been separated into three clinically meaningful phases. The exudative phase occurs immediately and lasts approximately 3 to 7 days. Pathologically, it is characterized by "diffuse alveolar damage," the cardinal features of which are (a) the accumulation of extravascular lung water, protein, and inflammatory cells (primarily neutrophils) in the interstitial and alveolar spaces, precipitates of which result in the characteristic intra-alveolar "hyaline membranes," (b) type 1 alveolar cell necrosis, and (c) intra-alveolar hemorrhage. The physiologic consequences of filling alveoli with edema and cellular debris are reduced alveolar ventilation, intrapulmonary shunting, and reduced lung compliance with increased work of breathing. The clinical consequences are a need for mechanical ventilatory support to reduce the work of breathing, a high FiO_2 to achieve an acceptable PaO_2, and positive airway pressure throughout the respiratory cycle to improve alveolar ventilation.

Overlapping with the late exudative phase is a proliferative phase, which usually lasts another 2 to 3 weeks, and is characterized by increased numbers of type 2 pneumocytes, clearing of alveolar edema and debris, improving gas exchange, and, eventually, liberation from the ventilator.

Finally, some patients may progress after 2 to 3 weeks to a clinically obvious fibrotic phase. These patients develop progressive interstitial and alveolar fibrosis, occasionally with large emphysematous bullae prone to rupture, and prolonged ventilator dependency with increased morbidity and mortality.

ARDS must be distinguished from cardiogenic pulmonary edema and other less common causes of diffuse pulmonary infiltrates due to differences in treatment. If the underlying cause of the acute pulmonary infiltrates is not certain, then x-ray computed tomography, bronchoalveolar lavage, or other diagnostic tests should be performed to exclude such entities as diffuse alveolar hemorrhage, acute interstitial pneumonia, disseminated cancer, acute eosinophilic pneumonia, miliary tuberculosis, and cryptogenic organizing pneumonia (Table 10.2). Although radiographically and physiologically similar, diffuse alveolar damage is not a prominent pathologic feature of these disease entities.

The evidence base for a particular strategy of mechanical ventilatory support for ALI/ARDS was greatly strengthened in 2000 by the landmark ARMA clinical trial, conducted by the National Institutes of Health ARDS Network. This trial demonstrated a 22% relative reduction in mortality when tidal volumes of 6 mL/kg of predicted body weight were used rather than more traditional volumes of 12 mL/kg. The lower tidal

TABLE 10.2	Conditions Mimicking Acute Lung Injury/Acute Respiratory Distress Syndrome
Cardiogenic pulmonary edema	Acute eosinophilic pneumonia
Diffuse alveolar hemorrhage	Miliary tuberculosis
Acute interstitial pneumonia	Cryptogenic organizing pneumonia
Hamman–Rich syndrome	Disseminated cancer

volumes are thought to prevent microscopic barotrauma to relatively normal alveoli, which can worsen the extent and/or severity of inflammatory pulmonary edema, an outcome sometimes described as *ventilator-induced lung injury.*

The other major, and still controversial, aspect of mechanical ventilatory support concerns the use of positive end-expiratory pressure (PEEP). PEEP increases the amount of aerated lung, thereby improving oxygenation by decreasing the shunt fraction, allowing a lower fraction of inspired oxygen to be used. However, it can also be associated with barotrauma and depressed cardiovascular function. Because of these potentially conflicting effects, another major clinical trial (ALVEOLI) was conducted by the ARDS Network to determine the relative benefit of high versus low PEEP. The results of this study showed no difference in outcomes between higher PEEP (mean, 13.2 cm H_2O) and lower PEEP (mean, 8.3 cm H_2O) levels. Thus, some recommend that the lowest level of PEEP be used to support oxygenation and to maintain an FiO_2 at or below 0.6. However, a recent meta-analysis of three trials examining lower versus higher levels of PEEP found a survival advantage in the subset of ARDS patients ($PaO_2/FiO_2 \leq 200$ mm Hg) who received higher levels of PEEP. Therefore, some experts favor higher (10–15 cm H_2O) rather than lower (5–10 cm H_2O) PEEP during the early phase of ALI/ARDS (Table 10.3).

Other ventilation strategies can be used as "rescue" therapies when oxygenation is inadequate despite the previously mentioned approach to ventilatory support, or when patients require unacceptable levels of FiO_2 or airway pressure. These include prone ventilation, inverse ratio ventilation, high-frequency ventilation, extracorporeal membrane oxygenation, or inhalational prostacyclin or nitric oxide (Table 10.4).

With the exception of glucocorticoids, no pharmacologic therapy has yet been shown to decrease the mortality of ALI/ARDS independent of treating the underlying cause. The benefit or harm of using glucocorticoids, however, appears to depend on dose, duration, and timing. In a prospective, randomized, double-blind, placebo-controlled clinical trial by Bone et al. in 1987 of very high-dose methylprednisolone (30 mg/kg every 6 hours for four doses) in 308 patients with sepsis, 88 developed ARDS. Of the patients who developed ARDS, significantly fewer reversed their ARDS

TABLE 10.3	Suggested Combinations of FiO_2 and PEEP in ARDS		
FiO_2	0.3	0.4	0.5	0.6
PEEP	5	5–8	8–10	10
FiO_2	0.7	0.8	0.9	1.0
PEEP	10–14	14	14–18	18–23

PEEP, positive end-expiratory pressure.

TABLE 10.4	**Rescue Therapies and Steroids in Acute Lung Injury/Acute Respiratory Distress Syndrome**[a]

Rescue therapies indicated when PaO$_2$, 55 mm Hg or SaO$_2$, 88% with
- FiO$_2$ $\geq$0.7 **or**
- PP >30 cm H$_2$O

Inhaled pharmacologic agents[b] (see Common Drug Dosages and Side Effects)
- Inhaled epoprostenol
- Inhaled nitric oxide
- Inhaled iloprost (prostaglandin I$_2$)

Prone ventilation
- Contraindications:
  - Open wounds/burns on the ventral body surface
  - Unstable fractures
  - Spinal instability
  - Increased intracranial pressure
  - Hemodynamic instability
- Caution if tracheostomy, chest tubes, obesity, ascites
- Maintain in prone position for 18–20 hr of every 24

Other adjunctive/salvage ventilator strategies
- Inverse ratio ventilation (inspiratory time > expiratory time)
- High-frequency ventilation
- Extracorporeal membrane oxygenation

Steroids
- 1–7 days but ideally $\leq$72 hr
  - Give methylprednisolone (or equivalent) 1 mg/kg IV bolus, then 1 mg/kg/day continuous IV infusion for 14 days.
  - If receiving paralytics, delay use until concomitant use of paralytic agents is not required.
  - If no clear physiologic or radiologic benefit in 3–5 days, discontinue.
  - After 14 days or successful patient extubation, decrease to 0.5 mg/kg/day IV and continue for 7 days, then decrease to 0.25 mg/kg/day IV and continue for 7 days, then stop.
- 7–14 days, if steroids were not started earlier
  - Benefit less certain, but in select cases may try the same protocol as above. If no clear physiologic or radiologic benefit in 3–5 days, discontinue.
- 14 days
  - Probably no role for steroid use in these cases (may cause increased mortality if used routinely in this time course). However, a trial may still be considered in select cases.

---

[a]PaO$_2$, arterial oxygen pressure in millimeters of mercury; SaO$_2$, oxygen saturation in percent; FiO$_2$, fraction inspired oxygen; PP, plateau pressure in centimeters of H$_2$O.
[b]These agents should not be given IV as they may worsen shunting by vasodilating capillaries in nonaerated alveoli.
IV, intravenously.

within 14 days of onset in the treatment group than in the placebo group (31% vs. 61%, respectively); mortality was also significantly higher in the methylprednisolone-treated group than in the placebo group (52% vs. 22%, respectively). Another prospective, randomized, double-blind, placebo-controlled clinical trial by Bernard et al. in 1987, using the same methylprednisolone dose in 99 patients with early ARDS, showed no difference in mortality or in the reversal of ARDS between the two groups after 45 days.

In contrast, a more recent prospective, randomized, double-blind, placebo-controlled clinical trial in 2007 by Meduri et al. of moderate-dose methylprednisolone (1 mg/kg for 2 weeks followed by a taper during 2 weeks) reported significantly reduced duration of mechanical ventilation (5 vs. 9.5 days; $p = 0.002$), length of intensive care unit (ICU) stay (7 vs. 14.5 days; $p = 0.007$), and pulmonary and extrapulmonary organ dysfunction in the methylprednisolone-treated group. There was also significantly reduced ICU mortality with a strong trend ($p = 0.07$) toward reduced hospital mortality. Finally, the corticosteroid treatment group also had a significantly lower rate of infections ($p = 0.0002$).

Two prospective, randomized, double-blind, placebo-controlled clinical trials of corticosteroid administration have also been conducted in patients with unresolving (>7 days) ARDS (one by the Meduri et al. group with 24 patients conducted at four medical centers, and the other by the multicenter National Institutes of Health-sponsored ARDS Network with 180 patients). Both studies showed significant improvements in ventilator-free , shock-free, and ICU-free days. The study by Meduri et al. reported improved ICU ($p = 0.002$) and in-hospital ($p = 0.03$) mortality, but the ARDS Network study did not. Indeed, in the latter study, there was a trend toward increased mortality in patients administered glucocorticoids >2 weeks after the onset of ARDS. Possible confounding factors in the latter study, however, include a greater use of paralytic agents in the treated group and a shortened course of therapy compared with the Meduri et al. protocol.

Overall, we believe data from these various studies support the use of moderate-dose steroids for all ARDS patients of duration <2 weeks (Table 10.4). Steroids should be withheld until it is certain that paralytic agents are not required concomitantly. Because physiologic and radiologic parameters appear to improve substantially within 3 to 5 days after beginning steroid use, it may be reasonable to discontinue steroids after this time in those patients who fail to show any significant response. In those who do respond, however, steroids should be continued for up to 4 weeks (Table 10.4).

Corticosteroids should not be *routinely* started in patients with unresolving ARDS more than 2 weeks after onset. However, they may be considered in selected cases; here again, a 3- to 5-day course should at least establish whether there will be physiologic or radiologic improvement before longer trials are considered.

The injured lung during ALI/ARDS is also highly vulnerable to worsening pulmonary edema by high pulmonary capillary pressures. However, until recently, fluid management during ALI/ARDS often emphasized the need to maintain intravascular volume to optimize hemodynamic performance, even at the risk of worsening pulmonary edema. Even though hemodynamic stability and organ perfusion need to be maintained, another trial by the ARDS Network from 2006 (FACTT) showed that minimizing pulmonary capillary pressures without compromising systemic organ perfusion could be accomplished, with a decreased duration of mechanical ventilation and ICU stay as the result (Algorithm 10.2). However, no mortality benefit was shown.

The FACTT study also showed no improvement in survival or organ function if hemodynamic management was guided with pulmonary artery catheters (PACs)

ALGORITHM 10.2 Fluid Management in Acute Lung Injury/ Acute Respiratory Distress Syndrome

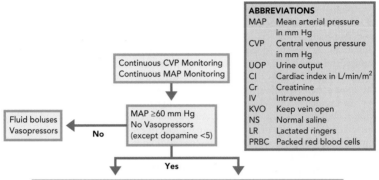

ABBREVIATIONS	
MAP	Mean arterial pressure in mm Hg
CVP	Central venous pressure in mm Hg
UOP	Urine output
CI	Cardiac index in L/min/m²
Cr	Creatinine
IV	Intravenous
KVO	Keep vein open
NS	Normal saline
LR	Lactated ringers
PRBC	Packed red blood cells

Continuous CVP Monitoring
Continuous MAP Monitoring

MAP ≥60 mm Hg
No Vasopressors
(except dopamine <5)

Fluid boluses
Vasopressors ← **No**

Yes

	Average UOP, <0.5 mL/kg/hr		Average UOP, ≥0.5 mL/kg/hr	
	CI <2.5 or cold, mottled extremities with capillary refill ≥2 seconds	CI ≥2.5 or no evidence of circulation impairment	CI <2.5 or cold, mottled extremities with capillary refill ≥2 seconds	CI ≥2.5 or no evidence of circulation impairment
CVP >13	1 Dobutamine * Furosemide	5 Furosemide	9 Dobutamine Furosemide	13 Furosemide
CVP 9–13	2 Dobutamine	6 Furosemide	10 Dobutamine	14 Furosemide
CVP 4–8	3 Fluid Bolus	7 Fluid Bolus	11 Fluid Bolus	15 Furosemide
CVP <4	4 Fluid Bolus	8 Fluid Bolus	12 Fluid Bolus	16 KVO

For Cell # 1, 5, 6 furosemide 20-mg IV bolus, or IV infusion at 3 mg/hr. **HOLD** if Cr >3, or Cr 0-3 with labs consistent with renal failure, or vasopressor/fluid bolus in last 12 hours.	Reassess in 1 hour; double furosemide dose hourly until UOP >0.5 mg/hr or maximum of 24 mg/hr or 160 mg bolus.
For Cell # 9, 13, 14, 15 furosemide 20-mg IV bolus, or IV infusion at 3 mg/hr. **HOLD** if Cr >3, or Cr 0-3 with labs consistent with renal failure, or vasopressor/fluid bolus in last 12 hours.	Reassess in 4 hours; if still in cell where furosemide is indicated give same dose if UOP >3 mL/kg/hr, double if ≤3 mL/kg/hr, to a maximum of 24 mg/hr or 160 mg bolus.
For Cell # 3, 4, 7, 8 give a NS, Plasmalyte, or LR bolus of 15 mL/kg, 1 U PRBCs, or 25 g 25% albumin.	Reassess in 1 hour. Administer up to 3 boluses in 24 hours if indicated by cell #.
For Cell # 11, 12 give a NS, Plasmalyte, or LR bolus of 15 mL/kg, 1 U PRBCs, or 25 g 25% albumin.	Reassess in 4 hour. Additional boluses at physician discretion
For Cell # 1, 2, 9, 10 Dobutamine, start at 5 mcg/kg/min	Increase by 5 mcg/kg/min until CI >2.5

* If furosemide not available can use bumetanide with a dose equivalency of 40:1 (lasix 40 mg = bumetanide 1 mg).

(Adapted from the 2006 FACTT trial, this complex algorithm may not be appropriate for all patients and in all clinical settings, and should be used with physician discretion and judgment.)

instead of with simple central venous pressure monitoring in patients with established ALI/ARDS, and PACs were associated with increased complications. Thus, the routine use of PACs for hemodynamic management of ALI/ARDS can no longer be recommended.

Numerous studies have examined the long-term outcome of patients who survive ALI/ARDS. In one study, the average stay in the ICU from ALI/ARDS was 25 days. At discharge, patients had lost 18% of their body weight, and had significant functional limitations. At 1 year, patients had persistent functional limitations due to muscle wasting and weakness. Lung volume and spirometric measurements in survivors were normal or near normal by 6 months to 1 year (defined as >80% of predicted amounts), and most patients did not require supplemental oxygen.

In summary, ALI/ARDS is a severe life-threatening form of pulmonary edema with characteristic clinical, radiologic, and physiologic consequences. Beyond treating the inciting event, current ALI/ARDS management centers on volume and pressure-limited lung protective ventilation, conservative fluid management, and the early use of moderate-dose corticosteroids. Rescue therapies are reserved for those patients who remain hypoxic despite steroids and optimal ventilator and fluid management. At 1 year, survivors often must endure some degree of functional disability from muscle weakness and wasting, but lung function measurements can be expected to approach normal values.

SUGGESTED READINGS

Bernard GR, Artigas A, Bringham KL, et al. The American-European Consensus Conference on ARDS: definitions, mechanism, relevant outcomes and clinical trial coordination. *Am J Respir Crit Care Med.* 1994;149:818–824.

The American-European Consensus Conference on ARDS was established in 1992 between the American Thoracic Society and the European Society of Intensive Care Medicine. The goals of the Committee were to form a uniform definition of ALI and ARDS, better define the mechanism of acute lung injury, identify risk factors, prevalence, and outcomes, and to promote clinical study coordination. The Committee's results are published in this landmark paper.

Bernard GR, Luce JM, Sprung CL, et al. High-dose corticosteroids in patients with the adult respiratory distress syndrome. *N Engl J Med.* 1987;317:1565–1570.

A prospective, randomized, double-blind, placebo-controlled trial of methylprednisolone therapy (30 mg per kilogram body weight every six hours for 24 hours) in 99 patients with ARDS. There were no differences in mortality or infectious complications between the groups.

Bone RC, Fisher CJ Jr, Clemmer TP, et al. Early methylprednisolone treatment for septic syndrome and the adult respiratory distress syndrome. *Chest.* 1987;92(6):1032–1036.

A prospective, randomized, double-blind, placebo-controlled study to determine if early treatment with methylprednisolone (MPSS) would decrease the incidence of ARDS in septic patients. Early treatment of septic patients with MPSS did not prevent the development of ARDS. Additionally, MPSS treatment impeded the reversal of ARDS and increased the mortality rate in patients with ARDS.

Briel M, Meade M, Mercat A, et al. Higher vs lower positive end-expiratory pressure in patients with acute lung injury and acute respiratory distress syndrome: systematic review and meta-analysis. *JAMA.* 2010;303:865–873.

Analysis of three trials comparing outcome in patients receiving higher PEEP versus lower PEEP levels. Overall, no difference in hospital survival was found. However, higher PEEP levels were associated with improved survival among the subgroup of patients with ARDS.

Herridge MS, Cheung AM, Tansey CM, et al. One-year outcomes in survivors of the acute respiratory distress syndrome. *N Engl J Med.* 2003;348:683–693.

This longitudinal study was conducted at four medical-surgical intensive care units in Toronto, Canada. At the time of discharge, patients had lost 18% of their body weight, with 71% returning to their baseline body weight by one year. Lung volume and spirometric measurements were normal by six months, defined as being within 80% predicted.

Meduri GU, Golden E, Freire AX, et al. Methylprednisolone infusion in early severe ARDS. Results of a randomized controlled trial. *Chest.* 2007;131:954–963.

Randomized, double blinded, placebo controlled trial of moderate dose methylprednisolone in early ARDS conducted in the surgical and medical intensive care units at 5 medical centers in Memphis, TN, randomizing patients 2:1 to methylprednisolone versus placebo (n = 63 vs. 28) and treating patients for up to 28 days, showing a significant reduction in duration of mechanical ventilation, length of ICU stay, and organ dysfunction in the treatment group.

Meduri GU, Headley AS, Golden E, et al. Effect of prolonged methylprednisolone therapy in unresolving acute respiratory distress syndrome. *JAMA.* 1998;280:159–165.

Randomized, double blinded, placebo controlled clinical trail conducted at 4 medical centers in Memphis, TN of 24 patients with ARDS that did not show improved lung injury scores by day 7 assigned 2:1 to receive methylprednisolone (initially 2 mg/kg/day and continued for 32 days) versus placebo. The study showed significant improvement in the primary outcomes of lung injury, MODS scores, and ICU and in-hospital mortality in the methylprednisolone treated patients.

The Acute Respiratory Distress Syndrome Network. Ventilation with lower tidal volumes as compared with traditional tidal volumes for acute lung injury and the acute respiratory distress syndrome. *N Engl J Med.* 2000;342:1301–1308.

The "ARMA" trial was conducted at 10 university centers in the ARDS Network. The trial enrolled patients with ALI/ARDS and compared ventilation with traditional tidal volumes (mean 11.8 ± 0.8 ml/kg PBW) versus low tidal volumes (mean 6.2 ± 0.8 ml/kg PBW). The trial was stopped after enrolling 861 patients after the lower tidal volume group had significantly lower mortality (31% vs. 39%).

The National Heart, Lung, and Blood Institute ARDS Clinical Trials Network. Higher versus lower positive end-expiratory pressures in patients with the acute respiratory distress syndrome. *N Engl J Med.* 2004;351:327–336.

The "ALVEOLI" trial was conducted by the ARDS Network at 23 affiliated centers. The trial compared mechanical ventilation with higher PEEP (mean 13.2 ± 3.5 cm H2O) versus lower PEEP (mean 8.3 ± 3.2) when tidal volumes of 6 ml/kg PBW were used. The trial was stopped after 549 patients were enrolled when no significant difference was found between the two groups for death.

The National Heart, Lung, and Blood Institute Acute Respiratory Distress Syndrome Clinical Trials Network. Efficacy and safety of corticosteroids for persistent acute respiratory distress syndrome. *N Engl J Med.* 2006;354:1671–1684.

The "LaSRS" trial was a double-blind randomized controlled clinical trial conducted by the ARDS Network at 25 affiliated centers. The study enrolled 180 patients with ALI/ARDS of at least 7–28 days duration and randomly assigned them to receive either methylprednisolone (2 mg/kg bolus then 0.5 mg/kg every 6 hours for 14 days, 0.5 mg/kg every 12 hours for 7 days, then tapered over four days), or placebo. The study found no difference in 60-day mortality between those treated with corticosteroids versus placebo (29.2% vs. 28.6%) but did identify significant physiologic and radiologic improvements favoring corticosteroids. Some have criticized the trial for too rapid withdrawal of steroids and for significant differences in use of paralytics between groups.

The National Heart, Lung, and Blood Institute Acute Respiratory Distress Syndrome (ARDS) Clinical Trials Network. Comparison of two fluid-management strategies in acute lung injury. *N Engl J Med.* 2006;354:2564–2575.

The "FACTT" trial was a randomized controlled clinical trial conducted by the ARDS Network at 20 affiliated centers. The study enrolled 1000 patients with ALI/ARDS of less than 48 hours duration and randomly assigned them to a conservative vs. liberal fluid management strategy for seven days. Patients were also randomly assigned to treatment guided by PAC vs. CVP monitoring (see the following citation). The study found no difference in 60 day mortality (25.5% vs. 28.4%) but did identify significant differences in ventilator time and ICU stay favoring the conservative fluid management strategy.

The National Heart, Lung, and Blood Institute Acute Respiratory Distress Syndrome (ARDS) Clinical Trials Network. Pulmonary artery versus central venous catheter to guide treatment of acute lung injury. *N Engl J Med.* 2006;354:2213–2224.

The "FACTT" study also yielded this paper based on outcome among the 1000 patients with ALI/ARDS who were randomly assigned to conservative versus liberal fluid management for seven days. Patients were randomly assigned to treatment guided by pulmonary vs. central venous catheter monitoring. The study found no difference between the PAC and CVP groups in 60-day mortality (27.4% vs. 26.3%).

Status Asthmaticus

Saad Ghafoor and Mario Castro

Asthma is a common disorder affecting approximately 34 million Americans. It is a chronic inflammatory disease of the airways characterized by airway hyperreactivity and inflammation, bronchoconstriction, and mucus hypersecretion. In 2007, asthma exacerbations resulted in nearly 13.3 million emergency department/physician office visits, 500,000 hospitalizations, and over 3000 deaths in the United States. In school-aged children, asthma accounts for nearly 13 million missed-school days per year. In adults, nearly 10.1 million days of work are missed because of asthma. The economic impact of asthma is estimated to be $19.7 billion annually.

Approximately 10% of patients hospitalized with asthma are admitted to the intensive care unit, and 2% are intubated. Mortality rates range from 0.5% to 3% in hospitalized patients. Morbidity and mortality from asthma disproportionately affect the economically disadvantaged, women, and minorities, especially African Americans and Hispanics from Puerto Rico. A recent study, the Nationwide Inpatient Sample from >80,000 U.S. hospital admissions for asthma, reported a hospital mortality rate of 0.5%. The majority of asthma-related deaths occurred in patients older than 35 years. The study found no significant differences in hospitalized mortality rates in regard to race, suggesting that the disproportionate affect on minorities may be the result of prehospital factors such as access to health care, inadequate preventive therapy, or delay in seeking medical treatment. Risk factors for death from asthma are listed in Table 11.1.

Clinically, patients present with dyspnea, cough, chest tightness, and wheezing. In severe asthma episodes, airway obstruction, respiratory muscle fatigue, and altered V/Q relationships can lead to hypercapnia and hypoxemic respiratory failure. This chapter will focus on the initial hospital and intensive care unit management, as well as ventilatory strategies for patients with status asthmaticus.

Status asthmaticus is defined as a prolonged severe episode of asthma that is unresponsive to initial standard therapy that may lead to respiratory failure. The episodes may be rapid onset (in a matter of hours) or, more typically, progress during several hours to days. The former is often referred to as *asphyxic* asthma and occurs in a minority of cases. Rapid-onset status asthmaticus is more common in men, and is oftentimes triggered by exposure to allergens, irritants, exercise, psychosocial stress, and inhaled illicit drugs. It may also develop after exposure to aspirin, nonsteroidal anti-inflammatory drugs, or β-blockers in susceptible individuals. This form of status asthmaticus represents a more "bronchospastic" pathophysiology, and is associated with rapid resolution with treatment. More commonly, asthma episodes develop during several hours to days, and may be triggered by viral or atypical infection. Airway

TABLE 11.1	Risk Factors for Death from Asthma

Lower socioeconomic status
Female gender
African American or Puerto Rican race
Smoking
"Labile asthma," high degree of variability in peak expiratory flow
Blood eosinophilia
Poor perception of dyspnea: alexithymia, a psychological trait characterized by
 difficulty in perceiving and expressing emotions and body sensations
History of sudden severe exacerbations (asphyxic asthma)
History of intubation for asthma
History of ICU admission for asthma
Two or more hospitalizations for asthma within the past year
Three or more ED visits for asthma in the past year
Hospitalization or ED visit for asthma within past month
Use of more than two canisters per month of inhaled short-acting β_2-agonists
Current use or recent withdrawal of oral corticosteroids
Poor perception of airflow obstruction
Comorbid cardiovascular disease
Sensitivity to Alternaria

ICU, intensive care unit; ED, emergency department.

obstruction in these cases is due to airway inflammation, bronchoconstriction, and mucus plugging.

In both forms, the pathologic processes result in airway obstruction and expiratory airflow limitation. Insufficient expiratory time results in air trapping, dynamic hyperinflation (DHI), and persistent positive end-expiratory alveolar pressure, also referred to as *intrinsic positive end-expiratory pressure* (iPEEP). This alters lung mechanics by increasing work of breathing while simultaneously placing the diaphragm at a mechanical disadvantage. The increased workload placed on the respiratory muscles results in increased O_2 consumption and CO_2 production, setting up a vicious cycle.

DHI adversely affects cardiovascular function because of the dramatic fluctuations in the intrathoracic pressure during inspiration and expiration (evident on physical examination as pulsus paradoxus). During inspiration, there can be exaggerated right ventricular filling and paradoxic interventricular septal motion, resulting in impaired left ventricular filling. During expiration, the increased intrathoracic pressure impairs ventricular diastolic filling, resulting in decreased cardiac output and compromised diaphragmatic blood flow, exacerbating metabolic acidosis and respiratory muscle fatigue. This downward spiral from the multiple pathophysiologic processes results in hypoxemic and hypercapnic respiratory failure (Algorithm 11.1).

Rapid evaluation of the patient presenting with status asthmaticus is essential, focusing on key points of the history such as duration of symptoms, potential inciting exposures, medication use, and previous history of severe attacks. Patients should be questioned regarding the presence of symptoms suggestive of comorbid, complicating, or similarly presenting conditions (Table 11.2). Key historical and physical examination findings are listed in Table 11.3.

ALGORITHM 11.1   Status Asthmaticus Pathophysiology

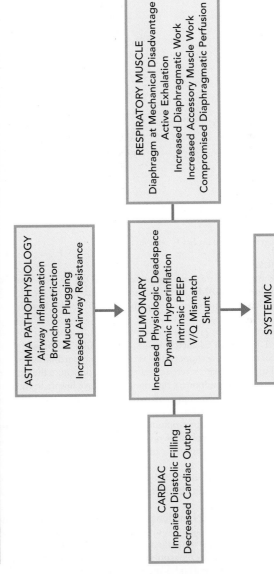

ASTHMA PATHOPHYSIOLOGY
Airway Inflammation
Bronchoconstriction
Mucus Plugging
Increased Airway Resistance

RESPIRATORY MUSCLE
Diaphragm at Mechanical Disadvantage
Active Exhalation
Increased Diaphragmatic Work
Increased Accessory Muscle Work
Compromised Diaphragmatic Perfusion

PULMONARY
Increased Physiologic Deadspace
Dynamic Hyperinflation
Intrinsic PEEP
V/Q Mismatch
Shunt

CARDIAC
Impaired Diastolic Filling
Decreased Cardiac Output

SYSTEMIC
Increased O_2 Consumption
Increased CO_2 Production
Normo/Hypoxemia
Hypo/Hypercapnea
Respiratory Acidosis
Metabolic Acidosis

PEEP, positive end-expiratory pressure.

69

TABLE 11.2	Differential Diagnoses to Consider

Upper airway obstruction
Tumor
Epiglottitis
Vocal cord dysfunction
Foreign body aspiration
Endobronchial lesion
Congestive heart failure
Gastroesophageal reflux
Obstructive sleep apnea
Tracheomalacia
Herpetic tracheobronchitis
Mitral stenosis
Adverse drug reaction
Aspirin sensitivity
    Angiotensin-converting enzyme inhibitor
    β_2-Adrenergic antagonist
    Inhaled pentamidine

TREATMENTS

Standard Treatment for All Patients

Oxygen
- Supplemental oxygen to maintain SaO_2 >92%.

Inhaled Bronchodilators
- β_2-agonists administered via metered dose inhalers (MDIs) or nebulized bronchodilators. They increase c-AMP mediated bronchodilation. Albuterol (2.5 to 5 mg) nebulization every 20 minutes (or four to eight puffs of MDI with spacer) within first hour.
- Alternatively, albuterol may be given as a continuous nebulization at a dose of 10 to 15 mg during 1 hour with telemetry monitoring. A 2009 Cochrane review of 165 randomized controlled trials supports the use of continuous nebulizations versus intermittent MDI in patients with severe acute asthma who present to the emergency department to increase their pulmonary functions and reduce hospitalization.
- Levalbuterol (1.25 mg) every 20 minutes within the first hour, then every 40 minutes alternatively, for three doses if needed.
- Initial treatment should include ipratropium 0.5 mg nebulized every 20 minutes, given concomitantly with albuterol (shown to improve airflow limitation in acute asthma exacerbations in first 36 hours). This antagonizes cGMP-mediated bronchoconstriction.
- In the case of intubated patients, bronchodilators should be given via MDI (e.g., albuterol) along the inspiratory circuit or between a Y-piece and the endotracheal tube.
- Long-acting β_2-agonists, salmeterol and formoterol, are not indicated for treatment of acute asthma. Long-acting β_2-agonists may be continued as add-on therapy in the hospitalized patient and in the outpatient setting.
- The administration of intravenous β_2-agonists is no more effective and potentially more toxic than delivery via aerosol and is therefore *not* recommended.

TABLE 11.3 Typical Physical Examination and Laboratory Findings in Asthma by Severity

Finding	Mild	Moderate	Severe	Respiratory arrest imminent
Breathless	Walking	Talking	At rest	
	Can lie down	Prefers sitting	Hunched forward	
Speaks in	Sentences	Phrases	Words	
Alertness	May be agitated	Usually agitated	Usually agitated	Drowsy or confused
Respiratory rate	Increased	Increased	>30 breaths/min	
Accessory muscle use and retractions	Usually not	Usually	Usually	
Wheeze	Moderate, often end-expiratory	Loud	Usually loud	Absent
Pulse (beats/min)	<100	100–120	>120	Bradycardia (<60)
Pulsus paradoxus	Absent (<10 mm Hg)	May be present (10–25 mm Hg)	Often present (>25 mm Hg)	Absence suggests respiratory muscle fatigue
PEF %predicted	>80%	60%–80%	<60%	
PaO_2	Normal	>60 mm Hg	<60 mm Hg	
$PaCO_2$	<45 mm Hg	<45 mm Hg	>45 mm Hg	
SaO_2	>95%	91%–95%	<90%	

PEF, peak expiratory flow.

Corticosteroids
- Initial dose of methylprednisolone, 125 mg intravenously once, or equivalent oral dose if the patient is able to tolerate oral administration. Corticosteroids decrease inflammatory response and upregulate β-receptors.
- Subsequently, methylprednisolone, 40 to 60 mg intravenously every 6–12 hours or equivalent dose given orally if there is no suspected impairment in gastrointestinal absorption.
- Consider tapering dose after 36 to 48 hours, depending on clinical response.

Additional Therapeutic Considerations
Antibiotics
- Not recommended routinely for uncomplicated asthma exacerbation.
- Justified if patients have fever, purulent sputum, or if there is evidence of pneumonia or bacterial sinusitis complicating the asthma exacerbation.

Magnesium
- Intra venous (IV) magnesium (2 g infused during 20 minutes) is relatively safe but does not appear to be more effective than standard therapy. Thought to antagonize calcium-mediated bronchoconstriction. No supporting data beyond administration of initial dose in emergency department (ED).
- Less data available regarding use of inhaled magnesium but may be added to inhaled bronchodilators.

Methylxanthines
- Not recommended for initial treatment in acute asthma.
- Equivalent bronchodilator properties as β_2-agonists but with increased potential of toxicity (tachyarrhythmia).

Epinephrine
- No proven advantage over inhaled bronchodilator therapy, but with added potential for toxicity, especially in hypoxemic patients.
- Consider in patients who do not respond or are unable to cooperate with intensive inhaled bronchodilator treatment.
- Dosing: 0.5 mg of a 1:1000 dilution given subcutaneously every 20 minutes up to 3 doses if needed.

Heliox
- The use of helium–oxygen (He–O_2) mixtures in severe obstructive airway disease is based on the decreased density of heliox compared with air, resulting in more laminar rather than turbulent airflow.
- Use either 60%:40% or 70%:30% heliox (He:O_2) mixtures.
- Limited data suggest improved delivery of aerosolized bronchodilators when given with heliox rather than oxygen.
- The use of heliox in the mechanically ventilated patient should only be considered in those institutions that have significant experience and familiarity with its use because of potential technical complications regarding volume and pressure monitoring with standard ventilators.

Ventilator Strategies

The goal of management in status asthmaticus is to unload the respiratory muscles, correct hypoxemia, provide adequate ventilation, and minimize lung injury, particularly from DHI, while treating the underlying airway inflammation and bronchoconstriction.

Noninvasive Ventilation
- Although the concept of treating acute asthma (an air trapping disease) with additional airway pressure at the end of expiration seem counterintuitive, a number of studies have indicated that it may actually reduce work of breathing during exacerbations of bronchospasm. Bilevel positive airway pressure (BiPAP) also enhances bronchodilatory effect of albuterol.
- Data regarding the use of noninvasive positive pressure ventilation (NIPPV) in severe asthma are limited.
- NIPPV with either continuous positive airway pressure or BiPAP may be considered as initial treatment of patients presenting to the emergency department with status asthmaticus who are alert, cooperative, and able to protect their airways while tolerating a full face mask.

TABLE 11.4	Initial Ventilator Settings in Status Asthmaticus
Parameter	Setting
Mode	Volume controlled
Minute ventilation	10 L
Tidal volume	7–8 mL/kg
Respiratory rate	12–14 breaths/min
Inspiratory flow rate	60–80 LPM
PEEP	0–5 cm H_2O
FiO_2	Titrate to keep SpO_2 >90%

LPM, liters per minute; PEEP, positive end-expiratory pressure.

- Initial BiPAP settings, inspiratory positive airway pressure (IPAP) of 8 and expiratory positive airway pressure (EPAP) of 5, and adjusted promptly to achieve patient comfort and compliance and decrease work of breathing (decreased respiratory rate, increased tidal volume) without exceeding IPAP of 15 and EPAP of 5.
- Aerophagia with subsequent vomiting and aspiration is potential complications of NIPPV, and patients should be closely monitored and kept fasting.
- Clinical improvement after initiation of NIPPV (decreased respiratory rate, improved air movement, decreased $PaCO_2$) should be documented shortly after initiation of NIPPV and pharmacologic treatment (within 30 minutes).
- Lack of improvement should prompt the clinician to the need for intubation and mechanical ventilation. Once deemed necessary, intubation should not be delayed.
- NIPPV is contraindicated in patients with decreased mental status and hemodynamic instability.

Invasive Ventilation

Ventilator strategies should concentrate on allowing adequate expiratory time to avoid DHI and barotrauma. Mechanical ventilation with volume-controlled ventilation is preferable. Suggested initial settings are listed in Table 11.4. A lung protective and permissive hypercapnia strategy should be employed, targeting a plateau pressure <30 cm H_2O. iPEEP should be monitored by performing an end-expiratory hold maneuver. The iPEEP is equal to total PEEP minus set PEEP (set on ventilator) (Fig. 11.1). The goal should be to maintain iPEEP <20 cm H_2O.

ADDITIONAL CONSIDERATIONS

Hypotension during or post-intubation is common in status asthmaticus because of multiple factors, including the application of positive pressure throughout the respiratory cycle in patients with pre-existing DHI and iPEEP, hypovolemia, and sedation. It should be managed with sedatives and liberal intravenous fluids (IVF) as well as the aforementioned ventilatory strategies to minimize DHI. If needed, with close monitoring of SpO_2, the patient can be disconnected from the ventilator circuit to allow adequate exhalation of trapped gas and decrease intrathoracic pressure.

Neuromuscular blockade should be considered in patients with status asthmaticus on mechanical ventilation who demonstrate considerable patient-ventilator dyssynchrony with unacceptably high plateau pressures and iPEEP despite adequate sedation and analgesia. Neuromuscular blocking agents should be given as

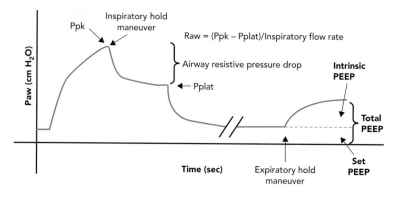

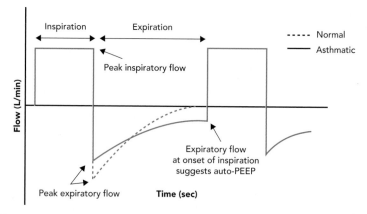

Figure 11.1. Intrinsic positive end-expiratory pressure (PEEP). Ppk, peak pressure; Pplat, plateau pressure.

intermittent boluses with neuromuscular (train of four) monitoring. Administration of neuromuscular blocking agents as continuous infusions should be avoided because of the increased risk of myopathy associated with concurrent corticosteroid use.

SUGGESTED READINGS

American Lung Association, Epidemiology & Statistics Unit, Research and Program Services. Trends in Asthma Morbidity and Mortality, November 2007.

Barr RG, Woodruff PG, Clark S, et al. Sudden-onset asthma exacerbations: clinical features, response to therapy, and a 2-week follow-up. Multicenter Airway Research Collaboration (MARC) investigators. *Eur Respir J.* 2000;15:266–273.

Brandstetter RD, Gotz VP, Mar DD. Optimal dosing of epinephrine in acute asthma. *Am J Hosp Pharm.* 1980;37:1326–1329.

British Thoracic Society & Scottish Intercollegiate Guidelines Network. British guideline on the management of asthma. April 2004. *Thorax.* 2003;58(Suppl 1):i1–i94.

Calverley PMA, Koulouris NG. Flow limitation and dynamic hyperinflation: key concepts in modern respiratory physiology. *Eur Respir J.* 2005;25:186–199.

Castro M. Near-fatal asthma what have we learned? *Chest*. 2002;121:1394–1395.

Cates CJ, Crilly JA, Rowe BH. Holding chambers (spacers) versus nebulisers for beta-agonist treatment of acute asthma. *Cochrane Database Syst Rev*. 2006;2:CD000052.

Camargo Jr CA, Spooner C, Rowe BH. Continuous versus intermittent beta-agonists for acute asthma. *Cochrane Database Syst Rev*. 2003;4:CD001115. DOI: 10.1002/14651858.

Dolan CM, Fraher KE, Bleecker ER, et al. Design and baseline characteristics of The Epidemiology and Natural History of Asthma: Outcomes and Treatment Regimens (TENOR) study: a large cohort of patients with severe or difficult-to-treat asthma. *Ann Allergy Asthma Immunol*. 2004;92:32–39.

Global Strategy for Asthma Management and Prevention. Global Initiative for Asthma (GINA). 2010. Available from: www.ginasthma.com. Accessed.

Guidelines for the Diagnosis and Management of Asthma—expert panel report 3. National Asthma Education and Prevention Program, National Institutes of Health, National Heart, Lung and Blood Institute. Available from: www.nhlbi.nih.gov/guidelines/asthma/ Accessed October 12, 2010.

Gupta D, Keogh B, Chung KF, et al. Characteristics and outcome for admissions to adult, general critical care units with acute severe asthma: a secondary analysis of the ICNARC case mix programme database. *Crit Care*. 2004;9:112–121.

Krishnan V, Diette GB, Rand CS, et al. Mortality in patients hospitalized for asthma exacerbations in the United States. *Am J Respir Crit Care Med*. 2006;174:633–638.

Levy BD, Kitch B, Fanta CH. Medical and ventilatory management of status asthmaticus. *Intensive Care Med*. 1998;24:105–117.

MacIntyre NR. Current issues in mechanical ventilation for respiratory failure. *Chest*. 2005;128:561–567.

McFadden ER. Acute severe asthma. *Am J Respir Crit Care Med*. 2003;168:740–759.

Oddo M, Feihl F, Schaller MO, et al. Management of mechanical ventilation in acute severe asthma: practical aspects. *Intensive Care Med*. 2006;32:501–510.

Pendergraft TB, Stanford RH, Beasley R, et al. Rates and characteristics of intensive care unit admissions and intubations among asthma-related hospitalizations. *Ann Allergy Asthma Immunol*. 2004;93:29–35.

Ram FSF, Wellington SR, Rowe B, et al. Non-invasive positive pressure ventilation for treatment of respiratory failure due to severe acute exacerbations of asthma (review). *Cochrane Database Syst Rev*. 2005;3:CD004360.

Rodrigo GJ, Castro-Rodriguez JA. Anticholinergics in the treatment of children and adults with acute asthma: a systematic review with meta-analysis. *Thorax*. 2005;60:740–746.

Rodrigo GJ, Rodrigo C. First-line therapy for adult patients with acute severe asthma receiving a multiple-dose protocol of ipratropium bromide plus albuterol in the emergency department. *Am J Respir Crit Care Med*. 2000;161:1862–1868.

Rodrigo GJ, Rodrigo C. Rapid-onset asthma attack: a prospective cohort study about characteristics and response to emergency department treatments. *Chest*. 2000;118:1547–1552.

Rodrigo GJ, Rodrigo C. The role of anticholinergics in acute asthma treatment: an evidence-based evaluation. *Chest*. 2002;121:1977–1987.

Rodrigo GJ, Rodrigo C, Pollack CV, et al. Use of helium-oxygen mixtures in the treatment of acute asthma: a systematic review. *Chest*. 2003;123:891–896.

Serrano J, Plaza V, Sureda B, et al. Alexithymia: a relevant psychological variable in near-fatal asthma. *Eur Respir J*. 2006;28:296–302.

Soroksky A, Stav D, Shpirer I, et al. A pilot prospective, randomized, placebo-controlled trial of bilevel positive airway pressure in acute asthmatic attack. *Chest*. 2003:123;1018–1025.

Turner MO, Noertjojo K, Vedal S, et al. Risk factors for near-fatal asthma. *Am J Respir Crit Care Med*. 1998;157:1804–1809.

Weiss KB, Sullivan SD. The health economics of asthma and rhinitis. *J Allergy Clin Immunol*. 2001;107:3–8.

Wenzel S. Severe asthma in adults. *Am J Respir Crit Care Med*. 2005;172:140–160.

World Health Organization. Global surveillance, prevention and control of chronic respiratory diseases: a comprehensive approach, 2007.

12 Acute Exacerbations of Chronic Obstructive Pulmonary Disease

Chad A. Witt and Marin H. Kollef

In the United States, more than 16 million adults have chronic obstructive pulmonary disease (COPD). COPD can manifest as predominantly chronic bronchitis or predominantly emphysema. In 2001, COPD accounted for more than 16 million office visits, 500,000 hospitalizations, and 110,000 deaths, making COPD the fourth leading cause of death in the United States, behind heart disease, cancer, and cerebrovascular disease. The number of patients with COPD is expected to rise with the aging of the population.

There are many definitions for what represents an acute exacerbation of COPD. The most widely used definition evaluates the severity of exacerbation based on three symptoms: (a) worsening dyspnea, (b) an increase in sputum purulence, and (c) an increase in sputum volume. Type 1 exacerbations (severe) have all three symptoms and type 2 exacerbations (moderate) exhibit two of the three symptoms. Type 3 exacerbations (mild) include one of the symptoms and at least one of the following: upper respiratory tract infection within the past 5 days, fever without apparent cause, increased wheezing, increased cough, or a 20% increase in respiratory rate or heart rate over baseline. Acute exacerbations can be triggered by infections (viral or bacterial) or environmental exposures; however, given that many patients have associated clinical conditions, such as congestive heart failure or extrapulmonary infections, defining which symptoms are secondary to acute exacerbations and which symptoms are secondary to other medical conditions is a clinical diagnosis. All patients who present with symptoms consistent with an acute exacerbation of COPD should undergo chest radiography to evaluate for evidence of pneumonia or pulmonary edema and measurement of arterial oxygen content by arterial blood glass analysis (Algorithm 12.1). Routine spirometric evaluation has not been shown to be beneficial in the setting of acute exacerbations of COPD and, therefore, is not recommended. Further evaluation should be dictated by the clinical scenario.

The medical management of acute exacerbations of COPD has been evaluated in numerous clinical trials. The treatment includes bronchodilator therapy, oxygen therapy, systemic corticosteroids, and antibiotics (Table 12.1). Although the exact duration of the treatment with systemic corticosteroids and antibiotics has not been defined, the benefit of the use of these agents has been demonstrated repeatedly.

Studies on bronchodilator therapy have shown that inhaled bronchodilators are superior to systemic bronchodilators, and that there is no advantage of nebulized treatment over metered-dose inhaler treatment. Bronchodilator therapy includes treatment

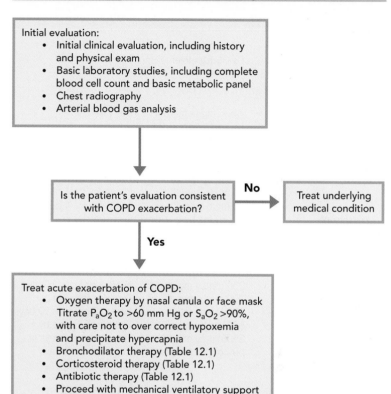

ALGORITHM 12.1 Initial Evaluation and Medical Management of Acute Exacerbations of Chronic Obstructive Pulmonary Disease (COPD)

Initial evaluation:
- Initial clinical evaluation, including history and physical exam
- Basic laboratory studies, including complete blood cell count and basic metabolic panel
- Chest radiography
- Arterial blood gas analysis

Is the patient's evaluation consistent with COPD exacerbation?

No → Treat underlying medical condition

Yes

Treat acute exacerbation of COPD:
- Oxygen therapy by nasal canula or face mask Titrate P_aO_2 to >60 mm Hg or S_aO_2 >90%, with care not to over correct hypoxemia and precipitate hypercapnia
- Bronchodilator therapy (Table 12.1)
- Corticosteroid therapy (Table 12.1)
- Antibiotic therapy (Table 12.1)
- Proceed with mechanical ventilatory support if needed (Algorithm 12.2).

with short-acting β_2-adrenergic receptor agonists and short-acting anticholinergic agents. Overall, the side effect profile of anticholinergic agents is favorable compared with β_2-adrenergic receptor agonists; thus, anticholinergic agents should be the first option. In addition, if the patient is not improving with maximum doses of anticholinergic treatment, the addition of a short-acting β_2-agonist has been shown to be beneficial.

Oxygen therapy has not been as rigorously studied because the benefit has been inferred. Oxygen should be administered by nasal canula or face mask to improve PaO_2 to >60 mm Hg or SaO_2 to 90% to 92%, with care not to increase oxygen tension to a high enough level to precipitate hypercapnia.

Corticosteroid treatment has been studied extensively, and the benefit of treating patients with acute exacerbations of COPD with systemic corticosteroids is clear. In the largest study comparing a 2-week course of corticosteroids to an 8-week course,

TABLE 12.1	Medications Commonly Used for Acute Exacerbations of Chronic Obstructive Pulmonary Disease	
Medication	Dose and route	Frequency
Bronchodilators		
Anticholinergic agent		
Ipratropium bromide	0.5 mg nebulized or 18–36 μg metered-dose inhaler	Every 4–6 hr
β_2-adrenergic receptor agonist		
Albuterol	2.5–5 mg nebulized 180 μg metered-dose inhaler	Every 4–6 hr
Corticosteroids		
Methylprednisolone	125 mg intravenously	Every 6 hr for 3 days then
	60 mg by mouth	Every day for 4 days then
	40 mg by mouth	Every day for 4 days then
	20 mg by mouth	Every day for 4 days
Prednisone	30–60 mg by mouth	Every day for 5–7 days or longer course with taper
Antibiotics		
Trimethoprim-sulfamethoxazole	160/800 mg by mouth	Every 12 hr for 5–10 days
Amoxicillin	250 mg by mouth	Every 6 hr for 5–10 days
Doxycycline	200 mg by mouth	First day followed by
	100 mg by mouth	Every 12 hr for 5–10 days
Azithromycin	500 mg by mouth	First day followed by
	250 mg by mouth	Every day for 4 days or
	500 mg by mouth	Every day for 3 days

there was no benefit to treating patients for 8 weeks compared with 2 weeks. Most patients will respond to treatment with corticosteroids for 5 to 10 days.

Treatment of acute exacerbations of COPD with antibiotics has been shown to be beneficial, especially in patients with moderate-to-severe exacerbations. The most commonly identified organisms from sputum in patients with acute exacerbations of COPD include *Streptococcus pneumoniae, Moraxella catarrhalis,* and *Haemophilus influenzae.* In patients with more severe disease, other Gram-negative bacteria, such as *Pseudomonas aeruginosa,* are identified with increasing frequency. Many antibiotics have been studied, including, but not limited to, amoxicillin, trimethoprim-sulfamethoxazole, tetracycline, clarithromycin, azithromycin, ciprofloxacin, levofloxacin, and moxifloxacin. There have been limited studies evaluating the use of newer, broader spectrum antibiotics compared with the older, narrower spectrum antibiotics, and to date there is no evidence that broader spectrum antibiotics decrease mortality. However, because of the concern of antibiotic resistance, broader spectrum agents, such as clarithromycin, azithromycin, levofloxacin, and moxifloxacin, are now frequently used. Given the lack of evidence to dictate the exact duration of treatment, patients are most commonly treated with antibiotics for 5 to 10 days.

ALGORITHM 12.2 Mechanical Ventilation in Acute Exacerbations of Chronic Obstructive Pulmonary Disease

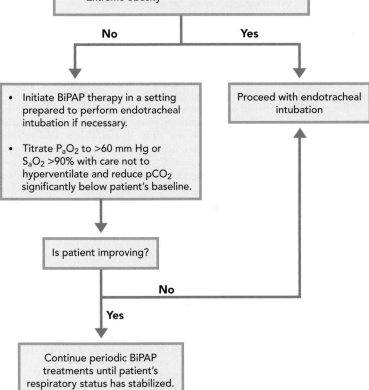

Are there reasons why patient cannot tolerate noninvasive ventilation?
- Acute respiratory failure
- Agitation or decreased mental status
- Hemodynamic instability
- Excessive secretions
- Structural abnormality precluding mask fitting
- Extreme obesity

No   **Yes**

- Initiate BiPAP therapy in a setting prepared to perform endotracheal intubation if necessary.

- Titrate P_aO_2 to >60 mm Hg or S_aO_2 >90% with care not to hyperventilate and reduce pCO_2 significantly below patient's baseline.

Proceed with endotracheal intubation

Is patient improving?

No

Yes

Continue periodic BiPAP treatments until patient's respiratory status has stabilized.

BiPAP, bilevel positive airway pressure.

There are other medical therapies that have been used to treat acute exacerbations of COPD, including mucolytic medications, chest physiotherapy, and methylxanthine bronchodilators. There is no evidence to support the use of these therapies, and, in fact, the latter two may be detrimental. No study has ever shown benefit of chest physiotherapy for acute exacerbations of COPD, and some studies have shown a transient decrease in forced expiratory volume in 1 second after treatment, thus raising the possibility that chest physiotherapy is harmful. Given the frequent and significant side effect profile of methylxanthines, and the lack of evidence demonstrating improved outcomes with these agents, the routine use of methylxanthines for acute exacerbations of COPD is not recommended.

In addition to the therapies already discussed, mechanical ventilatory support is an important treatment modality in patients with severe acute exacerbations of COPD (Algorithm 12.2). In patients with increasing respiratory distress, demonstrated by clinical deterioration, worsening hypercapnia and respiratory acidosis, worsening hypoxemia, and increasing dyspnea, mechanical ventilatory support may be temporarily necessary. Multiple studies have shown that noninvasive, positive-pressure ventilation is beneficial in patients with acute exacerbations of COPD. This strategy decreases the likelihood of needing endotracheal intubation, as well as possibly improving survival. In patients with altered mental status, acute respiratory failure, hemodynamic compromise, and extreme obesity, proceeding directly to endotracheal intubation and mechanical ventilation may be necessary.

Initial ventilator settings in patients with COPD should take into account this patient population's need for a long expiratory phase. Appropriate initial ventilator settings would be volume assist control, rate 10 to 12 breaths/min; tidal volume, 8 mL/kg; positive end-expiratory pressure (PEEP) of 0 to 5 cm H_2O; and an adequate FiO_2 to keep the hemoglobin saturation near 92%. These patients require high flows (peak flow 75 to 90 L/min) to allow for an inspiratory to expiratory ratio of 1:4 if possible. The initial settings should be adjusted by assessing the patient's comfort level and synchrony with the ventilator and by arterial blood gas analysis. The patient should not be ventilated for a "normal" arterial blood gas, and hypercapnia close to the patient's baseline level should be allowed.

It is also important to monitor the patient for the development of auto-PEEP while receiving mechanical ventilation. This can be detected by monitoring ventilator waveforms and the capnograph tracing. Auto-PEEP can occur with inadequate flows, excessive tidal volume, and high respiratory rates and can result in a reduction of venous return and systemic hypotension. Auto-PEEP also makes it more difficult for the patient to trigger the ventilator, and extrinsic PEEP can be added to offset this effect. In addition, patients with COPD on mechanical ventilator support should receive adequate deep venous thrombosis and stress ulcer prophylaxis. Nutritional support is vitally important in these patients, but should not contain excessive carbohydrates, as this will increase CO_2 production.

SUGGESTED READINGS

Bach PB, Brown C, Gelfand SE, et al. Management of acute exacerbations of chronic obstructive pulmonary disease: a summary and appraisal of published evidence. *Ann Intern Med.* 2001;134:600–620.
  Review of studies guiding management of acute exacerbations of COPD including evidence for or against oxygen therapy, bronchodilators, corticosteroids, antibiotics, and non-invasive ventilation.

Brochard L, Mancebo J, Wysocki M, et al. Noninvasive ventilation for acute exacerbations of chronic obstructive pulmonary disease. *N Engl J Med.* 1995;333:817–822.

Randomized study showing that noninvasive ventilation for acute exacerbations of COPD reduced the need for endotracheal intubation, reduced hospital stay, and reduced in-hospital mortality.

Lightowler JV, Wedzicha JA, Elliot MW, et al. Non-invasive positive pressure ventilation to treat respiratory failure resulting from exacerbations of chronic obstructive pulmonary disease: Cochrane systematic review and meta-analysis. *BMJ.* 2003;326:185–189.

Systematic review of randomized controlled trials showing that the use of non-invasive positive pressure ventilation should be first line therapy to decrease the need for endotracheal intubation and decrease mortality in patients with acute exacerbations of COPD.

McCrory DC, Brown C, Gelfand SE, et al. Management of acute exacerbations of COPD: a summary and appraisal of published evidence. *Chest.* 2001;119:1190–1209.

Review of available data on the evaluation, risk stratification, and management of patients with acute exacerbation of COPD.

Niewoehner D, Erbland M, Deupree RH, et al. Effect of systemic glucocorticoids on exacerbations of chronic obstructive pulmonary disease. *N Engl J Med.* 1999;340:1941–1947.

Randomized controlled trial showing clinical benefit of systemic glucocorticoids for acute exacerbations of COPD, as well as showing that there was no benefit to an 8 week course of corticosteroids over a 2 week course.

Nouira S, Marghli S, Boukef R, et al. Standard versus newer antibacterial agents in the treatment of severe acute exacerbation of chronic obstructive pulmonary disease: a randomized trial of trimethoprim-sulfamethoxazole versus ciprofloxacin. *Clin Infect Dis.* 2010;15:143–149.

Randomized controlled trial demonstrating that trimethoprim-sulfamethoxazole was not inferior to ciprofloxacin in the treatment of acute exacerbations of COPD.

Saginer A, Aytemur ZA, Cirit M, et al. Systemic glucocorticoids in severe exacerbations of COPD. *Chest.* 2001;119:726–730.

Randomized trial showing that patients receiving 10 days of glucocorticoid treatment instead of 3 days had significant improvements in arterial oxygen tension, FEV_1, and dyspnea on exertion.

Snow V, Lascher S, Mottur-Pilson C, et al. Evidence base for management of acute exacerbations of chronic obstructive pulmonary disease. *Ann Intern Med.* 2001;134:595–599.

Review of evidence concerning risk stratification, diagnostic testing, and therapeutic interventions for management of acute exacerbation of COPD.

Stoller J. Acute exacerbations of chronic obstructive pulmonary disease. *N Engl J Med.* 2002;346:988–994.

Review of treatment of acute exacerbations of COPD, including medical management and ventilatory support.

13 Sleep-Disordered Breathing in the Intensive Care Unit

Tonya D. Russell

Sleep has a range of effects on respiratory physiology in healthy patients, as outlined in Table 13.1. In patients with underlying comorbidities, such as severe chronic obstructive pulmonary disease or neuromuscular disease, these changes in respiratory physiology can lead to compromise of the patient's cardiopulmonary status. In addition, there are sleep-related breathing disorders that can lead to respiratory failure in which the main pathophysiology occurs during sleep, such as obstructive sleep apnea, central sleep apnea (CSA), and sleep-related obesity hypoventilation.

Apneic events during sleep can either be obstructive or central in nature. Obstructive events are associated with ongoing respiratory effort, while there is no respiratory effort present with central apneas. Obstructive sleep apnea occurs when there is narrowing of the upper airway during sleep due to excessive soft tissue or structural abnormalities, resulting in limitation or cessation of airflow that can be associated with arousals or oxygen desaturations. Obstructive sleep apnea has been associated with increased risk of excessive daytime somnolence, hypertension, stroke, and heart failure. The prevalence of obstructive sleep apnea–hypopnea syndrome (OSAHS) has been estimated to be 4% of men and 2% of women. CSA can occur in the setting of severe heart failure (Cheyne–Stokes respirations), stroke, or narcotic use. The severity of obstructive sleep apnea can be quantified by the number of events per hour (apnea–hypopnea index) or by the severity of sleepiness, as shown in Table 13.2.

Obesity hypoventilation syndrome (OHS) is frequently used to describe hypoventilation during sleep occurring in obese patients, which results in daytime hypercapnia. The prevalence of OHS is not clear, and the definition of OHS in the literature is variable. However, the American Academy of Sleep Medicine Task Force has made recommendations for diagnostic criteria for sleep hypoventilation syndrome, of which OHS is a part, as shown in Table 13.3. It is apparent that hypercapnia can occur in the setting of severe OSAHS alone, sleep-related hypoventilation without apneic or hypopneic events (OHS), or in combination.

Obstructive sleep apnea and obesity hypoventilation should be considered in patients with hypercapnic respiratory failure who have signs and symptoms as listed in Table 13.4. CSA should also be considered if there is a history of congestive heart failure, stroke, or narcotic use. In patients with hypercapnia solely related to obstructive sleep apnea, continuous positive airway pressure (CPAP), at a pressure that resolves the obstructive events, should correct the hypercapnia. However, in patients in whom

TABLE 13.1	Effects of Sleep on Respiratory Physiology

Decreased hypoxic ventilatory response
Decreased hypercapnic ventilatory response
Increased muscle hypotonia
Increased airway resistance
Increased arousal threshold from events related to increased airway resistance
(NREM > REM)

NREM, nonrapid eye movement; REM, rapid eye movement.

TABLE 13.2	Severity of Obstructive Sleep Apnea	

Severity	AHI[a]	Level of impairment[b]
Mild	5–15	Sedentary activities requiring minimal attention (i.e., watching television, reading, passenger in a car)
Moderate	15–30	Activities requiring some attention (i.e., meetings, concerts)
Severe	>30	Activities requiring active attention (i.e., conversation, eating, driving)

[a]AHI (apnea–hypopnea index), number of apneas and hypopneas per hour; apnea is defined as cessation of airflow; hypopnea is defined as $\geq$30% reduction in airflow associated with 4% oxygen desaturation; all events must be at least 10 seconds.
[b]Extent of daytime somnolence.

TABLE 13.3	Diagnostic Criteria for Sleep Hypoventilation Syndrome[a]

Signs and symptoms	Monitoring
Cor pulmonale	Increase in $PaCO_2$ during sleep >10 mm Hg from awake supine values
Pulmonary hypertension	
Unexplained excessive daytime somnolence	Oxygen desaturations during sleep not associated with apneas or hypopneas
Erythrocytosis	
Waking hypercapnia ($PaCO_2$ >45 mm Hg)	

[a]Must meet at least one criterion from each column.

TABLE 13.4	Signs and Symptoms of Obstructive Sleep Apnea–Hypopnea Syndrome and Obesity Hypoventilation Syndrome

Obesity
Snoring
Awakening snorting or gasping
Witnessed apneas
Excessive daytime somnolence
Morning headaches
Large neck circumference
Unrefreshing sleep
Poorly controlled hypertension
Craniofacial abnormalities (micrognathia, retrognathia, macroglossia)
Nocturnal oxygen desaturations
Hypercapnia not explained by other etiology
Hypothyroidism

there is a component of sleep-related hypoventilation, bilevel positive airway pressure (BiPAP) is usually required. Treatment of CSA requires BiPAP with a set of back-up respiratory rate.

Unfortunately, there is not much guidance in the literature for empirically picking pressures for CPAP or BiPAP in the setting of sleep-disordered breathing and sleep-related hypoventilation. In the outpatient setting, a split sleep study is performed, in which the first part of the study allows for the diagnosis of the sleep-disordered breathing and the second part of the study allows for the titration of CPAP or BiPAP. If an inpatient sleep study is available, this would be the best way to establish a diagnosis of OSAHS, CSA, or OHS, and the best way to determine the necessary pressures required to treat the disorder. However, if a patient requires initiation of therapy without the benefit of a sleep study, it should be initiated in a closely monitored setting such as an intensive care unit or step-down unit.

Patients who are morbidly obese or have very severe obstructive sleep apnea will frequently require high pressures to resolve the sleep-disordered breathing. If the empiric pressure is too low, then the apnea events or hypoventilation may not be fully resolved, leading to prolonged hypoxemia. Severe hypoxemia has been reported to occur during the empiric use of CPAP. If the empiric pressure is too high, then the patient may experience other complications related to positive pressure, as outlined in Table 13.5, which may decrease the patient's ability to comply with CPAP or BiPAP.

TABLE 13.5	Common Complications and Side Effects of Continuous Positive Airway Pressure or Bilevel Positive Airway Pressure

Nasal/oral dryness
Eye dryness
Mask leak
Aerophagia/gastric distention
Skin irritation

ALGORITHM 13.1 Proposed Evaluation and Treatment Guideline for Intensive Care Unit Patients Suspected of Having Severe Obstructive Sleep Apnea–Hypopnea Syndrome (OSAHS), Central Sleep Apnea (CSA), or Obesity Hypoventilation Syndrome (OHS)

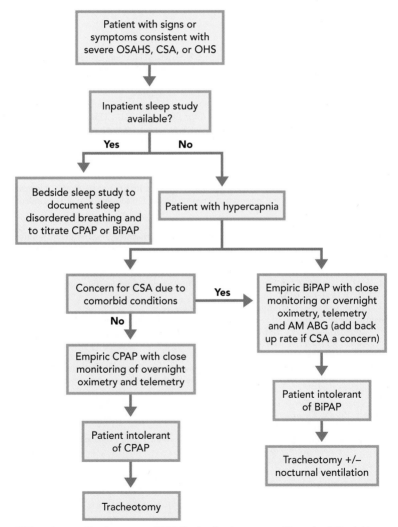

CPAP, continuous positive airway pressure; BiPAP, bilevel positive airway pressure; AM, morning; ABG, arterial blood gas.

In patients who cannot tolerate CPAP or BiPAP, tracheotomy is the gold standard for treatment of obstructive sleep apnea because it allows for the area of upper airway obstruction to be bypassed. However, some morbidly obese patients may require custom tracheotomy tubes in order to fully resolve the obstruction. In addition, if there is a component of CSA or sleep-related hypoventilation not solely due to OSAHS, then nocturnal ventilation through the tracheotomy tube is required. Algorithm 13.1 demonstrates a proposed algorithm for the evaluation and treatment of patients in the intensive care unit who are suspected of having severe obstructive sleep apnea or sleep-related hypoventilation.

SUGGESTED READINGS

American Academy of Sleep Medicine Task Force. Sleep related breathing disorders in adults: recommendations for syndrome definitions and measurement techniques in clinical research. *Sleep.* 1999;22:667–689.
  Reviews recommended definitions for sleep-disordered breathing.
Berger KI, Ayappa I, Chatr-Amontri B, et al. Obesity hypoventilation syndrome as a spectrum of respiratory disturbances during sleep. *Chest.* 2001;120:1231–1238.
  Retrospective review of 23 patients with daytime hypercapnia and excessive daytime somnolence.
Douglas NJ. Respiratory physiology: control of ventilation. In: Kryger MH, Roth T, Dement WC, eds. Principles and practices of sleep medicine. Philadelphia, PA: WB Saunders, 2000:221–228.
  Review of respiratory physiology in sleep.
Krieger J. Respiratory physiology: breathing in normal subjects. In: Kryger MH, Roth T, Dement WC, eds. Principles and practices of sleep medicine. Philadelphia, PA: WB Saunders, 2000:229–241.
  Review of respiratory physiology in sleep.
Kreiger J, Weitzenblum E, Monassier JP, et al. Dangerous hypoxaemia during continuous positive airway pressure treatment of obstructive sleep apnoea. *Lancet.* 1983;322:1429–1430.
  Report of a patient with severe hypoxemia occurring with empiric CPAP use for obstructive sleep apnea.
Meoli AL, Casey KR, Clark RW, et al. Hypopnea in sleep disordered breathing in adults. *Sleep.* 2001;24:469–470.
  Reviews recommended definitions of apnea and hypopnea.
Shamsuzzaman AS, Gersh BJ, Somers VK. Obstructive sleep apnea—implications for cardiac and vascular disease. *JAMA.* 2003;290:1906–1914.
  Report of MEDLINE review of 154 peer-reviewed studies assessing cardiovascular complications associated with obstructive sleep apnea.
Thorpy M, Chesson A, Sarkis D, et al. Practice parameters for the treatment of obstructive sleep apnea in adults: the efficacy of surgical modification of the upper airway. *Sleep.* 1996; 19:152–155.
  Reviews indications and efficacy of surgical treatment of obstructive sleep apnea.
Young T, Palta M, Dempsey J, et al. The occurrence of sleep disordered breathing among middle-aged adults. *N Engl J Med.* 1993;328:1230–1235.
  A random sample of state employees of Wisconsin who underwent polysomnograms to evaluate the prevalence of sleep-disordered breathing.

14 Pulmonary Hypertension and Right Ventricular Failure in the Intensive Care Unit

Murali M. Chakinala

Decompensated right ventricular failure (DRVF) is a less common cause of shock, which is frequently under diagnosed, and recognizing its presence requires vigilance for a constellation of symptoms and signs. The treatment of this condition also differs somewhat from the routine shock management guidelines as elucidated elsewhere in this book. Most often, DRVF occurs in the setting of chronic pulmonary hypertension (i.e., mean pulmonary artery (PA) pressure ≥ 25 mm Hg) with an inciting acute illness that converts a compensated right ventricle (RV) into DRVF and a hemodynamically unstable emergency.

PATHOPHYSIOLOGY OF RV FAILURE

The RV is a thin-walled chamber that empties by sequential contraction into a low-resistance, high-capacitance pulmonary vascular circuit over the entire period of RV systole. Despite a three to fourfold increase in cardiac output, there is no increase in pulmonary pressure and RV workload, thanks to pulmonary vasodilation and recruitment of pulmonary vasculature. But when faced with an acute rise in afterload (e.g., massive pulmonary embolism), the RV can decompensate rapidly, leading to shock (Algorithm 14.1). But in the setting of chronic pulmonary hypertension, the RV has an innate but limited ability to undergo myocardial hypertrophy, thus reducing wall tension and maintaining contractility for a finite period of time. Even then, a hypertrophied and compensated RV can deteriorate rapidly in the setting of acute pressure overload (Algorithm 14.1).

CAUSES OF DRVF

Table 14.1 lists causes of acute RV failure. Table 14.2 lists the etiology of acute on chronic decompensation in patients with known pulmonary hypertension.

ALGORITHM 14.1 Pathophysiology of Decompensated Right Ventricular Failure

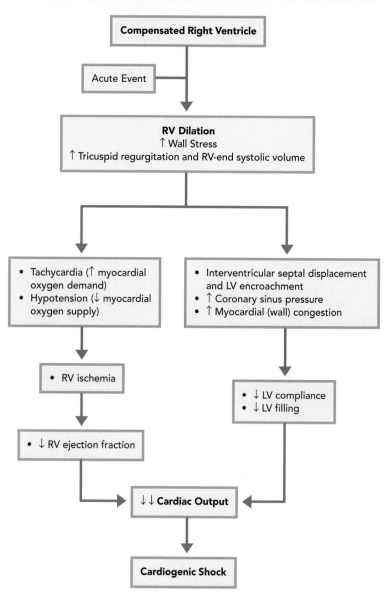

RV, right ventricular; LV, left ventricular.

TABLE 14.1	Etiology of Right Ventricular (RV) Failure

Left ventricular dysfunction
RV infarct or perioperative injury
Cardiac tamponade (mimicker of RV failure)
Tricuspid valve disease (regurgitation, stenosis)
Acute massive pulmonary embolus (thrombus, fat, air, or amniotic fluid)
Acute lung injury/adult respiratory distress syndrome
Sickle cell chest syndrome
Congenital heart disease (e.g., atrial septal defect, anomalous pulmonary
   venous return, Ebstein's anomaly)
Acute decompensation of chronic pulmonary arterial hypertension (Table 14.2)

DIAGNOSIS OF DRVF

Clinical Presentation

DRVF typically manifests as shock due to a low flow state. A history of pulmonary hypertension raises the possibility for an acute on chronic decompensation due to any of the causes listed in Table 14.2. Signs and symptoms of DRVRF are shown in Table 14.3.

Diagnostic Testing

Radiology
Plain radiographs may show enlarged central pulmonary arteries with peripheral pruning if chronic pulmonary hypertension is present. Chronic RV enlargement manifests with filling of the retrosternal space. Right-sided pleural effusions rarely may be present, but pleural effusions typically indicate left ventricular (LV) dysfunction. If an acute pulmonary embolism is suspected, lower extremity Doppler examinations and either ventilation–perfusion scan or pulmonary embolism protocol computed tomography should be obtained.

Electrocardiogram
Table 14.4 shows the RV changes that can be seen by electrocardiography.

TABLE 14.2	Causes of Acute Hemodynamic Instability in Chronic Pulmonary Arterial Hypertension

Acute medication failure (e.g., noncompliance, interruption of parenteral
   vasodilator therapy)
Dietary or fluid indiscretion
Increased metabolic demands (e.g., infection, fever, environmental heat,
   pregnancy)
Venous thromboembolism (submassive or massive)
Induction of general anesthesia
Surgery (left-sided valvular repair, pulmonary thromboendarterectomy, lung
   transplantation, lobectomy, or pneumonectomy)
Dysrhythmias
Endocrinopathies (e.g., thyroid disorders, adrenal insufficiency)

TABLE 14.3	Signs and Symptoms
Symptoms	Signs
Syncope, dizziness	Decreased pulses
RUQ pain	Cool extremities
Abdominal distention	Lower extremity edema
Weight gain	Elevated jugular venous pulsation (without
Early satiety	auscultatory crackles)
	Right-sided S3
	Pulsatile liver
	Hepatojugular reflux
	Ascites

RUQ, right upper quadrant.

Laboratory Data

In keeping with a low-output state, typical laboratory values of tissue/organ hypoperfusion may be encountered, including anion gap metabolic acidosis, elevated lactate, (pre-renal) blood urea nitrogen to creatinine ratio, and low urine sodium. Hepatic congestion results in elevated liver enzymes and hyperbilirubinemia. RV strain can result in significantly elevated B-type natriuretic peptide, while an elevated troponin I level would indicate RV infarction.

Echocardiography

Cardiac echocardiography is arguably the most useful examination in this scenario by establishing RV failure and preserved left-sided cardiac function. Table 14.5 lists echocardiographic findings in DRVF. It provides rapid and important data for diagnosing RV failure, elucidating precipitating causes, and triaging patients into three groups: RV failure with elevated PA pressures, RV failure without elevated pressures, and pericardial disease (Algorithm 14.2).

Pulmonary Artery Catheter

A complementary diagnostic tool in the management of DRVF is the pulmonary artery catheter (PAC). Indications for use of a PAC include differentiating "pump failure" from other causes of shock or assisting with management of DRVF (i.e., optimizing volume status, use of inotropes, and assessing response to pulmonary vasodilators). Challenges to using PAC in DRVF include difficulty introducing the catheter,

TABLE 14.4	Electrocardiographic Changes in Right Ventricular Failure

Sinus tachycardia
Atrial dysrhythmias (e.g., fibrillation, flutter, reentry tachycardia)
Right axis deviation
Right atrial enlargement
Right ventricular hypertrophy
Right bundle branch block
Qr pattern in lead V1
S1 Q3 T3 pattern

TABLE 14.5	Echocardiographic Findings in Right Ventricular (RV) Failure

RV hypertrophy (in chronic pulmonary hypertension)
RV dilation and hypokinesis
> *McConnell's sign* – akinesis of mid-RV free wall with preserved apical wall function is a specific (~95%) sign of acute pulmonary embolism

Paradoxic septal motion due to RV pressure overload
Right atrial enlargement
D-shaped left ventricle and late systolic left ventricular filling
Pericardial effusion
Tricuspid regurgitation
Elevated pulmonary arterial systolic pressure
Pulmonary artery dilatation
Dilated inferior vena cava or lack of inspiratory collapse
Markers of RV function:
> Reduced tricuspid annular plane systolic excursion (TAPSE: normal $\geq$2.5 cm)
> Elevated Tei index (normal $\leq$0.3)

increased risk of PA rupture from "overwedging" the distal balloon tip, and poor tolerance of arrhythmias. The characteristic pattern of DRVF includes elevated central venous, RV, and PA pressures with reduced cardiac output, stroke volume, and mixed venous oxygen saturation. With end-stage RV failure or in the setting of RV infarction, the PA pressure may not be elevated as the RV is unable to generate enough force to eject blood into the pulmonary vasculature. The PA occlusion pressure is typically low but may be elevated as LV compliance worsens. Cardiac output should be measured by the Fick method as tricuspid regurgitation or intracardiac shunts make thermodilution method unreliable. Lastly, one should place more emphasis on trends gleaned from PAC readings rather than on absolute values.

TREATMENT OF ACUTE DECOMPENSATED RV FAILURE

The treatment of acute DRVF (Algorithm 14.3) includes the following:

- Identify and correct precipitating factors
- Correct hypoxemia
- Reverse hypotension and restore circulation
- Treat volume overload and RV encroachment.

Identify and Correct Precipitating Factors

In patients with known pulmonary hypertension and chronic RV dysfunction, identification of precipitating factors (Table 14.2) must be sought and corrected. Maintain a high index of suspicion for occult infection in patients with chronic indwelling venous catheters; empiric therapy to treat bacteremia is appropriate. Sepsis will be poorly tolerated but fluid resuscitation has to be tempered by not aggravating RV dilation and LV compression. Atrial tachyarrhythmias should be slowed with digoxin, amiodarone, or cardioversion. Beta-blockers or verapamil should not be used because of their negative inotropic effects. Bradycardias may require temporary pacing as the situation demands.

ALGORITHM 14.2   Diagnostic Pathway in Suspected Right Ventricular (RV) Failure

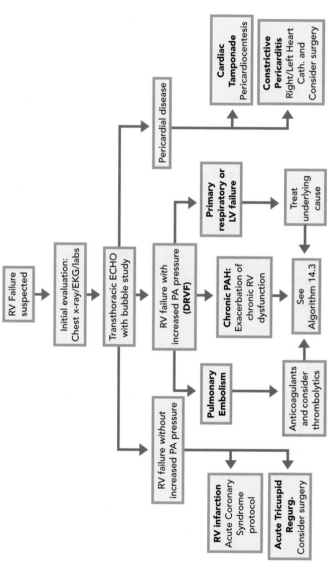

EKG, electrocardiogram; labs, laboratory findings; DRVF, decompensated right ventricular failure; LV, left ventricular; PAH, pulmonary arterial hypertension; PA, pulmonary artery; Cath., catheterization.

ALGORITHM 14.3 Management of Decompensated Right Ventricular (RV) Failure

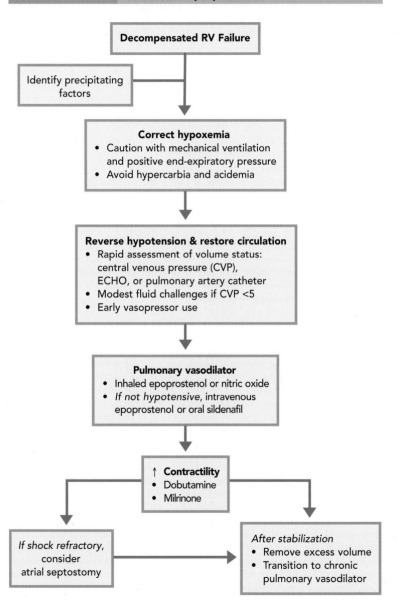

ECHO, echocardiography.

Correct Hypoxemia

Oxygen is the most potent pulmonary vasodilator, and liberal oxygen administration will minimize hypoxic vasoconstriction and improve cardiac output. If positive pressure ventilation is needed, employ the lowest plateau pressures, through low tidal volume and positive end-expiratory pressure, in order to limit RV afterload (from intra-alveolar vessel compression) and decreases in venous return, while still maintaining adequate oxygenation and avoiding respiratory acidosis. Hypotension and poor ventilation during intubation can also have profound hemodynamic consequences. Once intubated, permissive hypercapnia should be avoided as hypoxic pulmonary vasoconstriction is augmented in hypercarbic conditions.

Lastly, bronchospasm and agitation are frequently overlooked causes of elevated PVR in ventilated patients and should be managed aggressively.

Reverse Hypotension and Restore Circulation

Factors governing RV stroke volume are the same as those for the LV: preload, afterload, and myocardial contractility. Treatment of DRVF encompasses all three parameters, and the PAC may assist.

Preload

Insufficient preload is generally not an issue in DRVF. If shock is due to decreased preload (i.e., central venous pressure <5 mm Hg), cautious volume challenges of crystalloid should be employed until central venous pressure is 10 to 12 mm Hg or serial cardiac output assessments should be monitored. Overexuberant volume administration can worsen RV distention and encroach on the LV, further reducing cardiac output and worsening hypotension.

Systemic Hypotension

A low systemic diastolic pressure coupled with elevated RV end-diastolic pressure (common in DVRF) narrows the myocardial perfusion gradient, leading to RV ischemia. Thus, vasopressors have an important role in restoring systemic blood pressure to maintain organ perfusion and minimize RV ischemia. While no agent is superior, norepinephrine has both inotropic and peripheral vasopressor properties without major pulmonary vascular constriction. Dopamine, which may result in marked tachycardia, is also a reasonable choice given its positive inotropic and peripheral vasoconstrictive effects. The lowest doses of pressors should be used to minimize tachycardia, dysrhythmias, myocardial oxygen consumption, and pulmonary vasoconstriction.

Afterload Reduction

Selective pulmonary arterial dilation is a critical therapeutic step in breaking the spiral of RV decompensation. Inhaled agents preferentially lower PVR with minimal decreases in systemic vascular resistance and also minimize ventilation–perfusion mismatching and hypoxemia. Two available agents are inhaled nitric oxide and epoprostenol. Inhaled nitric oxide up to 40 ppm is administered via face mask or endotracheal tube, but methemoglobin levels must be followed. Inhaled epoprostenol (5,000–20,000 ng/mL) as a continuous nebulization is a cheaper alternative. Once cardiac output and blood pressure have improved, the patient can be transitioned to more conventional and longer-term options (e.g., parenteral or longer-acting inhaled prostacyclin analogues). Nonselective vasodilators such as nitroprusside, nitrates, hydralazine, and calcium channel antagonists must be avoided as they preferentially cause peripheral vasodilation and aggravate hypotension.

Contractility

In *normotensive* patients with persistently unmet peripheral metabolic needs, the next step is addition of an inotrope. There is no ideal inotrope that increases RV contractility without worsening systemic blood pressure. Options include dobutamine at 2–5 μg/kg/min or the longer-acting milrinone, which requires dosage reduction in renal insufficiency.

Treat Volume Overload and RV Encroachment

Once circulation is restored and the patient has stabilized, excess volume can then be removed. Severe right heart failure can be associated with diuretic resistance due to poor intestinal absorption, decreased glomerular filtration rate with poor renal arterial perfusion, renal venous congestion from elevated central venous pressures, and intense neurohormonal activation. A suggested stepwise approach is

1. Loop diuretic (e.g., furosemide and bumetanide) by intravenous (IV) bolus or continuous infusion. The latter maintains a continuous renal threshold of drug with constant diuresis and less ototoxicity.
2. If loop diuretic is insufficient, a thiazide diuretic (e.g., chlorothiazide [IV or PO] or metolazone (PO) can be added.
3. Spironolactone is effective to counter the intense neurohormonal pathway and can be added unless hyperkalemia is present.
4. Finally, mechanical fluid removal with continuous venovenous hemodialysis (CVVHD) may be appropriate.

SURGICAL INTERVENTIONS

Atrial septostomy, which is the percutaneous creation of a right-to-left shunt in the inter-atrial septum, allows for right-sided decompression and improved left-sided filling. Although right-to-left shunting results in oxygen desaturation, this is counterbalanced by improved cardiac output and total oxygen delivery. Septostomy is a risky procedure with associated morbidity and mortality that should only be performed at experienced centers.

GENERAL MEASURES

1. Control agitation
2. Suppress fevers
3. Place filters on IV catheters to prevent air embolization if intracardiac shunt present
4. Deep venous thrombosis prophylaxis
5. Minimize Valsalva maneuvers (e.g., constipation)
6. Caution with colloid infusions but consider transfusion if anemic and oxygen delivery severely compromised.

SUGGESTED READINGS

DeMarco T, McGlothin D. Managing right ventricular failure in PAH. *Adv Pulm Hypertens.* 2005;14(4):16–26.
    A review article with excellent flowcharts, algorithms, and detailed pathophysiology and therapeutic discussion.

Lahm T, McCaslin C, Wozniak T, et al. Medical and surgical treatment of acute right ventricular failure. *J Am Coll Cardiol.* 2010;56:1435–1446.
  Excellent review of the clinical features of DRVF, including comprehensive treatment strategy.
Mebazaa A, Karpati P. Acute right ventricular failure—from pathophysiology to new treatments. *Intensive Care Med.* 2004;30:185–196.
  A clinical case based review.
Piazza G, Goldhaber S. The acutely decompensated right ventricle: pathways for diagnosis & management. *Chest.* 2005;128:1836–1852.
  A detailed review article focusing on pathophysiology, diagnosis, and treatment of this increasingly common condition.
Taichman DB, Jeffery ME. Management of the acutely ill patient with pulmonary arterial hypertension. In: Mandel J, Taichman D, eds. Pulmonary vascular disease. Philadelphia, PA: Saunders Elsevier, 2006:254–265.
  A textbook chapter that discusses issues to consider when caring for patients with PAH in the ICU.

Pulmonary Embolism

Hannah C. Otepka and Roger D. Yusen

Intensive care unit (*ICU*) patients typically have multiple risk factors for deep vein thrombosis (*DVT*) and pulmonary embolism (*PE*) that include acute illness, comorbidities, immobilization, advanced age, and hypercoagulable states. These risk factors make venous thromboembolism (*VTE*) a frequent diagnosis in the ICU. Of patients who receive care for or develop PE in the ICU, many will have *submassive* PE (i.e., signs of right ventricular [*RV*] dysfunction without arterial hypotension or cardiogenic shock), and a smaller but significant proportion will have *massive* PE (i.e., RV dysfunction with arterial hypotension or cardiogenic shock).

DIAGNOSIS [Algorithm 15.1]

PE often has nonspecific *signs and symptoms* (e.g., tachycardia, tachypnea, dyspnea, pleuritic chest pain, hemoptysis, hypoxemia, presyncope, syncope, and hypotension) which frequently overlap with other conditions that occur in ICU patients.

The *differential diagnosis* list for patients with signs and symptoms of PE includes sepsis, hypovolemia, acute lung injury (e.g., pneumonia, aspiration, and transfusion-associated lung injury [*TRALI*]), heart failure, acute coronary syndrome, cardiac tamponade, decompensated pulmonary arterial hypertension, constrictive cardiac disease, valvular heart disease, and aortic dissection. Patients in the ICU often have multiorgan dysfunction, and PE may occur in conjunction with illnesses such as myocardial dysfunction or sepsis. Clinicians frequently underdiagnose PE because it mimics other diseases and *vice versa*. Prompt diagnosis and appropriate treatment will reduce mortality and recurrence rates.

Diagnostic Modalities

Pretest probability influences the diagnostic workup of patients with suspected PE, and its incorporation into the interpretation of diagnostic tests improves their accuracy. However, clinical probability scores (e.g., Wells Prediction Score, Geneva Score and pulmonary embolism severity index [PESI]) usually trend toward an intermediate to high pretest probability in the ICU setting. Nonspecific diagnostic tests, such as *D-dimer* assay (many false positives), have a low accuracy in the ICU setting, and waiting for the result may delay necessary additional diagnostic tests or treatments. Chest radiography (*CXR*), electrocardiogram (*EKG*), and arteriol blood gas (*ABG*) may prove useful for assisting in determining pretest probability and evaluating for other causes of a patient's illness, but they do not confirm or rule out the diagnosis of PE. *Cardiac biomarkers* assist with prognosis, though they have low diagnostic accuracy. Since many disorders on the differential diagnosis list fall into the category

ALGORITHM 15.1 Diagnostic Evaluation for Suspected Acute Pulmonary Embolism (PE) in the Intensive Care Unit (ICU)

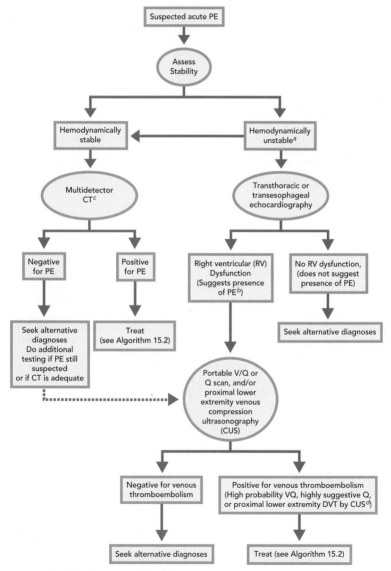

[a] search for alternative and concomitant diagnoses.
[b] try to confirm presence of PE with additional testing.
[c] if contraindication to intravenous (IV) contrast exist, consider V/Q scan, CUS, or MR angiography.
[d] proximal lower extremity DVT serves as a surrogate for PE in the appropriate clinical setting.

of life threatening, the clinical suspicion of PE should lead to expeditious objective diagnostic testing.

Multidetector helical computed tomography (CT) scan with contrast (PE protocol) has become the gold standard test for evaluating patients with suspected PE, and it may assist with the detection of alternative or concomitant diagnoses. CT scan may also help to quantify the severity of PE by assessing for *RV* dysfunction and evaluating the clot burden. The accuracy of CT for diagnosis of PE decreases with poorer scan quality and for smaller and more peripheral clots. Contraindications to CT include contrast allergy, severe renal dysfunction, or inability to safely travel out of the ICU. Patients with a contraindication to CT or inadequate CT results should undergo other testing that may include ventilation/perfusion (*V/Q*) scan, lower extremity venous compression ultrasonography (*CUS*), or echocardiography (ECHO).

Radionuclide scintigraphy (V/Q scan) allows for testing in the ICU because of its portability. A patient who has an abnormal CXR will often have an indeterminate V/Q result, and such a result warrants further testing. Because of the high likelihood of obtaining a nondiagnostic V/Q result, and since chest CT may reveal alternative or additional diagnoses, chest CT should remain the first-choice diagnostic test for evaluating patients in the ICU that have suspected PE.

CUS may diagnose DVT at the bedside in the ICU. Proximal lower extremity DVT may serve as a surrogate for PE in the appropriate clinical setting.

ECHO, another portable modality, may detect right-sided cardiac thrombus or signs of right heart dysfunction associated with PE (a surrogate for PE). Findings on ECHO may suggest an etiology other than PE for the signs and symptoms, and it may exclude mimics of PE that include acute myocardial infarction, pericardial tamponade, aortic dissection, pulmonary arterial hypertension, and heart failure. A patient with possible massive PE should urgently undergo ECHO. If transthoracic ECHO does not provide good images or if other indications exist, a clinician may prefer to use transesophageal ECHO. Findings on ECHO to suggest PE include RV dilation and hypokinesis; increase in RV/LV (left ventricle) diameter ratio; pulmonary artery dilation; tricuspid regurgitation; paradoxical septal motion; interventricular septal shift toward the LV; and *McConnell's sign,* defined by hypokinesis of the free wall of the RV with normal motion of the apex.

Stability Assessment

Cardiovascular stability helps to determine the diagnostic workup for suspected PE in an ICU setting (Algorithm 15.1). Stable patients should undergo evaluation with CT if contraindications do not exist. Unstable patients should undergo tests based on their likelihood of ruling in or ruling out diagnoses, their availability, and the ability to get rapid results. Patients with hemodynamic instability should undergo rapid risk stratification to assess for RV dysfunction (i.e., CT or ECHO) and stress/injury (i.e., brain natriuretic peptide [BNP] and cardiac troponin). If a patient cannot transport out of the ICU for diagnostic testing due to unacceptable risk or other reasons, the patient should undergo bedside testing (e.g., ECHO, portable V/Q scan, Q scan, or lower extremity venous CUS). For patients who have a cardiac arrest, bedside ECHO might also assist with decision making about interventions such as thrombolytic therapy.

PROGNOSIS

Hemodynamic status remains the most important prognostic factor for patients with acute PE. Massive PE accounts for 5% of all cases of PE and has a short-term mortality of at least 15%. During the first 30 days after diagnosis of PE, *RV* failure causes approximately half of the deaths. The degree of hemodynamic instability in patients with acute PE predicts in-hospital mortality. Mortality rises as the severity of the PE-associated cardiovascular dysfunction worsens (i.e., RV dysfunction without arterial hypotension, arterial hypotension, cardiogenic shock, and cardiopulmonary resuscitation).

Prognostic indicators may assist with decision making regarding escalation of therapy (*see treatment*). Elevated BNP and troponin in the setting of PE suggest RV stress/injury has occurred, and abnormal test results portend a poor prognosis even in the hemodynamically stable patient. On ECHO or CT, patients with RV thrombus or RV dysfunction have a higher mortality compared to those without these findings.

TREATMENT [Algorithm 15.2]

Clinicians should make their treatment decisions for PE based on confidence in the diagnosis of PE, hemodynamic status, degree of RV dysfunction/injury, bleeding risk, prognosis, and patient preferences. In patients who have a high clinical probability and acceptable bleeding risk, clinicians should initiate anticoagulation upon the initial suspicion of PE and prior to completion of any diagnostic tests. Satisfactory "exclusion" of the diagnosis PE should lead to prompt discontinuation of anticoagulation, unless otherwise indicated, and initiation of VTE prophylaxis. Confirmation of PE should lead to continuation or prompt initiation of anticoagulation if not contraindicated. Confirmation of PE in the setting of a contraindication to anticoagulation or a recurrence in the setting of therapeutic doses of anticoagulation should lead to placement of an inferior vena cava (*IVC*) filter (*see below*). *Hemodynamically unstable patients* with PE should undergo stabilization and resuscitation (*see SHOCK chapter*). Vasopressors/inotropes may lead to improved stability, and resuscitation should include cautious fluid management. Clinicians should use supplemental oxygen and ventilatory support as deemed necessary. Prompt risk stratification will assist with further decisions regarding escalation of care (i.e., thrombolytic therapy or embolectomy).

Anticoagulation

Anticoagulation acts to prevent new clot formation and decrease risk for recurrent VTE. Anticoagulants that have efficacy for the treatment of PE demonstrated in clinical trials include unfractionated heparin (UFH), low-molecular-weight heparin (LMWH), and fondaparinux (*see PHARMACOLOGY chapter for dosing, side effects, and complications*). However, most studies of anticoagulants excluded ICU patients. Since patients in the ICU often have higher than average bleeding risks, a relatively high rate of undergoing invasive procedures, and a higher chance of receiving thrombolytic therapy, intravenous (IV) UFH may be the preferred anticoagulant because of its bioavailability via the IV route, relatively short half-life, insignificant renal clearance, and reversibility. However, general guidelines suggest using LMWH instead of UFH for nonmassive PE.

Thrombolytic Therapy

Thrombolytic agents convert plasminogen to plasmin and lead to clot lysis. Thrombolytics may improve short-term physiologic measures that include pulmonary perfusion, RV function, and blood pressure. The high risk of death in patients with PE and associated hypotension or shock may indicate the need for aggressive treatment (i.e., thrombolysis). Studies do not support the use of thrombolytic agents in

ALGORITHM 15.2   Treatment of Confirmed Acute PE in the ICU

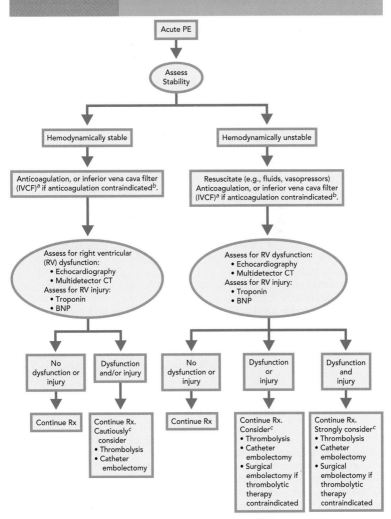

^aTemporary or permanent IVCF.
^bAnticoagulate after IVCF placement once contraindication to anticoagulation resolves.
^cIf contraindication do not exist.

most patients with acute symptomatic PE. In the absence of large randomized clinical trials that demonstrate the benefit of thrombolytic therapy on mortality, the American College of Chest Physicians (*ACCP*) guidelines recommended the use of thrombolytic therapy for (1) patients with acute symptomatic PE and hemodynamic instability that do not have major contraindications owing to bleeding risk (evidence strength Grade 1B) and (2) selected high-risk patients without hypotension and low risk of bleeding

TABLE 15.1	Contraindications to Thrombolytic Therapy

Absolute contraindications[a]
   Active internal bleeding
   Known bleeding diathesis
   History of intracranial hemorrhage
   Known intracranial neoplasm, arteriovenous malformation, or aneurysm
   Nonhemorrhagic stroke within the past 3 months
   Significant head trauma with the past 3 months
   Intracranial or intraspinal surgery within the past 3 months
   Severe uncontrolled systemic hypertension
   Suspected aortic dissection

Relative contraindications
   Recent internal bleeding
   Recent major surgery (see above) or organ biopsy
   Recent trauma (see above), including cardiopulmonary resuscitation
      (especially if prolonged)
   Recent blood vessel puncture at noncompressible site
   Platelet count less than $100,00/mm^3$
   Diabetic retinopathy or other hemorrhagic ophthalmic conditions
   Pregnancy
   Acute pericarditis
   Endocarditis
   Significant hemostatic defects
   Current use of long-acting anticoagulant with therapeutic dose or level
   Advanced age (e.g., greater than 75 years)
   For streptokinase/anistreplase, prior exposure (more than 5 days ago) or prior
      associated allergic reaction
   Any other condition in which bleeding would be difficult to manage

[a]Some absolute contraindications (except concurrent intracranial hemorrhage) might not be
"absolute" in the most extreme circumstances.

(evidence strength Grade 2B). However, some data suggest that thrombolytic therapy combined with long-term anticoagulation, compared to standard anticoagulation, has a higher risk of all-cause death among hemodynamically stable patients. More controversial indications for thrombolytic therapy for PE in normotensive patients consist of RV dysfunction, severe hypoxemia, extensive embolic burden, saddle embolism, free floating RA/RV thrombus, and presence of patent foramen ovale.

General contraindications to thrombolytic administration include active, recent, or high risk for bleeding (Table 15.1). Compared to UFH, thrombolytics may increase the major bleeding rate by 50–100%, from about 6–12% to about 9–22%.

Types of thrombolytics include *fibrin-specific* agents (recombinant tissue plasminogen activator [rtPA] [i.e., alteplase], recombinant plasminogen activator [i.e., reteplase], and modified human tissue plasminogen activator [i.e., tenecteplase]) and *nonselective agents* (urokinase and streptokinase). Three thrombolytic agents are currently approved by US Food and Drug Administration (*FDA*) for the use in patients with acute PE: alteplase, urokinase, and streptokinase. Studies have not demonstrated the superiority of one type of thrombolytic agent over another. Clinicians in the United

States commonly use alteplase because of its FDA-approved indication for treatment of PE and its relatively short 2-hour infusion time for the 100 mg dose.

Most guidelines recommend that clinicians discontinue anticoagulant therapy prior to initiating thrombolytic therapy. After completion of thrombolytic therapy, to prevent recurrent VTE the clinician should reinitiate anticoagulation without a bolus when the aPTT has decreased to less than twice the normal control value.

In a situation where the clinician would like to give thrombolytic therapy, but a contraindication exists, the patient should undergo assessment for *catheter or surgical embolectomy*. Catheter embolectomy lacks strong supporting data at this time, and surgical embolectomy carries a high mortality.

IVC Filters
Studies have demonstrated a decreased risk of PE and an increased risk of DVT, without a significant effect on mortality, associated with IVC filter placement. Guidelines recommend that patients should undergo (temporary or permanent) IVC filter placement if they have a contraindication to or develop VTE on therapeutic doses of anticoagulation. If and when a reversible (e.g., bleeding) contraindication to anticoagulation resolves, patients with IVC filters should undergo a standard course of anticoagulation. For patients with massive PE, guidelines recommend consideration of (permanent) IVC filter placement. Patients with temporary IVC filters should have them removed according to manufacturer and treatment guidelines. Limited data exist regarding the efficacy and safety of temporary IVC filters in medical ICU patients who have acute PE.

Risks of Treatment
Bleeding
In general, ICU patients have a high risk of major bleeding because of coagulopathies, liver or renal insufficiency, comorbidities, increased risk for stress ulcers, and invasive procedures. Concomitant use of antiplatelet agents increases the risk of bleeding.

Major bleeding should lead to the immediate discontinuation of all forms of anticoagulation, appropriate monitoring, and supportive measures. Many scenarios may require blood product transfusion. Some scenarios require reversal of anticoagulant therapy.

Heparin-Induced Thrombocytopenia (HIT)
Clinicians should consider the possibility that HIT has occurred in patients who develop VTE in the setting of absolute or relative thrombocytopenia. Patients receiving UFH should undergo monitoring for *HIT* by following the platelet count. Patients with PE and suspected or confirmed HIT should not receive UFH, LMWH, or warfarin until the HIT has resolved. Such patients should undergo treatment with a direct thrombin inhibitor such as *argatroban* or *lepirudin*.

SUGGESTED READINGS

Kearon C, Kahn SR, Agnelli G, et al. Antithrombotic therapy for venous thromboembolic disease: American College of Chest Physicians Evidence-Based Clinical Practice Guidelines (8th Edition). *Chest.* 2008;133:454S–545S.
The premier guideline for antithrombotic therapy for patients with venous thromboembolism.
Konstantinides S, Geibel A, Heusel G, et al; Management Strategies and Prognosis of Pulmonary Embolism-3 Trial Investigators. Heparin plus alteplase compared with heparin alone in

patients with submassive pulmonary embolism. *N Engl J Med.* 2002;347:1143–1150.

A randomized controlled trial of thrombolytic therapy for patients with submassive pulmonary embolism.

PIOPED investigators. Value of ventilation/perfusion scan in acute pulmonary embolism: results of the prospective investigation of the pulmonary embolism diagnosis (PIOPED). *JAMA.* 1990;263:2753–2759.

The largest study of the diagnostic test characteristics of V/Q scan for the evaluation of patient with suspected acute pulmonary embolism.

Stein PD, Fowler SE, Goodman LR, et al; for the PIOPED II Investigators. Multidetector computed tomography for acute pulmonary embolism (PIOPED II). *N Engl J Med.* 2006; 354:2317–2327.

The largest study of the diagnostic test characteristics of CT scan for the evaluation of patients with suspected acute pulmonary embolism.

Todd JL, Tapson VF. Thrombolytic therapy for acute pulmonary embolism: a critical appraisal. *Chest.* 2009;135(5):1321–1329.

A comprehensive review of thrombolytic therapy for patients with acute PE.

16

Pleural Disorders in the Intensive Care Unit

Alexander C. Chen

Disorders of the pleura are found often in the intensive care unit (ICU). In some instances, pleural processes may be the primary cause of patients' critical illness; in most cases, pleural disorders are recognized as secondary processes related to patients' underlying illness. This chapter reviews the pathophysiology of these disorders and provides guidelines for managing these conditions in the ICU.

PLEURAL EFFUSIONS

The pleural space is a potential space between the visceral pleura, which covers the outer surface of the lung, and the parietal pleura, which lines the inside of the chest wall. In this space, there is a small amount of fluid present that functions to mechanically couple the lung to the chest wall and lubricate the interface of the visceral and parietal pleura. Pleural fluid normally results from the filtration of blood through high-pressure systemic blood vessels, and is drained from the pleural space through lymphatic openings in the parietal pleura that drain into parietal lymphatic vessels. In different disease states, fluid may originate from the interstitial spaces of the lungs, the intrathoracic lymphatics, the intrathoracic blood vessels, or the peritoneal cavity.

A pleural effusion is defined as an abnormal collection of fluid in the pleural space. Effusions occur when the rate of fluid formation exceeds the rate of fluid absorption. The most common causes of pleural effusions are shown in Table 16.1. Pleural effusions are commonly classified as being either exudative or transudative. An exudative pleural effusion implies that there is a disease process that is affecting the pleura directly, causing the pleura and/or its vasculature to be damaged. A transudative pleural effusion results when the pleura itself is healthy and implies that a disease process is affecting hydrostatic and/or oncotic factors that either increase the formation of pleural fluid or decrease the absorption of pleural fluid. Deciding if the pleura is injured or intact helps in formulating a concise differential diagnosis for potential causes (Table 16.2).

There are certain nonspecific signs and symptoms that may indicate the presence of a pleural effusion, but these are often difficult to ascertain in the ICU. Chest pain, particularly when sharp and made worse with breathing, can result from inflamed pleura in the presence of an effusion. Dyspnea is also common as the effusion can affect the mechanics of the diaphragm, cause a restrictive ventilatory defect, and/or cause compressive atelectasis leading to hypoxemia. The history can also help to reveal the cause of the effusion. For example, a patient with a fever and cough productive of sputum might have pneumonia causing the effusion. On physical examination, signs

TABLE 16.1	Common Causes of Pleural Effusions

1. CHF, 36%
2. Pneumonia, 22%
3. Malignancy, 14%
4. Pulmonary embolism, 11%
5. Other infections, 7%
6. Other causes, 10%

CHF, congestive heart failure.

that an effusion is present include dullness to percussion over the effusion, loss of fremitus, decreased breath sounds, crackles/egophony immediately above the effusion, and asymmetric diaphragmatic excursion with inspiration.

The majority of ICU patients will have their pleural effusion detected first by chest x-ray. Although a posterior–anterior (PA) and lateral chest x-ray is the preferred image, ICU patients typically have portable x-rays. Blunting of the costophrenic angle and a meniscus sign are the most common findings when an effusion is present. On the lateral chest x-ray, as little as 175 mL of fluid can be detected, while on the PA film it takes approximately 500 mL of fluid. Portable films are less sensitive, and often do not show the meniscus sign. Signs on the portable chest x-ray include loss of the diaphragm silhouette and increased basilar opacity with gradation over the entire hemithorax (more opaque at the base than the apex). Once a pleural effusion is detected radiographically, a lateral decubitus chest x-ray (where the dependent side is the side of the effusion) can quantitate the volume of fluid present and determine if the effusion is free-flowing or loculated. If the fluid is free-flowing, fluid can be detected as a straight line between the chest wall and lower border of the lung. Measurement of the distance between the chest wall and the lower border of the lung can give an idea of how much fluid is present. It is generally accepted that if this distance is >1 cm, then the amount

TABLE 16.2	Pathophysiological Causes of Pleural Effusions	
How pleura are affected	Example	Exudate/ transudate
Pleura damaged		
• Local disease in pleural space	• Malignancy	• Exudate
• Local disease adjacent to pleural space	• Pneumonia, PE, subdiaphragmatic abscess	• Exudate
• Systemic diseases that affect the pleural surface	• Autoimmune disease (lupus, rheumatoid arthritis)	• Exudate
Pleura intact		
• Systemic disease that does not directly affect the pleural surface	• CHF, myxedema, cirrhosis	• Transudate

PE, pulmonary embolism; CHF, congestive heart failure.

ALGORITHM 16.1 Evaluation of the Unknown Effusion

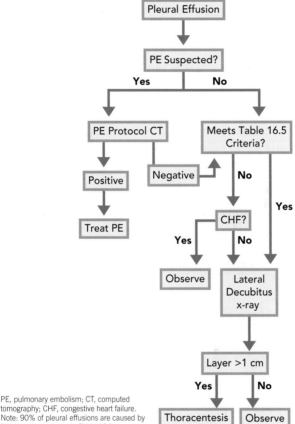

PE, pulmonary embolism; CT, computed tomography; CHF, congestive heart failure.
Note: 90% of pleural effusions are caused by five processes shown in Table 16.1.

of fluid is significant. Diagnostic evaluation of the effusion from this point is discussed in Algorithms 16.1 and 16.2.

Other imaging modalities can also detect, quantify, and sometimes even characterize the pleural effusion. Chest computed tomography (CT) is a useful imaging tool in assessing pleural effusions and can help the clinician diagnose not only the presence of the effusion but also delineate possible causes. Different techniques yield different information, so it is important to select the appropriate technique:

- Noncontrast CT scans can give a better idea of the amount of fluid within the pleural space, whether the fluid is loculated, and can detect abnormalities in the lungs that can be obscured by the effusion on standard chest x-ray.
- Standard contrast CT scans also assess the pleural surface for abnormalities that might suggest empyema or pleural malignancy.

ALGORITHM 16.2 Evaluation and Management of Pleural Fluid after Thoracentesis

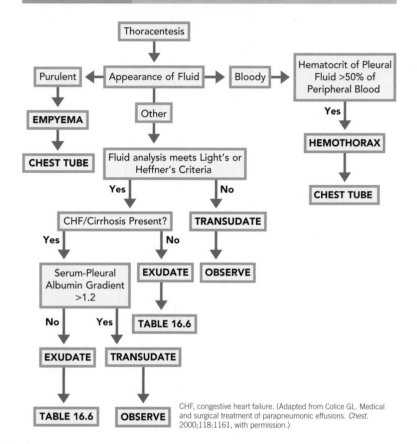

CHF, congestive heart failure. (Adapted from Colice GL. Medical and surgical treatment of parapneumonic effusions. *Chest.* 2000;118:1161, with permission.)

- CT scans with contrast given by pulmonary embolism protocol can detect a pulmonary embolism as the cause of the effusion, but do not provide information about the pleural surface beyond that of a noncontrast CT.

CT scans cannot be done at bedside, a big disadvantage when dealing with a patient who is not stable enough to travel out of the ICU.

Ultrasound is beneficial for multiple reasons. It gives a real-time image that can be done at the bedside and used not only for diagnosis that an effusion is present but also guide diagnostic and therapeutic interventions (i.e., thoracentesis and tube thoracostomy). Ultrasound can detect whether the fluid is loculated or free-flowing, and can give clues as to whether the fluid is transudative, exudative, or even whether it is an empyema.

ALGORITHM 16.3 **Management of Parapneumonic Effusions**

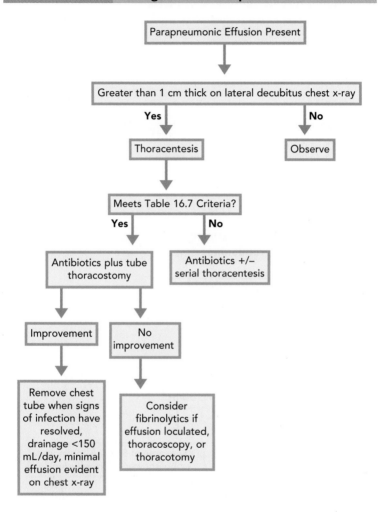

Once a pleural effusion is identified, it is important to attempt to diagnose the etiology of the effusion by obtaining a sample of the fluid for analysis. This is most often done by a thoracentesis. Thoracenteses can be safely performed as long as there is >1 cm of layered fluid on the lateral decubitus chest x-ray, even in patients receiving mechanical ventilation. One can remove a small amount of fluid for analysis or as much as 1,500 mL per drainage of fluid for both diagnostic and therapeutic goals (Algorithms 16.2 through 16.4). The most common criteria used to separate exudates from transudates are Light's criteria (Table 16.3). Heffner's criteria (Table 16.4) can also differentiate exudate from transudate. Heffner's criteria have a similar

TABLE 16.3 | **Light's Criteria**

- Pleural fluid to serum protein ratio >0.5
- Pleural fluid to serum LDH ratio >0.6
- Pleural fluid LDH >2/3 upper limit of normal for serum LDH

LDH, lactate dehydrogenase.

TABLE 16.4 | **Heffner's Criteria**

- Pleural fluid protein >2.9 g/dL
- Pleural fluid LDH >0.45 upper limit of normal

LDH, lactate dehydrogenase.

ALGORITHM 16.4 | **Management of Recurrent Malignant Effusions**

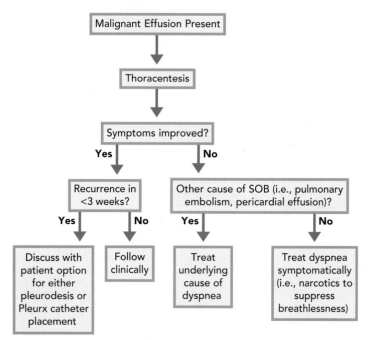

SOB, shortness of breath. (Adapted from Antunes G, et al. BTS guidelines for the management of malignant pleural effusions. *Thorax.* 2003;58(Suppl II): ii30, with permission.)

TABLE 16.5	Indications for Thoracentesis

1. Pleural effusion of unknown etiology
2. Fever in setting of long-standing pleural effusion
3. Air-fluid level in the pleural space
4. Rapid change in size of effusion
5. Concern that empyema is developing

sensitivity (98.4%), as Light's criteria (97.9%) do not require simultaneous blood work to be drawn. Other specific tests (Tables 16.5 and 16.6) can help determine a specific diagnosis.

As many as 20% of pleural effusions remain undiagnosed even after extensive investigation, and it is often unclear as to what the appropriate management of these effusions is in these situations. These idiopathic effusions with no clinical or radiologic evidence of malignancy will often resolve spontaneously without further therapy. In the ICU setting, as long as the patient does not clinically deteriorate, a conservative approach may be preferred when a diagnosis cannot be made after initial evaluation. If the patient continues to deteriorate despite serial thoracenteses, thoracoscopy can be considered as the next step to assess the pleural effusion.

SPECIAL SITUATIONS

Parapneumonic Effusion

A parapneumonic effusion is defined as any pleural effusion associated with bacterial pneumonia, lung abscess, or bronchiectasis. Parapneumonic effusions progress through different stages and, depending on when the patient presents, the treatment of the effusion will be different. The main distinction is whether the effusion is uncomplicated or complicated. Complicated effusions and empyemas will not resolve on their own and will require tube thoracostomy. As shown in Algorithm 16.3 and Table 16.7,

TABLE 16.6	Diagnostic Tests to Consider in Evaluation of Pleural Effusions
Diagnostic test	Type of effusion
1. Cytology	1. Malignant effusion
2. Gram stain or culture positive	2. Infectious effusion
3. AFB positive; pleural fluid ADA >70 U/L	(i.e., bacterial, fungal)
4. Rheumatoid arthritis cells	3. Tuberculous effusion
5. Chylomicrons present; pleural fluid triglycerides >110 mg/dL	4. Rheumatoid effusion
6. Salivary amylase present in pleural fluid	5. Chylothorax
7. Pleural creatinine/serum creatinine >1	6. Esophageal rupture
	7. Urinothorax

AFB, acid-fast bacillus; ADA, adenosine deaminase

TABLE 16.7	Indication for Tube Thoracostomy in Parapneumonic Effusions

1. Radiographic
   - Pleural fluid loculation
   - Effusion filling more than half of hemithorax
   - Air-fluid level present
2. Microbiologic
   - Pus in pleural space
   - Positive gram stain for microorganisms
   - Positive pleural fluid cultures
3. Chemical:
   - Pleural fluid pH <7.2
   - Pleural fluid glucose <60

radiographic, microbiologic, and chemical characteristics of the effusion will dictate whether thoracentesis with antibiotics alone will be sufficient to treat the effusion, or whether a chest tube must be inserted to effectively treat the effusion. If the chest tube is not effective in draining the fluid, intrapleural fibrinolytics might be required to break up the loculations and allow effective drainage of the infected fluid. If fibrinolytics are unsuccessful, the patient may require more invasive therapy, including thoracoscopy with breakdown of adhesions or thoracotomy with decortication.

Malignant Effusion

Malignant pleural effusions occur from a number of causes. Pleural metastases occur causing increased permeability of the pleura, and lymphatic obstruction can occur, which impairs drainage of pleural fluid through regional lymphatics. Table 16.8 shows the most common malignancies associated with pleural effusions. When these effusions occur, they are often large and lead to significant symptoms in the patient. Often, drainage of the effusion with thoracentesis alone is not sufficient as the effusion frequently recurs. Other management options include insertion of a chest tube followed by pleurodesis, which can obliterate the pleural space and prevent the effusion from recurring. Alternatively, insertion of a long-term indwelling catheter will allow the

TABLE 16.8	Most Common Primary Tumors of Malignant Effusions
Primary malignancy	Rate (%)
Lung	38
Breast	17
Lymphoma	12
Unknown primary	11
GU tract	9
GI tract	7

GU, genitourinary; GI, gastrointestinal.

TABLE 16.9	Causes of Hemothoraces
Causes	Examples
Traumatic	Penetrating trauma (gunshot wound), blunt trauma (usually with displaced rib fracture)
Nontraumatic	Metastatic malignant pleural disease, complication of anticoagulant therapy for pulmonary emboli
Iatrogenic	Perforation of a central vein from percutaneous catheter placement, following thoracentesis, following pleural biopsy

patient to drain the effusion at home and is a viable option that decreases hospitalizations and increases the quality of life of the patient. Additionally, these indwelling catheters can be attached to pleurevac systems and used as chest tubes to support patients through their period of critical illness. Once in place, these catheters can be managed similar to traditional tube thoracostomies. Management of this type of effusion is outlined in Algorithm 16.4.

Hemothorax

A hemothorax is the presence of blood in the pleural space such that the ratio of pleural fluid hematocrit to blood hematocrit is >0.5. This can be a serious condition and may result in ICU admission for treatment. Hemothoraces can be due to traumatic, nontraumatic, or rarely from iatrogenic causes (Table 16.9). Diagnosis is made after a thoracentesis returns bloody fluid (Algorithm 16.2). It should be noted that even a small amount of blood can make pleural fluid appear bloody; therefore, the fluid's hematocrit needs to be compared with peripheral blood hematocrit to confirm the presence of a hemothorax. Initial treatment of hemothoraces of all causes is tube thoracostomy. If bleeding is voluminous and persists, transfusion and surgical intervention may be required.

Pneumothorax

A pneumothorax is the presence of air in the pleural space. When this occurs, it can be an acute emergency that requires immediate attention. A pneumothorax can be spontaneous or traumatic. Spontaneous pneumothoraces are either primary, if no other disease process is present, or secondary, if there is an underlying disease process such as chronic obstructive pulmonary disease. Traumatic pneumothoraces include iatrogenic causes that may occur following a procedure (i.e., central line placement) or barotrauma. Primary spontaneous and traumatic pneumothoraces can often be treated effectively with observation or tube thoracostomy. Secondary spontaneous pneumothoraces typically require tube thoracostomy and may also require pleurodesis for definitive treatment.

Tension pneumothorax is the most serious consequence of a pneumothorax. This occurs when a one-way valve process develops, which allows air to enter the pleural space during inspiration but not leaves during expiration. As the air builds up in the pleural space, the lung and intrathoracic vasculature become compressed,

ALGORITHM 16.5 Management of Pneumothorax

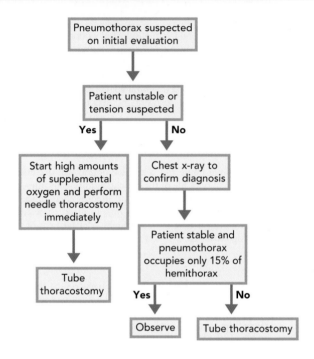

leading to dyspnea, hypoxemia, and hemodynamic compromise. Physical examination may reveal absent breath sounds on the side of the pneumothorax and/or shift of the trachea to the contralateral side of the pneumothorax. Tension pneumothorax should be suspected in unstable patients with absent breath sounds over one hemithorax, in mechanically ventilated patients who suddenly decompensate, in patients with known previously stable/improving pneumothorax who suddenly decompensate, or in patients who become unstable during or after a procedure known to cause a pneumothorax. Algorithm 16.5 gives further information on the evaluation and management of pneumothoraces. Table 16.10 covers the indications for removal of the chest tube.

TABLE 16.10 Indications for Removal of Chest Tube

1. Pneumothorax resolved
2. No air leak present in chest tube
3. Lung remains expanded after chest tube placed on water seal for 24 hours

If concern remains, chest tube can be clamped for 4–8 hours followed by chest radiograph; if lung expanded, then it is safe to remove the chest tube.

SUGGESTED READINGS

Abrahamian FM. Pleural effusions. Available at: http://www.emedicine.com/emerg/topic 462.htm. Accessed October 24, 2006.

Antunes G, Neville E, Duffy J, et al. BTS guidelines for the management of malignant pleural effusions. *Thorax.* 2003;58(Suppl II):ii29–ii38.

Colice GL, Curtis A, Deslauriers J, et al. Medical and surgical treatment of parapneumonic effusions: an evidence-based guideline. *Chest.* 2000;118:1158–1171.

Fartoukh M, Azoulay E, Galliot R, et al. Clinically documented pleural effusions in medical ICU Patients: how useful is routine thoracentesis. *Chest.* 2002;121:178–184.

Ferrer JS, Munoz XG, Orriols RM, et al. Evolution of idiopathic pleural effusion: a prospective, long-term follow-up study. *Chest.* 1996;109:1508–1513.

Heffner JE, Brown LK, Barbieri CA. Diagnostic value of tests that discriminate between exudative and transudative pleural effusions. *Chest.* 1997;111:970–980.

Lichtenstein DA, Meziere G, Lascols N, et al. Ultrasound diagnosis of occult pneumothorax. *Crit Care Med.* 2005;33:1231–1238.

Light RW. Pleural diseases. 4th ed. Philadelphia, PA: Lippincott Williams & Wilkins, 2001.

Mattison LE, Coppage L, Alderman DF, et al. Pleural effusions in the medical ICU: prevalence, causes, and clinical implications. *Chest.* 1997;111:1018–1023.

Tu C-Y, Hsu W-H, Hsia T-C, et al. Pleural effusions in febrile medical ICU patients: chest ultrasound study. *Chest.* 2004;126:1274–1280.

Vives M, Porcel JM, Vicente de Vera M, et al. A study of Light's criteria and possible modifications for distinguishing exudative from transudative pleural effusions. *Chest.* 1996;109:1503–1507.

17 Weaning of Mechanical Ventilation

Chad A. Witt

The gradual withdrawal of mechanical ventilation is termed *weaning*. Weaning can be divided into two components: (a) *liberation* refers to no longer requiring mechanical ventilatory support and (b) *extubation/decannulation* refers to the removal of the endotracheal or tracheostomy tube. Because of well-described complications of mechanical ventilation, such as infection and airway trauma, it is important to proceed with liberation and extubation as quickly as the patient will tolerate.

The first step in weaning a patient off mechanical ventilation is to determine whether the patient is ready for a spontaneous breathing trial. For patients to tolerate a spontaneous breathing trial, several requirements must be met. Most importantly, the cause of the patient's initial respiratory failure must be significantly improved or resolved. Additionally, the patient must be awake and able to cooperate, hemodynamically stable, and able to cough and protect the airway. Patients who are intubated on mechanical ventilation should be evaluated for readiness to undergo a spontaneous breathing trial on a daily basis (Algorithm 17.1). Protocols driven by nurses and respiratory therapists have been shown to improve the efficiency of the weaning process. Computer-driven protocols have also been associated with decreased duration of mechanical ventilation and intensive care unit (ICU) length of stay.

There are multiple weaning strategies and spontaneous breathing trial protocols. Spontaneous breathing trials can be performed with different ventilator modalities, including pressure support ventilation, continuous positive airway pressure (CPAP), or the T-tube technique. Using pressure support ventilation, a pressure support of 5 to 10 cm of H_2O is delivered to help the patient overcome the resistance of the endotracheal tube, usually accompanied by a positive end-expiratory pressure (PEEP) of 5 cm of H_2O. During a CPAP trial, 5 cm of H_2O of CPAP is provided. Lastly, the T-tube technique provides oxygen flow without any pressure support or CPAP during the trial. Determining success or failure of spontaneous breathing trials performed using the T-tube technique has been studied rigorously, and the most useful measure is the rapid shallow breathing index, defined as the respiratory rate/tidal volume (breaths/minute/liter). A rapid shallow breathing index of <100 breaths/min/L during a spontaneous breathing trial indicates that a patient is more likely to be successfully extubated. It should be kept in mind that there will be extubation failures in patients who are deemed ready by all objective evaluations (reported reintubation rates 11% to 23.5%), and it is these patients who may benefit most from early tracheostomy.

Difficult-to-wean patients are those who do not wean from mechanical ventilation within 48 to 72 hours of resolution of their underlying disease process. In such patients,

ALGORITHM 17.1 **Readiness to Liberate and Wean from Mechanical Ventilation**

Is the patient ready for a spontaneous breathing trial?
- Evidence for reversal of the underlying cause of respiratory failure
- Patient is awake, alert, and cooperative
- Adequate oxygenation (e.g., PEEP $\leq$ 5 cm H_2O; PaO_2 > 60 mm Hg with FiO_2 < 0.50)
- Hemodynamically stable: on no vasopressor or inotropic agents or stable minimal doses of vasopressors or inotropes; no evidence of myocardial ischemia; HR <140 beats per minute.
- Afebrile (T <38.0°C)
- pH and $PaCO_2$ appropriate for patient's baseline respiratory status

Yes   No

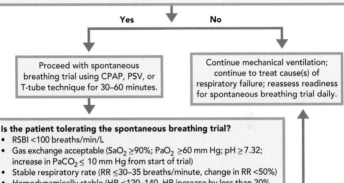

Proceed with spontaneous breathing trial using CPAP, PSV, or T-tube technique for 30–60 minutes.

Continue mechanical ventilation; continue to treat cause(s) of respiratory failure; reassess readiness for spontaneous breathing trial daily.

Is the patient tolerating the spontaneous breathing trial?
- RSBI <100 breaths/min/L
- Gas exchange acceptable (SaO_2 $\geq$90%; PaO_2 $\geq$60 mm Hg; pH $\geq$ 7.32; increase in $PaCO_2$ $\leq$ 10 mm Hg from start of trial)
- Stable respiratory rate (RR $\leq$30–35 breaths/minute, change in RR <50%)
- Hemodynamically stable (HR <120–140, HR increase by less than 20%, SBP >90 mm Hg and <180 mm Hg, change in SBP <20%)
- No significant change in mental status, evidence of anxiety, or agitation
- No diaphoresis or signs of increased work of breathing (use of accessory muscles, paradoxical breathing)

No

Yes

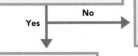

Is the patient ready to be extubated?
- Is the patient's airway patent?
- Can the patient protect his/her airway?
- Can the patient clear his/her secretions?

No

Continue mechanical ventilation, consider causes for weaning failure (Table 17.1), and consider evaluation for tracheostomy.

Yes

Proceed with extubation

Abbreviations:
PaO_2:	arterial partial pressure of oxygen
FiO_2:	fraction of inspired oxygen
PEEP:	positive end expiratory pressure
HR:	heart rate
T:	temperature
$PaCO_2$:	arterial partial pressure of carbon dioxide
CPAP:	continuous positive airway pressure
PSV:	pressure support ventilation
RSBI:	rapid shallow breathing index
SaO_2:	arterial oxygen saturation
RR:	respiratory rate
SBP:	systolic blood pressure

TABLE 17.1	Issues to Be Considered When Weaning Efforts Fail

Weaning parameters (see Algorithm 17.1)

Endotracheal tube
Use the largest tube possible
Consider use of supplemental pressure-support ventilation during spontaneous breathing trial
Suction secretions

Arterial blood gases
Avoid or treat metabolic alkalosis
Maintain PaO_2 at 60–65 mm Hg to avoid increased shunt in patients with chronic CO_2 retention
For patients with CO_2 retention, keep $PaCO_2$ at or above the baseline level

Nutrition
Ensure adequate nutritional support
Avoid electrolyte deficiencies
Avoid excessive calories

Secretions
Clear regularly
Avoid excessive dehydration

Neuromuscular factors
Avoid neuromuscular-depressing drugs (neuromuscular blockers, aminoglycosides, clindamycin) in patients with muscle weakness
Avoid unnecessary corticosteroids

Obstruction of airways
Use bronchodilators when appropriate
Exclude foreign bodies within the airway

Wakefulness
Avoid oversedation
Wean in morning or when patient is most awake

Adapted from *The Washington manual of medical therapeutics.* 31st ed. Philadelphia, PA: Lippincott Williams & Wilkins, 2004:192.

the acronym "WEANS NOW" has been developed as a set of factors to be considered in difficult-to-wean patients (Table 17.1).

SUGGESTED READINGS

Calfee C, Matthay M. Recent advances in mechanical ventilation. *Am J Med.* 2005;118:584–591.
    Review of mechanical ventilation, including noninvasive ventilation, ventilating patients with acute respiratory distress syndrome, and weaning of mechanical ventilation.
Kollef MH. Critical care. In: Green GB, Harris IS, Lin GA, Moylan KC, eds. The Washington manual of medical therapeutics. 31st ed. Philadelphia, PA: Lippincott Williams & Wilkins, 2004:192.
    "WEANS NOW" acronym for the difficult to wean patient.

Kollef MH, Shapiro SD, Silver P, et al. A randomized, controlled trial of protocol-directed versus physician-directed weaning from mechanical ventilation. *Crit Care Med.* 1997;25(4):567–574.

Randomized, controlled trial showing that protocol-guided weaning of mechanical ventilation performed by nurses and respiratory therapists is effective, and resulted in earlier extubation than physician-directed weaning.

Lellouche F, Mancebo J, Jolliet P, et al. A multicenter randomized trial of computer-driven protocolized weaning from mechanical ventilation. *Am J Respir Crit Care Med.* 2006;174(8):894–900.

Randomized trial demonstrating that duration of mechanical ventilation and length of ICU stay were decreased by using a computer-driven weaning protocol versus physician-controlled weaning according to local guidelines.

MacIntyre N. Evidence-based guidelines for weaning and discontinuing ventilatory support: a collective task force facilitated by the American College of Chest Physicians; the American Association for Respiratory Care; and the American College of Critical Care Medicine. *Chest.* 2001;120:375–396.

Evidence-based review and guidelines for weaning, including spontaneous breathing trials, weaning protocols, and the use of tracheostomy for failure to wean.

Manthous CA, Schmidt GA, Hall JB. Liberation from mechanical ventilation: a decade of progress. *Chest.* 1998;114:886–901.

Review of current practices and advances in assessment of readiness for liberation, weaning strategies, and extubation.

Meade M, Guyatt G, Cook D, et al. Predicting success in weaning from mechanical ventilation. *Chest.* 2001;120:400–424.

Meta-analysis of sixty three studies evaluating predictors of successful weaning, including the rapid-shallow breathing index.

Rumbak MJ, Newton M, Truncale T, et al. A prospective, randomized, study comparing early percutaneous dilational tracheotomy to prolonged translaryngeal intubation (delayed tracheotomy) in critically ill medical patients. *Crit Care Med.* 2004;32(8):1689–1694.

Prospective, randomized trial showing the benefit of early tracheotomy over prolonged translaryngeal intubation.

Tobin M. Advances in mechanical ventilation. *N Engl J Med.* 2001;334:1986–1996.

Review of mechanical ventilation strategies, including modes of ventilation, use of positive end-expiratory pressure, and discontinuation of mechanical ventilation.

18 Noninvasive Positive Pressure Ventilation

Michael Lippmann

Noninvasive positive pressure ventilation (NPPV) delivers mechanically assisted breaths using tight-fitting nasal or facial masks obviating the need for endotracheal intubation. The assisted ventilation is usually pressure-cycled either via pressure support ventilation (PSV) or bilevel positive airway pressure (BiPAP). Although NPPV can be used successfully in a number of clinical situations, there are specific contraindications to its use (Table 18.1) and it should not delay clinically indicated tracheal intubation and invasive ventilation. Additionally, NPPV is a supportive therapy and patients require prompt treatment of the underlying medical conditions leading to the respiratory failure.

Thorough patient assessment is critical prior to initiation of NPPV. NPPV is not indicated in patients with cardiac or respiratory arrest; nonrespiratory organ failure; impaired consciousness; unstable cardiac rhythm; hemodynamic instability; severe upper gastrointestinal bleeding; inability to protect upper airway or clear secretions; and facial surgery, trauma, or deformity.

Clinical trials and subsequent meta-analyses demonstrate that NPPV is beneficial in the management of chronic obstructive pulmonary disease (COPD) exacerbations, cardiogenic pulmonary edema, in immunocompromised patients with acute respiratory failure, and in selected patients with hypoxemic respiratory failure (Table 18.2). Patients with these conditions should receive a trial of NPPV if emergent intubation is not indicated, there are no contraindications and qualified personnel are available to initiate the trial. Patients whose pH and PCO_2 improve after a short trial have better outcomes. Worsening gas exchange, increasing tachypnea, hemodynamic instability, or mental status changes necessitate tracheal intubation and invasive mechanical ventilation. Algorithm 18.1 provides an algorithmic approach to initiating NPPV in a patient with an exacerbation of COPD.

The American Association for Respiratory Care recommends that patients with COPD exacerbations be started on NPPV if they have no contraindications and meet two or more of the following criteria: respiratory distress with moderate to severe dyspnea, arterial pH <7.35 with $PaCO_2$ >45, and respiratory rate ≥25 breaths/min. In these patients, NPPV decreases intubation, mortality, complications, treatment failure, and length of stay. Patients with less severe derangements in function do not benefit from NPPV and tend to tolerate it poorly. Patients with a Glasgow Coma Scale <11, pH <7.25, and respiratory rate >30 breaths/min are more likely to fail trials of NPPV.

TABLE 18.1	Contraindications to NPPV	
Cardiac or respiratory arrest		Unstable cardiac rhythm
Nonrespiratory organ failure		Facial surgery, trauma, or deformity
Severe encephalopathy		Upper airway obstruction
Severe UGI bleeding		Inability to protect airway
Hemodynamic instability		Inability to clear secretions
High risk for aspiration		

NPPV, noninvasive positive pressure ventilation.

In cardiogenic pulmonary edema, NPPV decreases preload by increasing thoracic pressure with consequent decrease in venous return and decreases afterload by decreasing intrathoracic transaortic pressure. The diminished work of breathing also lowers myocardial oxygen demands. A meta-analysis of 21 randomized controlled trials involving 1071 patients showed NPPV significantly decreased mortality and decreased the need for intubation. Early concerns that use of BiPAP is associated with an increased risk of myocardial infarction were not confirmed in larger, more recent trials.

A randomized study of immunocompromised patients with acute respiratory failure demonstrated that patients receiving NPPV had lower rates of endotracheal intubation, serious complications, and all cause mortality when compared to patients randomized to receive usual care.

NPPV appears beneficial in selected patients with hypoxemic respiratory failure. Randomized studies demonstrate reductions in mortality, need for intubation, intensive care unit (ICU) stay, and serious complications including sepsis and nosocomial pneumonias. The benefit appears to be greatest in patients whose arterial PCO_2 are >45 mm Hg.

NPPV appears to decrease the incidence of respiratory failure when applied immediately after extubation especially in patients with COPD and hypercapnia during spontaneous breathing trials pre-extubation. NPPV does not prevent reintubation when applied after a recently extubated patient develops respiratory failure. In this population, patients randomized to receive a trial of NPPV demonstrated an increase in all-cause mortality when compared to patients receiving standard medical therapy.

Physicians initiating NPPV must select the mode of ventilation, the patient interface, and ventilator settings. Most studies have applied NPPV using pressure-controlled ventilators that supply variable levels of inspiratory positive airway pressure

TABLE 18.2	Indications for NPPV
COPD exacerbations	
Cardiogenic pulmonary edema	
Hypoxemic respiratory failure in immunocompromised hosts with pulmonary infiltrates	
Weaning adjunct in COPD	

Note: Supported by randomized controlled trial data.
COPD, chronic obstructive pulmonary disease; NPPV, noninvasive positive pressure ventilation.

ALGORITHM 18.1 Initiation of NPPV in a Patient with a COPD Exacerbation

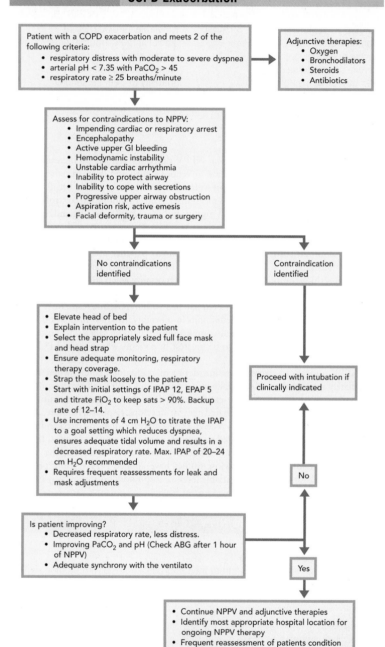

Patient with a COPD exacerbation and meets 2 of the following criteria:
- respiratory distress with moderate to severe dyspnea
- arterial pH < 7.35 with $PaCO_2$ > 45
- respiratory rate ≥ 25 breaths/minute

Adjunctive therapies:
- Oxygen
- Bronchodilators
- Steroids
- Antibiotics

Assess for contraindications to NPPV:
- Impending cardiac or respiratory arrest
- Encephalopathy
- Active upper GI bleeding
- Hemodynamic instability
- Unstable cardiac arrhythmia
- Inability to protect airway
- Inability to cope with secretions
- Progressive upper airway obstruction
- Aspiration risk, active emesis
- Facial deformity, trauma or surgery

No contraindications identified

Contraindication identified

- Elevate head of bed
- Explain intervention to the patient
- Select the appropriately sized full face mask and head strap
- Ensure adequate monitoring, respiratory therapy coverage.
- Strap the mask loosely to the patient
- Start with initial settings of IPAP 12, EPAP 5 and titrate FiO_2 to keep sats > 90%. Backup rate of 12–14.
- Use increments of 4 cm H_2O to titrate the IPAP to a goal setting which reduces dyspnea, ensures adequate tidal volume and results in a decreased respiratory rate. Max. IPAP of 20–24 cm H_2O recommended
- Requires frequent reassessments for leak and mask adjustments

Proceed with intubation if clinically indicated

No

Is patient improving?
- Decreased respiratory rate, less distress.
- Improving $PaCO_2$ and pH (Check ABG after 1 hour of NPPV)
- Adequate synchrony with the ventilato

Yes

- Continue NPPV and adjunctive therapies
- Identify most appropriate hospital location for ongoing NPPV therapy
- Frequent reassessment of patients condition

(IPAP) to assist inspiration, and a lower level of expiratory positive airway pressure (EPAP) to unload inspiratory muscles and potentially recruit closed airways. This bilevel ventilation is generally well tolerated and decreases the work of breathing and improves gas exchange more effectively than PSV that applies only positive inspiratory pressure.

Full facial masks are associated with improved physiologic parameters when compared to nasal masks likely due to decreased air leak through the mouth and bypass of the high resistance nasal passages that decrease airflow for any given inspiratory pressure. Patients tend to tolerate nasal masks better however, and they tend to be associated with less abdominal distension. Regardless of the interface, appropriate fit is key to assuring patient comfort and assures effective ventilatory support. Air leaks due to poorly fitting masks impair detection of inspiratory effort leading to patient-ventilator dyssynchrony. Patients also receive less inspiratory volume and are at risk of excessive drying of the corneas. Overly tight masks lead to skin necrosis. Careful adjustment of the ventilator settings and mask fit improves patient tolerance.

Patients receiving NPPV require close monitoring with frequent clinical assessment. Most patients will be admitted to ICUs, although studies have shown that carefully selected patients can be treated in less acute settings. Patients must be assessed for mental status, respiratory rate, use of accessory muscles, chest wall movement, coordination of respiratory effort with the ventilator, and overall comfort. Pulse oximetry monitors oxygen saturation but does not measure $PaCO_2$ and does not replace arterial blood gas analysis in evaluating a patient's response to NPPV.

SUGGESTED READINGS

Antonelli M, Conti G, Esquinas A, et al. A multiple-center survey on the use in clinical practice of noninvasive ventilation as a first-line intervention for acute respiratory distress syndrome. *Crit Care Med.* 2007;35:18.

Prospective, multiple-center cohort study of NPPV as a first-line intervention in patients with early ARDS. NPPV improved gas exchange and avoided intubation in 79 patients (54%). Avoidance of intubation was associated with less ventilator-associated pneumonia (2% vs. 20%; p < .001) and a lower intensive care unit mortality rate (6% vs. 53%; p < .001).

Antonelli M, Conti G, Rocco M, et al. A comparison of non-invasive positive pressure ventilation and conventional ventilation in patients with acute respiratory failure. *N Engl J Med.* 1998;339:429.

In a prospective, randomized trial of noninvasive positive-pressure ventilation versus endotracheal intubation with conventional mechanical ventilation in patients with hypoxemic acute respiratory failure who required mechanical ventilation, noninvasive ventilation was as effective as conventional ventilation in improving gas exchange and was associated with fewer serious complications and shorter stays in the intensive care unit.

Bauadouin S, Blumenthal S, Cooper B, et al. Non-invasive ventilation in acute respiratory failure. *Thorax.* 2002;57:192–211.

Recommendations of the British Society Standard of Care Committee regarding use of non-invasive ventilation.

Brochard L, Mancebo J, Wysocki M, et al. Noninvasive ventilation for acute exacerbations of chronic obstructive pulmonary disease. *N Engl J Med.* 1995;333:817.

A prospective, randomized study comparing noninvasive pressure support ventilation delivered through a face mask with standard treatment in 85 patients admitted to five intensive care units over a 15-month period. In selected patients with acute exacerbations of chronic obstructive pulmonary disease, noninvasive ventilation can reduce the need for endotracheal intubation, the length of the hospital stay, and the in-hospital mortality rate.

Esteban A, Frutos-Vivar F, Ferguson ND, et al. Noninvasive positive-pressure ventilation for respiratory failure after extubation. *N Engl J Med.* 2004;350:2452.

> *Multicenter, randomized trial in 221 patients who developed recurrent respiratory failure after extubation. The trial was stopped early after an interim analysis. The rate of death in the intensive care unit was higher in the noninvasive-ventilation group than in the standard-therapy group (25% vs. 14%; relative risk, 1.78; 95% CI, 1.03–3.20; p = 0.048), and the median time from respiratory failure to reintubation was longer in the noninvasive-ventilation group (12 hours vs. 2 hours 30 minutes, p = 0.02).*

Nava S, Ambrosino N, Clini E, et al. Noninvasive mechanical ventilation in the weaning of patients with respiratory failure due to chronic obstructive pulmonary disease: A random-ized, controlled trial. *Ann Intern Med.* 1998;128:721.

> *Multicenter, randomized trial in 50 patients with COPD who failed an initial SBT. These patients were then randomized to two methods of weaning: (1) extubation and application of noninvasive pressure support ventilation by face mask and (2) invasive pressure support ventilation by an endotracheal tube. Noninvasive pressure support ventilation during weaning reduced weaning time, shortens the time in the intensive care unit, decreases the incidence of nosocomial pneumonia, and improves 60-day survival rates.*

Vital FM, Saconato H, Ladeira MT, et al. Non-invasive positive pressure ventilation (CPAP or bilevel NPPV) for cardiogenic pulmonary edema. *Cochrane Database Syst Rev.* 2008;16: CD005351.

> *A meta-analysis of 21 studies comparing NPPV with standard medical care alone. NPPV significantly reduced hospital mortality (RR 0.6, 95% CI 0.45 to 0.84) and endotracheal intubation (RR 0.53, 95% CI 0.34 to 0.83)*

19 Acute Myocardial Infarction

Jeremiah P. Depta and Andrew M. Kates

Acute myocardial infarction (AMI) is a common diagnosis among hospitalized and critically ill patients. Each year there are approximately 610,000 new AMI and 310,000 recurrent AMIs in the United States. Despite improved survival during the last several decades, roughly one in five patients admitted with AMI will die within 1 year.

In the patient presenting with chest discomfort, rapid assessment of the patient's symptoms is crucial in determining the likelihood of acute coronary syndrome (ACS). Patients with ACS typically complain of moderate-to-severe chest discomfort that lasts more than 20 minutes. Atypical presentations are more common in patients with diabetes, advanced age, and in female patients. A prompt electrocardiogram (ECG) and cardiac-specific serum biomarkers (such as troponin and creatine kinase-MB [CK-MB] isoenzyme) are needed to distinguish between ST-segment elevation ACS (STE-ACS), non-ST segment elevation ACS (NSTE-ACS), and noncardiac chest discomfort. The diagnosis of *MI* is supported by evidence of cardiac myocyte death as evidenced by elevated cardiac-specific serum biomarkers. Patients who present with ACS and STE on ECG have actively infarcting myocardium and are often termed *ST-elevation myocardial infarction* (STEMI) or STE-ACS. Patients without STEs are further stratified into unstable angina (UA) or non-STEMI (NSTEMI) based on the absence or presence of elevated serum cardiac biomarker tests, respectively. The goal of the initial evaluation for the ACS patient is prompt diagnosis of STEMI or NSTEMI/UA with concurrent treatment of the patient's ischemia.

ST ELEVATION ACUTE CORONARY SYNDROME

STE-ACS results from sudden occlusion of a coronary artery, which almost exclusively is the product of plaque rupture in an atherosclerotic coronary artery. The resultant cascade of events involves platelet activation/aggregation and ultimately thrombus formation. One in three patients with STE-ACS does not survive with nearly half of the deaths in the first hour due to ventricular arrhythmias. The extent of cardiac myocyte death worsens with ischemic time and correlates strongly with cardiac morbidity and mortality, leading to the oft-quoted phrase, "time is muscle." As such, mechanical and medical therapies are designed to reestablish blood flow in the shortest time possible.

Algorithm 19.1 is our recommended management pathway that combines established benchmark goals and treatment options (Table 19.1) for the patient with STE-ACS/STEMI. Importantly, mechanical support with an intra-aortic balloon pump

PATIENT
GOAL: Time of symptom onset to calling EMS ≤ 5 min.[a]

TRANSPORT
GOAL: EMS on the scene ≤ 8 min.
Consider prehospital fibrinolysis (if available).

MEDICAL FACILITY—3D'S—DATA, DECISION, DRUGS
DATA—Focused history and physical exam.
GOAL: ECG ≤ 10 min
STEMI = ischemic symptoms with;
1) ≥1 mm ST elevation in two contiguous leads **OR**
2) New LBBB

- If inferior MI (leads II, III, avF)→ right-sided ECG (rV4) for right ventricular MI
- If ST-depression in precordial leads→ posterior ECG (V7, V8, V9) for posterior MI

DECISION—PRIMARY PCI

GOAL: Medical Contact-to-balloon time ≤90 min

Preferred over fibrinolytics if available

Also preferred when:
- Severe congestive heart failure
- Cardiogenic shock
- Unstable ventricular arrhythmias
- Contraindication to fibrinolytic therapy
- Late presentation (>3 hr of symptoms)
- The diagnosis of STEMI is in doubt

DECISION—FIBRINOLYTIC THERAPY

GOAL: Medical Contact-to-needle time ≤30 min

Preferred when:
- Lack of available PCI facility
- Delay in transport to PCI facility
- Contraindication to PCI

Absolute contraindications to fibrinolytics:
Prior hemorrhagic stroke
Ischemic stroke <3 months
Known intracranial malignant neoplasm
Known cerebral vascular lesion
Active bleeding or bleeding diathesis
Known or suspected aortic dissection
Closed head or facial trauma <3 months

DECISION—PCI AFTER FIBRINOLYSIS

If a patient has received fibrinolytics at a non-PCI-capable facility and is a high-risk STEMI, then immediate transfer to a PCI-capable facility should be arranged

Relative contraindications to fibrinolytics:
BP > 190/110
CPR > 10 min
Ischemic stroke >3 months
INR > 2.0
Recent internal bleeding within 2–4 weeks
Noncompressible vascular puncture
Pregnancy
Recent major surgery

Continued on next page

Continued on next page

DRUGS—Unless contraindicated, all patients receive:
- Aspirin 162–325 mg chewed
- Metoprolol 5 mg IV every 5 minutes × 3 doses unless patient has any contraindications[b]
- IV nitroglycerin, started at 10 μg/min & titrated for symptoms[c]
- Consider morphine sulfate 2–4 mg IV for chest pain unresponsive to nitrates
- Anticoagulant therapy:
    Unfractionated heparin: 60 U/kg IV bolus, max 4000 U; then 12 U/kg/hr, max 1000 U/hr
    OR,
    Enoxaparin (Lovenox): If < 75 years, then 30 mg IV bolus then 15 min later by 1 mg/kg SQ;
    If ≥ 75 years, then omit IV bolus and inject 0.75 mg/kg SQ avoid if Cr > 2.0
- Antiplatelet Therapy:
    If there is a high suspicion for CAD that may require CABG (i.e., diabetes or known multi-vessel CAD) then withhold a loading dose until the anatomy is defined:
    Clopidogrel (Plavix) 300–600 mg PO loading dose
    OR,
    Prasugrel (Effient) 60 mg PO loading dose for patients at the time of PCI only, don't use if body weight < 60 kg, history of stroke/TIA, age ≥ 75 years, or increased risk of bleeding

---

DRUGS—PRIMARY PCI
Use of and selection of a GP-IIb/IIIa inhibitor should be determined at the time of PCI by the interventional cardiologist

REPERFUSION—PRIMARY PCI
GOAL: Restoration of TIMI 3 flow (i.e., complete perfusion)

Advantages of PCI over fibrinolytics:
1) Superior restoration of coronary flow
2) Defines anatomy
3) Fewer complications
4) Treatment of thrombus AND plaque

Table 19.1 TNKase dosing

Weight (kg)	TNKase (mg)
<60	30
60–69	35
70–79	40
80–89	45
≥90	50

DRUGS—FIBRINOLYTIC
Regimens include:
Reteplase (Retavase) + UFH **(Preferred for age ≥75)**
    Reteplase 10 U IV bolus over 2 min and repeat 10 U IV bolus 30 min later.
    UFH IV as listed above.

Tenecteplase (TNKase) + Enoxaparin **(Preferred for age <75 years and/or >4 hr of symptoms if no PCI available)**
    TNKase dose is based on weight (see **Table 19.1**)
    Enoxaparin 30 mg IV push followed by 1 mg/kg SQ.

1/2 dose Reteplase + Abciximab + 1/2 dose UF heparin **(Preferred for age <75 years or those with large anterior MI's)**
    Reteplase 5 U IV bolus over 2 min and repeat 5 U IV bolus 30 min later
    Abciximab 0.25 mg/kg IV bolus then 0.125 μg/kg/min (max 10 mcg/min)
    UFH 60 U/kg IV bolus, max 4000 U; then 7 U/kg/hr infusion, max 1000 U/hr)

REPERFUSION—THROMBOLYSIS

Considered successful if:
1) Complete resolution of chest pain
2) ST segment elevation improvement >50%

If unsuccessful or the development of hemodynamic or electrical instability, consider transfer to center capable of rescue PCI

BPM, beats per minute; BP, blood pressure; CABG, coronary artery bypass grafting; CAD, coronary artery disease; CPR, cardiopulmonary resuscitation; Cr, creatinine; ECG, electrocardiogram; EMS, emergency medical services; GP, glycoprotein; HR, heart rate; INR, international normalized ratio; IV, intravenous; LBBB, left bundle branch block; MI, myocardial infarction; PCI, percutaneous coronary intervention; PO, by mouth; SBP, systolic blood pressure; SQ, subcutaneous; STEMI, ST-elevation myocardial infarction; TIA, transient ischemic attack; TIMI, thrombolysis in myocardial infarction; UFH, unfractionated heparin. [a]Patients who have taken SL nitroglycerin should call 911 if symptoms do not improve or worsen within 5 minutes of taking one SL nitroglycerin. [b]Signs of heart failure; evidence of a low cardiac output; increased risk of cardiogenic shock (age >70 years, SBP <120 mm Hg, HR <60 bpm, or sinus tachycardia >120 bpm, and increased time since onset of symptoms); or relative contraindications to beta-blockers (PR interval >0.24 seconds, 2nd- or 3rd-degree heart block, active asthma, or reactive airway disease). [c]Caution if suspected inferior MI, SBP <90 mm Hg, HR <50 bpm or >100 bpm, or phosphodiesterase inhibitors for erectile dysfunction in past 24–48 hours.

(IABP) or a percutaneous ventricular assist device (such as Impella 2.5 or 5.0) should be considered in the patient with hemodynamic or rhythm instability, severe heart failure, or cardiogenic shock.

NON-ST-ELEVATION ACUTE CORONARY SYNDROME

The initial step in evaluating patients with NSTE-ACS is risk stratification aimed at preventing major adverse cardiac events, defined as death, nonfatal MI, and stroke. A useful and well-validated method for risk stratification is the Thrombolysis In Myocardial Infarction (TIMI) risk score. Patients with a higher score are more likely to suffer from major adverse cardiac events than those with a lower score. All patients should receive medical management tailored to their level of risk and, importantly, should be considered for diagnostic angiography with an intent to perform percutaneous coronary intervention (PCI). High-risk patients benefit from early revascularization therapies. Our recommended algorithm for the treatment of patients with NSTE-ACS is shown in Algorithm 19.2.

HOSPITAL CARE OF THE ACS PATIENT

Patients with ACS are at an increased risk for recurrent MI and death, both during hospitalization and after discharge. Each hospitalization (as well as office visit) provides a venue to work with patients to reduce the risk of these events. One thoughtful way to organize the various in-hospital and postdischarge treatments is the "ABCDE" list (Table 19.2). These items should be considered an acute treatment guide as well as a discharge checklist for any patient admitted with ACS.

Classifying Myocardial Infarctions

It is important to recognize the different types of MIs as their management may differ from the recommendations for STE- and NSTE-ACS (Table 19.3). The classic MI due to ischemia from an unstable coronary plaque that leads to thrombus formation that may (STE-ACS) or may not completely occlude blood flow (NSTE-ACS) is termed a Type 1 MI. A Type 2 MI occurs with increased demand or decreased supply of myocardial oxygen. Typically, patients with Type 2 MIs have fixed coronary artery atheromas that do not cause ischemia at rest, but can induce ischemia at times of increased oxygen utilization (tachycardia, surgery, severe hypertension) or decreased oxygen delivery (anemia, hypoxia, hypotension, sepsis). Intraoperative MIs are typically due to myocardial oxygen supply–demand mismatch and often manifest postoperatively as elevated cardiac biomarkers. Our recommended algorithm for the treatment of Type 2 MI is shown in Algorithm 19.3.

Two unique forms of Type 2 MIs are stress-induced ("Takotsubo") and sepsis-induced cardiomyopathy. Both syndromes are driven by an excess of catecholamines and can be difficult to differentiate from ACS. Patients with these syndromes manifest ischemic ECG changes, focal-wall motion abnormalities including a depressed left ventricular ejection fraction (LVEF), and elevated cardiac biomarkers. Patients with suspected stress-induced cardiomyopathy should undergo diagnostic angiography that may be normal or show only mild CAD. Patients should be evaluated by transthoracic echocardiogram (TTE) or cardiac MRI to evaluate LV function as well as LV outflow tract obstruction. Management includes adrenergic-blocking agent (i.e., nonselective beta-blockers with alpha blocking activity), afterload reduction with ACE inhibitors,

ALGORITHM 19.2 Risk-Stratification and Treatment Algorithm for Non-ST-Segment Elevation Myocardial Infarction

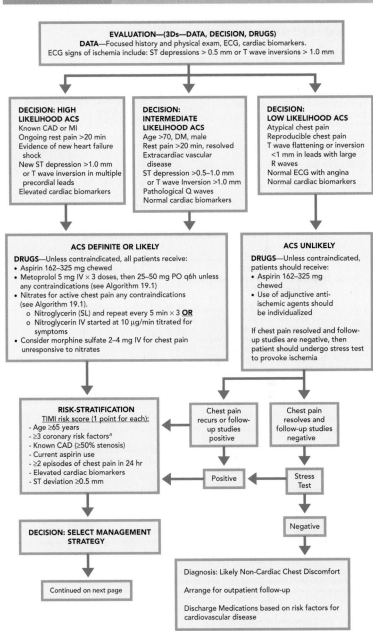

EVALUATION—(3Ds—DATA, DECISION, DRUGS)
DATA—Focused history and physical exam, ECG, cardiac biomarkers.
ECG signs of ischemia include: ST depressions > 0.5 mm or T wave inversions > 1.0 mm

DECISION: HIGH LIKELIHOOD ACS
Known CAD or MI
Ongoing rest pain >20 min
Evidence of new heart failure shock
New ST depression >1.0 mm or T wave inversion in multiple precordial leads
Elevated cardiac biomarkers

DECISION: INTERMEDIATE LIKELIHOOD ACS
Age >70, DM, male
Rest pain >20 min, resolved
Extracardiac vascular disease
ST depression >0.5–1.0 mm or T wave Inversion >1.0 mm
Pathological Q waves
Normal cardiac biomarkers

DECISION: LOW LIKELIHOOD ACS
Atypical chest pain
Reproducible chest pain
T wave flattening or inversion <1 mm in leads with large R waves
Normal ECG with angina
Normal cardiac biomarkers

ACS DEFINITE OR LIKELY
DRUGS—Unless contraindicated, all patients receive:
• Aspirin 162–325 mg chewed
• Metoprolol 5 mg IV × 3 doses, then 25–50 mg PO q6h unless any contraindications (see Algorithm 19.1)
• Nitrates for active chest pain any contraindications (see Algorithm 19.1).
  o Nitroglycerin (SL) and repeat every 5 min × 3 **OR**
  o Nitroglycerin IV started at 10 µg/min titrated for symptoms
• Consider morphine sulfate 2–4 mg IV for chest pain unresponsive to nitrates

ACS UNLIKELY
DRUGS—Unless contraindicated, patients should receive:
• Aspirin 162–325 mg chewed
• Use of adjunctive anti-ischemic agents should be individualized

If chest pain resolved and follow-up studies are negative, then patient should undergo stress test to provoke ischemia

RISK-STRATIFICATION
TIMI risk score (1 point for each):
- Age ≥65 years
- ≥3 coronary risk factors[a]
- Known CAD (≥50% stenosis)
- Current aspirin use
- ≥2 episodes of chest pain in 24 hr
- Elevated cardiac biomarkers
- ST deviation ≥0.5 mm

Chest pain recurs or follow-up studies positive

Chest pain resolves and follow-up studies negative

Positive

Stress Test

DECISION: SELECT MANAGEMENT STRATEGY

Negative

Continued on next page

Diagnosis: Likely Non-Cardiac Chest Discomfort

Arrange for outpatient follow-up

Discharge Medications based on risk factors for cardiovascular disease

DECISION: SELECT MANAGEMENT STRATEGY

Favors Invasive Strategy:
Recurrent chest pain despite maximal medical therapy
Elevated cardiac biomarkers
New ST-segment depression
Signs of heart failure
New or worsening mitral regurgitation
Hemodynamic instability
Sustained ventricular tachycardia
Prior CABG
High risk score (e.g., TIMI 5–7)
PCI within 6 months
Reduced LV ejection fraction

Favors Conservative Strategy:
Low risk score (e.g., TIMI 0–2)
Patient or physician preference
Risk of revascularization outweighs benefits

Calculated TIMI Score	14-day Risk of MACE
0 or 1	5%
2	8%
3	13%
4	20%
5	28%
6 or 7	41%

INVASIVE STRATEGY
(i.e., Diagnostic catheterization with intent to perform PCI)

Early invasive strategy (i.e., requiring immediate catheterization) should be considered in patients with:
• Refractory chest discomfort despite vigorous medical therapy
• Hemodynamic or rhythm instability

CONSERVATIVE STRATEGY

DRUGS—Unless contraindicated, all patients should receive the following regardless of the strategy:
• Anticoagulant therapy:
  Unfractionated heparin: 60 U/kg IV bolus, max 4000 U; then 12 U/kg/hr, max 1000 U/hr
  OR,
  Enoxaparin (Lovenox): If <75 years, then 30 mg IV bolus followed 15 min later with
  1 mg/kg SQ q12h (or q24h if CrCl < 30); If >75 years, then omit IV bolus and inject
  0.75 mg/kg SQ avoid if Cr > 2.0
  OR,
  Fondaparinux (Arixtra): 2.5 mg SQ daily (avoid if CrCl < 30)
  OR,
  Bivalirudin (Angiomax): 0.1 mg/kg IV bolus; then 0.25 mg/kg/h
• Dual antiplatelet therapy:
  *For the invasive strategy, If there is a high suspicion for CAD that may require CABG
  (i.e., diabetes or known multi-vessel CAD) then consider withholding therapy and starting
  a GP IIb/IIIa inhibitor until the anatomy is defined:*
  Clopidogrel (Plavix) 300–600 mg PO loading dose then 75 mg daily
  For patients undergo PCI, you may consider Prasugrel (Effient) 60 mg PO loading dose
  at the time of PCI then 10 mg daily (see Algorithm 19.1 for contraindications)

Continued on next page

Continued on next page

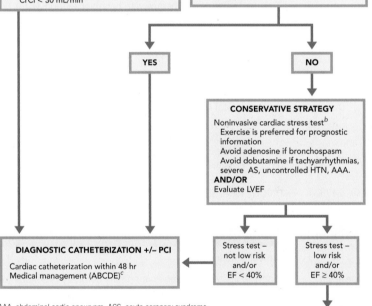

INVASIVE STRATEGY
(i.e., Diagnostic catheterization with intent to perform PCI)

Addition of a GP IIb/IIIA Inhibitor should be considered in patients who:
- Have refractory chest discomfort despite vigorous medical therapy
- Are high risk with positive troponins
- Have a delay to angiography >48 hr

Eptifibitide (Integrillin) 180 µg/kg bolus (max 22.6 mg), then 2 µg/kg/min (max 15 mg/hr) infusion. Can reduce infusion to 1 µg/kg/min if CrCl < 50 ml/min
OR
Tirofiban (Aggrastat) 0.4 µg/kg/min for 30 min, then 0.1 µg/kg/min infusion. Can reduce bolus and infusion to half-dose for CrCl < 30 mL/min

CONSERVATIVE STRATEGY

Any events necessitating catheterization?
- Hemodynamic instability
- Rhythm instability
- Recurrent symptoms despite medical therapy
- Heart failure

YES   **NO**

CONSERVATIVE STRATEGY

Noninvasive cardiac stress test[b]
   Exercise is preferred for prognostic information
   Avoid adenosine if bronchospasm
   Avoid dobutamine if tachyarrhythmias, severe AS, uncontrolled HTN, AAA.
AND/OR
Evaluate LVEF

DIAGNOSTIC CATHETERIZATION +/− PCI

Cardiac catheterization within 48 hr
Medical management (ABCDE)[c]

Stress test – not low risk and/or EF < 40%

Stress test – low risk and/or EF ≥ 40%

CONSERVATIVE STRATEGY

Medical management (ABCDE)[c]

AAA, abdominal aortic aneurysm; ACS, acute coronary syndrome; BPM, beats per minute; CABG, coronary artery bypass grafting; CAD, coronary artery disease; CP, chest pain; CrCl, creatinine clearance; CVA, cerebrovascular accident; DM, diabetes mellitus; ECG, electrocardiogram; GP, glycoprotein; HR, heart rate; HTN, hypertension; IV, intravenous; LVEF, left ventricular ejection fraction; MACE, major adverse cardiac events; MI, myocardial infarction; PAD, peripheral arterial disease; PCI, percutaneous coronary intervention; PO, by mouth; SBP, systolic blood pressure; SQ, subcutaneous; TIMI, thrombolysis in myocardial infarction. [a]Coronary risk factors include diabetes mellitus, cigarette smoking, hypertension (>140/90 mm Hg or on antihypertensive medication), low HDL cholesterol (<40 mg/dL), family history of premature CAD (male first-degree relative ≤55 years old or female first-degree relative ≤65 years old), and age (men ≥45 years old; women ≥55 years old). [b]Diagnostic accuracy of various stress tests are exercise treadmill: men—68% sensitive, 77% specific, women—61% sensitive, 70% specific; exercise, adenosine thallium—88% sensitive, 77% specific; exercise or dobutamine echo—76% sensitive, 88% specific. [c]See Table 19.2

TABLE 19.2	ABCDE as an Inpatient Treatment Guide and Discharge Checklist for Patients with ACS	
A	Antiplatelet	Aspirin indefinitely. Clopidogrel (or prasugrel) for at least 1 year Consider PPI prophylaxis in patients with risk factors for or history of PUD/GI bleeding
	Anticoagulation	Heparin or enoxaparin during hospitalization
	ACE inhibitor (ACE-I)	Consider if EF ($\leq$40%), heart failure with preserved EF, DM, CRI, or HTN
	Angiotensin receptor blocker	For ACE-I intolerant patients
	Aldosterone receptor blocker	For patients with EF < 40% with DM or heart failure who are already on an ACE-I and beta-blocker; caution in patients with hyperkalemia or CRI
B	Beta-blocker	All patients unless contraindicated.
	Blood pressure	Goal <140/90; for CRI or DM, goal is <130/80 (maximize therapy with beta-blocker and ACE-I before adding additional anti-HTN medications.)
C	Cigarette cessation	Complete cessation. Nicotine replacement, oral medications, counseling
	Cholesterol	Statin therapy regardless of LDL; Goal LDL <70 mg/dL. Goal HDL >40 mg/dL
D	Diet	If BMI >25, initial goal is to reduce weight by 10%
	Diabetes	Goal Hgb A1c <7.0%
E	Exercise	Thirty minutes of aerobic activity a minimum of 5 days/week Referral for cardiac rehabilitation
	Ejection fraction	Measurement of ejection fraction prior to discharge

BMI, body mass index; CRI, chronic renal insufficiency; DM, diabetes mellitus; EF, ejection fraction; Hgb, hemoglobin; HTN, hypertension; GI, gastrointestinal; PPI, proton pump inhibitor.

TABLE 19.3	Classification of Different Types of Myocardial Infarction
	Clinical scenario
Type 1	Spontaneous MI secondary to a primary coronary event due to plaque instability
Type 2	MI secondary to myocardial oxygen supply–demand mismatch
Type 3	Sudden cardiac death
Type 4a	MI secondary to PCI (*Note:* Cardiac biomarkers must be 3 × ULN)
Type 4b	MI secondary to stent thrombosis
Type 5	MI associated with CABG (*Note:* Cardiac biomarkers must be 5 × ULN)

CABG, coronary artery bypass grafting; MI, myocardial infarction; PCI, percutaneous coronary intervention; ULN, upper limit of normal.

diuretics as needed, and serial TTEs to monitor for persistence of ventricular dysfunction. Patients with a severely depressed LVEF or the presence of an LV thrombus will also need short-term oral anticoagulation. The majority of patients who overcome the inciting event or medical illness fully recover.

COMPLICATIONS AFTER MYOCARDIAL INFARCTION

Postinfarction complication rates have fallen dramatically since the advent of early reperfusion strategies. Nevertheless, many patients, including those with large infarction, silent infarction, late presentation, and delayed or incomplete reperfusion, remain at high risk for severe complications. The mnemonic FEAR AMI is a logical way to remember these potential life-threatening complications. The following sections discuss the individual letters of this mnemonic.

Failure

LV dysfunction is the single most powerful predictor of survival following an MI. Clinical symptoms of LV dysfunction range from mild heart failure (e.g., rales or S3) to cardiogenic shock. The severity of LV dysfunction correlates with the size of the infarct, advanced age, and other clinical risk factors such as diabetes. Treatment of post-MI LV dysfunction is determined by its severity and includes supplemental oxygen, diuretic therapy, afterload reduction with vasodilators (e.g., nitroglycerin or nitroprusside), and/or inhibition of the renin-angiotensin system, and digitalis in selected patients with atrial fibrillation. Patients who develop cardiogenic shock warrant insertion of a pulmonary artery catheter (PAC) and may require beta-agonists (e.g., dobutamine and dopamine), a phosphodiesterase inhibitor (e.g., milrinone), and/or vasopressor therapy. Early use of an IABP or percutaneous ventricular assist device is essential.

Right ventricular (RV) dysfunction occurs in about 10% of patients with inferior or posterior MIs and should be suspected in patients who develop hypotension with standard medical therapy for MI with an elevated jugular venous pulse in the absence of pulmonary edema. PAC will reveal a high central venous pressure and low pulmonary capillary wedge pressure (PCWP). Management includes intravenous fluids for preload and the use of dobutamine to maintain an appropriate cardiac index.

Embolism and Effusions/Pericarditis

Up to 20% of all patients and 60% of patients suffering a large anterior wall MI will develop a mural thrombus. Echocardiography should be performed in all patients with an MI to determine the presence of a mural thrombus or akinetic segments that predispose to thrombus formation. Systemic anticoagulation with heparin should be initiated to bridge the patient to at least 3 to 6 months of oral anticoagulation.

Post-MI pericardial effusions are rarely life threatening. However, when tamponade physiology is present then a hemorrhagic effusion from a ventricular rupture must be considered. The presence of an effusion on echocardiogram is a reason to withhold anticoagulation in the post-MI period to avoid contributing to a hemopericardium. If anticoagulation cannot be stopped, heightened vigilance for this complication is warranted.

Post-MI pericarditis can present in the first days and up to 6 weeks after the infarct. This complication is due to local pericardial irritation, usually by a transmural infarct. Pericarditis must be distinguished from recurrent ischemia. Pericarditis pain is often worse with deep inspiration, improves with sitting forward, radiates

ALGORITHM 19.3 **Management Algorithm for Type 2 Myocardial Infarction.**

EVALUATION—(3D's—DATA, DECISION, DRUGS)

DATA—Focused history and physical exam, assess cardiac risk factors, ECG, cardiac biomarkers.
ECHO recommended to assess focal wall motion abnormalities or new cardiomyopathy (e.g., myocarditis)

DECISION—Risk stratify patient based on above
Trend cardiac biomarkers every 6 hr until downtrending
IMPORTANT: Treat and correct the underlying cause for oxygen mismatch

DRUGS—Unless contraindicated, all patients receive:
- Aspirin 162–325 mg chewed
- Metoprolol 5 mg IV × 3 doses, then 25–50 mg PO q6h unless any contraindications (See STEMI algorithm)
- Nitrates for active chest pain any contraindications (see STEMI algorithm).
  o Nitroglycerin (SL) and repeat every 5 min × 3 **OR**
  o Nitroglycerin IV started at 10 µg/min titrated for symptoms
- Consider morphine sulfate 2–4 µg/mg IV for chest pain unresponsive to nitrates

For certain higher risk patients, consider:
- Anticoagulant therapy:
  Unfractionated heparin: 60 U/kg IV bolus, max 4000 U; then 12 U/kg/hr, max 1000 U/hr
  OR,
  Enoxaparin (Lovenox): 1 mg/kg SQ q12h (or q24h if CrCl < 30)

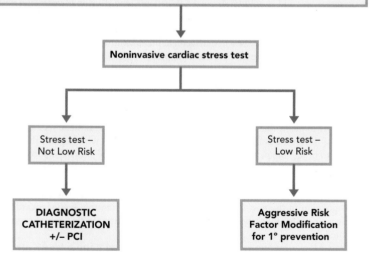

Noninvasive cardiac stress test

Stress test – Not Low Risk

Stress test – Low Risk

DIAGNOSTIC CATHETERIZATION +/– PCI

Aggressive Risk Factor Modification for 1° prevention

to the scapulae, and can be associated with characteristic ECG findings. Pain is treated with high-dose aspirin 650 mg every 4 to 6 hours, especially in early pericarditis.

Dressler syndrome is a type of postinfarction pericarditis that occurs 1 to 8 weeks after the infarct. It is thought to be immune mediated and is best treated with high-dose aspirin. Glucocorticosteroids and other nonsteroidal anti-inflammatory agents are avoided in the first month after infarction because of the potential to impair ventricular healing, leading to increased rates of ventricular rupture.

Arrhythmia

The management of many common arrhythmias is discussed elsewhere (see Chapter 20). Several infarction-specific arrhythmias are presented here.

Accelerated idioventricular rhythm is considered a "reperfusion rhythm," as it is often seen immediately after a successful reperfusion. No treatment is warranted for this arrhythmia when seen in the setting of reperfusion.

Ventricular tachycardia is often the terminal rhythm in the peri-infarct period and is associated with increased mortality when occurring in the first 48 hours of hospitalization. Aggressive restoration of sinus rhythm is achieved through the use of antiarrhythmic medications (amiodarone, lidocaine) and/or synchronized direct current cardioversion. Because hypokalemia and hypomagnesemia have been associated with development of sustained ventricular tachycardia, it is important to correct potassium (K) and magnesium (Mg) levels in the setting of an infarction (K >4 mEq/L and Mg >2 mEq/L). In contrast, nonsustained ventricular tachycardia (NSVT) is not associated with an increased risk of death during the index hospitalization or during the first year after infarction and suppressive treatment of asymptomatic NSVT is not routinely recommended in the post-MI patient.

Infarction can cause block at any level of the conduction system. The location of the infarct has an important influence on the patient's prognosis and treatment of conduction disease. In general, right coronary artery infarct is associated with proximal (atrioventricular [AV] nodal) conduction disease. This AV block is usually transient and often does not warrant transvenous pacemaker placement in the absence of symptoms. One exception is symptomatic AV block in the setting of RV infarction, as restoration of AV synchrony can improve RV filling and thus, cardiac output. Left anterior descending/septal infarct is associated with distal (infranodal) conduction disease and is potentially life threatening. Immediate pacing efforts should be pursued. Additional features of AV conduction disease are shown in Table 19.4 Acute treatment is discussed in Chapter 20.

Rupture and Regurgitation

The clinical presentation of a ventricular rupture is often striking and usually life threatening. The rupture can be in the ventricular free wall, ventricular septum, or papillary muscle (Table 19.5).

Ventricular free-wall rupture presents with hypotension and signs of cardiac tamponade. Any clinical suspicion warrants immediate use of echocardiography as well as PAC for prompt diagnosis. Emergent surgery is usually the only chance for survival.

Ventricular septal rupture (VSR) should be suspected in patients with a new pansystolic murmur or palpable thrill with signs of worsening biventricular failure. Echocardiography is needed to detect and localize the VSR. PAC is useful to assess for an increase in the oxygen saturation in right ventricle ("step-up") that is characteristic of a VSR. PAC can also be used to calculate a shunt fraction. All patients with a VSR

TABLE 19.4 Features of Ischemia-Related Atrioventricular Conduction Disease

	Proximal conduction disease	Distal conduction disease
Compromised artery	Right coronary/posterior descending (90%)	Septal perforators of left anterior descending
Site of block	Intranodal	Infranodal
Site of infarction	Inferoposterior	Anteroseptal
Type of AV block	1st degree or Mobitz I	Mobitz II or 3rd degree
Duration of AV block	Transient (2–3 days)	Variable
Mortality rate	Low, unless CHF or hypotension	High, because of extensive infarct
Temporary pacemaker	Rare	Early consideration, especially for anterior infarct and bifascicular block
Permanent pacemaker	Almost never	Indicated if high-grade block in His–Purkinje system or associated bundle branch block

should be considered for early surgical therapy. IABP and/or the use of nitroprusside can be used to bridge patients to surgery by reducing the shunt.

Mitral regurgitation (MR) is a common complication of MI occurring in almost half of all patients. Ischemic MR may be caused by mitral annular dilatation in LV dysfunction, papillary muscle dysfunction, or papillary muscle rupture. Typically, MR is transient and asymptomatic and does not warrant further intervention. However, MR secondary to papillary muscle rupture may cause severe MR and should be suspected in patients with a new pansystolic murmur in the setting of heart failure or hemodynamic compromise. Notably, some patients with severe MR in this setting may not have a prominent murmur. Echocardiography (TTE and TEE) is essential for the diagnosis and determining the etiology of MR. PAC reveals large v waves on the PCWP tracing. For patients with suspected papillary muscle rupture, immediate surgery is indicated with the use of nitroprusside or IABP in the setting of hypotension to stabilize the patient until surgery.

Aneurysm

True LV aneurysms complicate <5% of acute infarctions. They are thought to be a consequence of a complete occlusion of the supplying coronary artery without significant collateral blood flow. As such, anteroapical aneurysms (due to left anterior descending artery occlusion) are four times more common than inferoposterior aneurysms.

LV aneurysms are associated with a sixfold increase in mortality, mainly resulting due to ventricular arrhythmias. LV aneurysms are often supported by fibrous tissue and, thus, rarely rupture. The characteristic ECG findings of LV aneurysms are Q waves with persistent ST elevations, although the diagnosis is best made by a noninvasive imaging study. Because of the risk of mural thrombus formation and systemic embolization, patients with an LV aneurysm are generally treated with long-term

TABLE 19.5	**Clinical Profile of Mechanical Complications of Myocardial Infarction**		
	Ventricular septal defect	Free-wall rupture	Papillary muscle rupture
Days post-MI	1–5	1–7	3–5
Anterior MI	66%	50%	25%
New murmur	90%	25%	50%
Palpable thrill	Yes	No	Rare
2-D Echo findings	Visualize defect	May have pericardial effusion	Flail or prolapsing leaflet
Doppler echo findings	Detect shunt		Regurgitant jet in LA
PA catheterization	Oxygen step-up in RV	Equalization of diastolic pressure	Prominent *c-v* wave in PCW tracing
Medical mortality	90%	90%	90%
Surgical mortality	50%	Case reports	40–90%

MI, myocardial infarction; LA, left atrium; PA, pulmonary artery; RV, right ventricle; PCW, pulmonary capillary wedge.
Modified from Labovitz AJ, et al. Mechanical complications of acute myocardial infarction. *Cardiovasc Rev Rep.* 1984;5:948.

anticoagulation with warfarin. In addition, as ST segments may remain elevated for some time after successful reperfusion, persistent ST elevation (>4 weeks after AMI) is generally required for the ECG diagnosis of LV aneurysm. Acute aneurysms lead to acute decompensated heart failure and cardiogenic shock and are managed with vasodilators and an IABP. ACE inhibitors can reduce progression of the aneurysm and should be initiated in the absence of hypotension. Chronic aneurysms lead to heart failure or arrhythmias and should be treated accordingly. For patients with refractory symptoms, surgery may be considered to repair a chronic aneurysm.

Distinct from an aneurysm is a pseudoaneurysm. Rather than involving layers of muscle, the myocardium perforates and, as such, this clinical entity can be thought of as a "contained rupture." It is most often seen with inferior infarctions, and treatment of choice is surgery. Both surgical and medical treatments carry a very high mortality due to the risk for spontaneous rupture.

Recurrent Myocardial Infarction

The complaint of chest pain after an MI may represent recurrent ischemia from incomplete revascularization, infarct extension, reinfarction, or postinfarction angina. Ischemia recurs in 20% to 30% of patients receiving thrombolytic therapy and up to 10% of patients after percutaneous revascularization. Serial cardiac biomarkers and ECGs can help identify at-risk patients. Troponins may not be useful given their persistent elevation beyond 1 week after an MI. Increases in CK-MB isoenzymes after downtrending may be a more diagnostic marker of reinfarction. Aggressive medical therapy with anti-ischemic medications (aspirin, heparin, nitrates, beta-blockers) is important to control symptoms. Revascularization should be considered in patients whose symptoms are refractory to medical therapy.

New postinfarct ST elevations can be caused by reinfarction, pericarditis, or dyskinetic/aneurysmal ventricular segments. Reinfarction due to stent thrombosis usually has a dramatic presentation with severe anginal pain refractory to medical therapy and evolving ST elevations on ECG. These findings warrant immediate revascularization efforts.

SUGGESTED READINGS

Anderson JL, Adams CD, Antman EM, et al. ACC/AHA 2007 guidelines for the management of patients with unstable angina/non-ST-elevation myocardial infarction. *J Am Coll Cardiol.* 2007;50:e1–e157.
  Invaluable consensus guidelines for patients with NSTE-ACS.
Antman EM, Anbe DT, Armstrong PW, et al. ACC/AHA guidelines for management of patients with STEMI. *J Am Coll Cardiol.* 2004;44:e1–e211.
  Invaluable consensus guidelines detailing the state-of-the-art for management of patients with STEMI.
Antman EM, Cohen M, Bernink PJ, et al. The TIMI risk score for unstable angina/non-ST elevation MI: a method for prognostication and therapeutic decision making. *JAMA.* 2000;284:835–842.
  One of several validations of the popular TIMI risk score for NSTE-ACS.
Antman EM, Hand M, Armstrong PW, et al. 2007 Focused update of the ACC/AHA 2004 guidelines for the management of patients with ST-elevation myocardial infarction. *J Am Coll Cardiol.* 2008;51:210–247.
  Invaluable consensus guidelines detailing the state-of-the-art for management of patients with STEMI.
Bybee KA, Prasad A. Stress-related cardiomyopathy syndromes. *Circulation.* 2008;118:397–409.
  Nice review on various types or stress-induced cardiomyopathies including their mechanism, diagnosis, and suggested management.
Kushner FG, Hand M, Smith SC, et al. 2009 Focused updates: ACC/AHA guidelines for the management of patients with ST-elevation myocardial infarction and ACC/AHA/SCAI guidelines on percutaneous coronary intervention. *J Am Coll Cardiol.* 2009;54:2205–2241.
  Invaluable consensus guidelines detailing the state-of-the-art for management of patients with STEMI.
Thygesen K, Alpert JS, White HD, et al. Universal definition of myocardial infarction. *Circulation.* 2007;116:2634–2653.
  Updated definitions for diagnosing myocardial infarction in different clinical settings.

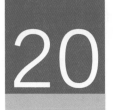

20 Cardiac Arrhythmias and Conduction Abnormalities

Sundeep Viswanathan and Marin Kollef

This chapter addresses the causes, recognition, and treatment of cardiac arrhythmias occurring in hospitalized and critically ill patients. Cardiac arrhythmias can disrupt cardiac output (CO) by impairing the heart rate (HR) and/or stroke volume (SV) according to the equation CO = HR × SV. The clinical presentation of cardiac arrhythmias varies widely, and they may present as (a) asymptomatic findings on an electrocardiogram (ECG) or telemetry, (b) symptoms without hemodynamic instability (e.g., palpitations, shortness of breath, syncope, or chest pain), (c) hemodynamic instability in conscious patients, or (d) cardiac arrest. Initial patient evaluation in hospitalized patients includes ensuring (a) adequate airway and breathing support; (b) continuous monitoring of cardiac rhythm, blood pressure, and oxyhemoglobin saturation; (c) adequate intravenous (IV) access; and (d) adequate support personnel. The cardiac rhythm should be analyzed by 12-lead ECG when possible, but initial treatment may be based on the rhythm seen on the intensive care unit bedside monitor or defibrillator. If time permits, the specific underlying rhythm should be identified, the cause sought, and therapy tailored accordingly. However, *cardiac arrest and severely symptomatic tachycardia and bradycardia require immediate treatment based on the advanced cardiac life support (ACLS) algorithms* shown later in this chapter (Algorithms 20.1 to 20.3).

TACHYARRHYTHMIAS

Tachycardia, defined as a HR >100 beats per minute, can be separated into (a) those that arise above the ventricles, termed *supraventricular tachycardias,* and (b) those that arise within the ventricles, termed *ventricular tachycardias (VTs).* Tachycardias can generally be distinguished on the basis of the HR, the width and morphology of the QRS complex, and the length of the PR interval. The approach to differentiating narrow and wide QRS complex tachycardias is outlined in Algorithms 20.4 and 20.5, respectively.

Supraventricular Tachycardias

Sinus tachycardia originates from the sinus node, and is not considered a primary arrhythmia. The ECG shows a normal P wave preceding each QRS complex, an upright P wave in lead II, and a downward P wave in lead aVL. Sinus tachycardia in

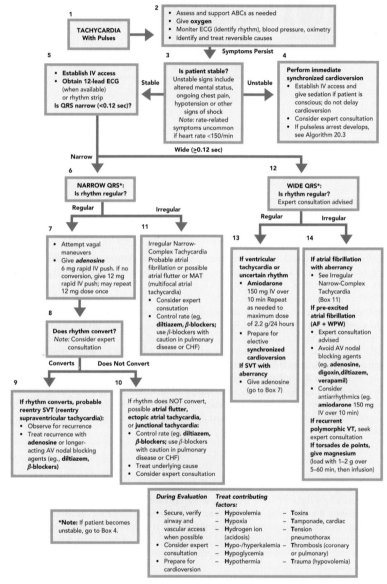

1

TACHYCARDIA
With Pulses

2
- Assess and support ABCs as needed
- Give **oxygen**
- Moniter ECG (identify rhythm), blood pressure, oximetry
- Identify and treat reversible causes

Symptoms Persist

5
- **Establish IV access**
- **Obtain 12-lead ECG**
  (when available)
  or rhythm strip
- **Is QRS narrow (<0.12 sec)?**

Stable

3
Is patient stable?
Unstable signs include altered mental status, ongoing chest pain, hypotension or other signs of shock
Note: rate-related symptoms uncommon if heart rate <150/min

Unstable

4
Perform immediate synchronized cardioversion
- Establish IV access and give sedation if patient is conscious; do not delay cardioversion
- Consider expert consultation
- If pulseless arrest develops, see Algorithm 20.3

Narrow

Wide (≥0.12 sec)

6
NARROW QRS*:
Is rhythm regular?

Regular   Irregular

12
WIDE QRS*:
Is rhythm regular?
Expert consultation advised

Regular   Irregular

7
- Attempt vagal maneuvers
- Give **adenosine**
  6 mg rapid IV push. If no conversion, give 12 mg rapid IV push; may repeat 12 mg dose once

11
Irregular Narrow-Complex Tachycardia Probable atrial fibrillation or possible atrial flutter or MAT (multifocal atrial tachycardia)
- Consider expert consutation
- Control rate (eg, **diltiazem, β-blockers;** use β-blockers with caution in pulmonary disease or CHF)

13
If **ventricular tachycardia or uncertain rhythm**
- **Amiodarone** 150 mg IV over 10 min Repeat as needed to maximum dose of 2.2 g/24 hours
- Prepare for elective **synchronized cardioversion**
If **SVT with aberrancy**
- Give adenosine (go to Box 7)

14
If **atrial fibrillation with aberrancy**
- See Irregular Narrow-Complex Tachycardia (Box 11)
If **pre-excited atrial fibrillation (AF + WPW)**
- Expert consultation advised
- Avoid AV nodal blocking agents (eg, **adenosine, digoxin,diltiazem, verapamil)**
- Consider antiarrhythmics (eg. **amiodarone** 150 mg IV over 10 min)
If **recurrent polymorphic VT,** seek expert consultation
If **torsades de points,** give magnesium (load with 1–2 g over 5–60 min, then infusion)

8
Does rhythm convert?
Note: Consider expert consultation

Converts   Does Not Convert

9
If rhythm converts, probable reentry SVT (reentry supraventricular tachycardia):
- Observe for recurrence
- Treat recurrence with **adenosine** or longer-acting AV nodal blocking agents (eg., **diltiazem, β-blockers)**

10
If rhythm does NOT convert, possible **atrial flutter, ectopic atrial tachycardia,** or **junctional tachycardia:**
- Control rate (eg. **diltiazem, β-blockers;** use β-blockers with caution in pulmonary disease or CHF)
- Treat underlying cause
- Consider expert consultation

During Evaluation
- Secure, verify airway and vascular access when possible
- Consider expert consultation
- Prepare for cardioversion

Treat contributing factors:
- Hypovolemia
- Hypoxia
- Hydrogen ion (acidosis)
- Hypo-/hyperkalemia
- Hypoglycemia
- Hypothermia

- Toxins
- Tamponade, cardiac
- Tension pneumothorax
- Thrombosis (coronary or pulmonary)
- Trauma (hypovolemia)

*Note: If patient becomes unstable, go to Box 4.

ECG, electrocardiogram; IV, intravenous; CHF, congestive heart failure; SVT, supraventricular tachycardia; AF, atrial fibrillation; WPW, Wolff–Parkinson–White; VT, ventricular tachycardia. (Adapted from 2005 American Heart Association Guidelines for Cardiopulmonary Resuscitation and Emergency Cardiovascular Care, Part 7.3: Management of Symptomatic Bradycardia and Tachycardia. *Circulation.* 2005;112(Suppl IV):IV-70, with permission.)

ALGORITHM 20.2 Advanced Cardiac Life Support Bradycardia Treatment Algorithm

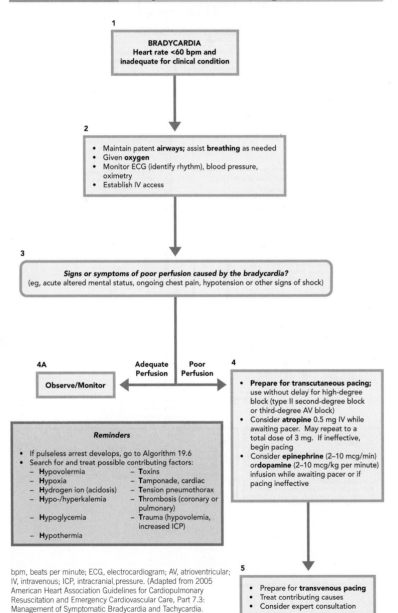

1

BRADYCARDIA
Heart rate <60 bpm and
inadequate for clinical condition

2
- Maintain patent **airways;** assist **breathing** as needed
- Given **oxygen**
- Monitor ECG (identify rhythm), blood pressure, oximetry
- Establish IV access

3

Signs or symptoms of poor perfusion caused by the bradycardia?
(eg, acute altered mental status, ongoing chest pain, hypotension or other signs of shock)

4A Adequate Perfusion   Poor Perfusion   **4**

Observe/Monitor

- **Prepare for transcutaneous pacing;** use without delay for high-degree block (type II second-degree block or third-degree AV block)
- Consider **atropine** 0.5 mg IV while awaiting pacer. May repeat to a total dose of 3 mg. If ineffective, begin pacing
- Consider **epinephrine** (2–10 mcg/min) or **dopamine** (2–10 mcg/kg per minute) infusion while awaiting pacer or if pacing ineffective

Reminders
- If pulseless arrest develops, go to Algorithm 19.6
- Search for and treat possible contributing factors:
  - **H**ypovolermia   – **T**oxins
  - **H**ypoxia   – **T**amponade, cardiac
  - **H**ydrogen ion (acidosis) – **T**ension pneumothorax
  - **H**ypo-/hyperkalemia   – **T**hrombosis (coronary or pulmonary)
  - **H**ypoglycemia   – **T**rauma (hypovolemia, increased ICP)
  - **H**ypothermia

5
- Prepare for **transvenous pacing**
- Treat contributing causes
- Consider expert consultation

bpm, beats per minute; ECG, electrocardiogram; AV, atrioventricular; IV, intravenous; ICP, intracranial pressure. (Adapted from 2005 American Heart Association Guidelines for Cardiopulmonary Resuscitation and Emergency Cardiovascular Care, Part 7.3: Management of Symptomatic Bradycardia and Tachycardia. *Circulation.* 2005;112(Suppl IV):IV-68, with permission.)

ALGORITHM 20.3 Advanced Cardiac Life Support Pulseless Arrest Algorithm

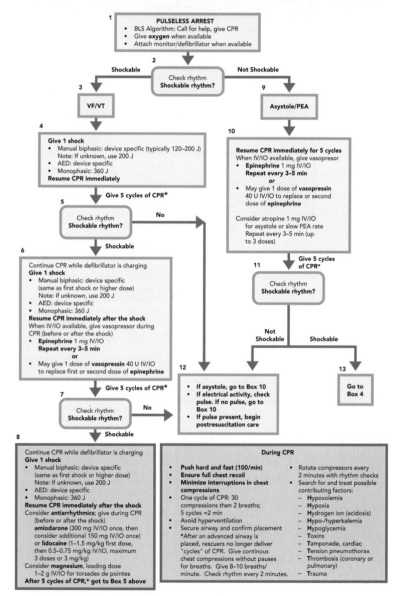

1

PULSELESS ARREST
- BLS Algorithm: Call for help, give CPR
- Give **oxygen** when available
- Attach monitor/defibrillator when available

2 Check rhythm **Shockable rhythm?**

Shockable → **3** VF/VT

Not Shockable → **9** Asystole/PEA

4
Give 1 shock
- Manual biphasic: device specific (typically 120–200 J)
  Note: If unknown, use 200 J
- AED: device specific
- Monophasic: 360 J
Resume CPR immediately

10
Resume CPR immediately for 5 cycles
When IV/IO available, give vasopressor
- **Epinephrine** 1 mg IV/IO
  Repeat every 3–5 min
  or
- May give 1 dose of **vasopressin** 40 U IV/IO to replace or second dose of **epinephrine**

Consider atropine 1 mg IV/IO for asystole or slow PEA rate Repeat every 3–5 min (up to 3 doses)

Give 5 cycles of CPR*

5 Check rhythm **Shockable rhythm?**

No →

Shockable ↓

6
Continue CPR while defibrillator is charging
Give 1 shock
- Manual biphasic: device specific (same as first shock or higher dose)
  Note: If unknown, use 200 J
- AED: device specific
- Monophasic: 360 J
Resume CPR immediately after the shock
When IV/IO available, give vasopressor during CPR (before or after the shock)
- **Epinephrine** 1 mg IV/IO
  Repeat every 3–5 min
  or
- May give 1 dose of **vasopressin** 40 U IV/IO to replace first or second dose of **epinephrine**

Give 5 cycles of CPR*

11 Give 5 cycles of CPR*
Check rhythm **Shockable rhythm?**

Not Shockable ↓   Shockable →

7 Check rhythm **Shockable rhythm?**

No →

12
- If asystole, go to Box 10
- If electrical activity, check pulse. If no pulse, go to Box 10
- If pulse present, begin postresuscitation care

13
Go to Box 4

Shockable ↓

8
Continue CPR while defibrillator is charging
Give 1 shock
- Manual biphasic: device specific (same as first shock or higher dose)
  Note: If unknown, use 200 J
- AED: device specific
- Monophasic: 360 J
Resume CPR immediately after the shock
Consider **antiarrhythmics**; give during CPR (before or after the shock)
amiodarone (300 mg IV/IO once, then consider additional 150 mg IV/IO once) or **lidocaine** (1–1.5 mg/kg first dose, then 0.5–0.75 mg/kg IV/IO, maximum 3 doses or 3 mg/kg)
Consider **magnesium**, loading dose 1–2 g IV/IO for torsades de pointes
After 5 cycles of CPR,* got to Box 5 above

During CPR
- **Push hard and fast (100/min)**
- **Ensure full chest recoil**
- **Minimize interruptions in chest compressions**
- One cycle of CPR: 30 compressions then 2 breaths; 5 cycles =2 min
- Avoid hyperventilation
- Secure airway and confirm placement
  *After an advanced airway is placed, rescuers no longer deliver "cycles" of CPR. Give continous chest compressions without pauses for breaths. Give 8–10 breaths/minute. Check rhythm every 2 minutes.
- Rotate compressors every 2 minutes with rhythm checks
- Search for and treat possible contributing factors:
  – Hypovolemia
  – Hypoxia
  – Hydrogen ion (acidosis)
  – Hypo-/hyperkalemia
  – Hypoglycemia
  – Toxins
  – Tamponade, cardiac
  – Tension pneumothorax
  – Thrombosis (coronary or pulmonary)
  – Trauma

BLS, basic life support; CPR, cardiopulmonary resuscitation; VF/VT, ventricular fibrillation/ventricular tachycardia; PEA, pulseless electrical activity; AED, automated external defibrillator; IV/IO, intravenous/intraosseous. (Adapted from 2005 American Heart Association Guidelines for Cardiopulmonary Resuscitation and Emergency Cardiovascular Care, Part 7.2: Management of Cardiac Arrest. *Circulation.* 2005;112(Suppl IV):IV-59, with permission.)

ALGORITHM 20.4 Approach to Differentiating Narrow QRS Complex Tachycardias

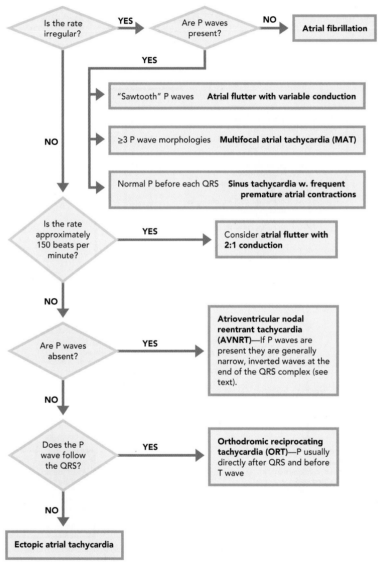

RBBB, right bundle branch block; LBBB, left bundle branch block; MAT, multifocal atrial tachycardia; PAC, premature atrial contraction; SVT, supraventricular tachycardia; ART, antidromic re-entrant tachycardia; DC, direct current; IV, intravenous.

ALGORITHM 20.5 Approach to Differentiating Wide QRS Complex Tachycardias

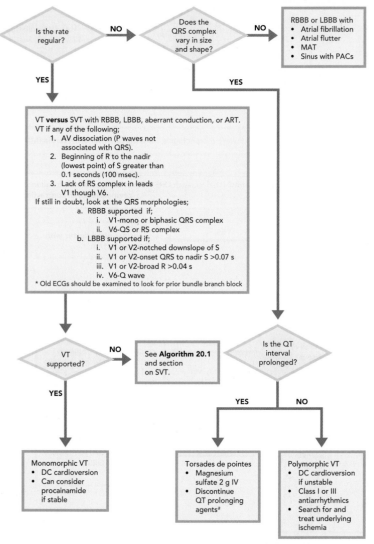

Wide complex tachycardias (except clear sinus tachycardia with aberrancy) should initially be assumed to be ventricular tachycardia (VT) and treatment urgency based on assessment of patient condition and hemodynamics (see text for details). [a]Agents that prolong the QT interval can be found online at http://www.arizonacert.org/medical-pros/drug-lists/drug-lists.htm

the intensive care unit can be a physiologic response to volume depletion, fever, pain, anxiety, shock, hypoxia, or in patients on vasopressor or inotropic support. Human's maximum heart rate (MHR) is age-dependent and roughly limited to 220 − age in years (e.g., in a 70-year-old man, MHR = 220 − 70 = 150).

Treatment of sinus tachycardia is directed at the underlying cause, which includes treating infections and fever, volume repletion, anxiolytics, and pain control. Rate-controlling agents are generally not indicated unless the rapid HR causes symptoms of low CO, such as in severe anxiety and pain. Reflex sinus tachycardia may be important to maintain adequate CO. Direct treatment of the tachycardia without treatment of the underlying cause may be deleterious.

Atrial fibrillation is a chaotic rhythm within the atria of 350–600 beats per minute without an appreciable P wave on ECG. All atrial beats are not conducted because of the refractory period in the atrioventricular (AV) node, and conduction is variably timed, resulting in an irregular ventricular rate. If the ventricular rate is greater than 100 beats per minute, a rapid ventricular response is said to be present. The associated rapid HR and the lack of atrial contribution to pumping blood can compromise CO, requiring immediate treatment. Loss of organized atrial contraction creates stasis of the blood pool within the atria, which may facilitate intracardiac thrombus formation and thromboembolism.

Atrial fibrillation is seen in patients with chronic cardiopulmonary disease. It can also be the presenting finding of the elderly with conduction disturbances, thyrotoxicosis, infection, pulmonary embolization, acute alcohol intoxication, pericarditis, and stress, and is common postoperatively. It is a rare presentation of acute myocardial infarction.

Typical *atrial flutter* is caused by a re-entrant rhythm localized to the right atrium, which generates impulses at a rate of approximately 300 beats per minute. The ventricular rate is frequently 150 beats per minute (half the atrial rate) due to 2:1 block within the AV node. In 3:1 block, every third beat is conducted, and the ventricular rate is approximately 100 beats per minute. A large portion of the atria is depolarized at once, causing a classic "sawtooth" appearance on the baseline of the ECG, with fairly narrow, negative flutter waves in the inferior leads (II, III, aVF). The ventricular rate may be regular, but can be irregular if conduction is variable (i.e., 2:1 alternating with 3:1). It is seen in patients with underlying heart disease and is also commonly seen in patients after open heart surgery. If left untreated, it may degrade to atrial fibrillation.

Treatment of atrial fibrillation and atrial flutter is outlined in Algorithm 20.6. Precipitating factors listed here should be sought and treated. Preoperative beta-blockers can reduce the incidence of postoperative atrial fibrillation/flutter. Thromboembolic risk management typically involves anticoagulation with IV heparin overlapping with Coumadin until the international normalized ratio (INR) is >2. Patients with contraindications to anticoagulation should be treated with aspirin if possible. Long-term anticoagulation therapy is beyond the scope of this chapter, but risk factors such as age, hypertension, heart failure, diabetes, and prior stroke portend to thrombus formation.

Paroxysmal supraventricular tachycardias (PSVT) are characterized by sudden onset and termination (hence, the name). The most common PSVT in adults is *atrioventricular nodal re-entrant tachycardia* (AVNRT). It is caused by a re-entrant electrical loop within the AV node. The rate generally varies from 120 to 250 beats per minute and is associated with a narrow QRS complex in the absence of aberrancy or an underlying bundle branch block. The atria and ventricles typically depolarize at virtually the same time, and thus the P waves are frequently not visible, obscured

ALGORITHM 20.6 — Treatment of Atrial Fibrillation and Atrial Flutter (see Chapter 87, Common Drug Dosages and Side Effects)

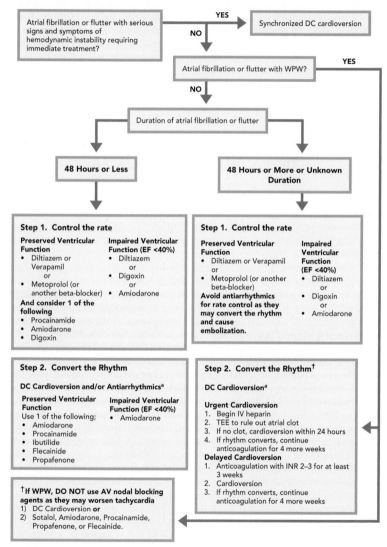

Atrial fibrillation or flutter with serious signs and symptoms of hemodynamic instability requiring immediate treatment?

YES → Synchronized DC cardioversion

NO ↓

Atrial fibrillation or flutter with WPW? **YES** →

NO ↓

Duration of atrial fibrillation or flutter

48 Hours or Less

48 Hours or More or Unknown Duration

Step 1. Control the rate

Preserved Ventricular Function
- Diltiazem or Verapamil
  or
- Metoprolol (or another beta-blocker)

And consider 1 of the following
- Procainamide
- Amiodarone
- Digoxin

Impaired Ventricular Function (EF <40%)
- Diltiazem
  or
- Digoxin
  or
- Amiodarone

Step 1. Control the rate

Preserved Ventricular Function
- Diltiazem or Verapamil
  or
- Metoprolol (or another beta-blocker)

Avoid antiarrhythmics for rate control as they may convert the rhythm and cause embolization.

Impaired Ventricular Function (EF <40%)
- Diltiazem
  or
- Digoxin
  or
- Amiodarone

Step 2. Convert the Rhythm

DC Cardioversion and/or Antiarrhythmics[a]

Preserved Ventricular Function
Use 1 of the following;
- Amiodarone
- Procainamide
- Ibutilide
- Flecainide
- Propafenone

Impaired Ventricular Function (EF <40%)
- Amiodarone

Step 2. Convert the Rhythm[†]

DC Cardioversion[a]

Urgent Cardioversion
1. Begin IV heparin
2. TEE to rule out atrial clot
3. If no clot, cardioversion within 24 hours
4. If rhythm converts, continue anticoagulation for 4 more weeks

Delayed Cardioversion
1. Anticoagulation with INR 2–3 for at least 3 weeks
2. Cardioversion
3. If rhythm converts, continue anticoagulation for 4 more weeks

[†]**If WPW, DO NOT use AV nodal blocking agents as they may worsen tachycardia**
1) DC Cardioversion **or**
2) Sotalol, Amiodarone, Procainamide, Propafenone, or Flecainide.

DC, direct current; WPW, Wolff–Parkinson–White; EF, ejection fraction; IV, intravenous; TEE, transesophageal echocardiogram; INR, international normalized ratio. [a]Premedicate when possible with a sedative (e.g., diazepam, midazolam, ketamine, and etomidate) and analgesic (e.g., fentanyl and morphine). Perform synchronized cardioversion with 100 J, 200 J, 300 J, 360 J biphasic energy or monophasic equivalent, starting with lowest energy level and increasing if needed. Perform asynchronous cardioversion if delays in synchronized cardioversion with worsening clinical status.

by the QRS complexes. If visible, they generally present as narrow inverted P waves at the end of the QRS complex, commonly described as a "pseudo R" in V1 and/or "a pseudo S" in lead II. AV nodal re-entrant tachycardia is not associated with any specific diseases, can occur at any age, and is more common in women.

PSVT may also be mediated by an accessory pathway between the atria and ventricles that bypasses the AV node. *Manifest* accessory pathways are seen on the sinus rhythm ECG as a delta wave of pre-excitation. The pre-excitation also causes a short PR interval because the accessory pathway does not have the delayed conduction of the AV node. Accessory pathways may conduct antegrade (forming the delta wave) or retrograde. *Concealed* accessory AV pathways only conduct retrograde, and are invisible in sinus rhythm. Either of these pathways may mediate an *orthodromic re-entrant tachycardia* in which the electrical impulse propagates antegrade through the AV node and retrograde (from ventricle to atrium) through the accessory pathway. The result is a narrow QRS complex tachycardia, typically with inverted retrograde P waves between the QRS and T wave (although the QRS may be wide because of aberrancy, e.g., bundle branch block or fascicular block).

The patient with visible pre-excitation (delta wave and short PR interval) in sinus rhythm and with palpitations (usually from paroxysmal orthodromic re-entrant tachycardia) is said to have *Wolff–Parkinson–White syndrome* (WPW). Patients with WPW are also prone to arrhythmias with antegrade conduction through the accessory pathway. These include *antidromic re-entrant tachycardia*, in which the excitation propagates antegrade through the accessory pathway and retrograde through the AV node. Atrial arrhythmias (including atrial fibrillation) may also conduct antegrade through the accessory pathway. The short refractory period of the accessory pathway may allow very rapid conduction of impulses to the ventricles, resulting in rapid "pre-excited atrial fibrillation" with ventricular rates up to 300 beats per minute, often resulting in hemodynamic instability requiring urgent intervention. Rapid conduction of atrial fibrillation through an accessory pathway may also induce ventricular fibrillation (VF). This is thought to be the pathogenesis of the rare sudden death that is associated with WPW.

Treatment of PSVT aims at aborting the re-entrant rhythm by blocking conduction through the AV node with vagal maneuvers (Valsalva, carotid massage, face immersion in cold water [diving reflex]) or adenosine given as a 6 mg IV bolus ($t_{1/2}$ approximately 10 seconds). A second 12-mg dose can be given after 1 to 2 minutes if the first was ineffective, and a third dose of 12 or 18 mg can be given if needed. If these treatments fail, the AV nodal blocking agents beta-blockers, calcium channel blockers, or digoxin should be used. Patients with WPW and pre-excited atrial fibrillation or flutter must be rapidly treated with direct current cardioversion or class IA, IC, or III drugs (e.g., procainamide, flecainide, and amiodarone), which slow myocardial conduction and prolong the refractory period, and not AV nodal blocking agents especially when the accessory pathway has a short anterograde refractory period capable of rapid ventricular conduction (Algorithm 20.6).

Ectopic atrial tachycardia occurs when there is automaticity at a single focus outside the sinoatrial (SA) node. A P wave precedes each QRS as in sinus tachycardia, but the P wave axis is altered. When increased automaticity occurs at three or more different atrial sites, which may include the SA node, it is termed *multifocal atrial tachycardia*, with the alternating foci causing at least three P wave morphologies on ECG. Both can be seen in cases of digitalis toxicity (which causes increased automaticity), severe cardiopulmonary disease, hypokalemia, hyperadrenergic states, and as a side effect of theophylline.

Treatment includes AV nodal blocking agents and removal of inciting agents/factors.

Ventricular Tachycardias

The two main tachyarrhythmias arising from the ventricles are **VF** and **VT**. VT may be monomorphic, if the QRS morphology is fixed, or polymorphic, if the QRS complex is variable. Polymorphic VT is more like VF than monomorphic VT in that it results in chaotic ventricular activation, often with hemodynamic instability, possibly leading to cardiac arrest and sudden death. Also like VF, it is more likely to occur in the setting of acute ischemia, infarct, or acute heart failure.

Monomorphic VT results from re-entrant electrical impulses within the ventricles or from a focal ventricular site with frequent spontaneous action potentials that propagate to the remainder of the ventricles. VT is characterized on ECG by a wide QRS complex (>0.12 seconds), and a rate usually between 100 and 200 beats per minute (although it may be higher). VT that lasts <30 seconds is termed *nonsustained VT* (NSVT), and sustained VT (just termed *VT*) if it lasts >30 seconds. The most common setting for monomorphic VT is in healed myocardial infarction. It occurs less commonly in acute ischemia and infarct. Importantly, monomorphic VT may occur in the absence of structural heart disease. The "idiopathic VTs" do not have a poor prognosis and may not cause hemodynamic instability, emphasizing the need to assess and treat the patient's condition, and not solely the ECG.

An important specific type of polymorphic VT is *torsades de pointes,* which is polymorphic VT associated with prolongation of the QT interval (in sinus rhythm) from numerous causes, including (a) drugs (especially tricyclic antidepressants, antipsychotics, certain antiarrhythmics, macrolides, and fluoroquinolone; see Web site in Algorithm 20.5); (b) electrolyte abnormalities (hypokalemia, hypomagnesemia, and hypocalcemia); and (c) congenital long QT syndromes. Torsades de pointes appears on ECG as a characteristic pattern of oscillating amplitude of the QRS, or "twisting," around the baseline. Torsades de pointes is generally symptomatic but may be nonsustained. If prolonged, hemodynamic instability, syncope, and/sudden death may result.

Wide complex tachycardias (except clear sinus tachycardia with aberrancy) should initially be assumed to be VT, and the urgency of treatment should depend on assessment of the patient and the hemodynamic situation. Distinguishing VT from SVT with a wide QRS is therefore of secondary importance. Mistaken diagnosis of "SVT with aberrancy" can result in mistreatment. The differential diagnosis of wide complex tachycardia is threefold: (a) VT, (b) SVT with aberrancy (typical bundle branch or fascicular blocks or atypical aberrancy), and (c) pre-excited supraventricular rhythm (including atrial fibrillation) in which case the ECG in sinus rhythm will typically feature a delta wave.

Algorithm 20.5 shows the ECG criteria that favor VT. Also, old ECGs should be examined for bundle branch blocks or ventricular pre-excitation syndromes. As previously mentioned, if the diagnosis of the wide complex rhythm is uncertain, it should be assumed to be VT, and treatment should proceed according to the patient's condition.

NSVT may occur in the setting of acute ischemia, and evaluation and treatment should be focused on the ischemia. Direct pharmacologic treatment (e.g., lidocaine and amiodarone) of NSVT in ischemia/infarct is not advisable. In the patient not suffering from active ischemia, NSVT is frequently asymptomatic and has little prognostic utility for malignant arrhythmia, especially in the absence of structural heart disease and ventricular dysfunction. Symptomatic NSVT may be treated pharmacologically, primarily to relieve symptoms.

Sustained VT generally causes symptoms by impairing CO, resulting in hypotension, loss of consciousness, and possibly cardiac arrest. It may also deteriorate into VF.

Treatment of symptomatic VT with a detectable pulse is *synchronous* direct current cardioversion (with sedation or anesthesia in the awake patient) or, if the VT is well tolerated, with an antiarrhythmic drug (such as procainamide, amiodarone, or lidocaine). Patients with hemodynamically compromising, pulseless monomorphic or polymorphic VT usually require immediate treatment with asynchronous defibrillation (see section "Cardiac Arrest"), followed by antiarrhythmic drugs if necessary.

Sustained torsades de pointes with hemodynamic collapse also requires asynchronous cardioversion. Treatment of torsades de pointes aims at correcting any underlying electrolyte abnormalities and stopping any drugs known to prolong the QT interval. Torsades de pointes is likely to recur if the inciting factors cannot be eliminated immediately. Magnesium sulfate given at 1 to 2 mg IV may have utility, particularly in hypomagnesemic patients. Lidocaine or phenytoin may also be suppressive. Torsades de pointes is frequently *bradycardia dependent,* and temporary pacing or isoproterenol infusion may be used to increase the HR and prevent recurrences.

VF is the result of chaotic electrical currents within the ventricles, preventing coordinated contractions. VF on ECG has a chaotic appearance without any discernible QRS complex. Untreated VF rapidly results in death. VF may be preceded by VT and is most commonly seen in patients with acute myocardial infarction.

Treatment is immediate asynchronous electrical defibrillation, followed by antiarrhythmic drugs when a stable rhythm returns (see section "Cardiac Arrest"). Also see treatment Algorithm 20.3.

BRADYARRHYTHMIAS

Bradycardia, defined as a HR of less than 60 beats per minute, occurs from (a) SA node dysfunction or (b) disturbances of the AV conduction system. Clinically significant bradycardia occurs when there is inadequate CO, generally associated with hypotension, and which may manifest as any or all of presyncope, syncope, fatigue, confusion, depressed level of consciousness, chest pain, shock, or congestive heat failure. Acute treatment aims at restoring adequate CO and identifying the underlying rhythm and its cause.

SA node dysfunction occurs in a number of pathophysiologic states seen in the intensive care unit including increased intracranial pressure, prolonged apneic periods in patients with the obstructive sleep apnea/hypopnea syndrome, myocardial infarction advanced liver disease, hypothyroidism, hypothermia, hypercapnia, acidemia, hypervagotonia, and certain infections. It may also be due to depression of the sinus node by drugs, including sympatholytics such as beta-blockers and clonidine, the cardioselective calcium channel blockers verapamil and diltiazem, parasympathomimetics, and antiarrhythmic drugs such as amiodarone. Sick sinus syndrome refers to intrinsic sinus node dysfunction with any of the previously mentioned clinical symptoms associated with the decrease in CO. An important variant of sick sinus syndrome is sinus bradycardia or prolonged sinus pause occurring after termination of atrial fibrillation or other atrial arrhythmias due to depression of SA node automaticity during the tachyarrhythmia, which may be slow to recover. Syncope is a common presentation of this variant, termed the *tachy-brady syndrome.*

Disturbances of the AV conduction system can occur in the atria, AV node, or His–Purkinje system. When there is complete block in any part of the AV conduction system (termed *third-degree AV block*), an escape pacemaker generally develops. When complete blockage occurs in the AV node, the His bundle escape pacemaker generally takes over at a rate of 40 to 60 beats per minute, and is associated with a narrow QRS complex (in the absence of an underlying bundle branch block or other aberrant conduction). Complete heart block distal to the AV node often results in an escape pacemaker originating from the more distal conduction system, usually with a rate between 25 and 45 beats per minute. These fascicular escape rhythms generate a QRS complex consistent with their origin (e.g., if the origin is in the right bundle, the QRS has a left bundle branch block pattern). If the conduction system fails, a rhythm from the ventricular myocardium may generate a heart beat, with a wide complex of ventricular origin. Thus, in general, the more distal the escape rhythm, the slower and less reliable it tends to be. Heart block with irregular fascicular escapes may require urgent temporary pacing. The ECG shows AV dissociation with nonconducted P waves that "march" out independently of the ventricular escape rhythm. There are many causes of third-degree heart block including acute myocardial infarction, idiopathic fibrosis, drug toxicity (e.g., digitalis, beta-blockers, and cardioselective calcium channel blockers), chronic cardiopulmonary disease, congenital heart disease, infiltrative diseases (sarcoidosis), infections/inflammatory diseases, collagen vascular diseases, trauma, and tumors.

First-degree AV block is not truly *block*, but is a PR interval >200 ms. It is in itself generally benign, but may result in symptoms if the degree of AV dyssynchrony is severe.

Second-degree AV block occurs when some atrial impulses fail to conduct to the ventricles. **Mobitz type I second-degree AV block** (Wenckebach block) is characterized on ECG by a variable (usually progressively prolonging) PR interval culminating in a nonconducted atrial beat. Mobitz I uncommonly progresses to complete heart block. When it does, the escape pacemaker of 40 to 60 beats per minute in the His bundle usually provides an adequate backup rate to maintain CO. Mobitz I block can be caused by drugs such as digoxin, beta-blockers, certain calcium channel blockers, ischemia (especially of the inferior wall), or in healthy individuals from hypervagotonia.

Mobitz type II second-degree AV block generally is due to disease in the His–Purkinje system and is characterized on ECG by a fixed PR interval with one or more nonconducting atrial impulses. It is more likely to progress to complete heart block than Mobitz 1, sometimes precipitously. The typical escape pacemaker rate of 25 to 45 arises in the more distal His–Purkinje system and has a wide QRS. The escape rhythm may not be sufficient to maintain CO and can progress rapidly to cardiac arrest and death. Mobitz II can occur from ischemia (especially anteroseptal infarcts), endocarditis, valvular or congenital heart disease, drugs such as procainamide, disopyramide, and quinidine, or idiopathic progressive cardiac conduction system diseases.

Treatment of clinically significant bradycardia follows the ACLS algorithm outlined in Algorithm 20.2, and aims at maintaining adequate CO. Atropine is first-line transient pharmacologic therapy, and is more successful in patients with sinus bradycardia or block within the AV node, rather than block in the more distal His–Purkinje system. Patients who remain clinically unstable require immediate transcutaneous or transvenous pacing. Reversible causes should be identified. In patients with sinus node dysfunction in which the cause is not reversible, permanent pacing can relieve symptoms. Permanent pacing is typically indicated in Mobitz II or third-degree AV block.

If symptoms of bradycardia are present in Mobitz I AV block, permanent pacing is indicated.

CARDIAC ARREST

Cardiac arrest refers to the cessation of a detectable noninvasive blood pressure and pulse. Cardiac arrest can be separated into three main types: (a) pulseless electrical activity (PEA), (b) VT and VF, and (c) asystole. All three fall under the overall heading of pulseless arrest outlined in Algorithm 20.3. Treatment of PEA and asystole is similar and centers on identifying reversible causes and pharmacologic intervention. VT and VF are treated with immediate electrical defibrillation. Studies have shown that the most important aspect of resuscitation remains CPR.

Treatment of cardiac arrest in an intensive care unit setting requires a team of nurses and physicians trained in ACLS. Ideally there should be an established and easily identifiable team leader responsible for continuously evaluating the patient's condition and the ECG, assimilating incoming data, and giving all orders. In addition, there should be a scribe, recording changes in condition, ECG and laboratory data, and therapies delivered. Initial patient evaluation follows the ABCs of cardiac arrest in a coordinated and overlapping fashion, ensuring adequate airway control, breathing (i.e., ventilation), and circulation. In nonintubated patients, an oral airway device should be placed and a bag-valve-mask should be used to deliver breaths. Intubation is performed when possible. Cardiopulmonary resuscitation (CPR) should begin immediately with chest compressions given at a rate of 100 compressions per minute at 1.5 to 2 inches depth, allowing full chest recoil between compressions. Patients should also be immediately connected to an automated external defibrillator (AED), or a manual defibrillator if an AED is not available. The defibrillator is connected to two pads or paddles placed on the chest wall, with one to the right of the sternum centered on the second intercostal space, and one on the left chest wall centered in the midaxillary line at the fifth intercostal space. IV access should be ensured for delivery of medications and fluids. Peripheral IV access is initially adequate. However, central IV access should be obtained as soon as possible via the femoral vein, subclavian vein, or internal jugular vein. Endotracheal intubation or central IV access should not interfere with CPR. Pulses are best monitored in the femoral artery, but the carotid arteries may be used. Once airway control is established and the patient is connected to an external defibrillator, the cardiac rhythm should be rapidly analyzed (Table 20.1).

Pulseless VT and VF

Confirmed VT and VF with hemodynamic collapse should be treated with *immediate* asynchronous defibrillation. Automated AED devices typically deliver escalating biphasic shocks at 200, 300, and 360 joules (J). Manual devices may generate monophasic or biphasic waveforms. If a manual biphasic device is used and the devices recommended dose scale is unknown, an initial dose of 200 J should be used, with subsequent shocks at the same or higher doses. If a monophasic device is used, the dose should be 360 J for all shocks. The patient's rhythm, blood pressure, and responsiveness must be continuously monitored with appropriate adjustment of therapy (e.g., continuation/discontinuation of CPR and infusion of new medications). If VT/VF persists or recurs after initial treatment, CPR should be resumed immediately after the first shock is given and continued for 2 minutes along with continuous ventilation via a mask airway or endotracheal tube. The rhythm and pulse should be reassessed 2 minutes after

TABLE 20.1	ACLS Pharmacotherapies: Dosing and Side Effects	
Medications	IV dosing	Side effects
Metoprolol	SVT: 2.5–5 mg IV Q5 min (max dose 15 mg over 15 min)	Hypotension, bradycardia, bronchoconstriction, CHF
Diltiazem	SVT: 0.25 mg/kg IV over 2 min, repeat bolus (after 15 min if response inadequate) 0.35 mg/kg IV over 2 min	Hypotension, bradycardia, CHF
Adenosine	SVT: Initial dose: 6 mg IV rapid push Repeat bolus (after 2 min if response inadequate)12 mg IV rapid push (Always flush with saline)	Flushing, headache, AV block, asystole
Digoxin	SVT: Initial loading dose: 0.25–0.5 mg IV slow push (reduce dose by 50% in renal failure), up to 1.5 mg in 24 hours	Atrial tachycardia with or without AV block, nausea, blurred vision
Epinephrine (1:10 000)	PEA/asystole: 1 mg IV Q3–5 min × 3 doses (higher doses or continuous infusions can be used to treat specific problems)	Tachyarrhythmias, chest pain, hypertension
Vasopressin	PEA/asystole: 40 units IV may replace first or second dose of epinephrine	Tachyarrhythmias, asystole, chest pain, hypertension
Atropine	Slow PEA/asystole: 1 mg IV Q3–5 min x 3 doses Bradycardia: 0.5–1 mg IV Q3–5 min, up to 0.04 mg/kg in 24-hr period	Anticholinergic side effects, tachyarrhythmias, hypotension
Dopamine	Hemodynamic support: 1–5 μg/kg/min, max dose 50 μg/kg/min	Vasoconstriction, arrhythmias, hypotension (at lower doses), chest pain
Norepinephrine	Hemodynamic support: 0.5–1 μg/min, max dose titrate to response	Vasoconstriction, arrhythmias, chest pain
Amiodarone	300 mg IV push, can redose if inadequate response 150 mg IV push	Hypotension, prolonged QT interval, bradycardia arrhythmias
Lidocaine	1–1.5 mg/kg IV over 2–3 min, may repeat 0.5–0.75 mg/kg IV Q10 min for total of 3 doses	Tachyarrhythmias, bradycardia, hypotension, AV block
Procainamide	20–50 mg/min until arrhythmia controlled	Hypotension, lupus-like syndrome, QRS widening
Magnesium	Torsades de pointes: 1–2 mg IV push over 5–20 min	Flushing, hypotension

the shock is given. Shocks should be repeated if patients remain in pulseless VT/VF and the CPR cycle repeated. When IV access is established, patients should be concomitantly treated with 1 mg IV epinephrine every 3 to 5 minutes. Vasopressin, 40 U IV, may also be substituted for the first or second dose. Studies comparing epinephrine and vasopressin given to hospitalized patients in cardiac arrest have shown no difference in survival. After the third shock is given, patients who remain in VF/VT should be considered for amiodarone or lidocaine at the doses shown in Algorithm 20.3. Careful evaluation for a treatable cause should be sought. If the rhythm on the monitor appears to be torsades de pointes, patients should be given IV magnesium sulfate. If a pulse becomes present at any point in treatment, the rhythm should be identified and appropriately treated according to Algorithms 20.1 and 20.2.

PEA and Asystole

PEA includes numerous pulseless rhythms such as bradyasystolic rhythms, idioventricular rhythms, and ventricular escape rhythms. PEA and asystole are not treated with electrical defibrillation. Treatment centers on well-delivered CPR and pharmacologic intervention as illustrated in Algorithm 20.3. Epinephrine should be given at 1 mg IV every 3 to 5 minutes and may be replaced with vasopressin 40 U for the first or second dose. If a slow rhythm is seen on the monitor, consider giving atropine 1 mg IV. If IV access is not available, the drugs may be given endotracheally, in which case the dose is generally doubled.

The five H's and five T's listed in Algorithm 20.3 are common conditions that may contribute to cardiac arrest. Airway control and ventilation can correct *hypoxemia*. IV fluids should be given at a wide open rate or via a rapid infuser to correct *hypovolemia*. If *hypoglycemia* is suspected, give 1 ampule (amp) of 50% dextrose, or 1 mg of intramuscular glucagon if IV access is not available. If *hypokalemia* or acidosis (*hydrogen ion*) are suspected, give 1 amp of sodium bicarbonate (50 mEq NaHCO$_3$). *Hypothermia* should be treated as outlined in Chapter 31. Cases of suspected cardiac *tamponade* should be treated with immediate pericardiocentesis (see Chapter 79). Suspected *tension* pneumothorax should be treated with rapid decompression by inserting a large-bore catheter (14- or 16-gauge) into the second intercostal space in the midclavicular line, or unilateral or bilaterally inserted thoracostomy tubes. Ischemia from coronary *thrombosis* should be rapidly identified and treated when patients are stabilized (see Chapter 18). If pulmonary thrombosis is suspected, fibrinolytics may be beneficial but are not recommended for routine use.

Cycles of CPR should continue until patients have palpable pulses and a detectable blood pressure or until resuscitation efforts have failed. There is no set period for when to stop resuscitation efforts. The decision to stop CPR is made by the medical team when a full trial at resuscitation has failed and the patient's chances of regaining a pulse and neurologic function are negligible. If patients do regain a pulse, the rhythm on the monitor should be identified and the patient treated accordingly. Blood pressure should be checked and hypotension should be treated with IV vasopressors and IV fluids. An arterial blood gas and other laboratory tests should be checked and abnormalities treated.

Postresuscitation hypothermia often occurs naturally after cardiac arrest. Active induction of hypothermia has also been evaluated in numerous randomized trials of patients with VF arrest and PEA/asystolic arrest occurring both in and out of the hospital. Patients were generally hemodynamically stable but comatose. They were cooled within minutes to hours to between approximately 32°C and 34°C, generally with cooling blankets. There were improved outcomes and metabolic end points in patients who were actively cooled. Thus, it is a current American Heart Association Class IIb recommendation for in-hospital cardiac arrest and non-VF arrest, and Class IIa for out-of-hospital VF arrest to cool hemodynamically stable but unconscious patients to between 32°C and 34°C for 12 to 24 hours after cardiac arrest. Patients with spontaneous hypothermia should not be actively rewarmed. Complications of cooling include coagulopathies and arrhythmias.

SUGGESTED READINGS

2005 American Heart Association Guidelines for Cardiopulmonary Resuscitation and Emergency Cardiovascular Care, Part 3: Overview of CPR, Part 4: Adult Basic Life Support, Part 5: Electrical Therapies, Part 6: CPR Techniques and Devices, Part 7: Advanced Cardiovascular Life Support. *Circulation.* 2005;112(Suppl IV):IV12–IV88. *Current recommendations from the AHA based on evaluation of current treatment evidence reviewed at the 2005 International Consensus Conference on Cardiopulmonary Resuscitation and Emergency Cardiovascular Care, and published in the supplement to Circulation.*

Aung K, Htay T. Vasopressin for cardiac arrest: a systematic review and meta-analysis. *Arch Intern Med.* 2005;165:17–24.
  Summation of evidence from five randomized trials comparing vasopressin and epinephrine in cardiac arrest showing no clear advantage of vasopressin over epinephrine.

Hypothermia After Cardiac Arrest Study Group. Mild therapeutic hypothermia to improve the neurologic outcome after cardiac arrest. *N Engl J Med.* 2002;346:549–556.
  Multicenter trial of patients resuscitated after cardiac arrest due to ventricular fibrillation who were randomly assigned to undergo therapeutic hypothermia or standard treatment with normothermia. The primary end point was a favorable neurologic outcome within 6 months after cardiac arrest, which was achieved by 55% of patients in the hypothermia group compared to 39% in the normothermia group. Mortality was 41% versus 55%, favoring the hypothermia group.

21 Aortic Dissection

Jay Shah and Alan C. Braverman

Aortic dissection is a life-threatening acute aortic syndrome that accounts for a small but significant proportion of cardiovascular system disease, with an incidence of approximately 5 to 30 per million people per year. It carries substantial morbidity and mortality, with a mortality rate up to 1% per hour within the first 24 to 48 hours. An algorithm for the immediate approach to the patient with aortic dissection is presented in Algorithm 21.1.

Classic aortic dissection results from a tear in the intimal layer of the aorta, allowing blood to enter the medial layer and propagate in an anterograde or retrograde direction, resulting in a second, "false" lumen. Additional intimal tears may occur, and allow reconnection with the true lumen. Variants of aortic dissection include aortic intramural hematoma (IMH) and penetrating atherosclerotic aortic ulcer (PAU), which together account for 10% to 20% of acute aortic syndromes (Figure 21.1). In aortic IMH, rupture of the vasa vasorum leads to hemorrhage in the medial layer without an intimal tear or communication with the aortic lumen. IMH of the aorta is generally treated in a similar fashion as aortic dissection, with emergency surgery for ascending aortic IMH and medical therapy for descending aortic IMH. PAU can arise when atherosclerotic lesions of the aorta develop ulcerations that penetrate the intimal and medial layers, and may form a false aneurysm that may lead to aortic dissection or rupture. Between these two variants of acute aortic syndromes, IMH is more likely to progress to classic aortic dissection and PAU is more common in the descending aorta. Once aortic dissection occurs, shear forces stemming from the rate of change in pressure (dP/dt) and mean blood pressure contribute to spread of the tear.

Several conditions predispose the aorta to dissection, most as a result of abnormalities in the arterial wall composition (Table 21.1). Approximately 75% of patients with aortic dissection have hypertension. Patients with bicuspid aortic valves or conditions, such as the Marfan syndrome, Loeys–Dietz syndrome, vascular Ehlers–Danlos syndrome, or familial thoracic aortic aneurysm/dissection, are particularly prone to aortic dilation and dissection. Cocaine or methamphetamine-induced hypertension, inflammatory conditions such as giant cell arteritis, or direct trauma from catheterization or aortic surgery can disrupt the aortic intima. Once the intima becomes injured, it is vulnerable to shear stresses and may progress to rupture or dissection.

There are several classification systems for aortic dissections, and involvement of the ascending aorta is the defining characteristic (see Figure 21.2). DeBakey types I and II and Stanford type A dissections involve the ascending aorta. DeBakey type III or Stanford type B dissections do not involve the ascending aorta. Classification of the anatomy is important because the decision regarding surgical or medical management

155

ALGORITHM 21.1 Algorithm for Aortic Dissection

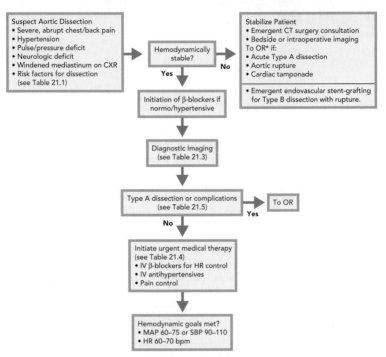

Suspect Aortic Dissection
• Severe, abrupt chest/back pain
• Hypertension
• Pulse/pressure deficit
• Neurologic deficit
• Windened mediastinum on CXR
• Risk factors for dissection
  (see Table 21.1)

Hemodynamically stable?

Yes / **No**

Stabilize Patient
• Emergent CT surgery consultation
• Bedside or intraoperative imaging
To OR* if:
• Acute Type A dissection
• Aortic rupture
• Cardiac tamponade

• Emergent endovascular stent-grafting for Type B dissection with rupture.

Initiation of β-blockers if normo/hypertensive

Diagnostic Imaging
(see Table 21.3)

Type A dissection or complications
(see Table 21.5)

Yes → To OR

No

Initiate urgent medical therapy
(see Table 21.4)
• IV β-blockers for HR control
• IV antihypertensives
• Pain control

Hemodynamic goals met?
• MAP 60–75 or SBP 90–110
• HR 60–70 bpm

CXR, chest x-ray; MAP, mean arterial pressure; SBP, systolic blood pressure; bpm, beats per minute; IV, intravenous.

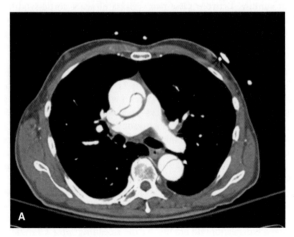

Figure 21.1. Types of acute aortic syndromes. **A:** Classic aortic dissection. (*continued*)

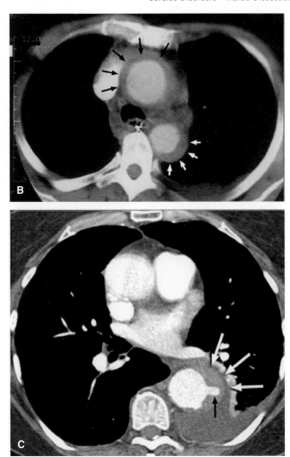

Figure 21.1. (*Continued*) **B:** Intramural hematoma (IMH) of the aorta. Black arrows indicate IMH in ascending aorta; white arrows denote crescentic IMH in descending aorta. **C:** Penetrating atherosclerotic ulcer (PAU) of the aorta (black arrow). White arrows point to associated contained hematoma. Modified from Braverman AC, Thompson RW, Sanchez LA. Diseases of the aorta. In: Bonow RO, Mann DL, Zipes DP, Libby P, eds. *Braunwald's heart disease,* 9th ed. Philadelphia, PA: Elsevier, 2011:1309–1338.

is dependent on the location of the dissection. Broadly, dissections of the ascending aorta (types I, II, and A) require immediate surgical repair, while those involving the descending aorta (type III or B) are initially treated medically.

The clinical presentation of aortic dissection may be quite variable, and one must maintain a high index of suspicion for the diagnosis. In contrast to the crescendo discomfort of angina pectoris, the pain of acute dissection is maximal at its onset, usually sudden and severe, and often described as a sharp, tearing pain in the chest, neck, or interscapular areas. In addition to the dissection itself, presenting symptoms

| TABLE 21.1 | Risk Factors for Aortic Dissection |

- Hypertension
- Thoracic
- Aortic
- Aneurysm
- Genetic disorders[a]
  - Marfan syndrome
  - Loeys–Dietz syndrome
  - Familial thoracic aortic aneurysm/dissection syndrome
  - Vascular Ehlers–Danlos syndrome
- Congenital conditions
  - Bicuspid aortic valve
  - Turner syndrome
  - Aortic coarctation
  - Supravalvular aortic stenosis
- Cocaine/amphetamine use
- Atherosclerosis/penetrating aortic ulcer
- Trauma—blunt or iatrogenic
  - Catheter-induced
  - Aortic valve surgery
  - Coronary artery bypass grafting
  - Deceleration injury (e.g., motor vehicle accident)
- Inflammatory conditions
  - Giant cell arteritis
  - Takayasu's arteritis
  - Behçet disease
  - Syphilitic aortitis

[a]First-degree relatives of patients with these conditions should be screened for aortic disease.

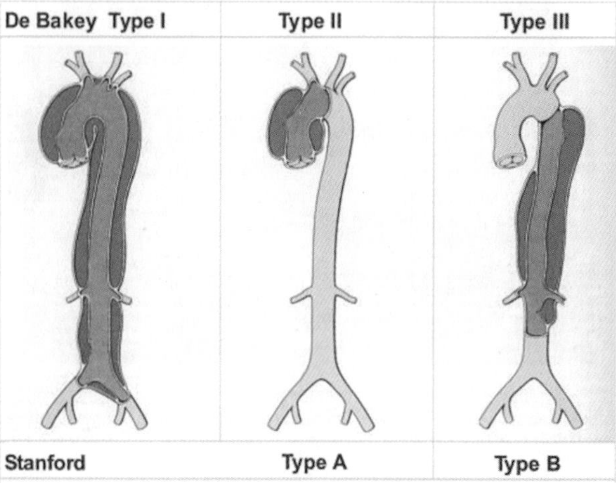

De Bakey

Type I	Originates in the ascending aorta, propagates at least to the aortic arch and often beyond it distally
Type II	Originates in and is confined to the ascending aorta
Type III	Originates in the descending aorta and extends distally down the aorta or, rarely, retrograde into the aortic arch and ascending aorta

Stanford

| Type A | All dissections involving the ascending aorta, regardless of the site of origin |
| Type B | All dissections not involving the ascending aorta |

Figure 21.2. Classification systems for aortic dissection: Stanford and DeBakey. (Adapted from Nienaber CA, Eagle KA. Aortic dissection: new frontiers in diagnosis and management. Part I: from etiology to diagnostic strategies. *Circulation.* 2003;108:628–635, with permission.)

TABLE 21.2	Complications of Aortic Dissection

- Aortic rupture
- Myocardial ischemia/infarction
- Neurologic deficits: stroke, coma, altered consciousness, syncope, paraplegia
- Malperfusion: coronary, mesenteric, limb, spinal cord, renal, hepatic
- Hypotension
- Hemothorax
- Cardiac tamponade
- Acute aortic regurgitation and congestive heart failure
- Subsequent aneurysm formation

may also be related to malperfusion or complications involving various organ systems. Physical examination should include a complete pulse exam and blood pressure in both arms and legs, as there may be pulse or pressure deficits. Cardiac auscultation may reveal an aortic regurgitation murmur. However, pulse differentials and an aortic regurgitation murmur are present in a minority of patients, and physical examination alone is not sufficient to rule out aortic dissection.

Significant morbidity and mortality from dissection is attributed to end-organ damage and aortic rupture (Table 21.2). Organ systems may be compromised by compression of branch vessels by an expanding false lumen, or direct extension of a dissection into the vessel. Cardiovascular and neurologic manifestations are two particularly devastating complications of aortic dissection. When the ascending aorta is involved, acute aortic regurgitation may lead to heart failure. Cardiac tamponade, aortic rupture, or myocardial infarction from coronary artery involvement may lead rapidly to hemodynamic shock and death. Dissection complicated by acute hemopericardium may lead to cardiac tamponade. Poor outcomes have been reported from pericardiocentesis secondary to further bleeding and acute decompensation. Therefore, pericardiocentesis should generally be avoided in favor of emergent surgery. Neurologic sequelae may result from acute dissection involving the carotid or vertebral arteries, as cerebral hypoperfusion may lead to syncope, altered mental status, and stroke. Transverse myelitis, myelopathy, paraplegia, or quadriplegia may result from spinal malperfusion. Mesenteric ischemia may occur, which may be difficult to diagnose and can be fatal.

Standard laboratory tests are of limited utility in evaluating aortic dissection, though the chest x-ray and the D-dimer may be useful. The chest radiograph may demonstrate a widened mediastinum or abnormal aortic contour. Pleural effusion may represent hemothorax, and displaced calcium at the aortic arch may also be present in dissection. Regardless, up to 10% to 20% of aortic dissections are associated with a normal chest radiograph. The D-dimer is another test that may be of assistance in the diagnosis; it is usually elevated in acute aortic dissection, and when normal, has been shown to have a high negative predictive value in the first 24 hours from symptom onset. Importantly, in IMH, the D-dimer may not be elevated, and in the setting of a high clinical index of suspicion, a negative D-dimer does not rule out an acute aortic syndrome. A clear role for the D-dimer in evaluation of aortic dissection has not been established.

Given the critical nature of aortic dissections, immediate diagnostic confirmation and definition of the extent of the dissection is imperative once it is suspected.

TABLE 21.3		Comparison of Diagnostic Imaging Modalities		
Test	Sensitivity (%)	Specificity (%)	Advantages	Disadvantages
TEE	98–99	94–97	Excellent evaluation of aortic root and descending thoracic aorta, aortic valve, and pericardium	Requires esophageal intubation; limited to thoracic aorta
CT	96–100	96–100	Widely and rapidly available; superior imaging of entire aorta, heart, branch vessels, and complications such as rupture and hemopericardium	Limited identification of the intimal tear/site of entry; nephrotoxic iodinated contrast required
MRI	>98	>98	Superior accuracy, sensitivity, and specificity for all types of dissection	Limited availability, time-consuming procedure, less monitoring during scan

The choice of imaging should be made on the basis of sensitivity, specificity, clinical stability, and operator availability and experience (Table 21.3). If the patient presents with hemodynamic instability or hypotension, rapid evaluation by transesophageal echocardiogram or computed tomography (CT) scan should be performed to assess for complications of dissection, including pericardial effusion, aortic regurgitation, or aortic rupture. CT is widely and rapidly available. Though CT scans require intravenous contrast dye, they offer superior imaging of the entire aorta, aortic arch, and branch vessels. Transesophageal echocardiogram requires an experienced operator and esophageal intubation to perform the procedure; however, it can be performed at the bedside, and visualizes the aortic valve, aortic root, and pericardium well. Because of the time delay and difficulties with hemodynamic monitoring, MRI is usually not the first test of choice.

When aortic dissection is suspected, immediate initiation of β-blocker therapy to reduce shear forces is paramount while pursuing confirmation of the diagnosis (Table 21.4). Blood pressure should be reduced to as low a level as possible without compromising organ perfusion. β-Blocker therapy is recommended to achieve a target heart rate <70 beats per minute. Nondihydropyridine calcium channel blockers (diltiazem, verapamil) may be considered if β-blocker therapy is contraindicated. Care should be taken to avoid vasodilators, such as sodium nitroprusside, in the absence of negative chronotropic medications, as they may induce reflex tachycardia, thereby increasing dP/dt, which may extend the dissection.

Emergent surgery is indicated with ascending aortic dissection because medical therapy alone is associated with a high risk of morbidity and mortality (Figure 21.3).

TABLE 21.4	Selected Pharmacologic Therapy[a]

1. Intravenous β-blocker (preferred negative inotrope)[b]
   - Esmolol: Give 500 μg/kg IV bolus, then continuous IV infusion at 50–200 μg/kg/min, titrated to effect. Short half-life allows rapid titration.
   - Labetalol: Give 20 mg IV over 2 min, then 40–80 mg IV every 15 min until adequate response (maximum 300 mg), then continuous IV infusion at 2–10 mg/min IV, titrated to effect.
2. Intravenous vasodilator (after initiation of β-blockade)
   - Sodium nitroprusside: Start continuous infusion with no bolus at 20 μg/min, titrate 0.5–5 μg/kg/min with a maximum of 800 μg/min. *Use only in presence of β-blockers.*
   - Caution: thiocyanate toxicity may occur in patients with renal impairment or prolonged infusions.
   - Enalaprilat: Give 0.625–1.25 mg IV, then increase by 0.625–1.25 mg every 6 hr to a maximum of 5 mg every 6 hr, titrated to effect.

[a]Goal of therapy is HR less than 70 beats per minute and blood pressure as low as possible without compromising organ perfusion.
[b]If contraindication to β-blockers, use diltiazem: 0.25 mg/kg IV over 2 min, then continuous IV infusion at 5–15 mg/hr, titrated to effect.

Surgery or endovascular repair in descending aortic dissection is reserved for complications such as end-organ ischemia, refractory pain, uncontrolled hypertension, rupture, or a rapidly expanding aortic diameter (Table 21.5). There is growing experience managing complications of descending aortic dissections with percutaneous interventional therapy using stent grafting to exclude intimal tears, and balloon fenestration of the

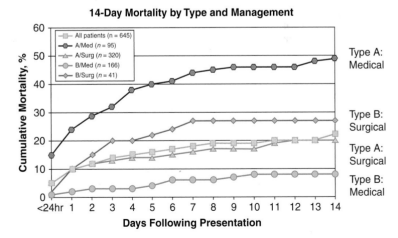

Figure 21.3. IRAD graph of outcomes after medical/surgical treatments for type A and B dissections. (Adapted from Hagan PG, Nienaber CA, Isselbacher EM, et al. The International Registry of Acute Aortic Dissection (IRAD): new insights into an old disease. *JAMA.* 2000;283:897–903, with permission.)

TABLE 21.5	Indications for Surgery[a]

- Type I, II, or A dissection
- Type III or B with
  - Rupture
  - Branch vessel compromise/organ ischemia
  - Refractory hypertension
  - Aneurysmal dilation
  - Refractory pain

---

[a]Or endovascular intervention for appropriate patients.

false lumen to relieve ischemia of a compromised branch vessel. These techniques and others continue to evolve the management of complex aortic dissections.

SUGGESTED READINGS

Braverman AC. Acute aortic dissection: clinician update. *Circulation.* 2010;122:184–188.
   Current review of diagnosis and management of acute aortic dissection.
Braverman AC, Thompson RW, Sanchez LA. Diseases of the aorta. In: Bonow RO, Mann DL, Zipes DP, Libby P, eds. Braunwald's heart disease, 9th ed. Philadelphia, PA: Elsevier, 2011:1309–1338.
   Comprehensive overview of entire spectrum of aortic disease.
Estrera A, Miller C, Lee T, et al. Acute type A intramural hematoma: analysis of current management strategy. *Circulation.* 2009;120:S287–S291.
   Nice review of management of Type A IMH.
Hagan PG, Nienaber CA, Isselbacher EM, et al. The International Registry of Acute Aortic Dissection (IRAD). New insights into an old disease. *JAMA.* 2000;283:897–903.
   The largest database of acute aortic dissection with emphasis on clinical presentation.
Mehta RH, Suzuki T, Hagan PG, et al. Predicting death in patients with acute type A aortic dissection. *Circulation.* 2002;105:200–206.
   IRAD study of 547 patients which develops a risk prediction tool in patients with acute type A aortic dissection.
Nienaber CA, Eagle KA. Aortic dissection: new frontiers in diagnosis and management. Part I: from etiology to diagnostic strategies. *Circulation.* 2003;108:628–635.
   A broad review of aortic dissection with emphasis on etiology and diagnostic methods of detecting aortic dissection.
Nienaber CA, von Kodolitsch Y, Petersen B, et al. Intramural hematoma of the thoracic aorta: diagnostic and therapeutic implications. *Circulation.* 1995;92:1465–1472.
   Describes clinical features and prognosis of a series of patients with aortic intramural hematoma.
Tsai TT, Nienaber CA, Eagle KA. Acute aortic syndromes. *Circulation.* 2005;112:3802–3813
   Outstanding review of the three different acute aortic syndromes, and key points for diagnosis, imaging, and management.
Tsai TT, Trimarchi S, Nienaber CA. Acute aortic dissection: perspectives from the International Registry of Acute Aortic Dissection (IRAD). *Eur J Vasc Endovasc Surg.* 2009;37(2):149–159.
   Update of IRAD database.
Von Kodolitsch Y, Schwartz AG, Nienaber CA. Clinical prediction of acute aortic dissection. *Arch Intern Med.* 2000;160:2977–2982.
   Proposes independent predictors of acute aortic dissection and creates a prediction model for facilitated estimation of the individual risk of dissection.

22 Acute Decompensated Heart Failure

Shane J. LaRue and Gregory A. Ewald

The combination of an increasing elderly population and successful reperfusion strategies for acute myocardial infarction (MI) has led to an epidemic growth in the number of patients with left ventricular dysfunction and heart failure (HF). It is estimated that there are 5 million Americans living with HF, with 500,000 new cases occurring each year. In fact, HF is the leading cause of hospitalization for patients age 65 or more years and costs nearly 40 billion dollars per year in the United States and is an estimated 1% to 2% of the entire health-care budget in Europe. The 1-year mortality from this condition approaches 50% for patients with advanced HF, corresponding to 300,000 deaths annually in the United States.

The management of chronic HF has improved substantially during the past decade. Successful approaches validated by clinical trials have become well established and are documented in numerous evidence-based guidelines. These approaches will not be detailed here but involve (a) modulation of neurohormonal activation, specifically the renin-angiotensin-aldosterone system (via angiotensin converting enzyme inhibitors [ACEIs], angiotensin receptor blockers [ARBs], and aldosterone antagonists) and sympathetic nervous system (via beta-blockers); (b) fluid management (via diuretics and sodium/water restriction); (c) reducing cardiac work and improving cardiac output (via hydralazine, nitrates, and digoxin); and (d) attempting to restore synchronized ventricular contraction and preventing sudden cardiac death (via implantation of biventricular pacemakers and cardiac defibrillators).

In contrast to chronic HF, the management of acute decompensated HF (ADHF) is not as well studied in randomized controlled trials, and evidence-based guidelines have only recently appeared. There are now three sets of guidelines that provide the clinician with recommendations for treating ADHF, with one from the European Society of Cardiology, one from the American College of Cardiology/American Heart Association, and another from the Heart Failure Society of America. Our approach to HF in the critical care setting is consistent with these guidelines and is summarized in this chapter.

Recognizing HF is an important first step, as previously existent HF may not have been diagnosed, or there may be acute HF in the setting of MI or acute cardiomyopathy. Typical patients have a history of coronary artery disease, MI, or HF with subjective complaints of paroxysmal nocturnal dyspnea, orthopnea, and dyspnea on exertion. Physical findings that correlate with HF include a third heart sound (S3) and signs of volume overload, such as jugular venous distention, hepatojugular reflux, pulmonary rales, and lower extremity edema. Chest radiography may show cardiomegaly or pulmonary venous congestion. Electrocardiogram findings are not specific but may show atrial fibrillation, ventricular hypertrophy, or evidence of prior MI.

It is important to remember that although HF is a clinical diagnosis, echocardiography, angiography, and invasive hemodynamic monitoring are useful to document systolic or diastolic dysfunction. The role of blood testing is limited in the diagnosis of HF, although B-type natriuretic peptide (BNP) levels can be helpful if the diagnosis is uncertain. In particular, patients with serum BNP <100 pg/mL are very unlikely to have decompensated HF, whereas values >500 pg/mL are consistent with the diagnosis, with the exception of patients on hemodialysis or with an estimated glomerular filtration rate <60 mL/min. In these patients, the BNP should not be used for diagnosis as it is typically elevated out of proportion to the degree of HF. Elevated serum creatinine and hepatic function tests may suggest poor end-organ perfusion secondary to reduced cardiac output.

It is critical to make an accurate assessment regarding the precipitating events for the patient's decompensated state. Common precipitants include myocardial ischemia, acute MI, hypertensive crisis, arrhythmias, sepsis, anemia, and decompensation of pre-existing HF secondary to medical or dietary nonadherence. Less common precipitating factors include acute myocarditis, peripartum cardiomyopathy, valvular heart disease (including infective endocarditis), cardiac tamponade, and thyrotoxicosis (Table 22.1).

Once the diagnosis of ADHF is confirmed, an initial algorithmic approach should focus on stabilizing the patient and performing noninvasive assessments of heart rhythm, oxygenation, hemodynamics, and volume status (Algorithm 22.1). This will guide therapies such as digoxin or amiodarone for atrial fibrillation with rapid ventricular response, vasodilators to reduce afterload and the work of the failing heart, or inotropes for the patient with inadequate end-organ perfusion.

Two classification schemes are frequently used for ADHF: the Killip and Forrester classifications, both of which were developed for ADHF in the setting of MI. The Forrester classification is useful with either noninvasive data (clinical perfusion status and evidence of pulmonary congestion) or invasive hemodynamic data (Algorithm 22.2). When an accurate clinical assessment of hemodynamic and volume status cannot be made, a pulmonary artery catheter (Swan-Ganz) can be useful to measure the cardiac index, pulmonary capillary wedge pressure (PCWP), and systemic vascular resistance (SVR), with the additional benefit of monitoring the response to therapy. However, this procedure is not without risks and thus should be reserved for selected cases and only performed by an experienced operator (see Chapter 76).

TABLE 22.1	Precipitants of Acute Decompensated Heart Failure
Common	Less common
Medical/dietary noncompliance	Peripartum cardiomyopathy
Acute myocardial infarction	Acute myocarditis
Hypertensive crisis	Infective endocarditis
Arrhythmias	Valvular heart disease
Sepsis	Cardiac tamponade
Anemia	Thyrotoxicosis

ALGORITHM 22.1   **Algorithmic Approach to Acute Decompensated Heart Failure**

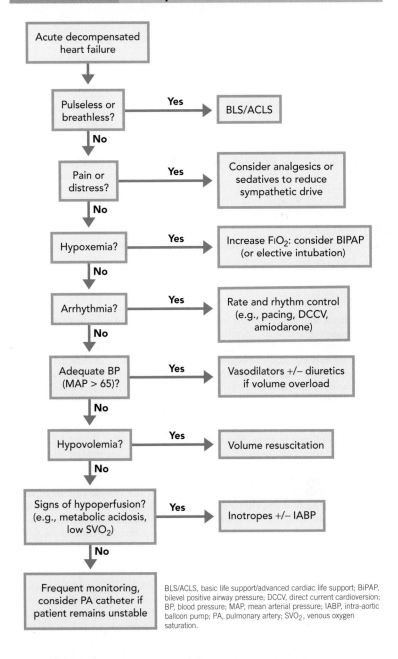

BLS/ACLS, basic life support/advanced cardiac life support; BiPAP, bilevel positive airway pressure; DCCV, direct current cardioversion; BP, blood pressure; MAP, mean arterial pressure; IABP, intra-aortic balloon pump; PA, pulmonary artery; SVO2, venous oxygen saturation.

ALGORITHM 22.2 Acute Decompensated Heart Failure Therapies by Clinical Presentation (Forrester Classification)

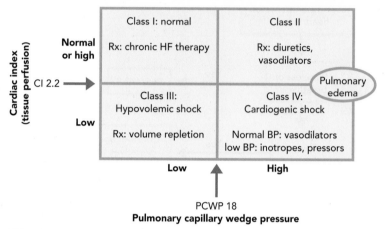

HF, heart failure; Rx, therapy; CI, cardiac index; BP, blood pressure; PCWP, pulmonary capillary wedge pressure.

TREATMENT

Most patients with ADHF present with volume overload and pulmonary congestion. The mainstays of therapy are diuretics and vasodilators, reserved for those patients with adequate cardiac output to maintain sufficient blood pressure (systolic blood pressure >85 to 90 mm Hg) and end-organ perfusion (Algorithm 22.2, Forrester Class II) prior to their initiation. These therapies are considered Class I recommendations and reduce the work that must be performed by the failing heart by reducing both preload and afterload while providing symptomatic relief. Initial therapy with intravenous (IV) diuretics has a relatively rapid effect, with reductions in right atrial pressure, PCWP, and PVR within 5 to 30 minutes. For patients requiring high doses of furosemide, a continuous drip may be more effective than boluses >1 mg/kg. Guidelines for practical diuretic use are shown in Table 22.2, and include adding thiazide diuretics for refractory cases. In selected patients with ADHF (such as MI with pulmonary edema), vasodilator therapy with IV nitroglycerin should be considered the first-line agent (Table 22.3). Nitroglycerin IV is a balanced arterial and venous vasodilator when given in appropriate doses, effectively reducing both preload and afterload without impairing tissue perfusion. At low doses, IV nitroglycerin induces venodilation (without significant coronary artery dilation), and may not effectively unload the failing heart. Therefore, IV nitroglycerin should be titrated aggressively (with careful blood pressure monitoring) in patients suffering from ADHF in the setting of myocardial ischemia. In other patients with pulmonary congestion in the setting of ADHF, the combination of IV nitroglycerin and IV loop diuretics provides rapid symptomatic relief and has been found to be more effective than high-dose diuretics alone.

Nesiritide is recombinant BNP that, like nitroglycerin, is a balanced arterial and venous vasodilator, but also promotes natriuresis in combination with loop diuretics.

TABLE 22.2	Diuretics for Acute Decompensated Heart Failure		
Severity of volume overload	Diuretic	Dose	Comments
Mild to moderate	Furosemide	20–40 mg PO or IV	Follow Na$^+$ and K$^+$
Severe	Furosemide	40–120 mg IV, or IV drip at 2–20 mg/hr	Up to every 6 hr for bolus dosing
Refractory to loop diuretics	Add metolazone 30 min prior to each furosemide dose	2.5–5 mg PO	Most helpful when CrCl <30 mL/min
Refractory to combination of loop and thiazide diuretics	Consider inotrope (dobutamine) if renal perfusion is inadequate. Consider renal replacement therapy if renal failure (HD or CVVHDF).		

PO, by mouth; IV, intravenously; CrCl, creatinine clearance; HD, hemodialysis CVVHDF, continuous venovenous hemodiafiltration.

Nesiritide decreases PCWP promptly and improves dyspnea in patients with ADHF. Nesiritide can be initiated most safely without a bolus at 0.01 μg/kg/min, with titration to a maximum dose of 0.03 μg/kg/min.

ACEIs and ARBs have an important role in the management of chronic HF, but their role in the setting of ADHF is less clear. Chronic ACEI or ARB therapy promotes afterload reduction, but may require dosage reduction or discontinuation in patients with ADHF to facilitate diuresis without impairment of renal function. Cautious initiation of ACEI or ARB therapy in the intensive care unit setting may be helpful with careful monitoring of renal function and electrolytes. The short-acting ACEI captopril (starting dose 6.25 to 12.5 mg every 6 to 8 hours) may be carefully titrated with each dose until a prespecified goal is met (systolic blood pressure <100 mm Hg, reduced SVR, or 300-mg daily dose). For patients with chronic HF, ACEIs or ARBs should be initiated approximately 48 hours after stabilization of an ADHF episode, most likely after transfer out of the critical care setting (Class I recommendation, level of evidence A).

TABLE 22.3	Vasodilators (all have potential for causing hypotension)		
Indication	Vasodilator	Dose (μg/min)	Comments
ADHF	Nitroglycerin	10–200	Headache, tachyphylaxis
ADHF	Nesiritide	0.01–0.03	Use bolus dosing with caution
Hypertensive crisis	Nitroprusside	0.5–5	Isocyanate toxicity

ADHF, acute decompensated heart failure.

Other medical therapies such as beta-blockers and calcium channel blockers have a limited role in the management of patients with ADHF. Beta-blockade is a mainstay of treatment for acute MI as well as for chronic HF, but patients presenting with MI and ADHF involving hypotension, or more than mild-to-moderate pulmonary congestion, have not been included in most of the relevant clinical trials. As such, IV metoprolol and other agents should be used with caution in this setting. Patients receiving chronic beta-blocker therapy may require a dose reduction, but beta-blockers should not be abruptly discontinued to avoid adverse events related to elevated catecholamine levels in patients with ADHF. Milrinone should be considered for these patients if they require inotropic support as it acts downstream from the beta-adrenergic receptor. Calcium channel blockers (including diltiazem, verapamil, and amlodipine) are contraindicated in patients with ADHF, secondary to their negative inotropic effects.

For patients in cardiogenic shock with hypotension and evidence of inadequate tissue perfusion (Algorithm 22.2, Forrester Group IV), dobutamine and milrinone are the inotropic agents of choice. Dobutamine is predominantly a beta-1 and beta-2 adrenergic receptor agonist, which augments both inotropy and chronotropy. There is frequently a reflex decrease in sympathetic tone that leads to lowered SVR, further augmenting cardiac output. In patients receiving chronic beta-blocker therapy or in patients in whom tachycardia is problematic, milrinone is an effective alternative to dobutamine. Milrinone is a type-III phosphodiesterase inhibitor with characteristics of both an inotrope and peripheral vasodilator. It has the disadvantage of renal clearance, and must be used with caution in patients with acute or chronic renal failure. The peripheral vasodilation of milrinone may also cause hypotension, particularly if it is given inappropriately in the setting of volume depletion (Algorithm 22.2, Forrester Class III). Dobutamine and milrinone increase myocardial oxygen demand and should be reserved for cases of documented or suspected cardiogenic shock and systemic hypoperfusion. They do not have a role for mild episodes of ADHF. The use of vasopressors (e.g., dopamine or norepinephrine) may also be necessary in urgent situations to maintain blood pressure while the patient is being stabilized, but they should be weaned quickly as they increase afterload, and may further reduce end-organ perfusion. Table 22.4 shows typical dosing of inotropic agents and vasopressors.

For patients who cannot be adequately stabilized with medical therapy, consideration should be given to mechanical support, particularly if the patient is a candidate for advanced HF therapies such as cardiac transplantation or mechanical circulatory support with a left ventricular assist device (LVAD). Acute dialysis, especially continuous venovenous hemodialysis, can be used for volume control of diuretic-refractory

TABLE 22.4	Inotropic Agents and Vasopressors		
Drug	Class	Dose (μg/kg/min)	Comments
Dobutamine	Inotrope	2.5–10	First line for ADHF
Milrinone	Inotrope/vasodilator	0.25–0.75	Useful with beta-blockade
Dopamine	Inotrope/vasopressor	5–50	Relatively weak agonist
Epinephrine	Inotrope/vasopressor	0.05–0.5	If refractory to dobutamine
Norepinephrine	Vasopressor	0.05–1	More appropriate for sepsis

ADHF, acute decompensated heart failure.

patients with renal failure. Intra-aortic balloon pump placement can provide mechanical afterload reduction, and augmented diastolic pressure to improve coronary artery filling in low-output states. Several temporary VADs have recently become available to provide less invasive mechanical circulatory support in the short term. The Tandem-Heart is a left atrial to femoral artery bypass system capable of providing up to 4 L/min of flow. It consists of an inflow cannula placed into the left atrium from femoral vein via trans-septal puncture, a continuous flow centrifugal (extracorporeal) pump, and an outflow cannula to the femoral artery. The Impella is an all-arterial percutaneous LVAD that utilizes a contained microaxial pump placed retrogradely across the aortic valve via the femoral artery. The catheter removes blood from the left ventricular cavity and pumps it into the ascending aorta. Two different sizes are available, capable of providing 2.5 and 5 L/min of flow, respectively. Finally, the CentriMag is a surgically implanted, temporary LVAD, which can be used to bridge severely decompensated HF patients to definitive therapy with LVAD or heart transplant. Pursuing more advanced mechanical therapy (e.g., LVAD support) or cardiac transplantation is an increasingly viable option for patients without irreversible end-organ damage who are at centers with the appropriate resources; thus early involvement of heart-failure and cardiac surgery specialists should be considered in such patients to facilitate institution of appropriate advanced therapy.

SUGGESTED READINGS

Cuffe MS, Califf RM, Adams KF Jr, et al. Short-term intravenous milrinone for acute exacerbation of chronic heart failure: a randomized controlled trial. *JAMA.* 2002;287:1541–1547.
> *This RCT highlights the dangers of routine inotrope use in ADHF and demonstrates that inotropic agents should be reserved for those patients with evidence of clinically significant hypoperfusion.*

Dickstein K, Cohen-Solal A, Filippatos G, et al. ESC guidelines for the diagnosis and treatment of acute and chronic heart failure 2008: the Task Force for the diagnosis and treatment of acute and chronic heart failure 2008 of the European Society of Cardiology. Developed in collaboration with the Heart Failure Association of the ESC (HFA) and endorsed by the European Society of Intensive Care Medicine (ESICM). *Eur J Heart Fail.* 2008;10:933–989
> *The 2005 ESC guidelines were the first to address the diagnosis and treatment of ADHF in a systematic fashion. The 2008 update cited here remains an excellent overview of the topic and the supporting scientific literature.*

Heart Failure Society of America. Executive summary: HFSA (Heart Failure Society of America) 2010 comprehensive heart failure practice guideline. *J Card Fail.* 2010;16:475–539.
> *While the ESC guidelines are dedicated specifically to ADHF, the 2010 HFSA guidelines represent a consensus-driven approach to establish best practices for diagnosis and treatment of HF, in general, including ADHF.*

Hunt S, Abraham W, Chin M, et al. 2009 Focused update incorporated into the ACC/AHA 2005 guidelines for the diagnosis and management of heart failure in adults. A report of the American College of Cardiology Foundation/American Heart Association Task Force on practice guidelines developed in collaboration with the International Society for Heart and Lung Transplantation. *J Am Coll Cardiol.* 2009;53:e1–e90.
> *The ACC/AHA practice guidelines regarding chronic heart failure provide a broad review of the data substantiating state-of-the art therapies for management of the heart failure patient. New to the 2009 update is a section (4.5) 'The Hospitalized Patient' which provides recommendations for evaluation and management of acute decompensated heart failure.*

Lloyd-Jones D, Adams R, Brown T, et al. Heart disease and stroke statistics–2010 update: a report from the American Heart Association. *Circulation.* 2010;121:e46–e215.
> *This AHA update details the extensive cardiovascular disease burden in the United States.*

McCullough PA, Nowak RM, McCord J, et al. B-type natriuretic peptide and clinical judgment in emergency diagnosis of heart failure: analysis from Breathing Not Properly (BNP) Multinational Study. *Circulation.* 2002;106:416–422.

This study is the most widely recognized trial validating the utility of serum BNP measurement for differentiating heart failure from other entities with similar presentations.

Publication Committee for the VI. Intravenous nesiritide vs nitroglycerin for treatment of decompensated congestive heart failure: a randomized controlled trial. [erratum appears in *JAMA.* 2002;288:577]. *JAMA.* 2002;287:1531–1540.

This trial demonstrates the utility of nesiritide for improving the hemodynamics of patients with ADHF.

Sarkar K, Kini A. Percutaneous left ventricular support devices. *Cardiol Clin.* 2010;28:169–184.

This review describes available percutaneous mechanical support devices. The authors also provide details of placement technique, complications, contraindications, and hemodynamics of each device.

23 Approach to Hypertensive Emergencies

Derrick R. Fansler and Daniel H. Cooper

Hypertensive emergencies have become a less frequent cause for admission to the intensive care unit (ICU) with the widespread availability of antihypertensive medications in the current medical era. Only 1% of patients with hypertension will present with a hypertensive emergency during their lifetime. Unfortunately, severe hypertension is still very common, so distinguishing a true hypertensive emergency from hypertensive urgency is key to guiding therapy. Therefore, the following terms are worth defining.

- *Hypertensive crisis:* A generic term for severe elevations in blood pressure that have the potential to cause target organ (heart, vasculature, kidneys, eyes, brain) damage. This includes both *hypertensive emergency* and *hypertensive urgency.*
- *Hypertensive urgency:* A severe elevation in blood pressure *without* evidence of acute and ongoing target organ damage (TOD).
- *Hypertensive emergency:* A severe elevation in blood pressure *with* evidence of acute, ongoing TOD.
  - *Hypertensive encephalopathy:* A specific hypertensive emergency characterized by irritability, headaches, and mental status changes caused by significant and often, rapid elevations in blood pressure.
  - *Accelerated-malignant hypertension:* A specific hypertensive emergency characterized by fundoscopic findings of papilledema and/or acute retinal hemorrhages and exudates.

Timely differentiation between hypertensive emergencies and urgencies is imperative so that patients with severely elevated blood pressure can be triaged to the appropriate level of care and monitoring (i.e., outpatient follow-up vs. inpatient ward vs. ICU) with the appropriate antihypertensive agents initiated (parenteral vs. oral) and the establishment of blood pressure lowering goals at the appropriate time interval (minutes-to-hours vs. days-to-weeks). In the absence of acute, progressive end-organ damage, elevated blood pressure alone does not require immediate, emergent therapy. The above definitions intentionally are devoid of any absolute blood pressure numbers because the level at which individuals develop TOD can vary depending on clinical substrate and the rapidity with which the blood pressure rises. For example, a patient with long-standing poorly controlled hypertension may tolerate a blood pressure in excess of 230/120 mm Hg without evidence of acute end-organ damage,

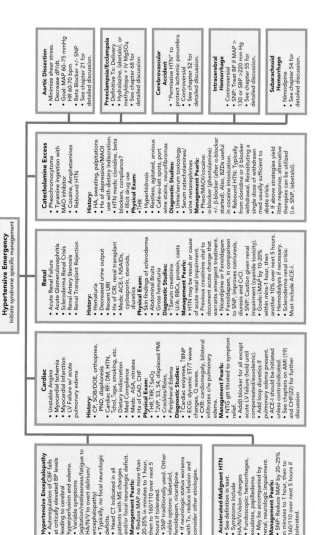

Figure 23.1. Management of specific hypertensive emergencies. CBF, cerebral blood flow; BP, blood pressure; HA headache; N, nauses; V, vomiting; MS, mental status; MAP, mean arterial pressure; SNP, sodium nitroprusside; Tx, treatment; HTN, hypertension; LV, left ventricle; CP, chest pain; SOB, shortness of breath; PND, paroxysmal nocturnal dyspnea; RF, risk factors; DM, diabetes mellitus; chol, cholesterol; ASA, aspirin; CAD, coronary artery disease; CHF, congestive heart failure; HR, heart rate; RR, respiratory rate; SaO_2, saturation arterial oxygen; JVP, jugular venous pressure; PMI, point of maximal impulse; BNP, brain natriuretic peptide; CXR, chest x-ray; IV, intravenous; NTG, nitroglycerin; gtt, drip (intravenous); ACEI, angiotensin-converting enzyme inhibitor; AMI, acute myocardial infraction; URI, upper respiratory infection; Hx, history; CRI, chronic renal insufficiency; NSAIDs, nonsteroidal anti-inflammatory drugs; CrCl, creatinine clearance; MAOI, monoamine oxidase inhibitor; pheo, pheochromocytoma; BZDs, benzodiazepines; dP/dt, rate of change in pressure; bpm, beats per minute.

ALGORITHM 23.1 General Approach to Hypertensive Emergencies

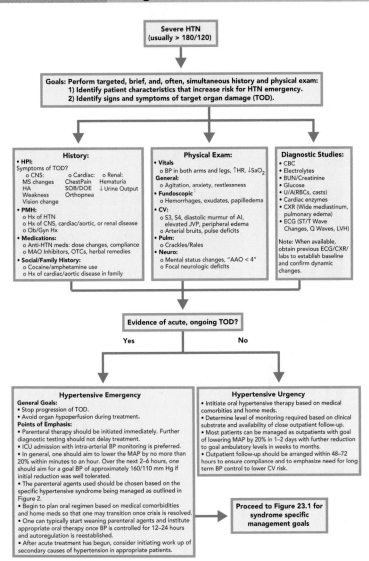

Severe HTN
(usually > 180/120)

Goals: Perform targeted, brief, and, often, simultaneous history and physical exam:
1) Identify patient characteristics that increase risk for HTN emergency.
2) Identify signs and symptoms of target organ damage (TOD).

History:
- **HPI:**
  Symptoms of TOD?
  - o CNS: o Cardiac: o Renal:
    MS changes   ChestPain   Hematuria
    HA   SOB/DOE   ↓ Urine Output
    Weakness   Orthopnea
    Vision change
- **PMH:**
  - o Hx of HTN
  - o Hx of CNS, cardiac/aortic, or renal disease
  - o Ob/Gyn Hx
- **Medications:**
  - o Anti-HTN meds: dose changes, compliance
  - o MAO Inhibitors, OTCs, herbal remedies
- **Social/Family History:**
  - o Cocaine/amphetamine use
  - o Hx of cardiac/aortic disease in family

Physical Exam:
- **Vitals**
  - o BP in both arms and legs, ↑HR, ↓SaO₂
  General:
  - o Agitation, anxiety, restlessness
- **Fundoscopic:**
  - o Hemorrhages, exudates, papilledema
- **CV:**
  - o S3, S4, diastolic murmur of AI,
    elevated JVP, peripheral edema
  - o Arterial bruits, pulse deficits
- **Pulm:**
  - o Crackles/Rales
- **Neuro:**
  - o Mental status changes, "AAO < 4"
  - o Focal neurologic deficits

Diagnostic Studies:
- CBC
- Electrolytes
- BUN/Creatinine
- Glucose
- U/A(RBCs, casts)
- Cardiac enzymes
- CXR (Wide mediastinum, pulmonary edema)
- ECG (ST/T Wave Changes, Q Waves, LVH)

Note: When available, obtain previous ECG/CXR/labs to establish baseline and confirm dynamic changes.

Evidence of acute, ongoing TOD?

Yes   No

Hypertensive Emergency
General Goals:
- Stop progression of TOD.
- Avoid organ hypoperfusion during treatment.
Points of Emphasis:
- Parenteral therapy should be initiated immediately. Further diagnostic testing should not delay treatment.
- ICU admission with intra-arterial BP monitoring is preferred.
- In general, one should aim to lower the MAP by no more than 20% within minutes to an hour. Over the next 2–6 hours, one should aim for a goal BP of approximately 160/110 mm Hg if initial reduction was well tolerated.
- The parenteral agents used should be chosen based on the specific hypertensive syndrome being managed as outlined in Figure 2.
- Begin to plan oral regimen based on medical comorbidities and home meds so that one may transition once crisis is resolved.
- One can typically start weaning parenteral agents and institute appropriate oral therapy once BP is controlled for 12–24 hours and autoregulation is reestablished.
- After acute treatment has begun, consider initiating work up of secondary causes of hypertension in appropriate patients.

Hypertensive Urgency
- Intitiate oral hypertensive therapy based on medical comborities and home meds.
- Determine level of monitoring required based on clinical substrate and availability of close outpatient follow-up.
- Most patients can be managed as outpatients with goal of lowering MAP by 20% in 1–2 days with further reduction to goal ambulatory levels in weeks to months.
- Outpatient follow-up should be arranged within 48–72 hours to ensure compliance and to emphasize need for long term BP control to lower CV risk.

Proceed to Figure 23.1 for syndrome specific management goals

HTN, hypertension; BP, blood pressure; HPI, history of present illness; EOD, end-organ damage; CNS, central nervous system; MS, mental status; HA, headache; SOB, shortness of breath; DOE, dyspnea on exertion; PMH, past medical history; Hx, history; Ob/Gyn, obstetrics/gynecology; MAO monoamine oxidase; OTC, over the counter; HR, heart rate; SaO₂, saturation arterial oxygen; AI, aortic insufficiency; CV cardiovascular; JVP, jugular venous pressure; "AAO <4", note awake, alert and oriented to either person, place, time, or situation; CBC, complete blood count; BUN, blood, urea, nitrogen; U/A, urinalysis; RBC, red blood cells; CXR, chest x-ray; ECG, electrocardiogram; LVH, left ventricular hypertrophy; ICU, intensive care unit; MAP, mean arterial pressure.

TABLE 23.1 Parenteral Agents Used in Hypertensive Emergencies

Drug	Dose	Onset/duration	Adverse effects[a]	Points of emphasis
Sodium nitroprusside	Initial: 0.25–0.50 μg/kg/min continuous infusion Maint: titrate to goal BP up to 8–10 μg/kg/min continuous infusion	Onset: Seconds Duration: 2–3 min after infusion is stopped	Thiocyanate and cyanide poisoning, nausea, vomiting, ↓BP	• Potent arterial and venous dilator with rapid onset and offset of effect. • Preferred agent for most HTN emergencies. • Use with beta-blocker if used in aortic dissection. • Administer via continuous infusion in ICU, guided by intra-arterial BP monitoring. • Caution in renal or hepatic impairment due to thiocyanate/cyanide accumulation. Signs of toxicity include metabolic acidosis, tremors, seizures, nausea, and vomiting. Thiocyanate levels >10 mg/dL should be avoided. • Avoid prolonged use (>24–48 hr) in all patients. Max level infusions should be used for no more than 10 min to limit toxicity. • Increases intracranial pressure but the simultaneous fall in SVR offsets this effect. Therefore, it is still recommended in hypertensive encephalopathy.
Labetalol	Bolus: 20 mg × 1, then 20–80 mg q 10 min to total dose 300 mg or Infusion: 0.5–2 mg/min	Onset: 5–10 min Duration: 3–6 hr	↓HR, HB, HF, bronchospasm, nausea, vomiting, flushing	• Combined alpha and beta-adrenergic blocker. • Can be given as IV bolus or IV infusion. Excessive BP drops are unusual. • Useful in most hypertensive emergencies but avoid in CHF and severe asthma. • Commonly used agent (along with hydralazine) in HTN in pregnancy.

Drug	Dose	Onset/Duration	Side Effects	Comments
Nitroglycerin	Initial: 5 μg/min Maint: titrate q3–5 min up to 100 μg/min	Onset: 2–5 min Duration: 5–15 min	Tolerance, HA, ↓BP, nausea, methemoglobinemia	• Similar to SNP, but causes mostly venodilation with only modest arteriolar dilation effects at higher doses. • Most useful in emergencies complicated by cardiac compromise (i.e., myocardial ischemia/infarct, LV failure/pulmonary edema). • Also indicated in management of postoperative HTN following CABG. • Avoid use with phosphodiesterase-5 inhibitors. • Tolerance will develop with prolonged use.
Hydralazine	Bolus: 10–20 mg q30 min until goal BP	Onset: 10–30 min Duration: 2–4 hr	↓BP, ↑HR, flushing	• Direct arteriolar vasodilator with no significant venous effects. • Caution in patients with CAD or aortic dissection given reflex sympathetic stimulation. Must use with beta-blocker in these patients. • Avoid in patients with increased ICP. • BP lowering response is less predictable than with above agents and, therefore, use should be limited to HTN in pregnancy if possible.
Enalaprilat	Initial: 1.25 mg × 1, then 1.25–5 mg q6hr	Onset: 15–30 min Duration: 6–12 hr	↓BP, renal failure, hyperkalemia	• The only available IV angiotensin-converting enzyme (ACE) inhibitor. • Response to agent is unpredictable and depends on plasma renin activity and volume status of patient. • Most useful as an adjunctive agent in patients with CHF or scleroderma renal crisis. • Contraindicated in pregnancy and in renal-artery stenosis.

(continued)

TABLE 23.1	Parenteral Agents Used in Hypertensive Emergencies *(Continued)*			
Drug	Dose	Onset/duration	Adverse effects[a]	Points of emphasis
Nicardipine	Initial: 5 mg/hr, increase by 2.5 mg/hr q20 min up to max dose, 15 mg/hr	Onset: 15–30 min Duration: 1–4 hr	↓BP, ↑HR, HF, HA nausea, flushing	• Dihydropyridine calcium channel blocker. • Can be used effectively in most emergencies, but should be avoided in acute heart failure. • Reflex tachycardia may be avoided with addition of beta-blocker.
Fenoldopam	Initial: 0.1 μg/kg/min Maint: titrate q15 min, up to 0.6 μg/kg/min	Onset: 3–5 min Duration: 30 min	↑HR, HA, nausea, flushing, hypokalemia	• Selective peripheral dopamine-1 receptor agonist causing primarily arterial vasodilation with rapid onset and relatively short offset of effect. • Shown to improve renal perfusion, therefore, useful in patients with renal impairment. • Contraindicated in patients with glaucoma.
Esmolol	Bolus: 500 μg/kg, repeat after 5 min Infusion: 50–100 μg/kg/min, up to 300 μg/kg/min	Onset: 1–5 min Duration: 15–30 min	↓HR, HB, HF, bronchospasm, nausea, vomiting, flushing	• Short-acting, cardioselective beta-adrenergic blocker. • If concern for significant adverse effects to beta-blockers, short duration of esmolol may be useful.
Phentolamine	Bolus: 5–10 mg, repeat q5–15 min Infusion: 0.2–5.0 mg/min	Onset: 1–2 min Duration: 10–20 min	↑HR, HA, nausea	• Alpha-adrenergic blocker, used primarily in syndromes associated with excess catecholamines (i.e., pheochromocytoma, tyramine ingestion while on MAOI).

[a]Either common or life-threatening adverse effects of these medications are listed. This does not represent a comprehensive list of all possible adverse effects.
↓BP, hypotension; ↓HR, bradycardia; ↑HR, tachycardia; HB, heart block; HF, heart failure; HA, headache; Maint, maintenance dose; SNP, sodium nitroprusside; LV, left ventricle; HTN, hypertension; ICP, intracranial pressure; SVR, systemic vascular resistance; CABG, coronary artery bypass grafting; IV, intravenous; MAO, monoamine oxidase inhibitor.

while the young healthy patient who acutely develops glomerulonephritis may become encephalopathic from hypertension at much lower pressures.

The approach to severely elevated blood pressure is outlined in Algorithm 23.1. It should be emphasized that when presented with these patients, one should perform a truncated history and physical exam that (1) quickly identifies patient characteristics that place the patient at risk for hypertensive emergencies and (2) searches for signs and/or symptoms of underlying TOD. If this rapid assessment reveals evidence for a true hypertensive emergency, then treatment should be initiated immediately, preferably in an ICU setting.

The goal of treating hypertensive emergency is to sufficiently lower arterial pressure to stop the progression of TOD without overcorrecting and causing organ hypoperfusion. This careful balance is best achieved with parenteral agents that have a rapid onset and short half-life, administered under the guidance of intra-arterial blood pressure monitoring in an ICU setting. Oral and sublingual agents should not be used as initial treatment for hypertensive emergency due to their variable effects with slower onset and longer half-life. Sodium nitroprusside can be rapidly titrated and is the preferred agent in most hypertensive emergencies. (Table 23.1 has details for agents used in hypertensive emergencies.) One must tailor therapy with syndrome-specific management, as outlined in Figure 23.1.

SUGGESTED READINGS

Calhoun DA, Oparil S. Treatment of hypertensive crisis. *N Engl J Med.* 1990;323:1177.
  A review of treatment options for the hypertensive crisis.
Choubanian AV, Bakris GL, Black HR, et al. Seventh report of the Joint National Committee on Prevention, Detection, Evaluation and Treatment of High Blood Pressure. *Hypertension.* 2003;42:1206–1252.
  JNC VII, a comprehensive expert review of hypertension, including sections dedicated to addressing approach to hypertensive emergencies.
Elliot WJ. Clinical features in the management of selected hypertensive emergencies. *Prog Cardiovasc Dis.* 2006;48:316–325.
  Concise review of definitions, epidemiology, pathophysiology, and syndrome-specific treatment options.
Kaplan NM. Hypertensive crises. In: Kaplan NM, ed. Kaplan's clinical hypertension, 9th ed. Philadelphia, PA: Lippincott Williams and Wilkins, 2006:311–324.
  A leader in hypertension provides his approach to management of hypertensive crises. Also embedded elsewhere in text are chapters that address HTN in pregnancy, catecholamine excess states, renal failure, etc. in greater detail.
Rehman SU, Basile JN, Vidt DG. Hypertensive emergencies and urgencies. In: Black HR, Elliot WJ, eds. Hypertension: A companion to Braunwald's heart disease. Philadelphia, PA: Saunders-Elsevier, 2007:517–524.
  A current review of approach to hypertensive urgencies and emergencies in a comprehensive text dedicated to addressing all aspects of hypertension, written by leaders in the field.

24 Electrolyte Abnormalities

Ahsan Usman and Seth Goldberg

DISORDERS OF WATER BALANCE

Hyponatremia and hypernatremia are primarily disorders of *water* balance (osmoregulation) or *water* distribution across the various fluid compartments in the body. The countercurrent mechanisms of the kidneys in concert with the hypothalamic osmoreceptors via antidiuretic hormone (ADH) secretion maintain a very finely tuned balance of water. When the serum osmolality becomes too dilute (<280 mOsm/kg), excess water is excreted by the kidneys as dilute urine. Conversely, when the serum osmolality becomes too concentrated (>290 mOsm/kg), ADH release and thirst result in water retention to bring the system back into balance. Defects in such handling of water present as hyponatremia or hypernatremia (Fig. 24.1).

Although it may seem that regulation of this plasma Na^+ concentration must have something to do with total Na^+ balance, osmoregulation is almost entirely mediated by changes in *water balance.* Thus, the effectors for *osmoregulation* (ADH and thirst, affecting water excretion and water intake) are very different from those involved in *volume regulation* (renin-angiotensin-aldosterone system, atrial natriuretic peptide, and the sympathetic nervous system) that affect sodium excretion (Fig. 24.2). ADH does play a small overlapping role in volume regulation, where it can maintain volume, but at the expense of osmolality.

The incidence of hyponatremia and hypernatremia in the intensive care unit (ICU) may each be 15% to 30%. Their significance lies not only in their direct clinical effects in the individual patient but also through their ability to predict mortality. The in-hospital mortality of patients with either hyponatremia or hypernatremia is approximately 30% to 40%, which is significantly greater than for normonatremic patients.

The most osmotically sensitive organ in the body is the brain. Therefore, it should not be surprising that symptoms of hyponatremia and hypernatremia predominantly involve the nervous system as water shifts into or out of neurons. Hyponatremia results in water entry, leading to cell swelling within the fixed cranial vault (with risk of herniation), while hypernatremia results in cell shrinkage and tearing of the brain away from the meninges (with risk of hemorrhage). The severity of clinical symptoms often depends on the *acuity* of the disturbance and not just the *magnitude*, as neurons have the capability to adapt to gradual changes over 48 hours. Hyponatremia and hypernatremia can present with similar symptomatology, and range from headache to confusion, stupor, or seizures and coma.

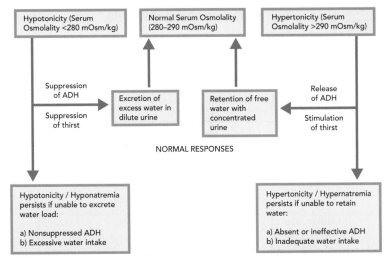

Figure 24.1. Regulation of osmolality. ADH, antidiuretic hormone.

Hyponatremia

When evaluating a patient for hyponatremia (Algorithm 24.1), one should first confirm that the low [Na$^+$] truly reflects a hypotonic state by checking the serum osmolality. When normal, "pseudohyponatremia" as a measurement artifact was likely present. When paradoxically *elevated*, a hypertonic disorder (e.g., hyperglycemia, mannitol, and glycine) accounts for water shifting out of cells, diluting the serum [Na$^+$]. If there

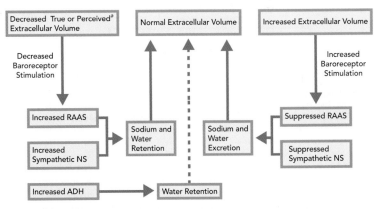

Figure 24.2. Regulation of extracellular volume. ADH, antidiuretic hormone; NS, nervous system; RAAS, renin–angiotensin–aldosterone system. ^{a}Decreased perceived extracellular volume occurs in decompensated congestive heart failure and cirrhosis, leading to a maladaptive sodium-avid state and edema.

ALGORITHM 24.1   Evaluation of Hyponatremia

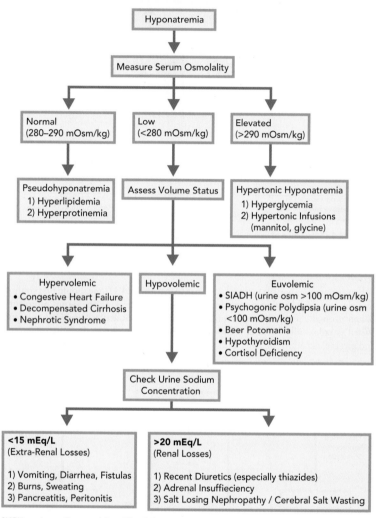

SIADH, syndrome of inappropriate antidiuretic hormone.

is indeed hypotonic hyponatremia, the patient's volume status can help determine if there is ADH from true hypovolemia, or from a perceived decrease in effective circulating volume leading to an edematous state. If the patient is euvolemic, the cause is either from "inappropriate" ADH secretion (nonosmotic, nonvolume mediated) or from hypotonic fluid loading (e.g., psychogenic polydipsia); these can be distinguished by the urine osmolality, which should be maximally dilute (<50 to 100 mOsm/kg) if ADH is appropriately suppressed.

Etiologies of Special Importance in the Critically Ill Patient

Hyperglycemia (Hypertonic Hyponatremia)

Glucose acts as an osmotically active solute because it is restricted to the extracellular fluid (ECF) in states of insulin deficiency. In the marked hyperglycemia of diabetic ketoacidosis (DKA) and hyperosmolar hyperglycemic states, the ECF hyperosmolarity (usually >290 mOsm/kg) causes water to shift from the intracellular fluid (ICF) compartment to the ECF, and dilutional hyponatremia ensues. The plasma [Na^+] falls by 2.4 mEq/L for every 100 mg/dL rise in the plasma [glucose] above normal.

Edematous States (Hypervolemic Hyponatremia)

Heart failure and cirrhosis result in a decreased "effective circulating volume." Given the primacy of volume preservation, the body's response to this perceived threat is to hold onto salt and water, with "nonosmotic" ADH release as part of the response. Thus, water excretion is submaximal. If the rise in total body water exceeds the increase in total body sodium, hyponatremia results. The degree of hyponatremia often correlates with the severity of the underlying condition.

Syndrome of Inappropriate ADH (Euvolemic Hyponatremia)

"Nonosmotic" release of ADH (either from the posterior pituitary or an ectopic source) also underlies the pathophysiology of the syndrome of inappropriate antidiuretic hormone (SIADH). However, these patients are euvolemic, indicating that a true or perceived volume deficit is not the stimulus for ADH production. The urine osmolality is inappropriately concentrated (>100 mOsm/kg) for the prevailing hypotonic state, indicating the "inappropriate" presence of ADH. Commonly associated conditions include neuropsychiatric disorders (e.g., meningitis, encephalitis, acute psychosis, cerebrovascular accident, and head trauma), pulmonary diseases (e.g., pneumonia, tuberculosis, positive pressure ventilation, and acute respiratory failure), malignant tumors (most commonly, small cell lung cancer), and physical/emotional stress and pain. Before making the diagnosis of SIADH, pharmacologic agents that enhance ADH action must be withdrawn:

- Nicotine, carbamazepine, antidepressants, narcotics, antipsychotic agents, and certain antineoplastic drugs may stimulate ADH release
- Chlorpropamide, methylxanthines, and nonsteroidal anti-inflammatory drugs (NSAIDs) potentiate the action of ADH
- Oxytocin and desmopressin acetate are ADH analogs.

Also, deficiencies of thyroid hormone or cortisol can present with euvolemic hyponatremia and should be ruled out.

Cerebral Salt Wasting (Hypovolemic Hyponatremia)

Neurosurgery and central nervous system trauma, especially subarachnoid hemorrhage, may be associated with excessive renal Na^+ excretion. Although poorly understood, the mechanism may involve the release of a brain natriuretic peptide and/or the loss of renal sympathetic tone. The loss of Na^+ results in volume depletion, which leads to the "nonosmotic" release of ADH. This volume depletion is the main feature that distinguishes cerebral salt wasting from SIADH. The hyponatremia, however, does not always correct with volume resuscitation, perhaps as a result of concomitant ADH release from the damaged brain. In some cases, the use of fludrocortisone can ameliorate the decline in [Na^+].

ALGORITHM 24.2 Treatment of Hyponatremia

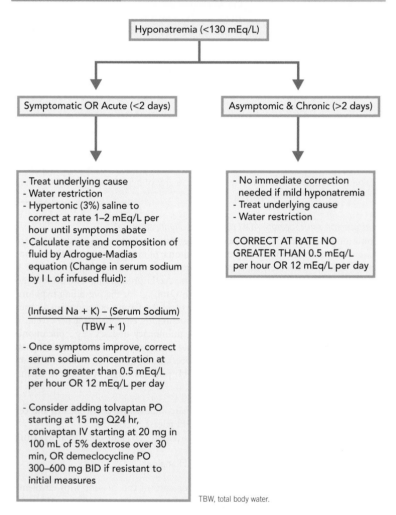

Hyponatremia (<130 mEq/L)

Symptomatic OR Acute (<2 days)

- Treat underlying cause
- Water restriction
- Hypertonic (3%) saline to correct at rate 1–2 mEq/L per hour until symptoms abate
- Calculate rate and composition of fluid by Adrogue-Madias equation (Change in serum sodium by I L of infused fluid):

$$\frac{(\text{Infused Na} + \text{K}) - (\text{Serum Sodium})}{(\text{TBW} + 1)}$$

- Once symptoms improve, correct serum sodium concentration at rate no greater than 0.5 mEq/L per hour OR 12 mEq/L per day

- Consider adding tolvaptan PO starting at 15 mg Q24 hr, conivaptan IV starting at 20 mg in 100 mL of 5% dextrose over 30 min, OR demeclocycline PO 300–600 mg BID if resistant to initial measures

Asymptomic & Chronic (>2 days)

- No immediate correction needed if mild hyponatremia
- Treat underlying cause
- Water restriction

CORRECT AT RATE NO GREATER THAN 0.5 mEq/L per hour OR 12 mEq/L per day

TBW, total body water.

Treatment

The hyponatremia in *hypertonic* or *isotonic* states is usually of little clinical significance as fluid shifts and neuronal swelling do not occur or are readily corrected. When true *hypotonic* hyponatremia occurs, the rate of correction depends on the acuity with which it developed and the degree of symptomatology exhibited by the patient. Overly rapid correction can precipitate central pontine myelinolysis (CPM). In its most complete form, CPM is characterized by flaccid paralysis, dysarthria, dysphagia, and death.

Algorithm 24.2 outlines the standard treatment of hyponatremia. When the process is acute (duration of <2 days) or when severe neurological dysfunction is

---

Box 24.1

Adrogue–Madias equation:

Change in $[Na^+]$ per liter = (infusate $[Na^+]$ + $[K^+]$ − Serum $[Na^+]$)/ (estimated total body water (kg) + 1)

Total body water = 60% of body weight

Infusate $[Na^+]$ for selected fluids:

3% Hypertonic saline: 513 mEq/L

Normal (0.9%) saline: 154 mEq/L

Ringer's lactate: 130 mEq/L (+4 mEq/L of potassium)

Half-normal (0.45%) saline: 77 mEq/L

5%-Dextrose (D5) water: 0 mEq/L

Example no. 1:

An obtunded 70 kg man presents with a serum $[Na^+]$ of 110 mEq/L. His clinician concludes that the $[Na^+]$ needs to be increased by 4 mEq/L in 2 hours using 3% hypertonic saline.

Expected change in $[Na^+]$ per liter of 3% saline = (513 − 110)/(42 + 1) = 9.37 mEq/L

Amount of fluid required to achieve desired change: 4/9.37 = 0.4 L (400 mL)

Rate of infusion: 400 mL/2 hr = 200 mL/hr

---

present, correction of the serum $[Na^+]$ can be 1 to 2 mEq/L per hour until symptoms improve, then slowed to no more than 0.5 mEq/L per hour. When the hyponatremia has been present for at least 2 days, correction should begin at no more than 0.5 mEq/L per hour, or no more than 12 mEq/L over a 24-hour period.

Most cases of hyponatremia can be corrected with free water restriction. When more urgent correction is needed, 3% hypertonic saline can be used cautiously to raise the $[Na^+]$. The Adrogue–Madias equation (Box 24.1) can be used to estimate the expected change in $[Na^+]$ after 1 L of infusion; this anticipated change needs to be spread out over a number of hours to prevent overly rapid correction. However, this equation (and others) does not take into account the ongoing urinary losses and are notoriously inaccurate. There is no substitute for measuring the serum $[Na^+]$ frequently (initially every 1 to 2 hours) to ensure a safe rate of correction.

Any saline solution that is hypertonic to the *urine* can increase the $[Na^+]$ when oral water intake is restricted. Addition of intravenous (IV) loop diuretics can promote further water excretion by blocking the concentrating ability of the kidney. However, administering a fluid with an osmolarity *less than urine osmolarity* may actually worsen the hyponatremia, even if the fluid's $[Na^+]$ is greater than the serum $[Na^+]$. For example, if a patient with a serum $[Na^+]$ of 110 mEq/L and urine osmolality persistently >500 mOsm/kg from SIADH is given normal saline to attempt to correct the hyponatremia, the 308 mOsm (154 Na^+ + 154 Cl^-) contained in the liter of fluid will be extracted and concentrated down into a smaller volume of urine, resulting in the retention of further free water and worsening of the hyponatremia.

ALGORITHM 24.3 Evaluation of Hypernatremia

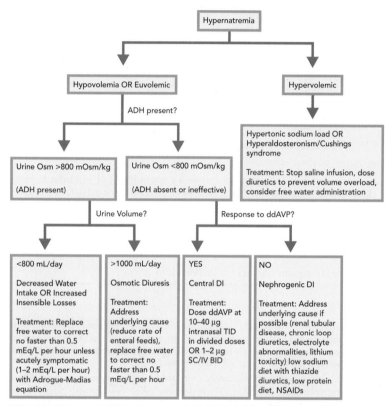

ADH, antidiuretic hormone; ddAVP, arginine vasopressin; DI, diabetes insipidus; NSAIDs, nonsteroidal anti-inflammatory drugs.

Hypernatremia

Hypernatremia is almost always the result of a relative water deficit (Algorithm 24.3). The three primary mechanisms are (a) decreased free water intake, (b) increased free water loss, or (c) excessive gain of hypertonic fluid.

Etiologies of Special Importance in the Critically Ill Patient

Decreased Water Intake

The most common etiology for hypernatremia in hospitalized patients is decreased free water intake. Although thirst is indeed a powerful stimulus, patients in certain circumstances may lack the ability to access or request water (nursing home resident with dementia or sedated, intubated patient in the ICU). Thus, even at maximal ADH release and urinary concentration (urine osmolality >800 mOsm/kg), hypernatremia may ensue.

Insensible Free Water Loss

In ambulatory adults at room temperature, hypotonic fluid loss occurs from the skin and respiratory tract, each at a rate of approximately 400 to 500 mL/day. However, insensible water losses greatly depend on the respiratory rate, body temperature, ambient temperature, and humidity. These variables make losses much more difficult to predict in the ICU patient who may be mechanically ventilated. In general, water losses increase by 100 to 150 mL/day for each degree of body temperature more than 37°C. Still, fluid losses from the skin can vary enormously (100 to 2000 mL/hr) with sweating or in the setting of severe burns. If these insensible losses are not matched in addition to calculated free water loss, hypernatremia will develop.

Diabetes Insipidus

As noted above, the appropriate renal response to hypernatremia is excretion of maximally concentrated urine (>800 mOsm/kg) under the control of ADH. These responses are diminished in diabetes insipidus (DI), where there is either impaired ADH secretion (central DI) or resistance to its effect at the kidney (nephrogenic DI), resulting in an inappropriately dilute urine. Central DI is typically the result of damage to the neurohypophysis from trauma, neurosurgery, granulomatous disease, neoplasms, vascular accidents, or infection. Nephrogenic DI can be classified into disorders associated with intrinsic renal diseases of the collecting duct where ADH acts (e.g., sickle cell nephropathy, polycystic kidney disease, obstructive nephropathy, and Sjogren syndrome), drugs (e.g., lithium, demeclocycline, amphotericin, and glyburide), electrolyte disorders (hypercalcemia and hypokalemia), and conditions that reduce renal medullary hypertonicity (e.g., excessive water intake and the chronic use of loop diuretics).

Osmotic Diuresis

Osmotic diuresis occurs when an osmolar load passes through the kidney, drawing out large amounts of water into the urine. This commonly results from poorly controlled diabetes mellitus and its associated glycosuria. IV mannitol, retained uremic toxins in recovering renal failure, or large enteral solute loads with high osmolar tube feeds can also result in an osmotic diuresis. This cause of hypernatremia can resemble DI with its large urine volumes, but is distinguished by measuring the increased number of osmoles excreted in the urine per day.

Primary Na^+ Gain

Critically ill patients often require the administration of large amounts of saline solutions, such as normal saline or sodium bicarbonate during cardiopulmonary resuscitation. Normally functioning kidneys have a large capacity to excrete this excess sodium load, and so iatrogenic hypernatremia is uncommon unless there is a concomitant urinary concentration defect.

Treatment

Hypernatremia treatment is outlined in Algorithm 24.3. The same principles as for hyponatremia apply here are well, since overly rapid correction (particularly if brain adaptation has occurred over 2 days) can result in dangerous fluid shifts. Excessive correction can result in water entering the cells, leading to cerebral edema and fatal brain herniation. Correction should be not faster than 0.5 mEq/L per hour unless acute symptoms are present or the disorder is of acute onset (<2 days), in which case correction can be 1 to 2 mEq/L per hour until symptoms abate.

The Adrogue–Madias equation (Box 24.2) used in correcting hyponatremia also applies to hypernatremia. The typical fluid used in 5% dextrose (D5W) containing no sodium, although in cases of concomitant volume depletion, normal saline or half-normal saline can be used initially to correct the volume deficit (note that even at an infusate $[Na^+]$ of 154 mEq/L, the serum sodium concentration would improve if it starts above this level, albeit slowly). One needs to be sure to include on-going water losses (sensible and insensible) to the amount being replaced. Once again, equations are not precise, and one must be sure to serially check the serum $[Na^+]$ to ensure overly rapid correction is avoided.

Box 24.2

Adrogue–Madias equation:

Change in $[Na^+]$ per liter = (infusate $[Na^+]$ + $[K^+]$ − serum $[Na^+]$)/ (estimated total body water (kg) + 1)

Total body water = 60% of body weight

Infusate $[Na^+]$ for selected fluids:

3% Hypertonic saline: 513 mEq/L

Normal (0.9%) saline: 154 mEq/L

Ringer's lactate: 130 mEq/L (+4 mEq/L of potassium)

Half-normal (0.45%) saline: 77 mEq/L

5%-Dextrose (D5) water: 0 mEq/L.

Example no. 2:

An 70 kg woman presents with lassitude and a serum $[Na^+]$ of 160 mEq/L. She is having 2 L or diarrhea and 1 L of urine output each day. The replacement fluid chosen is 5% dextrose in water.

Expected change in $[Na^+]$ per liter of 5% dextrose = (0 − 160)/(42 + 1) = −3.72 mEq/L

One liter would need to be given over 7 to 8 hours to correct at a rate of 0.5 mEq/L (3.72/0.5 = 7.44)

Rate of infusion: 1000 mL over 8 hr = 125 mL/hr

Then, to account for on-going water losses: (3000 mL per day)/24 = 125 mL/hr

Total fluid to be given: 125 + 125 = 250 mL/hr

Note some are more familiar with the calculation of the "free water deficit." This calculation can yield a similar answer, although it does not directly account for the rate of correction or fluid used.

Free water deficit: TBW [(Serum $[Na^+]$/140) − 1] = 42[(160/140) − 1] = 6 L

If one was to correct this to 140 mEq/L with 5% dextrose, the change in 20 mEq/L would need to occur over roughly 40 to 48 hours to avoid overly rapid correction. Adding back the 3 L/day of on-going losses, or 6 L over these 2 days, the total to be replaced is 12 L over 48 hours, or 250 mL/hr.

DISORDERS OF VOLUME BALANCE

In contrast to the regulation of water balance (osmoregulation) that is reflected by serum *sodium concentration,* control of the ECF volume depends on *total body sodium* (Fig. 24.2). Volume-depleted states result from total body sodium loss, while edematous states reflect total body sodium gain. As long as osmoregulatory mechanisms remain intact, the serum [Na$^+$] and serum osmolality remain normal.

True volume depletion, sensed by baroreceptors, results in the activation of the renin-angiotensin-aldosterone system, sympathetic nervous system, and, to some degree, ADH to promote the retention of salt and water. Urinary sodium excretion is low (often <15 mEq/L). In congestive heart failure or decompensated cirrhosis, the "effective circulating volume" is diminished, and these same responses occur. However, instead of correcting the underlying state, this excess salt and water retention results in edema formation, ascites, and still the salt-avid state persists, to the point that it has become maladaptive.

Treatment of these edema-forming conditions is often centered on the underlying cause. Loop diuretics and potassium-sparing diuretics (spironolactone) in combination with salt and water restriction can alleviate the swelling. Renal function must be followed carefully as overzealous diuresis can precipitate a drop in the glomerular filtration rate and is particularly worrisome in the case of hepatorenal syndrome in decompensated cirrhosis. When advanced congestive heart failure compromises renal perfusion, diuresis may paradoxically improve renal function as cardiac performance is enhanced. These disorders are further covered in Chapters 22 and 47.

DISORDERS OF POTASSIUM CONCENTRATION

The total body potassium in a normal adult is approximately 3000 to 4000 mEq, of which 98% is intracellular. Perturbations in the serum [K$^+$] therefore are generally the result of transcellular shifts, and do not accurately reflect the total body K$^+$ deficit or excess. Potassium excretion is primarily accomplished by the kidneys, at the level of the collecting duct under the influence of aldosterone. This process is coupled to sodium resorption, and therefore volume repletion and blood pressure elevation. Aldosterone activity on the collecting duct also stimulates H$^+$ excretion, and thus the acid–base status of the patient often offers a clue to the underlying cause of potassium disorders.

Hypokalemia

Hypokalemia can result from (a) shifting of potassium into cells, (b) renal wasting, or (c) extrarenal losses (Algorithm 24.4). Calculating the transtubular K$^+$ gradient (TTKG) may help distinguish renal from extrarenal losses, although clues from the history will often suffice. The TTKG is calculated as (urine [K$^+$] x serum osmolality)/(serum [K$^+$] × urine osmolality), and reflects potassium losses in the urine. The TTKG should be <3 *in the setting of hypokalemia,* reflecting renal conservation; a level greater than this suggests inappropriate renal wasting of potassium.

Symptoms of hypokalemia seldom occur unless the potassium concentration is <3.0 mEq/L, with more acute changes having greater effect. Neuromuscular fatigue, weakness, cramps, constipation, or ileus may occur and even progress to rhabdomyolysis or ascending paralysis when the potassium concentration falls to 2.0 mEq/L. Although the ECG does not correlate well with [K$^+$], progressive changes may be seen in the individual patient. Moderate hypokalemia may have T-wave flattening,

ALGORITHM 24.4 Evaluation of Hypokalemia

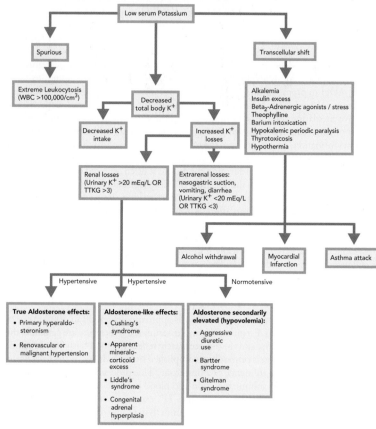

TTKG; transtubular K^+ gradient, WBC; white blood cell count.

ST-segment depression, and the appearance of U-waves. Severe hypokalemia shows decreased voltage, PR-interval prolongation, and QRS widening.

Etiologies of Special Importance in the Critically Ill Patient
Transcellular Shifts
Movement of K^+ into cells may transiently decrease the plasma $[K^+]$ without altering total body K^+ content. The magnitude of the change is relatively small, often <1 mEq/L, but may exaggerate hypokalemia from other causes. Triggers of intracellular shift include alkalemia, insulin activity, and catecholamine excess. The refeeding syndrome, where nutritional support is initiated after a prolonged period of starvation, is a classic scenario where a transcellular shift exacerbates the hypokalemia in a patient with deficient stores.

Renal Wasting

Increased potassium loss in the kidney can be the result of increased urine flow (e.g., loop or thiazide diuretic use, and osmotic diuresis) or an elevated aldosterone state (usually with concomitant metabolic alkalosis). The presence of volume overload and hypertension suggests that the aldosterone (or aldosterone-like) effect is driving the underlying process (primary hyperaldosteronism, apparent mineralocorticoid excess, Liddle syndrome). When euvolemia and normal blood pressures are present, the aldosterone effect is secondary (or reactive) in response to a volume-depleted state (Bartter syndrome, Gitelman syndrome, diuretic use).

Extrarenal K^+ Loss

Gastrointestinal fluids (e.g., saliva, stomach secretions, and diarrhea) have significant K^+ content and therefore excessive enteral losses will result in hypokalemia. When vomiting is the primary cause, there is often a concomitant metabolic alkalosis from the acid loss. However, metabolic acidosis typically prevails when diarrhea is the prominent cause, from the bicarbonate loss.

Treatment

Treatment of hypokalemia is outlined in Algorithm 24.5. Rapid correction of hypokalemia is required when symptoms or ECG changes are present. In these cases and when patients are unable to take oral medications, IV repletion is appropriate. Otherwise it is generally safer to correct hypokalemia via the enteral route, and larger doses can be administered orally. Potassium chloride (KCl) is typically the preparation of choice regardless of the route of administration as it promotes more rapid correction of hypokalemia and concomitant metabolic alkalosis than the other preparations.

ALGORITHM 24.5 Treatment of Hypokalemia

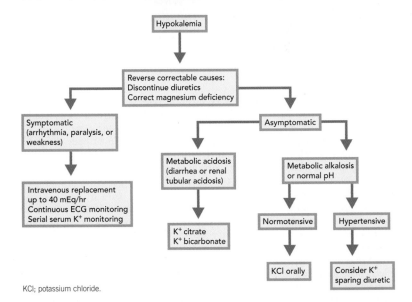

KCl; potassium chloride.

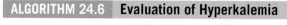
ALGORITHM 24.6 Evaluation of Hyperkalemia

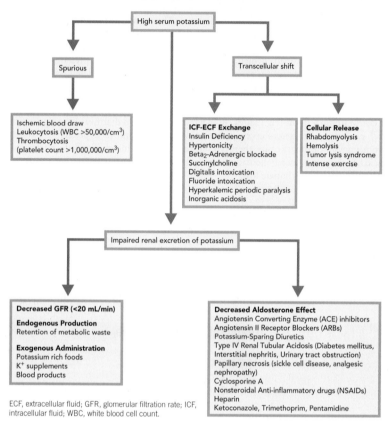

ECF, extracellular fluid; GFR, glomerular filtration rate; ICF, intracellular fluid; WBC, white blood cell count.

Potassium bicarbonate or citrate may be useful in cases associated with metabolic acidosis (e.g., chronic diarrhea, renal tubular acidosis). Hypomagnesemia should be sought in all hypokalemic patients and corrected prior to or concurrently with K^+ repletion. A decrement of 1 mEq/L represents an estimated total body deficit of 200 to 400 mEq. However, the serum $[K^+]$ should be monitored frequently during therapy as this total body deficit is difficult to estimate accurately.

Hyperkalemia

There are three main mechanisms of hyperkalemia (Algorithm 24.6): (a) transcellular shifts, (b) reduced glomerular filtration, (c) or effective aldosterone deficiency. Sustained hyperkalemia almost always requires decreased renal function as normal kidneys have a tremendous capacity for K^+ excretion.

Symptoms of hyperkalemia are more pronounced when acute. Neuromuscular effects may manifest as weakness that can progress to flaccid paralysis and hypoventilation. As with hypokalemia, ECG changes do not correlate well with hyperkalemia, although progressive changes are seen within the individual. Moderate hyperkalemia shows peaked T-waves with increased amplitude. More severe $[K^+]$ elevations cause prolonged PR-intervals and QRS duration, atrioventricular delays, and loss of P-waves. Profound hyperkalemia causes progressive widening of the QRS complex and merging with the T-wave to produce sine waves; ventricular fibrillation and asystole may ultimately occur.

Etiologies of Special Importance in the Critically Ill Patient

Transcellular Shifts

The movement of K^+ from the ICF to the ECF may transiently increase the plasma $[K^+]$ without altering total body K^+ content, often amplifying the hyperkalemia resulting from other causes. Potential causes of extracellular shift include insulin deficiency, ECF hyperosmolarity, inorganic acidemia, and cell breakdown (e.g., rhabdomyolysis, hemolysis, and tumor lysis syndrome). DKA may promote hyperkalemia through relative insulin deficiency, despite the presence of total body potassium depletion. Medications that cause extracellular shifts include nonselective beta-blockers, digitalis, and succinylcholine. The hyperkalemia that occurs with succinylcholine is usually small (0.5 mEq/L) and brief (resolving within 10 to 15 minutes), but it can be significantly accentuated in patients with massive trauma, burns, or neuromuscular disease.

Reduced Glomerular Filtration

Diseased kidneys respond to progressive insufficiency with increased potassium excretion per functioning nephron. This compensation is typically adequate until the glomerular filtration rate falls to the point of oliguria. Thus, when hyperkalemia develops in a nonoliguric patient, there is usually a second contributing mechanism or the renal injury is severe and acute. Diminished distal tubular fluid delivery, as occurs in volume depletion (prerenal azotemia), is a common contributing mechanism in the critically ill patient.

Effective Aldosterone Deficiency

Medications typically account for the relative hypoaldosterone state that contributes to hyperkalemia in the ICU patient. Heparin, ketoconazole, angiotensin-converting enzyme (ACE) inhibitors, and angiotensin II receptor blockers (ARBs) decrease aldosterone production. Spironolactone and eplerenone are competitive aldosterone antagonists, while amiloride, triamterene, trimethoprim, and pentamidine all block sodium resorption (and thus potassium excretion) at the collecting duct where aldosterone would exert its effect. NSAIDs inhibit renin secretion, a process that is several steps upstream of aldosterone release; these medications can also decrease glomerular filtration in volume-depleted states through the inhibition of local vasodilatory prostaglandins.

Treatment

Hyperkalemia treatment is outlined in Table 24.1. The presence of symptoms or ECG changes associated with hyperkalemia necessitates the prompt initiation of measures capable of rapidly lowering the serum $[K^+]$. Calcium serves to stabilize the cardiac myocyte membrane but does not actually reduce the $[K^+]$; therefore it is given simultaneously with other therapies that shift potassium into the cell (insulin and albuterol) and promote its excretion (sodium polystyrene sulfonate, diuretics, and hemodialysis). The use of sodium bicarbonate to shift potassium intracellularly is falling out of favor given its comparatively weak effect in the absence of an inorganic metabolic acidosis. Dialytic therapies are generally reserved for cases of severe hyperkalemia not responsive to medical management.

TABLE 24.1 Acute Therapies for the Management of Hyperkalemia

Treatment	Dosing	Onset/duration	Magnitude of [K⁺] decline	Comments
Ca^{2+}	1 g of 10% calcium gluconate or calcium chloride infused IV over 2–3 min; may repeat if no improvement in ECG by 5 min	Immediate onset, lasting 30–60 min	None	Calcium chloride should be administered via a central vein to decrease risk of extravasation and skin necrosis
Insulin	10 U of regular insulin IV (with one ampule of D50 IV if not significantly hyperglycemic)	Onset at 15 min, lasting 6–8 hr	~1 mEq/L	Watch for hypo- or hyperglycemia (if dextrose given); the latter can offset insulin's K^+ lowering effect
Albuterol	10–20 mg given by nebulized inhalation over 15 min OR 0.5 mg in 100 mL of 5% dextrose infused IV over 15 min	Onset at 10–30 min, lasting 3–6 hr	1–1.5 mEq/L	Tachycardia and variable effects on blood pressure may result; hyperglycemia may worsen and offset some K^+ lowering effect
$NaHCO_3$	2–4 mEq/min in drip (3 ampules $NaHCO_3$ in sterile water or 5% dextrose) until bicarbonate normalized	Onset at 4 hr, lasting >6 hr	0.5–0.75 mEq/L	Not effective unless concurrent inorganic metabolic acidosis; watch for volume overload and may lower serum ionized [Ca^{2+}] and make more susceptible to arrhythmias
Loop +/– thiazide diuretics	Widely variable dose depends on GFR	Onset at 30–60 min, lasting 4–6 hr (duration prolonged in renal insufficiency)	Variable depending on diuretic response	Avoid in volume-depleted states until euvolemia restored
Sodium polystyrene sulfonate	25–50 g mixed in 100 mL 20% sorbitol PO OR 50 g in 200 mL 30% sorbitol per rectum	Onset at 1–2 hr, lasting 4–6 hr	0.5–1 mEq/L	Caution with use in the postoperative patient because of risk of intestinal necrosis; watch for worsening volume overload or hypernatremia from exchanged [Na^+]
Hemodialysis	Variable, based on starting [K^+]	Immediate onset, lasting until dialysis completion	Variable, based on dialysis dose and dialysate [K^+]	Watch for post-treatment K^+ rebound beginning immediately after dialysis completion

IV, intravenous; ECG, electrocardiogram; GFR, glomerular filtration rate; PO, by mouth

Another important component of therapy is to limit exogenous potassium intake. Each 8-ounce can of high-protein tube feeds contains approximately 10 mEq of K^+, and a single unit of packed red blood cells with a prolonged storage time may contribute approximately 5 mEq.

DISORDERS OF CALCIUM CONCENTRATION

The extracellular calcium concentration is tightly maintained and reflects the coordinated action of multiple hormones: parathyroid hormone (PTH), 1,25-OH vitamin D (calcitriol), and to a lesser extent, calcitonin. Approximately 99% of body calcium is in bone with most of the remaining 1% in the ECF. The total plasma calcium concentration consists of three fractions:

• Approximately 45% circulates as the physiologically active ionized (or free) calcium
• About 40% is bound to albumin, with greater binding in alkalemia
• The remaining 15% is bound to multiple organic and inorganic anions such as sulfate, phosphate, lactate, and citrate.

The ionized Ca^{2+} concentration, which must lie within a narrow range (4.6 to 5.1 mg/dL) for optimal neuromuscular function, is under exquisitely tight minute-to-minute control by PTH. PTH increases serum $[Ca^{2+}]$ by stimulating bone resorption, calcium reclamation in the kidney, and renal conversion of 25-OH vitamin D to its more active form, 1,25-OH vitamin D, which then promotes intestinal calcium absorption (Fig. 24.3)

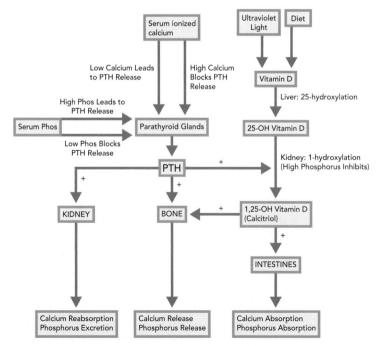

Figure 24.3. Regulation of calcium and phosphorus. PTH, parathyroid hormone.

ALGORITHM 24.7 Evaluation of Hypocalcemia

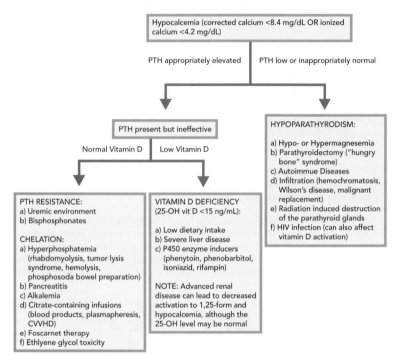

CVVHD, continuous venovenous hemodialysis; HIV, human immunodeficiency virus; PTH, parathyroid hormone.

Disorders of Ca^{2+} concentration are common among critically ill patients. Low ionized $[Ca^{2+}]$ has been observed in up to 88% of ICU patients. Furthermore, the presence of hypocalcemia serves as a marker of disease severity and patient mortality.

Hypocalcemia

Since the vast majority of calcium is stored in bone, hypocalcemia (corrected calcium <8.4 mg/dL or ionized calcium <4.2 mg/dL) reflects a defect in transferring this calcium into the ECF (Algorithm 24.7). Evaluation of such disorders always starts with measuring the PTH level, which should be elevated (even levels in the "normal" range are inappropriate in the setting of hypocalcemia). If the PTH level is appropriately elevated, then there is either resistance to its function at the level of bone, inadequate vitamin D activity, or chelation from the circulation.

Symptoms of hypocalcemia include circumoral or distal paresthesias and tetany. Latent tetany may be induced through several maneuvers. Trousseau's sign is positive when carpal spasm is induced after inflating a blood pressure cuff around the arm above systolic pressure for three minutes. Cvostek's sign is present when perioral muscle twitching is elicited with tapping the area of the facial nerve anterior to the ear. Acute, severe hypocalcemia may present with confusion, seizures, or bradycardia. ECG findings include QT interval prolongation, bradycardia, or complete heart block.

Etiologies of Special Importance in the Critically Ill Patient

Pseudohypocalcemia

Approximately 45% of serum Ca^{2+} exists in its free ionized form. Changes in serum albumin and serum anions alter total measured serum $[Ca^{2+}]$ without affecting the clinically relevant ionized $[Ca^{2+}]$. Hypoalbuminemia is very common in the ICU setting because albumin concentrations fall during the systemic inflammatory response and with large-volume fluid resuscitation. The total measured serum $[Ca^{2+}]$ is lowered in such situations, but ionized $[Ca^{2+}]$ remains within the normal range. It is recommended that the ionized $[Ca^{2+}]$ always be measured in this setting, since the equation for correction (adding back 0.8 mg/dL to the measured calcium for each 1 mg/dL drop in albumin from 4 mg/dL) does not correlate well.

Chelation

An increase in the availability of any anion that combines readily with Ca^{2+} may cause hypocalcemia as ionized Ca^{2+} is chelated. The release of negatively charged fatty acids in severe pancreatitis or the spillage of large amount of phosphate in rhabdomyolysis or hemolysis can result in hypocalcemia. Tremendous deposition into bone after parathyroidectomy is termed the "hungry bone" syndrome and can persist for months. Chelation by citrate-containing fluids, such as blood products in massive transfusions or anticoagulants in some forms of continuous dialysis and plasmapheresis, can occur in the critically ill patient.

Sepsis

Hypocalcemia occurs commonly in sepsis, particularly when involving a Gram-negative organism. Indeed, in one study, ionized calcium reduction was found in 30% of cases of Gram-negative septicemia and in none of those cases caused by Gram-positive bacteria. The pathogenesis is incompletely understood, but most patients have elevated PTH and low calcitriol levels. Elevated levels of procalcitonin have been found in many of these patients, suggesting that this hormone precursor may exert a hypocalcemic effect in the critically ill population.

Treatment

The management of symptomatic hypocalcemia or that associated with ECG abnormalities should be prompt and aggressive. IV Ca^{2+} replacement should be initiated in such situations. Treatment is outlined in Table 24.2.

Hypomagnesemia, if present, must be treated first for effective correction, as this electrolyte can impair PTH release. If the cause of low $[Ca^{2+}]$ is marked hyperphosphatemia, it is important to limit calcium replacement to those cases in which cardiac and neurologic symptoms are significant, since overaggressive correction may result in rebound hypercalcemia and metastatic calcification. In cases of profound hypocalcemia, clearance of the chelating species through the early initiation of hemodialysis with higher Ca^{2+} dialysate should be considered. For hypocalcemia occurring in the setting of profound sepsis or other shock states, therapy-guiding evidence is lacking. Although increases in cardiac contractility and blood pressure have been observed by Ca^{2+} administration, some animal data exist that suggest reperfusion injury and mortality may be worsened.

Asymptomatic hypocalcemia may be managed with oral calcium supplements along with vitamin D or its active metabolite, calcitriol, to increase intestinal absorption. Supplemental calcium should be administered between meals and away from other medications (particularly thyroid hormone and iron) to maximize absorption.

TABLE 24.2	Treatment of Hypocalcemia

General guidelines of therapy:
1. If ECG changes or symptoms present, begin IV replacement:
   a. Consider early initiation of hemodialysis when caused by hyperphosphatemia or hyperoxalemia
   b. Bolus 2 g $MgSO_4$ IV over 15 min if known hypomagnesemia or empirically if renal function is normal
   c. Bolus 2 g calcium gluconate (20 mL or 2 ampules of 10% calcium gluconate; 1 g = 93 mg elemental Ca^{2+}) in 50–100 mL of 5% dextrose or saline IV over 10–15 min
   d. Begin continuous Ca^{2+} infusion: Dilute 6 g of calcium gluconate (or 2 g, 20 mL, or 2 ampules of 10% calcium chloride[a]; 1 g = 272 mg elemental Ca^{2+}) in 500 mL of 5% dextrose or saline and infuse at 0.5–1.5 mg elemental Ca^{2+}/kg/hr
   e. Follow ionized $[Ca^{2+}]$ or corrected $[Ca^{2+}]$ Q 6 hours and continue infusion until $[Ca^{2+}]$ normalizes
   f. Overlap with PO replacement
2. Dose 1–2 g elemental Ca^{2+} PO TID to QID, separate from meals
3. Can add 0.25–4 μg/d calcitriol AND/OR ergocalciferol especially in vitamin D-deficient states
4. Can add salt restriction and hydrochlorothiazide if hypercalciuria occurs

[a]Although calcium gluconate may be given peripherally, calcium chloride should only be administered through a central vein.

Hypercalcemia

As with hypocalcemia, hypercalcemic disorders (corrected calcium >10.3 mg/dL or ionized calcium >5.2 mg/dL) are first evaluated by determining the PTH status (Algorithm 24.8). Levels should be maximally suppressed, and thus, even "normal" levels are inappropriately high, suggesting a hyperparathyroid state. If the PTH level is indeed suppressed, hypercalcemia can still result from nutritional vitamin D overdose or excess formation of 1,25-OH vitamin D (sarcoidosis, granulomatous disease, or lymphoma). Malignancy can lead to hypercalcemia through production of a PTH-like substance (PTH-related peptide, PTHrP) or lytic destruction of bone with release of calcium into the circulation. Hypercalcemia itself, through its action in the kidneys, can induce significant volume depletion.

Symptoms of hypercalcemia can occur at levels >12 mg/dL and tend to be more severe with rapid elevations. Polyuria is common, leading to a volume-depleted state. Gastrointestinal symptoms are common, with anorexia, constipation, and abdominal pain, with pancreatitis a rare secondary complication. Neurologic symptoms include weakness, fatigue, confusion, stupor, or coma. The ECG may reveal a shortened QT interval or variable degrees of atrioventricular block.

Etiologies of Special Importance in the Critically Ill Patient

Humoral Hypercalcemia of Malignancy

Certain malignancies, particularly squamous cell lung cancer, cancers of the head and neck, esophagus, genitourinary tract, and pheochromocytomas, may produce a hormone that differs from PTH but retains its biologic activity. This PTHrP is not detected

ALGORITHM 24.8   Evaluation of Hypercalcemia

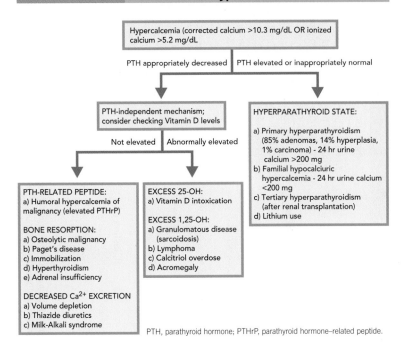

PTH, parathyroid hormone; PTHrP, parathyroid hormone–related peptide.

by standard PTH measurements and must be ordered separately when suspected. In most cases of humoral hypercalcemia of malignancy, patients usually have advanced disease.

Osteolytic Hypercalcemia of Malignancy
In this separate form of cancer-associated hypercalcemia, cytokines produced by tumor cells stimulate osteoclast bone resorption. Hypercalcemia and hyperphosphatemia occur only with extensive bone involvement by tumor, and the serum alkaline phosphatase is often significantly elevated. PTH is appropriately suppressed. The most frequently associated malignancies include breast carcinoma, non-small cell lung cancer, myeloma, and lymphoma.

Excess Calcitriol Production
Excess unregulated vitamin D activation can be produced by granulomatous disease, such as sarcoidosis, as well as the lymphocytes of some Hodgkin's and non-Hodgkin's lymphomas. These cells possess intrinsic 1-alpha hydroxylase activity, leading to excessive calcitriol production. The elevation in $[Ca^{2+}]$ is usually less severe than in humoral hypercalcemia of malignancy.

Immobilization
Complete bedrest can result in hypercalcemia after several days. There is increased osteoclast activity as well as diminished bone formation, with resultant hypercalcemia.

TABLE 24.3 Treatment of Hypercalcemia

Treatment	Dosing	Onset/duration	Comments
Isotonic saline	Bolus isotonic saline until euvolemic (may require up to 3–4 L), then adjust rate to achieve urine output of 100–150 mL/hr	Onset at 2–4 hr	Watch for signs of volume overload; loop diuretics may help with calcium excretion, but should be held until volume deficits have first been corrected
Calcitonin	4–8 IU/kg IM or SC q6–12h	Onset at 4–6 hr; tachyphylaxis develops after 2–3 d	Lowers serum Ca^{2+} 1–2 mg/dL; side effects include flushing, nausea, and, rarely, allergic reactions
Bisphosphonates	Zoledronate 4 mg IV over 15 min OR pamidronate 60–90 mg IV over 2–4 hr	Onset at 2 d with peak effect at 4–6 d; lasts 2–4 wk	Decrease infusion rate of pamidronate or lower zoledronate dose in renal insufficiency
Denosumab	60–120 mg SC	Onset within 3 days half-life of 25 days	Watch for hypocalcemia, risk for infection
Gallium nitrate	100–200 mg/m²/d continuous infusion for up to 5 d	Onset after 2 d; lasts 1–2 wk	Significant risk of nephrotoxicity and is contraindicated if creatinine >2.5 mg/dL
Glucocorticoids	Prednisone 20–60 mg/d (or equivalent glucocorticoid dose)	Onset in 5–10 d	Effective only in cases of granulomatous disease and hematologic malignancies
Hemodialysis	Variable based on starting [Ca^{2+}]	Immediate onset, lasting until dialysis completion	Useful for cases of severe hypercalcemia (>16 mg/dL) and when diuretic-resistant volume overload prohibits saline administration

General guidelines of therapy:
1. Correct volume depletion FIRST, with isotonic normal saline
2. If ECG changes or severe symptoms are present, begin the most rapidly acting therapies in combination
3. If rapid improvement is not seen (or anticipated due to the underlying condition), consider adding the longer acting treatments (bisphosphonates) early since their effects are delayed

It is usually more severe when renal function is impaired. Remobilization, when possible, leads to improvement and eventual resolution of the hypercalcemia.

Treatment

Hypercalcemia treatment is outlined in Table 24.3. Rapidly acting therapies for hypercalcemia are warranted if severe symptoms are present or with $[Ca^{2+}] > 12$ mg/dL. First, the anticalciuric effect of hypovolemia should be corrected with IV isotonic fluid boluses. Continuing maintenance IV saline after achieving euvolemia further promotes Ca^{2+} excretion. Loop diuretics add little to the calciuretic effect of saline administration and may prevent adequate volume restoration. However, they are useful if signs of hypervolemia develop. Calcitonin and hemodialysis against a low Ca^{2+} dialysate can also lower the serum $[Ca^{2+}]$ within hours.

While initiating the previously mentioned acute therapies, it is often necessary to simultaneously start more long-term measures of Ca^{2+} control. Usually, this consists of administering an IV bisphosphonate, which decreases Ca^{2+} resorption from bone by osteoclasts. In situations of calcitriol excess and when hypercalcemia occurs as a result of hematologic malignancies such as multiple myeloma, the administration of glucocorticoids is effective for lowering the serum $[Ca^{2+}]$ and can be used alone or with bisphosphonates.

DISORDERS OF PHOSPHORUS CONCENTRATION

Approximately 85% of total body phosphorus (as PO_4^{3-}) is in bone, and most of the remainder is within cells, as the major intracellular anion. As only 1% of total body phosphorus is in the ECF, the serum PO_4^{3-} concentration may not reflect total body phosphorus stores. In addition to its importance in bone formation, phosphorus is an integral component of adenosine triphosphate (ATP) and thus critical for normal cellular metabolism. Furthermore, its presence in the red blood cell as 2,3-bisphosphoglycerate makes it important in the regulation of hemoglobin oxygen affinity and therefore tissue oxygen delivery.

Phosphorus balance is determined primarily by PTH, active vitamin D (calcitriol), and insulin. PTH lowers $[PO_4^{3-}]$ through urinary excretion. Calcitriol increases $[PO_4^{3-}]$ by enhancing intestinal phosphorus absorption. Finally, insulin lowers serum levels by shifting PO_4^{3-} into cells. Hypophosphatemia has been found to occur in 29% of surgical ICU patients. Because renal failure is its major predisposing factor, hyperphosphatemia is common in the medical ICU.

Since many of the regulators of phosphorus are the same as those involved in calcium homeostasis, there is considerable overlap in the maintenance of an appropriate balance. In order to adequately assess phosphorus disorders, one must take into account the concurrent calcium concentration. This is summarized in Table 24.4 for the more common etiologies.

Hypophosphatemia

When evaluating a patient with hypophosphatemia, one should first rule out severe vitamin D deficiency and primary hyperparathyroidism (Algorithm 24.9). The remaining causes include gastrointestinal losses (e.g., phosphate binders, malnutrition, and diarrhea), transcellular shifts (e.g., insulin, refeeding syndrome, and respiratory alkalosis), or renal wasting. Losses by the kidney can be distinguished by the finding of a

TABLE 24.4 Interpretation of Calcium and Phosphorus Values

Ca^{2+}	PO_4^{3-}	PTH	Diagnosis
↑	↓	↑	Primary hyperparathyroidism
↑	↓	↓	Humoral hypercalcemia
↑	↑	↓	Osteolytic malignancy (myeloma)
↑	↑	↓	Vitamin D excess, granulomas, lymphomas
↓	↑	↓	Hypoparathyroidism, Mg^{2+} disorders
↓	↑	↑	PTH resistance (pseudohypoparathyroidism)
↓	↑	↑	CKD (secondary hyperparathyroidism)
↓	↓	↑	Severe vitamin D deficiency

CKD, chronic kidney disease.

high fractional excretion of phosphorus, an inappropriate response to the prevailing hypophosphatemia.

Symptoms typically occur only when there is total body PO_4^{3-} depletion and the serum $[PO_4^{3-}]$ is <1 mg/dL. Muscular weakness (including the diaphragm) can be seen, while paresthesias, seizures, stupor, or coma may develop when severe.

ALGORITHM 24.9 Evaluation of Hypophosphatemia

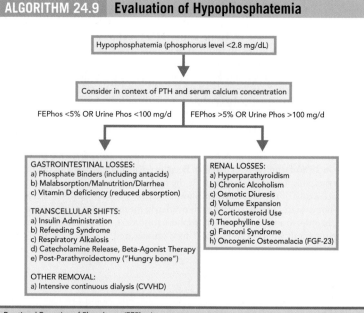

CVVHD, continuous venovenous hemodialysis; FEPhos, fractional excretion of phosphorus; FGF-23, fibroblast growth factor-23; PTH, parathyroid hormone.

Etiologies of Special Importance in the Critically Ill Patient

Intracellular Shift

Respiratory alkalosis is a very common cause of redistributive hypophosphatemia as the intracellular rise in pH stimulates glycolysis and the subsequent phosphorylation of various intermediates in the pathway. The marked anabolism that occurs during the abrupt reversal of negative caloric states with dextrose-containing IV fluids or total parenteral nutrition (refeeding syndrome) similarly shifts PO_4^{3-} to the ICF and can occur after as little as 2 days of nutritional restriction. The accompanying surge in insulin further promotes the intracellular translocation.

Renal Wasting

Hyperparathyroidism from any cause increases renal PO_4^{3-} excretion. Chronic alcohol consumption also causes renal PO_4^{3-} wasting by an unknown mechanism. This, in combination with the usually poor nutritional status of these patients, leads to a total body PO_4^{3-} deficit. With possible contributions from intracellular shift from the respiratory alkalosis of liver failure, the increased adrenergic tone of withdrawal, and the refeeding syndrome occurring with dextrose infusions, profound hypophosphatemia can manifest in the hospitalized alcoholic patient.

Increased renal tubular fluid flow from any cause can also lead to urinary PO_4^{3-} wasting. This can be seen with aggressive volume expansion or with osmotic diuresis, such as that which occurs with the glycosuria of DKA. Furthermore, insulin therapy in DKA shifts PO_4^{3-} into cells and may worsen the hypophosphatemia.

Oncogenic osteomalacia involves tumor production of fibroblast growth factor-23 (FGF-23), a hormone that induces phosphorus loss in the urine. FGF-23 is a newly recognized hormone in normal phosphorus homeostasis, but can lead to renal phosphorus wasting when overproduced through nonregulated ectopic production from tumors.

Continuous Hemodialysis

Conventional intermittent hemodialysis is only able to remove phosphorus inefficiently from the intravascular space, and thus rarely leads to hypophosphatemia on its own. However, with more aggressive continuous hemodialysis modalities, there is a state of constant negative efflux that can result in significant hypophosphatemia. Patients on continuous venovenous hemodialysis (CVVHD) should have their phosphorus levels checked every 12 to 24 hours, and if hypophosphatemia develops, the administered dialysis dose (dialysate flow rate) may need to be reduced in addition to standard treatment measures.

Treatment

Hypophosphatemia treatment is outlined in Table 24.5. Mild hypophosphatemia (1.9 to 2.5 mg/dL) is common in the hospitalized patient and is often simply caused by transcellular shifts, requiring no specific treatment except correction of the underlying cause. Severe, symptomatic hypophosphatemia (<1.0 mg/dL), however, may require IV PO_4^{3-} therapy. Although the rapid administration of large doses of IV PO_4^{3-} (0.8 mmol/kg over 30 min) to critically ill patients has been shown to be safe and effective, care must be taken with parenteral therapy to avoid hyperphosphatemia, which may lead to hypocalcemia and metastatic calcification in tissues. In the presence of renal insufficiency, IV PO_4^{3-} should be given at lower doses (33% of usual doses in severe renal failure) and with even greater care. IV repletion can be transitioned over to oral therapy when the $[PO_4^{3-}]$ is > 1.5 mg/dL. Enteral replacement may result

TABLE 24.5 Treatment of Hypophosphatemia

1. If symptomatic, or intolerant to PO, begin IV replacement (reduce doses in setting of renal insufficiency):
   a. Severe ($\leq$1 mg/dL): dose 0.6 mmol/kg IBW IV^a over 6 hr; if hypotension ensues, suspect hypocalcemia and discontinue infusion
   b. Moderate (1–1.8 mg/dL): dose 0.4 mmol/kg IBW IV^a over 6 hr
   c. Mild (1.9–2.5 mg/dL): dose 0.2 mmol/kg IBW IV^a over 6 hr
2. If asymptomatic, dose 0.5–1 g elemental phosphorus PO bid-tid; this should correct most deficits by 1 wk
   a. Neutra-phos: 250 mg (8 mmol) phosphorus and 7 mEq each of Na$^+$ and K$^+$
   b. Neutra-phos K: 250 mg phosphorus and 14 mEq K$^+$
   c. K-phos neutral: 250 mg phosphorus with 13 mEq Na$^+$ and 1.1 mEq K$^+$
3. Treat vitamin D deficiency, if present

^{a}Two IV preparations exist: use potassium phosphate if normal renal function and [K$^+$] <4 mEq/L; use sodium phosphate if renal function is impaired or [K$^+$] >4 mEq/L.

in diarrhea and nausea. Because of the need to replenish intracellular stores, 24 to 36 hours of repletion may be required. There has been no demonstrated clear benefit to aggressive repletion of PO$_4{}^{3-}$ in asymptomatic hypophosphatemia. Studies of PO$_4{}^{3-}$ therapy in the treatment of DKA, for instance, have shown no improved outcomes, and may even suggest increased morbidity, primarily through resultant hypocalcemia.

Hyperphosphatemia

When evaluating hyperphosphatemia (Algorithm 24.10), vitamin D levels and PTH activity should be assessed. The kidneys possess a remarkable ability to excrete phosphorus, but retention may result if there is acute or chronic renal damage. Chronic kidney disease often leads to secondary hyperparathyroidism (elevated PTH with increased phosphorus and variable calcium concentrations). When increased intake or transcellular shifts are responsible for hyperphosphatemia, the urinary excretion is often quite high to attempt to correct the imbalance.

Symptoms of hyperphosphatemia primarily relate to the concomitant hypocalcemia that results. Metastatic calcification of soft tissue, vasculature, cornea, kidney, and joints can occur. Calciphylaxis is skin ischemia and necrosis that can occur in patients with chronic kidney disease, resulting from calcium and phosphorus deposition within small blood vessels and subsequent thrombosis.

Etiologies of Special Importance in the Critically III Patient
Transcellular Shifts
Since the majority of phosphorus is sequestered intracellularly, any process that leads to widespread cell destruction (e.g., rhabdomyolysis, hemolysis, and tumor lysis syndrome) can lead to impressive hyperphosphatemia. The calcium concentration is often decreased as it complexes with the circulating phosphorus. Metabolic acidosis, especially lactic acidosis and DKA (with its concomitant relative insulin deficiency), can also result in phosphorus shifting out of cells.

ALGORITHM 24.10 Evaluation of Hyperphosphatemia

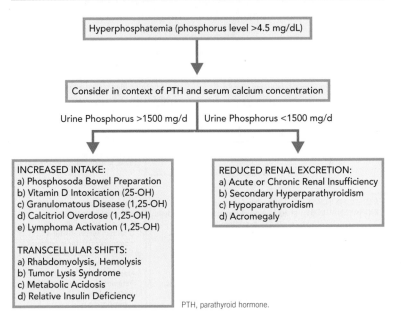

PTH, parathyroid hormone.

Treatment

Treatment of hyperphosphatemia is outlined in Table 24.6. Saline diuresis may help in excreting some of the excess phosphorus in the acute overload state. Acetazolamide is particularly effective at encouraging phosphorus elimination. If these conservative measures are unsuccessful and the underlying cause is not rapidly reversible, dialysis may become necessary for very severe hyperphosphatemia. For cases where chronic kidney disease is the cause, dietary restriction combined with oral phosphate binders is recommended.

TABLE 24.6 Treatment of Hyperphosphatemia

General guidelines of therapy:
1. Correct underlying cause (if normal renal function and phosphate handling is achieved, hyperphosphatemia will usually correct within 12 hr)
2. Consider forced saline resuscitation with addition of acetazolamide (15 mg/kg Q4 hr)
3. When severe, especially when renal insufficiency is not rapidly reversible, consider hemodialysis or continuous renal replacement therapy
4. When chronic, use phosphate binders (noncalcium based if concomitant hypercalcemia) and dietary restriction

ALGORITHM 24.11   Evaluation of Hypomagnesemia

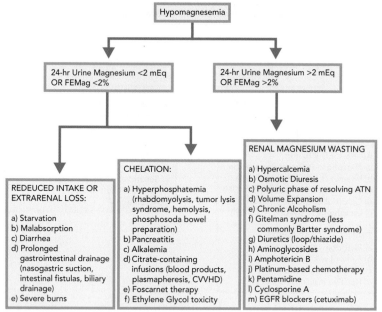

ATN, acute tubular necrosis; CVVHD, continuous venovenous hemodialysis; EGFR, epithelial growth factor receptor; FEMag, fractional excretion of magnesium.

DISORDERS OF MAGNESIUM CONCENTRATION

Approximately 60% of body magnesium is in bone, and most of the remainder is within cells. Only 1% of the total magnesium is in the ECF. Mg^{2+} is not exchanged easily across the cell membrane, and therefore there is little buffering of fluctuations in the serum Mg^{2+} concentration. Furthermore, the $[Mg^{2+}]$ is a poor predictor of intracellular and total body stores. Unlike calcium and phosphorus, there are no known hormones specifically delegated to the regulation of Mg^{2+} balance. The main determinant of Mg^{2+} balance is the serum $[Mg^{2+}]$ itself; hypomagnesemia stimulates renal tubular resorption of Mg^{2+}, whereas hypermagnesemia inhibits this process.

Hypomagnesemia

Hypomagnesemia occurs commonly in the ICU. As an important participant in most processes involving calcium flux and a cofactor in reactions consuming ATP, Mg^{2+} is critical for many biologic processes. Algorithm 24.11 describes the primary etiologies of hypomagnesemia. Urinary losses in renal wasting have a fractional excretion of magnesium >2%. This is calculated as (urine Mg^{2+} × serum creatinine)/(0.7 × serum Mg^{2+} × urine creatinine). Also, there may be gastrointestinal losses, reduced intake, or chelation (similar process as in hypocalcemia).

Symptoms of hypomagnesemia generally do not occur until the [Mg^{2+}] is <1 mEq/L. Lethargy, confusion, ataxia, nystagmus, tremor, fasciculations, tetany, and seizures may occur. Atrial and ventricular arrhythmias may be seen, particularly in patients on digoxin. The ECG may show prolonged PR and QT intervals with widened QRS complexes and U-waves. Torsades de pointes is the classically associated arrhythmia with hypomagnesemia. There may be concurrent hypokalemia and hypocalcemia (particularly in alcoholic patients), and may contribute to the overall clinical picture.

Etiologies of Special Importance in the Critically Ill Patient

Gastrointestinal Loss
Intestinal secretions have significant Mg^{2+} content, with more magnesium present in lower intestinal fluids. Fistulas, prolonged gastrointestinal drainage, or diarrhea can therefore lead to negative Mg^{2+} balance.

Renal Wasting
Chronic alcoholism may lead to renal tubular dysfunction, resulting in inappropriate Mg^{2+} wasting. This is exacerbated by the malnutrition that is often present. Numerous drugs have similarly been associated with urinary Mg^{2+} wasting. Prolonged dosing of aminoglycosides may cause renal tubular damage with characteristic Mg^{2+} wasting and polyuria. The development of hypomagnesemia may even be delayed until after completion of therapy and the tubular transport defect can persist for months. Other common offenders are the platinum-based chemotherapies such as cisplatin and carboplatin. A newer anticancer drug, cetuximab, is an epithelial growth factor (EGF) receptor antagonist and can cause hypomagnesemia by its effects on the distal convoluted tubule.

Chelation
Because Mg^{2+} is an ion with similar charge and size as Ca^{2+}, similar causes of hypocalcemia from chelation can also result in hypomagnesemia, although usually to a lesser degree. This phenomenon has been described, for instance, in cases of severe acute pancreatitis. Hypomagnesemia worsens the hypocalcemia in this setting through its inhibition of PTH release.

Treatment

Hypomagnesemia treatment is outlined in Table 24.7. The route of Mg^{2+} repletion depends on whether clinical manifestations from Mg^{2+} deficiency are present and not on the actual [Mg^{2+}]. Asymptomatic hypomagnesemia without ECG abnormalities can be treated orally, even if the deficiency is severe, unless malabsorption is present. Oral therapy avoids the abrupt increase in [Mg^{2+}] that occurs with IV repletion and which then increases renal excretion of part of the administered dose. The major side effect of enteral therapy is diarrhea. In scenarios with chronic urinary Mg^{2+} wasting, potassium-sparing diuretics like amiloride can be administered to reduce renal losses. Symptomatic hypomagnesemia should be treated parenterally, often with continued oral or IV replacement for 3 to 7 days to replenish intracellular stores. Deep tendon reflexes should be tested frequently during aggressive parenteral dosing as hyporeflexia implies the development of hypermagnesemia. Reduced doses and more frequent monitoring must be used even in mild renal insufficiency.

TABLE 24.7 | Treatment of Hypomagnesemia

General guidelines of therapy:
1. If ECG changes or symptoms present, begin IV replacement (reduce doses in renal insufficiency):
   a. 1–2 g $MgSO_4$ (1 g $MgSO_4$ = 96 mg elemental Mg^{2+} = 8 mEq Mg^{2+}) IV over 15 min, followed by an infusion of 6 g $MgSO_4$ in 1 L IV fluid over 24 hr
   b. Continuous infusion may be required for 3–7 d to replenish total body stores; follow $[Mg^{2+}]$ q24h (more frequently if renal insufficiency present) and adjust infusion to maintain $[Mg^{2+}] < 2.5$ mEq/L
   c. Check deep tendon reflexes often to detect developing hypermagnesemia
2. If asymptomatic and no ECG changes:
   a. For mild hypomagnesemia: 240 mg PO elemental[a] Mg^{2+} per d in divided doses
   b. For severe hypomagnesemia: up to 720 mg PO elemental[a] Mg^{2+} per d in divided doses
   c. If PO not possible or diarrhea present: 2–6 g IV $MgSO_4$ infused at 1 g/hr or less
3. For chronic hypomagnesemia from renal wasting, consider high-dose amiloride

[a]Magnesium oxide = 0.6 mg elemental Mg^{2+} per mg.

ALGORITHM 24.12 | **Evaluation and Treatment of Hypermagnesemia**

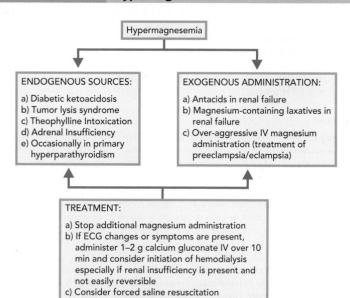

Hypermagnesemia

The kidneys have a remarkable capacity to excrete excess magnesium, and therefore it is uncommon to see hypermagnesemia unless concomitant renal insufficiency is present. Symptoms are typically seen only if the serum $[Mg^{2+}]$ is >4 mEq/L, and patients present with neuromuscular manifestations including hyporeflexia (usually the first sign of magnesium toxicity), weakness, and lethargy that can progress to somnolence and paralysis. With diaphragmatic involvement, this can lead to respiratory failure. Cardiac manifestations include hypotension, bradycardia, and cardiac arrest. The ECG may show prolonged PR, QRS, and QT intervals when the magnesium is 5 to 10 mEq/L. With more severe hypermagnesemia (>15 mEq/L), complete heart block or asystole may ensue.

The diagnostic differential is summarized in Algorithm 24.12. Treatment is focused on the cardiac manifestations, with administration of calcium gluconate to stabilize the myocardium. Exogenous magnesium should be discontinued and dialysis may be needed if renal insufficiency is present and not easily reversible (Algorithm 24.12).

SUGGESTED READINGS

Adrogue H, Madias N. Aiding fluid prescription for the dysnatremias. *Intensive Care Med.* 1997;23:309–316.
> *The original paper first presenting the use of the Adrogue–Madias equation for planning initial therapy in the dysnatremias. The concepts underlying the equation and its derivation are presented. Several examples with a comparison to the prior approach are also given.*

Allon M, Shanklin N. Effect of bicarbonate administration on plasma potassium in dialysis patients: interactions with insulin and albuterol. *Am J Kidney Dis.* 1996;28:508–514.
> *The time course of the acute therapies for hyperkalemia are studied and compared. This is one of several papers confirming the relative ineffectiveness of bicarbonate in the acute treatment of hyperkalemia.*

Amanzadeh J, Reilly RF. Hypophosphatemia: an evidence-based approach to its clinical consequences and management. *Nat Clin Pract Nephrol.* 2006;2:136–148.
> *An excellent review of the effects of hypophosphatemia and its treatment based on the available clinical data.*

Fraser CL, Arieff AI. Epidemiology, pathophysiology, and management of hyponatremic encephalopathy. *Am J Med.* 1997;102:67–77.
> *Review describing the pathophysiology of hyponatremia and factors linked with neurologic compromise based on case-control associations. Management guidelines differing from the traditional are offered. Includes a bibliography with most of the papers of significance on this topic.*

Kraft MD, Btaiche IF, Sacks GS. Treatment of electrolyte disorders in adult patients in the intensive care unit. *Am J Health Syst Pharm.* 2005;62:1663–1682.
> *An extensive topic review on the presentations and management of all of the electrolyte abnormalities touched upon here. Whenever possible, clinical studies are cited by an extensive bibliography.*

Palevsky PM, Bhagrath R, Greenberg A. Hypernatremia in hospitalized patients. *Ann Intern Med.* 1996;124:197–203.
> *Describes the incidence of in-hospital hypernatremia and clinical characteristics, pathophysiologic mechanisms, and outcomes for a cohort of hypernatremic patients.*

Palmer BF. Hyponatremia in patients with central nervous system disease: SIADH versus CSW. *Trends Endocrinol Metab.* 2003;14:182–187.
> *A good review on the difficult topic of cerebral salt wasting.*

Rose B, Post T. Clinical physiology of acid-base and electrolyte disorders. 5th ed. New York: McGraw-Hill, 2001.

A textbook which thoroughly describes the renal handling of sodium, potassium, and water, including normal physiology and pathophysiology. Many classic experiments in renal physiology are presented throughout the text to illustrate the described principles.

Zivin JR, Gooley T, Zager RA, et al. Hypocalcemia: a pervasive metabolic abnormality in the critically ill. *Am J Kidney Dis.* 2001;37:689–698.

A study which defines the high incidence of hypocalcemia in a diverse population of the critically ill. Associations with increased illness severity are highlighted.

25 Metabolic Acid–Base Disorders

Peter Juran and Steven Cheng

Acid–base disorders are commonly encountered in the critical care setting. A stepwise approach to the evaluation of these disorders helps delineate underlying causes, compensatory mechanisms, and the correct approach to management. This chapter reviews the diagnosis and management of metabolic acidosis and alkalosis. Respiratory acidosis and alkalosis are discussed separately (see Chapter 26).

The average individual generates a daily production of approximately 15,000 mmol of carbon dioxide (CO_2) and 50 to 100 mEq of hydrogen ions (H^+) from the catabolism of carbohydrates, fats, and proteins. An appropriate response to this acid load is essential because the range of extracellular H^+ concentration compatible with life (150 to 15 nmol/L and respective pH of 6.8 to 7.8) is fairly narrow. Disorders of the acid–base system and the appropriate management are best understood by examining the equation for the bicarbonate–carbon dioxide buffer system:

$$H_2O + CO_2 \leftrightarrow H_2CO_3 \leftrightarrow H^+ + HCO_3^-$$

The enzyme carbonic anhydrase catalyzes the reaction of water (H_2O) and carbon dioxide (CO_2) to form carbonic acid (H_2CO_3). Carbonic acid dissociates into bicarbonate (HCO_3^-) and a hydrogen ion (H^+). The physiologic pH is thus balanced by respiratory processes, which adjust the partial pressure of CO_2 (PCO_2), and metabolic processes, which modulate the generation and excretion of bicarbonate and hydrogen ions in the kidney.

When acid–base homeostasis is disturbed by a metabolic acidosis or alkalosis, respiratory compensation is required to attenuate the degree of change in pH. In metabolic acidosis, this compensation begins immediately, although the full degree of compensation (a decrease in PCO_2 of 1.2 mm Hg for each 1 mEq/L decrease in the serum bicarbonate) may not be completely attained for 12 to 24 hours. In metabolic alkalosis, the appropriate respiratory response is a 0.7 mm Hg increase in the PCO_2 for each 1 mEq/L increase in the serum bicarbonate (Table 25.1). However, the hypoventilation required for an increase in PCO_2 is often not possible for critically ill patients with underlying cardiac and pulmonary disorders.

The clinical identification of metabolic acid–base disorders, the evaluation of respiratory compensation, and the detection of mixed disorders require a careful systemic approach of the following steps (Algorithm 25.1).

TABLE 25.1	Expected PCO₂ and Respiratory Compensation for Metabolic Acidosis and Alkalosis
Metabolic acidosis	PCO_2 is >10 mm Hg in a single disorder $PCO_2 = -1.2$ mm Hg for every 1 mEq/L fall in $[HCO_3^-]$ (below 24 mEq/L)
Metabolic alkalosis	PCO_2 is <60 mm Hg in a single disorder $PCO_2 = +0.7$ mm Hg for every 1 mEq/L rise in $[HCO_3^-]$ (above 24 mEq/L)

1. Determine the underlying abnormality—metabolic acidosis and/or metabolic alkalosis.
2. Determine the contributing factors and concomitant disorders (anion gap acidosis $\pm$ nonanion gap acidosis $\pm$ metabolic alkalosis)
3. Evaluate the appropriateness of respiratory compensation.
4. Determine the likely cause of the disorder and whether or not urgent intervention is necessary.

METABOLIC ACIDOSIS

Acidemia is the most common acute metabolic acid–base disturbance presenting in the critical care setting. The four main mechanisms used in an attempt to maintain homeostasis in this setting are as follows:

1. Extracellular buffering primarily via HCO_3^-
2. Intracellular and bone buffering (buffers up to 55% to 60% of the acid load)
3. Renal excretion of H^+ and regeneration of bicarbonate
4. Removal of CO_2 by alveolar ventilation.

Metabolic acidosis may present as a single disturbance or as a more complex combined disorder due to various simultaneous processes with different effects on acid–base homeostasis. Double and triple metabolic disorders often reflect a metabolic alkalosis occurring with an anion-gap acidosis (as can occur during diabetic ketoacidosis and vomiting) and/or a nonanion gap acidosis. Inappropriate respiratory compensation in any of these situations may add the additional component of respiratory acidosis or alkalosis.

Anion Gap Acidosis

The anion gap is a way of reflecting "unmeasured" anions in the blood (as opposed to the "measured" chloride and bicarbonate anions typically identified in basic chemistry laboratory results). It can be calculated with the equation:

Anion Gap = [Serum Sodium (Na^+) − (Serum Chloride (CL^-) + Serum HCO_3^-)]

Normal values are between 8 and 12 mEq/L. An anion gap greater than this simply suggests that the patient has been exposed to an "unmeasured" anion, which increases the anion gap. For example, the accumulation of lactate, beta-hydroxybutyrate, and acetoacetate—all of which are "unmeasured" anions—increases the anion gap. Thus,

ALGORITHM 25.1 Approach to Metabolic Acidosis and Alkalosis

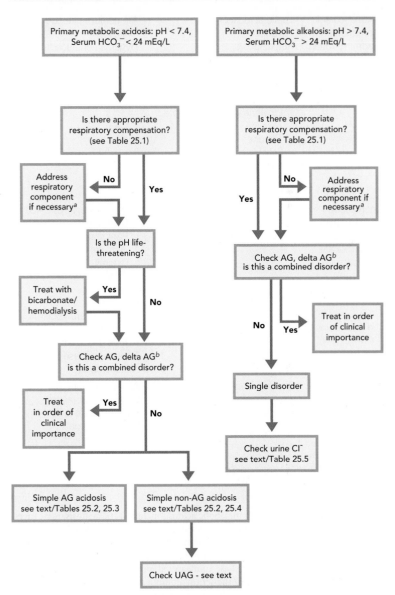

AG, anion gap; UAG, urine anion gap. [a]May require intubation and mechanical ventilation for patients with life-threatening acid–base disturbances unable to fully hyper- or hypoventilate appropriately. [b]See text for details.

TABLE 25.2	Causes of Anion Gap and Nonanion Gap Metabolic Acidosis	
Mechanism	Increased anion gap acidosis[a]	Normal anion gap acidosis

Increased acid production or administration	Lactic acidosis—lactate, D-lactate
	Ketoacidosis
	Massive rhabdomyolysis
	Intoxications:
	    Methanol/formaldehyde—formate
	    Ethylene glycol—glycolate, oxalate
	    Toluene—hippurate
	    Salicylates
	    Paraldehyde—organic anions
	    L-5 oxoprolinuria
		Ammonium chloride ingestion
		Hyperalimentation fluids/saline infusion

Increased bicarbonate loss or loss of bicarbonate precursors		GI losses (negative UAG)
		    Diarrhea
		    Pancreatic, biliary, intestinal fistulas
		    Ostomy
		    Cholestyramine
		    Sevelamer
		Renal losses
		    Carbonic anhydrase inhibitors
		    Type 2 (proximal) RTA
		Treatment phase of ketoacidosis

Decreased acid excretion (positive UAG)	Chronic renal failure	Acute renal failure Chronic renal failure Type 1 (distal) RTA Hypoaldosteronism (type 4 RTA)

GI, gastrointestinal; UAG, urine anion gap; RTA, renal tubular acidosis.
[a]See Table 25.3 for further discussion.

common causes of an anion gap metabolic acidosis include lactic acidosis, toxic ingestions, ketoacidosis, rhabdomyolysis, and renal failure (Tables 25.2 and 25.3).

Of note, the normal range for the anion gap reflects the presence of physiologic unmeasured anions, such as albumin, in nonpathologic states. However, conditions that alter the concentrations of these unmeasured anions also alter the anion gap. For example, a 1 g/dL decrease in the serum albumin would be expected to decrease the anion gap by 2.5 to 3 mEq/L. It is important to adjust the anion gap for these changes in order to properly detect an anion gap acidosis that may be present despite a calculated anion gap that appears within the normal range of 8 to 12 mEq/L. The

TABLE 25.3 Causes and Treatment of Anion Gap Metabolic Acidosis

Condition	Cause and symptoms	Treatment	Comments

Lactic acidosis
Pyruvate
↕
Lactate
	Increased lactate production
	1. Increased pyruvate production: enzymatic defects in glycogenolysis or gluconeogenesis.
	2. Decreased pyruvate utilization: enzymatic defects in pyruvate dehydrogenase or carboxylase.
	3. Increased conversion of pyruvate to lactate:
	  Increased metabolic rate
	  Grand mal seizure
	  Severe exercise
	  Hypothermic shivering
	  Shock/cardiac arrest/acute pulmonary edema
	  Severe hypoxemia
	CO poisoning[a]
	  Cyanide intoxication[a]
	Decreased lactate utilization
	  Hypoperfusion
	  Alcoholism[a]
	  Liver disease
		Correction of the underlying disorder and reversal of circulatory failure is the primary therapy. Role of sodium bicarbonate administration is controversial; may be indicated if severe acidosis–pH <7.1 or loss of buffering capacity (bicarbonate <5 mEq/L). Hemodialysis may be indicated in resistant cases.
		Alternative therapies (clinical efficacy and safety for these have not been demonstrated in randomized controlled human studies).
		Tham (tromethamine)–inert amino alcohol that buffers acids without generating CO_2. Renally excreted and may produce hyperkalemia, hypoglycemia, and respiratory depression in anuric/oliguric patients.
		Carbicarb: equimolar mixture of sodium carbonate and sodium bicarbonate. Diminished risk of hypercapnia and intracellular acidosis compared with sodium bicarbonate.
		Dichloroacetate: activates pyruvate dehydrogenase and increases oxidation of pyruvate thus decreasing its conversion to lactate.
			Caution with bicarbonate therapy in the following settings:
			Volume overload
			Postrecovery metabolic alkalosis
			Hypernatremia
			Increased CO_2 production and possible retention in setting of circulatory failure with worsening of mixed venous PCO_2
			Intracellular acidosis
			Reduction in ionized calcium and worsening of cardiac contractility.

(Continued)

TABLE 25.3 Causes and Treatment of Anion Gap Metabolic Acidosis (*Continued*)

Condition	Cause and symptoms	Treatment	Comments
Propylene glycol toxicity[a]	Converts to pyruvate and lactate. Vehicle for lorazepam and other agents, and continuous infusion may result in lactate accumulation and increased osmolar gap.	Discontinue infusion.	
Ketoacidosis (see Chapter 28)	In the setting of insulin deficiency. Symptoms include vomiting, abdominal pain, severe volume depletion/dehydration.	Insulin and fluids—acidosis will improve with insulin-induced metabolism of ketoacids and regeneration of serum HCO_3^-.	
Salicylate toxicity[a]	Toxicity when plasma level >40–50 mg/dL (therapeutic, 20–35 mg/dL). Mixed metabolic acidosis and respiratory alkalosis. Increased ketoacid and lactate production. Diagnosis—plasma salicylate level.	Reduce salicylate levels to avoid neurotoxicity. Alkalinization of plasma to a pH > 7.45–7.5 converts salicylate to ionized form that lowers CNS levels. Alkalinization of urine decreases renal tubular reabsorption of ionized salicylate. Consider hemodialysis for plasma concentration >80 mg/dL.	If respiratory alkalosis is the primary disturbance, then further alkalinization is not necessary.
Methanol[a] ↕ Formaldehyde ↕ Formic acid	Minimal lethal dose is 50–100 mL. Symptoms include weakness, headache, blurred vision, and blindness. Diagnosis—plasma methanol assay.	The treatment for both methanol and ethylene glycol is identical. Prompt treatment is necessary and includes: Oral charcoal Sodium bicarbonate	Simultaneous use of both ethanol and fomepizole is not recommended as fomepizole increases the half-life of ethanol.

Ethylene glycol[a] → Glycolic and oxalic acid	Component of antifreeze and solvents. Symptoms include neurologic and cardiopulmonary abnormalities, flank pain, and renal failure. Envelope- and needle-shaped oxalate crystals may be visible in the urine. Diagnosis—plasma ethylene glycol assay.	Administration of ethanol or fomepizole competes with or inactivates metabolism, respectively, of parent compound and prevents formation of toxic metabolites. Administration of folic acid, thiamine, and pyridoxine. Hemodialysis for removal of toxic metabolites and parent compound.
L-5 oxoproline toxicity	High anion gap acidosis in children secondary to congenital glutathione synthetase deficiency. Acquired oxoprolinuria associated with acetaminophen and other medications. Renal dysfunction and sepsis predispose. Diagnosis—negative toxicity screening and high plasma and urine levels of 5-oxoproline/urine organic acid screen.	Treatment primarily includes cessation of the offending agent. N-acetylcysteine may be beneficial; restoration of glutathione stores reduces L-5 oxoproline levels.
D-Lactic acidosis Glucose bacterial overgrowth in the colon D-Lactate	Associated with short gut syndrome and overproduction of D-lactate. Symptoms: episodic anion gap acidosis (usually occurring after high-carbohydrate meals) and neurologic abnormalities including cerebellar ataxia, confusion, slurred speech. Diagnosis: enzymatic assay for D-lactate.	Treatment includes sodium bicarbonate administration and antimicrobial agents.

[a]See Chapter 32.

serum osmolal gap may also be of value when a toxic ingestion (ethanol, methanol, ethylene glycol) is a suspected cause of an anion gap acidosis (Table 25.3). An increased osmolal gap is an otherwise nonspecific finding and may be seen in other forms of anion gap acidosis. The normal osmolal gap is approximately 10 mOsm/kg.

$$\text{Osmolal gap} = \text{Measured serum osmolality} - \text{calculated serum osmolality}$$

$$\text{Calculated serum osmolality} = 2[Na^+] + [BUN]/2.8 + [glucose]/18$$

Nonanion Gap Acidosis

Nonanion gap acidosis occurs in the setting of bicarbonate loss, but without the presence of an additional pathologic anion. In a nonanion gap acidosis $[Cl^-]$ is increased to maintain electroneutrality and the calculated anion gap remains normal. The differential of nonanion gap acidosis includes gastrointestinal losses versus a renal etiology (Table 25.2).

The urine anion gap (UAG) is used to discern the source of bicarbonate loss in a nonanion gap acidosis when the cause is not clinically evident.

$$\text{UAG} = (\text{Urine } [Na^+] + \text{Urine } [K^+]) - (\text{Urine } [Cl^-])$$

The UAG is normally zero or slightly positive. In the setting of a nonanion gap acidosis, the appropriate renal response would be to increase ammonium excretion, as NH_4Cl, which causes the UAG to become negative, usually ranging from -20 to -50 mEq/L. This is seen in nonrenal causes of nonanion gap acidosis, such as severe diarrhea. In conditions with impaired renal acid excretion, such as chronic kidney disease and distal renal tubular acidosis (RTA), the UAG will remain positive or become only slightly negative. The UAG has no utility in the setting of hypovolemia, oliguria, low urine $[Na^+]$, or in anion gap acidosis.

Renal Tubular Acidosis

These disorders are characterized by a hyperchloremic metabolic acidosis resulting from diminished capacity of the kidney to accommodate the acid load. A diagnosis of RTA cannot be made in the setting of acute renal failure or with moderate-to-severe chronic kidney disease. Although RTA is generally a chronic condition and rarely causes acute critical illness, the identification of a RTA in the critical care setting is important as it may point clinicians toward underlying conditions that are associated with the various forms of RTA. Distal (type 1) RTA is associated with drugs such as amphotericin and autoimmune conditions such as lupus and Sjogren syndrome. Proximal (type 2) RTA is associated with multiple myeloma and may manifest with profound wasting of other solutes that are typically reabsorbed in the proximal tubule, such as glucose and phosphorus. And type 4 RTA, which is due to hyporeninemic hypoaldosteronism, is a commonly seen manifestation of diabetes and is closely linked to hyperkalemia. A detailed discussion of this topic is beyond the intent of this manual (Table 25.4).

Treatment

Treatment of the various disorders is outlined in Table 25.3. The primary goal in treating metabolic acidosis is reversal of the underlying process. Administration of bicarbonate is controversial, as some clinical parameters may actually worsen with correction of the acidosis. However, partial correction should be considered in the

TABLE 25.4 Renal Tubular Acidosis (RTA)

	Distal (type 1) RTA	Proximal (type 2) RTA	Hyporeninemic hypoaldosteronism (type 4) RTA
Causes	Idiopathic, familial, Sjogren syndrome, hypercalciuria, rheumatoid arthritis, sickle cell anemia, SLE, amphotericin	Idiopathic, multiple myeloma, carbonic anhydrase inhibitors, heavy metals (lead, mercury), amyloidosis, hypocalcemia, and vitamin D deficiency	Diabetes, ACE inhibitors, tubulointer-stitial nephritis, NSAIDS, heparin, adrenal insufficiency, obstructive uropathy, K$^+$-sparing diuretics
Defect	Impaired distal tubular H$^+$ excretion (distal acidification)	Impaired proximal tubular bicarbonate absorption ± associated glycosuria, aminoaciduria, phosphaturia	Aldosterone deficiency or resistance
Plasma HCO$_3^-$	Variable; usually more severe acidosis with level <10 mEq/L.	Less severe acidosis than distal RTA; usually 12–20 mEq/L	Usually >15 mEq/L
Urine pH during acidemia[a]	>5.3	Variable; >5.3 if serum HCO$_3^-$ is above the reabsorptive threshold. The excessive bicarbonate "spills out" into the urine causing a high urine pH. <5.3 if serum HCO$_3^-$ is below threshold	Usually <5.3
Plasma K$^+$	Usually low; usually corrects with alkali therapy	Low; usually worsened by bicarbonaturia seen with alkali therapy	High
UAG	Positive	Variable; not helpful	Positive
Associated conditions	Renal stones/nephrocalcinosis	Rickets/osteomalacia/Fanconi syndrome	None
Treatment	Alkali therapy: sodium citrate/potassium citrate/sodium bicarbonate	Alkali therapy: higher doses are needed because of bicarbonaturia. Thiazide diuretics may be tried in resistant cases	Treat the cause of hypoaldosteronism/low potassium diet/loop diuretics

[a]In metabolic acidosis with intact renal acid excretion, urine pH should be <5–5.3.

SLE, systemic lupus erythematosus; ACE, angiotensin-converting enzyme; NSAIDs, nonsteroidal anti-inflammatory drugs; UAG, urine anion gap.

Modified from Rose B, Post T. Clinical physiology of acid-base and electrolyte disorders. 5th ed. New York: McGraw-Hill, 2001.

setting of life-threatening metabolic acidosis (pH <7.1) or when the serum bicarbonate is low enough (i.e., <10 to 12 mEq/L) that loss of effective respiratory compensation would result in life-threatening acidosis. For example; the pH is approximately 7.2, the serum bicarbonate is 8 mEq/L, and the PCO_2 is appropriately compensated at 20 mm Hg. If respiratory compensation becomes inadequate and the PCO_2 increases to 55 mm Hg, the pH will suddenly decrease to approximately 6.9. To decrease the risk of either a further drop in the serum bicarbonate or a sudden inability to achieve appropriate respiratory compensation, a serum bicarbonate target of 10 to 12 mEq/L is recommended.

One caveat is the administration of bicarbonate in the setting of severe circulatory failure. This may result in an apparent improvement in acidosis as measured by the arterial blood gas, but an actual worsening of the overall acidosis if a venous blood gas is obtained (given delayed elimination of the CO_2 produced as a result of the administered bicarbonate). Thus, both arterial and venous values should be monitored when bicarbonate is administered in this setting. Continuous or intermittent hemodialysis may also be used to correct severe, refractory acidosis particularly if the patient cannot accommodate the volume associated with administration of intravenous bicarbonate-containing fluids. In the setting of a combined metabolic and respiratory acidosis, correction of the respiratory acidosis component should be addressed prior to administration of bicarbonate or initiation of hemodialysis.

Bicarbonate Deficit

The amount of bicarbonate required to correct a metabolic acidosis can be estimated from the following formula:

Total body weight (kg) $\times [0.4 + (2.4/[HCO_3^-])]$ = apparent volume of distribution

Apparent volume of distribution $\times$ target change in $[HCO_3^-]$ = mEq of $NaHCO_3$

For example, to increase the serum bicarbonate to 12 mEq/L in a 60-kg patient with a serum bicarbonate level of 5 mEq/L:

60 kg $\times [0.4 + 2.4/5]$ = apparent VD of 53 L

53 $\times$ target change in $[HCO_3^-](12 - 5 = 7$ mEq/L) = 371 mEq

Thus, in a static situation, almost 400 mEq of $NaHCO_3$ would need to be administered in an attempt to increase the $[HCO_3^-]$ to 12 mEq/L. This calculation is obviously an approximation and does not take into account ongoing bicarbonate losses or continued acid production. A standard ampule of sodium bicarbonate contains 50 mEq in 50 mL, given as an intravenous bolus or mixed with 5% dextrose containing sterile water.

METABOLIC ALKALOSIS

Most cases of metabolic alkalosis encountered in the intensive care unit are induced by loss of gastric secretions from gastric suctioning or vomiting, or from diuretic therapy. Other causes include bicarbonate administration, the posthypercapnic state, and citrate associated with centrifugal plasma exchange, massive transfusion, or fresh-frozen plasma administration. The condition is often aggravated by renal insufficiency, which delays bicarbonate excretion. Metabolic alkalosis may be the primary disorder, but likewise can be associated with an anion gap or nonanion gap acidosis as well as with a respiratory acidosis or alkalosis. Of note, however, is that a slight increase in the calculated anion gap can occur in some cases of metabolic alkalosis, often related to an

TABLE 25.5	Chloride-Responsive and Chloride-Resistant Metabolic Alkalosis
Chloride responsive (urinary Cl⁻ ≤25 mEq/L)	Chloride resistant (urinary Cl⁻ >25 mEq/L)
Loss of gastric H⁺-vomiting or gastric suction	Mineralocorticoid excess: primary hyperaldosteronism, Cushing or Liddle syndromes, exogenous steroid use, licorice ingestion
Prior loop/thiazide diuretic use	
Chloride-losing diarrhea: villous adenoma/some cases of factitious diarrhea due to laxative abuse	Active loop/thiazide diuretic use
	Bartter or Gitelman syndromes
Cystic fibrosis (high sweat Cl⁻)	Alkali load: exogenous bicarbonate infusion, citrate-containing blood products, antacids (milk-alkali syndrome)
Posthypercapnia	
	Severe hypokalemia
Treatment includes administration of 0.9% or 0.45% NaCl and repletion of potassium stores.	Treatment is disease-specific and includes repletion of potassium stores.

increased albumin concentration resulting from a contracted volume state. Metabolic alkalosis can be broadly categorized into a chloride-responsive or chloride-resistant process (Table 25.5).

Common Causes of Metabolic Alkalosis

Gastric Secretion Loss

Loss of gastric secretions occurs from removal of gastric contents by tube drainage or from vomiting. Normally, hydrogen ions released into the stomach reach the duodenum, where they stimulate pancreatic bicarbonate secretion into the gastrointestinal tract, maintaining acid–base balance. When gastric contents are lost, bicarbonate is not secreted, resulting in increased plasma bicarbonate and metabolic alkalosis. Self-induced vomiting is often denied by patients with eating or factitious disorders, and a low urine chloride supports the diagnosis.

Contraction Alkalosis

Contraction alkalosis occurs in the setting of excessive loss of chloride-rich, bicarbonate-free fluid. This is most commonly seen with the use of loop or thiazide diuretics, but can also occur with gastric losses or with cystic fibrosis (high sweat [Cl⁻]). As a result of "contraction" of the extracellular volume, there is a relative increase in the bicarbonate concentration. Despite the relative intravascular volume depletion, there is an obligate urinary loss of sodium with bicarbonate in this setting. Therefore, urine chloride concentration is usually a better predictor of the volume status in this form of metabolic alkalosis than urine sodium.

Posthypercapnic Alkalosis

Chronic respiratory acidosis is associated with an appropriate compensatory increase in the serum bicarbonate concentration. Sudden normalization of a chronically elevated PCO_2 via mechanical ventilation can result in an acute, potentially lethal increase in the pH. Therefore, the PCO_2 should not be decreased rapidly in the setting of a well-compensated chronic respiratory acidosis.

Refeeding Syndrome

Patients fed a high-carbohydrate diet after a prolonged fast can acutely develop metabolic alkalosis. Intracellular hydrogen ion shift is the proposed mechanism. Refeeding may also be independently associated with hypophosphatemia.

Severe Hypokalemia

Severe hypokalemia via multiple renal mechanisms causes hydrogen ion secretion and bicarbonate reabsorption. The ensuing metabolic alkalosis is refractory to treatment until potassium stores are replaced.

Milk-Alkali Syndrome

Milk-alkali syndrome results from a chronic high calcium intake (usually in the form of calcium-containing antacids) and is usually associated with renal insufficiency.

Treatment

Intravenous sodium chloride fluid administration will reverse chloride-responsive metabolic alkalosis (Table 25.5). Response to treatment can be monitored via urine pH and urine chloride concentration. Concomitant hypokalemia may also play a critical role in the maintenance of metabolic alkalosis, as it increases tubular secretion of H^+ and reabsorption of bicarbonate. Patients with hypokalemia and alkalosis may have a profound total body potassium deficit, and treatment of this will be necessary in the correction of metabolic alkalosis. If the patient is able to take medication by mouth, oral supplementation is preferred with potassium chloride 40 mEq every 4 to 6 hours. Alternatively, if the patient is unable to take medication enterally, intravenous infusion of potassium chloride at a rate of 10 mEq/hr with close monitoring of serum potassium may be initiated.

Acetazolamide can be considered in cases of worsening metabolic alkalosis associated with volume overload complicated by the need for continued attempts at diuresis (nonchloride responsive). Acetazolamide inhibits carbonic anhydrase, the enzyme that catalyzes the conversion of carbon dioxide and water into carbonic acid, causing renal excretion of hydrogen ions and retention of bicarbonate. Decreased bicarbonate excretion from carbonic anhydrase inhibition causes a metabolic acidosis to counter the alkalosis. Acetazolamide has minimal diuretic effects as a single agent, but can have additive effects when combined with loop and/or thiazide diuretics if the serum bicarbonate concentration is elevated.

In cases of severe, refractory alkalosis (usually associated with bicarbonate administration in the setting of renal failure), hydrochloric acid infusion through a central line is rarely needed, but can be used. Other alternatives include the use of intermittent hemodialysis with the bicarbonate bath decreased to the lowest allowable value (limited bicarbonate gradient available with most systems) or a continuous hemofiltration modality using primarily a nonbicarbonate, noncitrate replacement fluid.

MIXED ACID–BASE DISORDERS

The delta anion gap is useful in determining the presence of other metabolic disturbances superimposed on a known anion gap acidosis. It is calculated as follows:

$$\text{Delta Anion Gap } (\Delta/\Delta): \frac{\Delta^*\text{AG (from normal, which is approximately 10)}}{\Delta^*\text{HCO}_3 \text{ (from normal, which is approximately 25 mEq/L)}}$$

$^*\Delta = \text{Change}$

The delta gap is based on the principle that the change in AG should roughly approximate the change in serum bicarbonate in a simple anion gap acidosis. A ratio of <1 occurs if the change in serum bicarbonate is larger than the change in the anion gap, and indicates that a nonanion gap acidosis may be present, causing the disproportionate fall in serum bicarbonate. A ratio >1 suggests a combined anion gap acidosis and metabolic alkalosis (which both raises the anion gap and attenuates the expected drop in serum bicarbonate from the anion gap acidosis).

Elucidation of double or triple acid base disturbances requires assessment of multiple metabolic parameters. Because complex acid–base disorders may at first manifest with several normal appearing lab values, a methodical evaluation of all data (including the calculation of anion gap and delta gap) should be done routinely. The following patterns are often suggestive of a combined acid base disturbance despite a "normal" pH:

Normal pH + ↓PCO_2 + ↓HCO_3: respiratory alkalosis plus metabolic acidosis

Normal pH + ↑PCO_2 + ↑HCO_3: respiratory acidosis plus metabolic alkalosis

Normal pH + normal PCO_2 + normal HCO_{3+} ↑AG: metabolic acidosis and alkalosis

SUGGESTED READINGS

Arroliga AC, Shehab N, McCarthy K, et al. Relationship of continuous infusion lorazepam to serum propylene glycol concentration in critically ill adults. *Crit Care Med.* 2004;32:1709–1714.
Prospective observational study evaluating the dose relationship between lorazepam infusion and propylene glycol accumulation.

Gauthier PM, Szerlip HM. Metabolic acidosis in the intensive care unit. *Crit Care Clin.* 2002;18:289–308.
An extensive review of diagnostic and therapeutic approach to metabolic acidosis with focus on critical care issues.

Gehlbach BK, Schmidt GA. Bench-to-bedside review: treating acid-base abnormalities in the intensive care unit—the role of buffers. *Crit Care.* 2004;8:259–265.
This review article extensively discusses the role of bicarbonate therapy as well as alternative therapies in lactic acidosis.

Judge BS. Differentiating the causes of metabolic acidosis in the poisoned patient. *Clin Lab Med.* 2006;26:31–48, vii.
Describes toxicities due to methanol, ethylene glycol, and other ingestions, their effects on acid base balance, diagnosis, and treatment.

Rose B, Post T. Clinical physiology of acid base and electrolyte disorders. 5th ed. New York: McGraw-Hill, 2001:615–619.
An extremely comprehensive text book describing pathophysiologic mechanisms, diagnoses, and treatment of metabolic acid–base disorders.

Tailor P, Raman T, Garganta CL, et al. Recurrent high anion gap metabolic acidosis secondary to 5-oxoproline (pyroglutamic acid). *Am J Kidney Dis.* 2005;46:e4–e10.
Case report and discussion of a common but underdiagnosed cause of high anion gap acidosis-5 oxoproline toxicity.

26 Respiratory Acid–Base Disorders

Andrew Labelle

Respiratory acid–base disorders are commonly seen in the intensive care unit, and can occur independently or coexist with metabolic acid–base disorders (see Chapter 24). Respiratory acid–base disorders are characterized by altered plasma carbon dioxide levels, measured on arterial blood gas (ABG) analysis as the partial pressure of carbon dioxide ($PaCO_2$). Respiratory acidosis is characterized by an elevated $PaCO_2$ and decreased pH, and respiratory alkalosis by a decreased $PaCO_2$ and elevated pH. The $PaCO_2$ in healthy adults is 35 to 45 mm Hg and the normal pH is 7.35 to 7.45. For calculation purposes, it is reasonable to use 40 mm Hg as the baseline $PaCO_2$ level and 7.4 as the baseline pH. In general, each *acute* 10 mm Hg change in the $PaCO_2$ causes a 0.08 change in the arterial pH. For example, in a patient with a plasma pH of 7.4, an acute increase in the $PaCO_2$ from 40 to 50 mm Hg would be expected to decrease the plasma pH from 7.4 to 7.32. An acute 10 mm Hg decrease in the $PaCO_2$ from 40 to 30 mm Hg would be expected to increase the pH from 7.4 to 7.48.

In respiratory acid–base disorders, the kidneys compensate for changes in the $PaCO_2$ by increasing the plasma bicarbonate (HCO_3^-) in respiratory acidosis, or decreasing the plasma HCO_3^- in respiratory alkalosis. Acute respiratory acid–base disorders result in small changes in the HCO_3^- concentration, and cellular buffering predominates. Chronic renal compensation occurs during days to weeks, and results in a larger change in plasma HCO_3^-. Table 26.1 shows the expected change in the plasma HCO_3^- level in acute and chronic respiratory acidosis and alkalosis. The serum HCO_3^- in a healthy adult is approximately 22 to 26 mEq/L. Thus, it is reasonable to use a level of 24 mEq/L for calculation purposes. Compensatory change in HCO_3^- is associated with a shift in the pH back toward normal. A normal pH is not achieved by compensation alone and *overcompensation does not occur.* Therefore, a mixed respiratory and metabolic disorder is present if the pH is normal and the $PaCO_2$ is altered. For example, a pH of 7.4 with a $PaCO_2$ of 60 mm Hg means that, in addition to the respiratory acidosis, a metabolic alkalosis is present that has moved the pH back to normal (see Step 4). Mixed acid–base disorders do not include the renal HCO_3^- compensation that occurs for acute and chronic respiratory acid–base disorder.

Evaluation of respiratory acid–base disorders can be relatively straightforward in patients with an isolated acute primary respiratory acidosis or alkalosis, such as occurs in a young patient with an acute asthma exacerbation or in an otherwise healthy patient with anxiety-induced hyperventilation, or more difficult when superimposed metabolic acid–base disorders are present in a critically ill patient. Further complicating evaluation is the change that occurs in the serum HCO_3^- in acute and chronic

TABLE 26.1	Expected [HCO$_3^-$] Change in Acute and Chronic Respiratory Acid–Base Disorders (Assume a Baseline [HCO$_3^-$] of 24 mEq/L)
Acute respiratory acidosis	[HCO$_3^-$] = +1 mEq/L for every 10 mm Hg increase in PaCO$_2$ above 40 mm Hg
Chronic respiratory acidosis	[HCO$_3^-$] = +3[a] mEq/L for every 10 mm Hg rise in PaCO$_2$ above 40 mm Hg
Acute respiratory alkalosis	[HCO$_3^-$] = −2 mEq/L for every 10 mm Hg decrease in PaCO$_2$ below 40 mm Hg
Chronic respiratory alkalosis	[HCO$_3^-$] = −4[a] mEq/L for every 10 mm Hg decrease in PaCO$_2$ below 40 mm Hg

[a]Some authors use 3.5 mEq/L for chronic respiratory acidosis and 5 mEq/L for chronic respiratory alkalosis.

respiratory acidosis and alkalosis. Algorithm 26.1 and steps 1 through 6 can aid in analyzing a respiratory acid–base disorder. However, these are general rules, and when evaluating a given ABG in a primary respiratory acid–base disorder, the patient's clinical history and physical examination have to be incorporated to arrive at the correct diagnosis (see step 5 for further explanation).

Respiratory acidosis results from hypercapnia induced by alveolar hypoventilation. The approach to hypercapnia and the differential diagnosis is outlined in Chapter 7, Algorithm 7.1 and includes disorders in any component of the ventilatory mechanism, such as the central or peripheral nervous system, neuromuscular junction, respiratory muscles, chest wall, pleura, upper airway, or lungs.

Respiratory acidosis treatment is directed at the underlying cause, outlined in various other chapters in this manual. In general, treatment is aimed at improving alveolar ventilation and includes bronchodilators for asthma and chronic obstructive pulmonary disease (COPD), bilevel positive airway pressure, mechanical ventilation (used with caution in patients with chronic respiratory acidosis with an elevated serum HCO$_3^-$ as rapid correction can cause a life-threatening metabolic alkalosis), reversal of drug effects, treatment of pulmonary edema, and addressing neuromuscular diseases. Sodium HCO$_3^-$ is not recommended in respiratory acidosis as it may worsen hypercapnia and pulmonary edema, or cause a metabolic alkalosis. Small doses of sodium HCO$_3^-$ can be considered in cases of severe acidosis (pH <7.1) with intractable hypercapnia.

Causes of respiratory alkalosis are listed in Table 26.2; the underlying pathophysiologic mechanism for each is alveolar hyperventilation. Respiratory alkalosis can be associated with a normal or elevated alveolar-arterial oxygen gradient (P[A-a]O$_2$ gradient, abbreviated A-a gradient, and is discussed in more detail in Chapter 7). In patients with an elevated A-a gradient, the differential diagnosis is the same as for patients with an elevated A-a gradient and hypoxia (see Algorithm 7.2). In patients with a normal A-a gradient, causes include central nervous system disorders such as tumors, encephalitis, anxiety, along with fever, hypoxia from altitude or severe anemia, hyperventilation in intubated patients on mechanical ventilatory support, endocrine disorders, and drugs.

As in respiratory acidosis, respiratory alkalosis treatment is directed at the underlying cause. Causes of hypoxia should be identified and treated. In mechanically

ALGORITHM 26.1 **Approach to Respiratory Acid–Base Disorders (see Steps 1 through 6)**

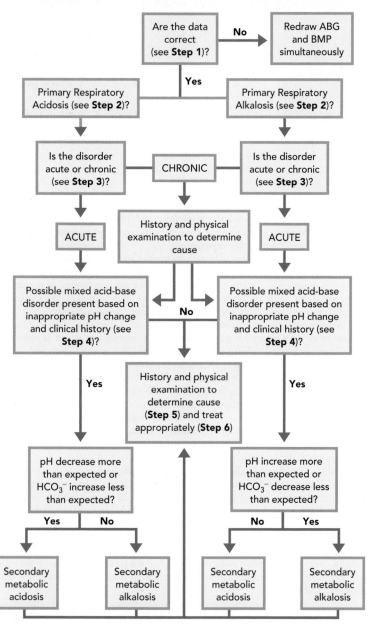

ABG, arterial blood gas; BMP, basic metabolic panel.

TABLE 26.2	Causes of Respiratory Alkalosis

Normal P(A-a)O$_2$ Gradient

Mechanical hyperventilation	Drugs
Central nervous system	Salicylates
Psychogenic hyperventilation	Progesterone
Fever	Catecholamines
Pain	Hypoxia
Encephalitis/meningitis	High altitude
Tumors	Severe anemia
Pregnancy	Endotoxinemia
Hyperthyroidism	Cirrhosis

Elevated P(A-a)O$_2$ gradient[a]

V/Q mismatch	Shunt

[a]The differential diagnosis of respiratory alkalosis with an elevated alveolar-arterial oxygen gradient (P(A-a)O$_2$) is the same as hypoxia with an elevated P(A-a)O$_2$ listed in Chapter 7, Algorithm 7.2. P[A-a]O$_2$, alveolar-arterial oxygen gradient; V/Q, ventilation/perfusion.

ventilated patients, minute ventilation should be decreased by decreasing the respiratory rate and/or tidal volume. In psychogenic hyperventilation, reassurance and anxiolytics can be used. In patients at high altitudes, acetazolamide can be used to induce a metabolic acidosis to compensate for the respiratory alkalosis.

Step 1—Obtain an ABG (see section on arterial cannulation) and ensure the [HCO$_3^-$] is accurate using the Henderson Equation.[a]

$$[HCO_3^- = 24 \times PaCO_2/[H^+]$$

H^1 concentration and corresponding pH	
pH	[H$^+$mEq/L]
7.10	79
7.20	63
7.30	50
7.40	40
7.50	32
7.60	25

Step 2—Determine the underlying abnormality, that is, a primary respiratory acidosis or alkalosis (metabolic acid–base disorders are discussed separately).

1. A primary respiratory acid–base disorder is present if the PaCO$_2$ is altered and the change in pH is in the opposite direction.

[a]Conversely, obtain ABG and basic metabolic panel simultaneously and compare [HCO$_3^-$] in the ABG and basic metabolic panel to ensure accuracy. They should agree within 2 mmol/L.

a. A respiratory acidosis is present if the $PaCO_2$ is >45 mm Hg and the pH is decreased.
b. A respiratory alkalosis is present if the $PaCO_2$ is <35 mm Hg and the pH is increased.

Step 3—Examine the pH, $PaCO_2$, and serum HCO_3^- to determine if the respiratory acid–base disorder is acute or chronic.

1. Each acute change in the $PaCO_2$ of 10 mm Hg will change the pH 0.08 (or 0.008 for each 1 mm Hg change) in the opposite direction.
2. Each partially metabolically compensated change in the $PaCO_2$ of 10 mm Hg will change the pH 0.03 to 0.08 in the opposite direction.
3. Each fully compensated change in the $PaCO_2$ of 10 mm Hg will change the pH approximately 0.03, *but not back to normal.*
4. Table 26.1 shows the expected metabolic compensation for acute and chronic respiratory acid–base disorders, which occurs through changes in serum HCO_3^-. Deviations in the serum HCO_3^- that are significantly less than or greater than expected suggest a superimposed metabolic acid–base disorder.

Step 4—Determine if a mixed respiratory and metabolic acid–base disorder is present.

1. A superimposed metabolic acid–base disorder is present if the change in pH is *more* than 0.08 in the *opposite* direction of each 10 mm Hg change in the $PaCO_2$.
a. A metabolic acidosis is superimposed on a respiratory acidosis if the decrease in pH is greater than expected based on the $PaCO_2$. For example, pH 7.1 and $PaCO_2$ 60 mm HG. The expected pH for an acute increase in the $PaCO_2$ to 60 mm Hg is 7.24. Thus, a superimposed metabolic acidosis is present.
b. A metabolic alkalosis is superimposed on a respiratory alkalosis if the increase in pH is greater than expected based on the $PaCO_2$. For example, pH 7.55 and $PaCO_2$ 30 mm Hg. The expected pH for an acute decrease in the $PaCO_2$ to 30 mm Hg is 7.48. Thus, a superimposed metabolic alkalosis is present.
2. A combined acidosis and alkalosis is present if the $PaCO_2$ is increased or decreased and the pH is normal (~7.4).
a. As stated, compensation back to normal does not occur. Therefore, a normal pH with an altered $PaCO_2$, regardless of metabolic compensation, supports a superimposed metabolic disorder.

Step 5—Correlate the above steps with the patients' clinical history and physical exam to arrive at the correct diagnosis.

For example, consider an ABG with pH 7.20, $PaCO_2$ 80, and plasma HCO_3^- 33 mEq/L. The primary disorder is a respiratory acidosis, evidenced by the decrease in pH and increase in $PaCO_2$ (Step 2). The expected plasma HCO_3^- would be 28 mEq/L if this were an acute acidosis, or 36 mEq/L if it were chronic (Step 3). If this were an acute change in the $PaCO_2$, the pH would be 7.08 (0.08 change in pH for each 10 mm Hg change in $PaCO_2$). Thus, this cannot be a simple acute respiratory acidosis (Step 4). However, there are multiple valid explanations for these ABG findings. One possibility is that it represents a partially compensated respiratory acidosis. Conversely, this could represent an acute respiratory acidosis with a superimposed metabolic alkalosis (explaining the higher than normal serum HCO_3^-). A final possibility is that it represents an acute respiratory acidosis on a compensated chronic respiratory acidosis. Thus, the patient's clinical history and physical exam must be incorporated to determine the correct interpretation. If the patient had severe, compensated COPD complicated by acute cardiogenic pulmonary edema, an acute respiratory acidosis on a chronic compensated respiratory acidosis would seem likely.

Step 6—Once the etiology has been determined, treat appropriately (see end of opening text).

SUGGESTED READINGS

Epstein SK, Singh N. Respiratory acidosis. *Respir Care.* 2001;46:366–383.
  Review of the pathophysiology, evaluation, and causes of respiratory acidosis.
Foster GT, Vazin ND, Sassoon CS. Respiratory alkalosis. *Respir Care.* 2001;46:384–391.
  Review of the pathophysiology, evaluation, and causes of respiratory alkalosis.
Kaufman D, Kitching AJ, Kellum JA. Acid-base balance. In: Hall JB, Schmidt GA, Wood LD, eds. Principles of critical care. 3rd ed online. New York: McGraw-Hill, 2002:1202–1208.
  Comprehensive textbook review of acid-base disorders.

27 Thyroid Disorders

William E. Clutter

HYPERTHYROIDISM

Major clinical findings in hyperthyroidism are listed in Table 27.1. Cardiac findings may be prominent including tachycardia, atrial fibrillation, heart failure, and exacerbation of coronary artery disease. Rarely, severe hyperthyroidism may be associated with fever and delirium, sometimes called "thyroid storm."

Major causes of hyperthyroidism are listed in Table 27.2. Graves' disease (which may also cause proptosis) is the most common.

When hyperthyroidism is diagnosed in a critically ill patient, plasma thyroid stimulating hormone (TSH) and free thyroxine (T_4) should be measured. Clinical hyperthyroidism suppresses TSH to <0.1 $\mu U/mL$, so a nonsuppressed plasma TSH excludes the diagnosis of hyperthyroidism. Plasma TSH may also be suppressed by severe nonthyroidal illness (about 10% of patients in intensive care units have plasma TSH <0.1 $\mu U/mL$) and by therapy with dopamine or high dose glucocorticoids. Thus, a suppressed plasma TSH alone does not establish the diagnosis.

If plasma TSH is suppressed and plasma free T_4 is elevated, the diagnosis of hyperthyroidism is established. If plasma free T_4 is not elevated, one of the other causes of suppressed plasma TSH listed earlier is more likely. Heparin therapy may artifactually increase plasma free T_4, so in heparin-treated patients, plasma total T_4 should be measured instead.

TABLE 27.1	Major Clinical Findings in Hyperthyroidism
Common	**Seen primarily in severe hyperthyroidism**
• Heat intolerance	• Heart failure
• Weight loss	• Exacerbation of coronary artery disease
• Palpitations	• Fever and delirium ("thyroid storm")
• Sinus tachycardia	
• Atrial fibrillation	
• Brisk tendon reflexes	
• Fine tremor	
• Lid lag	
• Proximal muscle weakness	

TABLE 27.2 Major Causes of Hyperthyroidism

Associated with increased radioactive iodine uptake
- Graves' disease
- Toxic multinodular goiter
- Thyroid adenoma

Associated with decreased radioactive iodine uptake
- Iodine-induced hyperthyroidism (due to amiodarone or iodine-containing contrast media[a])
- Painless thyroiditis
- Subacute thyroiditis
- Factitious hyperthyroidism (ingestion of thyroid hormone)

[a]Iodine excess can cause both hyper- and hypo-thyroidism depending on the patients' underlying thyroid function and basal iodine consumption.

Treatment

The etiology of hyperthyroidism determines the best long-term therapy, but differential diagnosis can be deferred in the critically ill patient. Emergency therapy (Table 27.3) is indicated when hyperthyroidism exacerbates heart failure or an acute coronary syndrome, or when thyroid storm is present. It includes rapid inhibition of thyroid hormone synthesis (and conversion of T_4 to tri-iodothyronine [T_3]) by the thionamide propylthiouracil (PTU), inhibition of thyroid hormone secretion by iodine, and inhibition of the cardiovascular effects of hyperthyroidism by beta-adrenergic antagonists. Hydrocortisone is usually recommended because it also inhibits T_4 conversion to T_3.

Some authors have advocated treatment of amiodarone-induced hyperthyroidism with glucocorticoids alone, but the regimen described above has a high success rate in this disorder.

Plasma free T_4 should be measured every 3 to 7 days. When free T_4 approaches the normal range, the doses of PTU and iodine should be gradually decreased. Iodine can usually be stopped at the time of hospital discharge, and radioactive iodine (RAI) therapy for Graves' disease or toxic multinodular goiter can be scheduled 2 to 3 weeks later. If long-term thionamide therapy is chosen instead of RAI, PTU should be stopped and methimazole used instead.

TABLE 27.3 Emergency Therapy of Hyperthyroidism

Propylthiouracil (PTU) 300 mg PO Q6h
Iodine (super saturated potassium iodide) 2 drops PO Q12h
Beta-antagonist, with the dose adjusted to control tachycardia; initially:
  Propranolol 40 mg PO Q6h, or
  Esmolol 500 μg/kg IV followed by 50 μg/kg/min IV
Hydrocortisone 50 mg IV Q8h

TABLE 27.4	Major Clinical Findings in Hypothyroidism
Common	Seen primarily in severe hypothyroidism
• Cold intolerance • Fatigue • Somnolence • Constipation • Weight gain • Slow tendon reflexes • Nonpitting edema (myxedema) • Dry skin	• Hypothermia • Bradycardia • Hypoventilation • Hypotension • Hyponatremia • Pericardial or pleural effusion

HYPOTHYROIDISM

Major clinical findings in hypothyroidism are listed in Table 27.4. Severe hypothyroidism may contribute to hypothermia, hypoventilation, bradycardia, hypotension and hyponatremia in the setting of concomitant critical illnesses.

Major causes of hypothyroidism are listed in Table 27.5. More than 90% of cases are primary hypothyroidism, most often iatrogenic or due to chronic autoimmune thyroiditis. Any pituitary or hypothalamic disorder can cause secondary hypothyroidism, but these disorders are usually clinically apparent because of other manifestations.

When the diagnosis of hypothyroidism is suspected in a critically ill patient, plasma TSH and free T_4 should be measured. Even mild primary hypothyroidism causes elevation of plasma TSH, so a normal plasma TSH excludes this diagnosis. Plasma TSH values >20 $\mu U/mL$ establish the diagnosis of primary hypothyroidism. Milder elevations of plasma TSH are usually due to primary hypothyroidism, but may also occur transiently during recovery from severe nonthyroidal illness.

If plasma free T_4 is low and plasma TSH is not elevated, the patient may have secondary hypothyroidism, but in a critically ill patient, this pattern of test results is more likely to be due to functional suppression of TSH and T_4 secretion by the nonthyroidal illness (the "euthyroid sick syndrome"). If the patient has clinical findings that may be due to hypothyroidism, empiric treatment with T_4 should be started

TABLE 27.5	Major Causes of Primary Hypothyroidism

• Chronic lymphocytic thyroiditis (Hashimoto's disease)
• Iatrogenic (after radioactive iodine therapy or thyroidectomy)
• Drugs
   ◦ Iodine excess (e.g., amiodarone, iodine-containing contrast media[a])
   ◦ Lithium
   ◦ Interferon-alpha
   ◦ Interleukin-2
• Iodine deficiency

[a]Iodine excess can cause both hyper- and hypo- thyroidism depending on the patients' underlying thyroid function and basal iodine consumption.

TABLE 27.6	**Emergency Therapy of Hypothyroidism**

Thyroxine 50–100 μg IV Q6–8h for 24 hr, then
Thyroxine 75–100 μg IV Q24h until oral intake is possible
Hydrocortisone 50 mg IV Q8h

and the diagnosis should be reassessed after recovery. Otherwise, the patient can be observed with periodic measurement of plasma TSH and free T_4 to determine whether the abnormalities resolve with recovery.

Treatment

Emergency therapy of hypothyroidism (Table 27.6) is indicated if the patient has clinical signs that could be contributed to by hypothyroidism, such as bradycardia, hypoventilation, hypothermia, or hypotension. Each of these abnormalities should also be treated in the standard fashion, since they are rarely due to hypothyroidism alone. Vital signs and cardiac rhythm should be monitored since the treatment can exacerbate underlying heart disease. Hydrocortisone may be given because adrenal failure may be associated with chronic autoimmune thyroiditis.

No clinical trials have determined the optimum method of emergency treatment of hypothyroidism, but this method rapidly alleviates T_4 deficiency while minimizing the risk of adverse events. There is no evidence to support treatment of the functional suppression of TSH and T_4 by nonthyroidal illness.

SUGGESTED READINGS

Adler SM, Wartofsky L. The nonthyroidal illness syndrome. *Endocrinol Metab Clin North Am.* 2007;36:657–672.
  Review of the pathophysiology, diagnosis, and management of the changes in thyroid function in nonthyroidal illness.
Cooper DS. Antithyroid drugs. *N Engl J Med.* 2005;352:905–917.
  Comprehensive review of thionamide drugs.
Kaptein EM, Beale E, Chan LS. Thyroid hormone therapy for obesity and nonthyroidal illnesses: a systematic review. *J Clin Endocrinol Metab.* 2009;94:3663–3675.
  The data do not support treatment of thyroid test abnormalities due to nonthyroidal illness.
Osman F, Franklyn JA, Sheppard MC, et al. Successful treatment of amiodarone-induced thyrotoxicosis. *Circulation.* 2002;105:1275–1277.
  Case series showing a high success rate with thionamide treatment alone.

28 Adrenal Insufficiency in Critical Illness

Timothy J. Bedient and Marin H. Kollef

An increase in circulating and tissue corticosteroid levels during critical illness is an important adaptive response. Normally, severe illness and stress stimulate the hypothalamic–pituitary–adrenal (HPA) axis, causing release of corticotropin releasing hormone (CRH) from the hypothalamus. CRH stimulates the anterior pituitary to release adrenocorticotropic hormone (ACTH or corticotropin), with ACTH causing increased cortisol production by the adrenal cortex's zona fasciculata. With acute illness such as severe infection, trauma, and burns, there is an increase in cortisol production by as much as a factor of six. Normally, circulating cortisol is bound to corticosteroid-binding globulin (CBG), with <10% in the free, bioavailable form. During acute illness, however, CBG levels decrease by as much as 50%, with unbound cortisol levels increasing. Although it is the unbound cortisol that is physiologically active, current laboratory assays only measure total cortisol. In a healthy, unstressed person, the HPA axis undergoes diurnal variation, but this is lost in critical illness. The major physiologic actions of circulating cortisol include increasing blood sugar levels; facilitating the delivery of glucose to cells during stress; facilitating normal cardiovascular reactivity to angiotensin II, epinephrine, and norepinephrine; contributing to the maintenance of cardiac contractility, vascular tone, and blood pressure; and anti-inflammatory and immunosuppressive effects.

Chronic adrenal insufficiency (Addison's disease) is a rare cause of intensive care unit admission and is distinct from the HPA axis dysfunction that occurs during critical illness, which has been termed *critical illness-related corticosteroid insufficiency* (CIRCI). CIRCI is characterized by an inappropriately low increase in cortisol during acute illness, also referred to as *relative adrenal insufficiency*. It is mediated in part by inflammatory cytokine inhibition of (a) CRH and ACTH release, (b) adrenal cortisol synthesis, and (c) glucocorticoid receptor translocation and transcription. In addition to CIRCI, adrenal insufficiency in critical illness may also be separated into two categories: *primary* if it is due to adrenal gland dysfunction, or *secondary* if it caused by central disruption of CRH or ACTH release. Causes of primary adrenal insufficiency in acute illness include direct injury to the adrenal glands from trauma, infarction, infection, malignancy, and hemorrhage; drug-induced suppression of cortisol synthesis; and autoimmune adrenalitis. Secondary causes include discontinuation of exogenous corticosteroids in patients on chronic immunotherapy, central nervous system malignancies, and head trauma. Causes of adrenal insufficiency are listed in Table 28.1.

TABLE 28.1	Causes of Adrenal Insufficiency
Cause	Example
Infection	Sepsis/septic shock HIV Cytomegalovirus *Staphylococcus aureus,* toxin-producing strain Fungal disorders (histoplasmosis, blastomycosis, cryptococcus) Tuberculosis
Medications	Suppressing release of corticotropin releasing hormone from the hypothalamus and pituitary: 　Corticosteroids 　Megestrol acetate Inhibition of enzymes involved in cortisol synthesis: 　Etomidate 　Ketoconazole 　Metyrapone Increased metabolism of cortisol: 　Rifampin 　Phenytoin
Malignancy	Adrenal metastases
Adrenal hemorrhage	Secondary to shock 　Anticoagulation 　Meningococcemia (Waterhouse–Friderichsen syndrome) 　Disseminated intravascular coagulation 　Antiphospholipid syndrome
Autoimmune	Addison's disease
Hypothalamic and pituitary disorders	Resulting in secondary adrenal insufficiency: 　Infection 　Pituitary tumor or metastases 　Infiltrative disorders (sarcoidosis, histiocytosis) 　Postpartum pituitary necrosis 　Trauma (blunt, radiation, surgical)

HIV, human immunodeficiency virus.

Signs and symptoms of corticosteroid insufficiency resulting from HPA dysfunction are listed in Table 28.2. In pre-existing hypoadrenalism, these findings may be present before the onset of acute illness. However, in critically ill patients, adrenal insufficiency should be suspected in all patients with hypotension that is unresponsive to intravenous (IV) fluid administration and who require vasopressor support.

Although it is well documented that acute illness increases cortisol through stimulation of the HPA axis, it is less clear what defines an adequate stress response to

TABLE 28.2	**Signs and Symptoms of Adrenal Insufficiency**
Sign	Symptoms
Cardiovascular	Hypotension that is usually not responsive to fluid administration requiring use of vasopressors; hyperdynamic hemodynamic profile is common; tachycardia unless severe hypothyroidism is also present
Metabolic/electrolyte	Hypoglycemia, hyponatremia, hyperkalemia, fever
Hematologic	Eosinophilia and anemia
Neuromuscular	Weakness, fatigue, myalgia, arthralgia, headache, memory impairment, depression
Gastrointestinal	Anorexia, diarrhea, nausea, salt craving, weight loss
Cutaneous	Vitiligo, alopecia

acute illness. In addition, although CIRCI should be considered in all critically ill patients, most of the studies have focused on patients with severe sepsis and septic shock. Previous studies have suggested that a random serum cortisol >25 to 34 μg/dL in critically ill patients makes relative adrenal insufficiency unlikely. However, recent studies have suggested that random cortisol measurements may have limited utility in the diagnosis of adrenal insufficiency, except in patients with a baseline cortisol <10 to 15 μg/dL, and have highlighted the diagnostic value of a cortisol increase of $\leq$9 μg/dL 60 minutes after stimulation with 250 μg of IV cosyntropin (synthetic ACTH) as making adrenal insufficiency likely in critical illness.

In a prospective inception cohort study performed by Annane et al. in 2000 of 189 patients with septic shock, it was noted that an intermediate or poor prognosis occurred in patients with a cortisol increase in response to cosyntropin of $\leq$9 μg/dL, with the highest mortality found in those patients who, in addition to a cosyntropin response of $\leq$9 μg/dL, had an initial cortisol >34 μg/dL. Another study by Annane et al. in 2006 of 101 patients with sepsis, 41 patients without sepsis, and 32 healthy controls, the overnight metyrapone stimulation test (Algorithm 28.1) was used to investigate the diagnostic value of the cosyntropin test, and found that adrenal insufficiency was likely if the baseline cortisol level was <10 μg/dL or change in cortisol after cosyntropin was $\leq$9 μg/dL, and unlikely when cosyntropin stimulated cortisol levels were $\geq$44 μg/dL and the change in cortisol after cosyntropin was $\geq$16.8 μg/dL. These diagnostic values were explored further in 2007 by Lipiner-Friedman et al. in the retrospective arm of the CORTICUS study group. This retrospective multicenter cohort study included 477 patients with severe sepsis and septic shock who had undergone an ACTH stimulation test on the first day of sepsis, and found that random cortisol levels $\geq$15 μg/dL, regardless of the cutoff, were not independent predictors of shock reversal, hospital mortality, or survival duration. However, patients with a baseline cortisol level <15 μg/dL or change in cortisol $\leq$9 μg/dL after cosyntropin had a longer duration of shock and a shorter survival time. Corticosteroids were used to treat 44% of patients and were associated with a strong reduction in the risk of dying (OR, 0.21; 98% CI, 0.08 to 0.52). Measuring serum cortisol 30 and 60 minutes after cosyntropin added no significant diagnostic value to checking cortisol at 60 minutes alone.

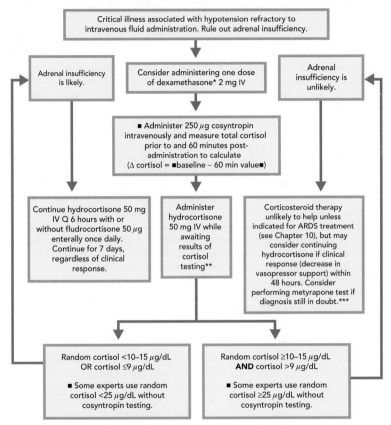

ALGORITHM 28.1 Diagnostic and Therapeutic Approach to Adrenal Insufficiency in the Critically Ill Patient

Critical illness associated with hypotension refractory to intravenous fluid administration. Rule out adrenal insufficiency.

Adrenal insufficiency is likely.

Consider administering one dose of dexamethasone* 2 mg IV

Adrenal insufficiency is unlikely.

■ Administer 250 μg cosyntropin intravenously and measure total cortisol prior to and 60 minutes post-administration to calculate (Δ cortisol = ■baseline − 60 min value■)

Continue hydrocortisone 50 mg IV Q 6 hours with or without fludrocortisone 50 μg enterally once daily. Continue for 7 days, regardless of clinical response.

Administer hydrocortisone 50 mg IV while awaiting results of cortisol testing**

Corticosteroid therapy unlikely to help unless indicated for ARDS treatment (see Chapter 10), but may consider continuing hydrocortisone if clinical response (decrease in vasopressor support) within 48 hours. Consider performing metyrapone test if diagnosis still in doubt.***

Random cortisol <10–15 μg/dL OR cortisol ≤9 μg/dL

■ Some experts use random cortisol <25 μg/dL without cosyntropin testing.

Random cortisol ≥10–15 μg/dL **AND** cortisol >9 μg/dL

■ Some experts use random cortisol ≥25 μg/dL without cosyntropin testing.

ARDS, acute respiratory distress syndrome; Δ cortisol, change in cortisol level in μg/dL.
*Dexamethasone does not interfere with the cosyntropin test and 2 mg IV is equivalent to approximately 50 mg of hydrocortisone.
**Administer only if dexamethasone was not given initially.
***Metyrapone blocks the conversion of 11-deoxycortisol to cortisol by CYP11B1 and causes a rapid fall in cortisol.
To test, give metyrapone orally at 30 mg/kg at midnight and measure 11-deoxycortisol and cortisol 8 hours later. A normal response is an 8 AM serum 11-deoxycortisol level of 7–22 μg/dL and serum cortisol <5 μg/dL. Serum 11-deoxycortisol <7 μg/dL indicates adrenal insufficiency. Patients who undergo metyrapone testing should receive at least 24 hours of corticosteroid replacement. *Metyrapone is not currently available for routine clinic use in the United States.*

Randomized studies have been performed to determine if corticosteroid replacement therapy is beneficial in patients with varying diagnostic definitions of adrenal insufficiency. In a placebo-controlled, randomized, double-blind study by Annane et al. in 2002, 300 patients with septic shock were randomized to receive hydrocortisone

50 mg every 6 hours and fludrocortisone 50 μg once daily for 7 days, or placebo, after undergoing a 250 μg cosyntropin test. Of the 229 patients with relative adrenal insufficiency (115 placebo and 114 corticosteroid), defined as an increase after cosyntropin of ≤ 9 μg/dL, there was significantly reduced mortality (73 patients vs. 60 patients, $p = 0.02$) and withdrawal of vasopressor therapy within 28 days (46 patients vs. 65 patients, $p = 0.001$) in the corticosteroid treated patients, without increasing adverse events. In the 70 patients who had a cosyntropin response ≥ 9 μg/dL, corticosteroid replacement therapy had no significant effect on the same outcomes and no trend toward efficacy. These data were supported by two meta-analyses examining glucocorticoids administration in severe sepsis and septic shock showing reduced mortality when glucocorticoids were given at similar dosages. Previous studies showing a survival disadvantage used higher-dose corticosteroids (23,975 mg vs. 1209 mg) administered for a shorter duration.

However, the preliminary results of the randomized arm of the CORTICUS study found no benefit to treating patients with septic shock, including the subgroup with a cosyntropin response ≤ 9 μg/dL. This study differed from the initial randomized study by Annane in 2002 in that patients in the CORTICUS study were randomized up to 72 hours after the onset of septic shock rather than within 8 hours, patients in the CORTICUS study included those with severe sepsis and septic shock rather than septic shock alone (i.e., could be included in the study without hypotension requiring vasopressors), received 11 days of corticosteroid replacement rather than 7 days, and were not given fludrocortisone. Additionally, the CORTICUS study lacked clinical equipoise resulting in a selection bias whereby patients least likely to benefit from corticosteroids were enrolled in the study. How this study will change clinicians' approach to treating adrenal insufficiency in septic shock has yet to be seen.

Glucocorticoids, however, may not be appropriate for all critically ill patients as highlighted in a case-control study by Britt et al. in 2006 in 100 patients (six with septic shock) in a burn trauma ICU who received steroids, compared with 100 matched control patients, showing that corticosteroid use was associated with increased infection rates, increased ICU and ventilator duration, and a trend toward increased mortality.

Based on these data, there are no definitive diagnostic criteria for relative corticosteroid insufficiency in critically ill patients. Some experts believe the supraphysiologic dose of cosyntropin used in an attempt to increase cortisol production from an already stimulated adrenal gland may be less important than the baseline cortisol alone. However, numerous studies have found benefit from corticosteroid replacement in patients with relative adrenal insufficiency defined by cosyntropin stimulated cortisol ≤ 9 μg/dL, and there is suggestion, at least in retrospective data, that baseline cortisol levels >10 to 15 μg/dL may be less important than adrenal reserves as measured with 250 μg cosyntropin stimulated serum cortisol levels at 1 hour.

Thus, although our understanding of relative adrenal insufficiency in the critically ill continues to evolve, nearly all evidence agrees that adrenal insufficiency is likely when the baseline cortisol is <10 to 15 μg/dL in critically ill patients, and that cosyntropin stimulation testing may have additional diagnostic value in identifying which patients are likely to respond to corticosteroid replacement, at least in the setting of volume unresponsive hypotension in patients with septic shock. We recommend that critically ill patients with shock unresponsive to IV fluids requiring vasopressor support be evaluated for adrenal insufficiency and treated as illustrated in Algorithm 28.1. Patients may be given dexamethasone 2 mg IV while waiting for cosyntropin testing results, as dexamethasone does not interfere with the cosyntropin test. Otherwise, patients should be started on hydrocortisone immediately following cosyntropin testing while waiting for the results. Once treatment is initiated, the cause of adrenal insufficiency can be explored further. Many patients with adrenal insufficiency related to critical illness can be expected to regain normal function of the HPA axis with recovery from their illness. Some experts, however, still use the random cortisol alone, feeling that adrenal insufficiency is unlikely when the random cortisol is ≥25 μg/dL and that cosyntropin testing has no additional diagnostic value. Certainly more studies are needed.

SUGGESTED READINGS

Annane A, Bellissant E, Bollaert PE, et al. Corticosteroids for severe sepsis and septic shock: a systematic review and meta-analysis. *BMJ.* 2004;329:480–489.
Meta-analysis of 16 randomized and quasi randomized trials involving 2063 patients with severe sepsis and septic shock showing that long courses (≥5 days) with low dose corticosteroids (≤300 mg hydrocortisone or equivalent) reduced 28 day and hospital mortality.

Annane D, Maxime V, Ibrahim F, et al. Diagnosis of adrenal insufficiency in severe sepsis and septic shock. *Am J Respir Crit Care Med.* 2006;174:1319–1326.
An update on the diagnosis of adrenal insufficiency using cosyntropin stimulation.

Annane D, Sebille V, Charpentier C, et al. Effect of treatment with low dose of hydrocortisone and fludrocortisone on mortality in patients with septic shock. *JAMA.* 2002;288:862–871.
A placebo controlled, randomized, double-blind study showing a 7-day treatment with low doses of hydrocortisone and fludrocortisone in patients with septic shock and relative adrenal insufficiency, significantly reduced the risk of death without an increase in adverse events.

Annane D, Sebille V, Troche G, et al. A 3-level prognostic classification in septic shock based on cortisol levels and cortisol response to corticotropin. *JAMA.* 2000;283:1038–1045.
A prospective inception cohort study evaluating the prognostic value of cortisol and the cosyntropin stimulation test in patients with septic shock.

Cooper MS, Stewart PM. Corticosteroid insufficiency in acutely ill patients. *N Engl J Med.* 2003;348:727–734.
A focused review on the pathogenesis and treatment of adrenal insufficiency in the critically ill.

Lipiner-Friedman D, Sprung CL, Laterre PF. Adrenal function in sepsis: The retrospective Corticus cohort study. *Crit Care Med.* 2007;35:1012–1018.
Retrospective cohort study from 20 European intensive care units examining the relationship between baseline and cosyntropin stimulated cortisol levels and mortality in patients with severe sepsis and septic shock showing that delta cortisol and not basal cortisol levels were associated with clinical outcomes.

Marik PE. Critical illness-related corticosteroid insufficiency. *Chest.* 2009;135:181–193.
Concise review of the causes, pathophysiology, diagnosis and treatment of adrenal insufficiency in critically-ill patients.

Marik PE, Pastores SM, Annane D, et al. Recommendations for the diagnosis and management of corticosteroid insufficiency in critically ill adult patients: consensus statements from an international task force by the American College of Critical Care Medicine. *Crit Care Med.* 2008;36:1937–1949.
Evidence-based guidelines for the diagnosis and medical management of adrenal insufficiency in critically ill patients. This guideline recommends that adrenal insufficiency in critical illness is best diagnosed by a delta cortisol (after 250 mcg cosyntropin) of <9 mcg/dL or a random total cortisol of <10 mcg/dL. Treatment with hydrocortisone (200–300 mg/day) is recommended for patients with septic shock who have responded poorly to fluid resuscitation and vasopressor agents.

Sprung CL, Annane D, Keh D, et al. Hydrocortisone therapy for patients with septic shock. *N Engl J Med.* 2008;358:111–124.

The prospective CORTICUS study which demonstrated that hydrocortisone did not improve survival or reversal of shock in patients with septic shock, either overall or in patients who did not have a response to corticotropin, although hydrocortisone hastened reversal of shock in patients in whom shock was reversed.

29 Diabetic Ketoacidosis and Hyperosmolar Hyperglycemic State

David A. Rometo, Marin H. Kollef, and Garry S. Tobin

Diabetic ketoacidosis (DKA) and hyperosmolar hyperglycemic state (HHS) are life-threatening hyperglycemic complications of diabetes mellitus (DM), and common reasons for admission to the intensive care unit. The annual incidence of DKA ranges from 4.6 to 8 episodes per 1,000 patients with DM, resulting in more than 500,000 hospital days per year. The annual incidence of HHS is lower than DKA and accounts for <1% of primary diabetic admissions. The mortality rate is 1% to 5% in DKA and 5% to 20% in HHS, with worse outcomes at extremes of age, and with the presence of coma, hypotension, and severe comorbidities. Precipitating factors include inadequate insulin treatment or noncompliance, new-onset DM, infections (most commonly pneumonia and urinary tract infections), cardiovascular events, cerebrovascular accident, pancreatitis, drugs, and pregnancy. DKA typically occurs in patients with type 1 DM, but does occur in patients with type 2 DM (as high as 1/3 of DKA cases). HHS is typically confined to patients with type 2 DM, often precipitated by loss of access to water in the elderly or chronically ill. DKA and HHS are the result of insulin deficiency in patients with DM. In both disorders, insulin deficiency causes increased hepatic glycolysis, gluconeogenesis, and impaired glucose utilization by peripheral tissues, leading to hyperglycemia. The hyperglycemia in both disorders causes an osmotic diuresis. Table 29.1 highlights the differences between DKA and HHS.

DIABETIC KETOACIDOSIS

DKA is characterized by hyperglycemia (blood glucose [BG] typically $\geq$250 mg/dL), anion gap metabolic acidosis (arterial pH $\leq$7.3), and ketosis (positive urine and plasma ketones), along with dehydration and electrolyte abnormalities in varying degrees. Common ketone assays use nitroprusside, measuring acetoacetate and acetone, but not beta-hydroxybutyrate. Prominent presenting symptoms include nausea/vomiting, abdominal pain, labored breathing (Kussmaul respirations), and polyuria. A mixed acid–base disorder may also be present, such as a concomitant severe contraction metabolic alkalosis elevating the serum bicarbonate level, masking the underlying metabolic acidosis.

In patients with DKA, the absolute lack of insulin causes an increase in counterregulatory hormones (cortisol, growth hormone, catecholamines, and glucagon),

TABLE 29.1	Initial Laboratory Values in DKA and HHS			
	DKA			
Value	Mild	Moderate	Severe	HHS
Plasma glucose (mg/dL)	>250	>250	>250	>600
Arterial pH	7.25–7.30	7–7.24	<7	>7.30
Serum bicarbonate (mEq/L)	15–18	10–14	<10	>15
Urine and serum ketones	Positive	Positive	Positive	Trace/small
Serum osmolarity (mOsm/L)	<320	<320	<320	330–380
Anion gap	>10	>12	>12	<12
Mental status	Alert	Alert/drowsy	Stupor/coma	Stupor/coma
Sodium (mmol/L)	125–135	125–135	125–135	135–145
Potassium (mmol/L)	Normal to ↑	Normal to ↑	Normal to ↑	Normal
Creatinine (mg/dL)	Slight ↑	Slight ↑	Slight ↑	Moderate ↑

DKA, diabetic ketoacidosis; HHS, hyperosmolar hyperglycemic state.

which promote lipolysis in adipose tissue and the release of free fatty acids. In the liver, the free fatty acids are converted to ketones. These patients suffer from a metabolic acidosis as a result of these circulating ketoacids. Ketone bodies contribute to the osmotic diuresis, and diuresis causes loss of sodium and potassium. Although initial laboratory values are variable, total body sodium and potassium are depleted.

While prompt management of DKA as described below is essential, finding and treating the precipitating cause should not be forgotten or delayed. Blood, urine, sputum cultures, chest x-ray, EKG, and empiric treatment based on clinical suspicion should be part of the initial management of DKA. One should evaluate the cause of abdominal pain if the symptom does not resolve with correction of dehydration and metabolic acidosis.

Treatment of DKA requires reversal of the hyperglycemia by administering insulin, and replacing the circulating and total body volume and electrolyte deficits (as outlined in Algorithm 29.1). Normal saline boluses for acute volume resuscitation, followed by $\frac{1}{2}$ NS replacement of the remaining fluid deficit, and later 5% dextrose containing fluids when glucose falls below 250 mg/dL is the mainstay of fluid therapy. Insulin should be given as an intravenous (IV) bolus, followed by continuous infusion. Hyperglycemia resolves faster than acidosis, and supraphysiologic insulin is needed to overcome hyperglycemia-induced insulin resistance to achieve euglycemia. After this is achieved, insulin is still required to drive peripheral ketone use, resolving the remaining acidosis. Therefore, BG should be kept between 150 and 200 mg/dL with 5% dextrose until the anion gap is closed. Intermediate or long-acting subcutaneous (SC) insulin must be given before insulin drip discontinuation. Failure to do this properly can lead to rebound hyperglycemia and DKA. The patient should be able to tolerate PO fluids, and dextrose containing IV fluids should be stopped at that time.

ALGORITHM 29.1 Management of Diabetic Ketoacidosis (DKA) and Hyperosmolar Hyperglycemic State (HHS)

INSULIN TREATMENT

1) Bolus 0.1–0.15 U/kg regular insulin intravenously (IV) (subcutaneous [SC]/intramuscular [IM] can be given if no IV access)
2) Start continuous IV insulin infusion via an infusion pump
   Standard infusion is 100 U **regular human insulin** (IV t $^1/_2$ 5–9 minutes) in 100 mL 0.9% NaCl.
   For **DKA** start at 0.1 U/kg/hr
   For **HHS** start at 0.05 U/kg/hr delay insulin in **HHS** until at least 1 L NS infused

BLOOD GLUCOSE MONITORING

1) Check initial blood glucose (BG) q1h. **Goal decrease in BG is 50–75 mg/dL/hr.**
2) Once stable (3 consecutive values decreased in target range), change BG monitoring to q2h. Resume q1h BG monitoring for each change in the insulin infusion rate (see below).
3) Add dextrose 5% to IV fluids when BG <250 mg/dL
   For DKA goal BG 150–200 mg/dL until anion gap closed.
   For HHS goal BG is 250–300 mg/dL until mental status improves.

CHANGING THE INSULIN INFUSION RATE

1) ↓ IV insulin by 50%/hr if BG decreases by >100 mg/dL/hr in any 1 hour period.*
2) ↑ insulin drip by 50%/hr if change in BG is <50 mg/dL/hr.
3) For **DKA and HSS**, when BG decreases to 250 mg/dL, insulin infusion may need to be decreased 50% to maintain glucose at target levels (see Blood Glucose Monitoring above).

Start SC insulin when:
1) Anion gap closed (DKA)
2) Serum bicarbonate increases to >15 mEq/L (DKA)
3) Patient able to eat
4) Mental status improves (HHS)

Stop the insulin drip after all of the following are done**
1) Give short acting insulin (aspart or lispro) SC at twice the hourly IV rate (e.g., if IV rate is 5 U/hr, give 10 U short acting insulin SC).
2) Give long acting insulin (NPH or glargine) SC at 0.2–0.3 U/kg (divided q8 for NPH), or home insulin dose.
3) Ensure patient has a meal and is eating.

*Lowering glucose >100 mg/dL/hr may cause osmotic encephalopathy.
**Failure to give SC insulin may result in rebound hyperglycemia and ketosis due to the short $t^1/_2$ of IV regular insulin (5–9 min).

Initially, insulin should be given IV. If IV administration cannot be achieved, an intramuscular or SC route is an option. However, this is a less reliable method to achieve the insulin levels needed in seriously ill patients. In adults, BG should be decreased by 50 to 100 mg/dL/hr. Decreasing the BG more than 75 to 100 mg/dL/hr can cause an osmotic encephalopathy (0.3% to 1% of DKA in children, extremely

ALGORITHM 29.1 **Management of Diabetic Ketoacidosis (DKA) and Hyperosmolar Hyperglycemic State (HHS) (*Continued*)**

FLUID MANAGEMENT*

Fluid replacement varies based on age, weight, hemodynamics, and comorbidities. A reasonable approach follows:

1) **Replace intravascular volume**
   Give 1 L 0.9% NaCl over 30–60 min. Give an additional 1–2 L q30–60 min until hemodynamically stable and urine output increased.
2) **Replace total body water deficit**
   Change to 0.45% NaCl and infuse at 150–500 mL/hr.
   When BG <250 mg/dL add dextrose 5% and decrease to 100–200 mL/hr.

*Fluid is replaced over 12–24 hr and patients are generally depleted 3–6 L in DKA and 8–12 L in HHS.
*Monitor urine output, heart rate, blood pressure, and respiratory status. Care must be taken in patients with congestive heart failure and kidney disease.

ELECTROLYTE MANAGEMENT

1) Check basic metabolic panel (BMP), arterial blood gas, magnesium (Mg^{2+}), and phosphorus (PO_4^{3-}).
2) Repeat BMP, Mg, PO_4^{3-} q2–4h depending on degree of electrolyte imbalance.

Potassium (K^+)
   K^+ ≥5.5 mEq/L: leave potassium supplement out of IVF
   K^+ 4–5.4 mEq/L: add 20 mEq KCl/L to IVF
   K^+ 3–3.9 mEq/L: add 40 mEq KCl/L to IVF
   K^+ <3 mEq/L: add 60 mEq KCl/L to IVF
   In DKA, if initial K^+ is <3.3 mEq/L, **DO NOT** give IV insulin until the serum K^+ is supplemented to >3.3 mmol/L due to the risk of severe hypokalemia.

Sodium (Na^+)
Hypoglycemia causes an artifactually low serum sodium, and the correct value must be calculated. Corrected Na^+ = Measured Na^+ [mmol/L] + (1.6 (Measured BG [mg/dL] − 100)/100)
Na^+ replaced with IV fluids initially as 0.9% NaCl for first 1–3 L and then as 0.45% NaCl (see Fluid Management).

Bicarbonate (HCO_3^-)
Usually in DKA only.
Replacement generally not necessary as insulin will reverse the HCO_3^- deficit with its inhibition of lipolysis.
Consider HCO_3^- in the following situations (see Chapter 24; metabolic acidosis):
   1) Severe acidosis with pH <7 (the HCO_3^- should be stopped once the pH is >7.1)
   2) Severe loss of buffering capacity when serum HCO_3^- <5–10 mEq/L
   3) Acidosis induced cardiac or respiratory distress
   4) Severe hyperkalemia

Magnesium and Phosphorus
   Severe hypomagnesemia and hypophosphatemia are not common complications of DKA and HHS (see Chapter 23 if they occur) and supplementation is usually not necessary.

PRECIPITATING FACTOR TREATMENT

The cause of the DKA or HHS should be sought and treated. Common precipitants include missed insulin therapy, infections such as pneumonia, sepsis, and urinary and upper respiratory tract infections, trauma, myocardial infarction, pregnancy, or as the initial presentation of DM.

rare in adults). Glucose lowering in the first 2 hours may be more rapid as a result of initial volume expansion.

Insulin and IV fluids will correct the acidosis in patients with DKA, but can rapidly produce hypokalemia as potassium shifts intracellularly. The patient is total body potassium deficient at presentation, even if serum potassium is elevated, unless chronic kidney disease is present. Successful treatment requires frequent monitoring and decision-making based on the patient's clinical condition, and laboratory data as it becomes available.

HYPEROSMOLAR HYPERGLYCEMIC STATE

HHS is characterized by hyperglycemia (BG typically 600 to 1,200 mg/dL), hyperosmolarity (serum osmolarity 320 to 380 mOsm/L), pronounced dehydration (hemodynamic instability, prerenal azotemia, decreased urine output), and neurologic sequelae ranging from mild lethargy to coma. HHS has an insidious onset, typically over weeks, with patients experiencing polyuria, polydipsia, weight loss, and neurologic changes including fatigue, confusion, or coma. Even in the absence of exogenous insulin, there is typically enough intrinsic insulin production by beta cells to suppress hepatic lipoprotein lipase and ketoacid production. In HHS the hyperglycemia is more pronounced than in DKA, resulting in greater diuresis. The resulting dehydration impairs renal function, decreasing glucose excretion, and worsening hyperglycemia. IV insulin should not be given until fluid resuscitation with 1 to 2 L of normal saline has been completed to prevent rapid hyperglycemia correction and hemodynamic collapse from intracellular fluid shifts. Patients with HHS are often more responsive to insulin than patients with DKA and a lower dose is often used. The BG should be kept slightly higher, generally between 250 and 300 mg/dL to allow gradual correction of intracranial fluid shifts. These levels should be maintained until the patient's mental status improves. When this happens, IV insulin can be converted to SC insulin as listed in Algorithm 29.1. Failure to give SC insulin when IV insulin is stopped can result in rebound hyperglycemia with worsening mental status in HHS. Of note, mental status has been shown to correlate with elevated serum osmolality at presentation, but not with acidosis. Stupor or coma while serum osmolality is <320 mOsm/L warrants immediate consideration of other causes of altered mental status.

CEREBRAL EDEMA

Cerebral edema is a serious complication of both DKA and HHS. This devastating consequence is observed more frequently in children than in adults. Symptoms include headache, altered mental status, or a sudden deterioration in mental status after an initial improvement. Bradycardia, hypertension, and papilledema can be seen. Cerebral edema usually develops 4 to 12 hours after the treatment has started, but can occur before the treatment has begun, or uncommonly, may develop as late as 24 to 48 hours after the start of the treatment. The risk factors for cerebral edema are excessive correction with free H_2O and a rapid decline in the BG. Effective osmolality and water deficit can be calculated to replete at an appropriate rate (Algorithm 29.1). Failure of the serum sodium to rise during the treatment is a clue to excess hydration with free H_2O. Prompt recognition and treatment with IV mannitol and corticosteroids is essential to prevent neurologic sequelae. Computed tomography imaging can show

TABLE 29.2 Treatment of Cerebral Edema Complicating DKA or HHS

- Initiate treatment as soon as cerebral edema is clinically suspected.
- Give mannitol 0.5–1 g/kg IV over 20 min and repeat if there is no initial response in 30 min to 1 hr.
- Reduce the rate of fluid administrated by one-third.
- Hypertonic saline (3%), 5–10 mL/kg over 30 min, may be an alternative to mannitol, especially if there is no initial response to mannitol.
- Elevate the head of the bed.
- Intubation for airway protection and impending respiratory failure. Hyperventilation to a PCO_2 <22 mm Hg has been associated with poor outcomes and is not recommended.
- After treatment for cerebral edema is initiated, a brain CT should be obtained to rule out other possible causes of intracerebral deterioration, especially thrombosis or hemorrhage.

DKA, diabetic ketoacidosis; HHS, hyperosmolar hyperglycemic state.

the presence of cerebral edema. Morbidity and mortality are high once cerebral edema is recognized (Table 29.2).

SUGGESTED READINGS

Faich GA, Fishbein HA, Ellis SE. The epidemiology of diabetic acidosis: a population based study. *Am J Epidemiol.* 1983;177:551–558.
  A 12-month epidemiologic study conducted from 1979–1980 of all acute care centers in Rhode Island which examined the incidence, mortality rates, precipitating factors, and cost for patients admitted with DKA.

Glaser N. Cerebral injury and cerebral edema in children with diabetic ketoacidosis: could cerebral ischemia and reperfusion injury be involved? *Pediatr Diabetes.* 2009;10:534–541.
  A concise review of the pathogenesis of cerebral edema in DKA and how this is related to treatment.

Kitabchi AE, Guillermo EU, Miles JM, et al. Hyperglycemic crises in adult patients with diabetes. *Diabetes Care.* 2009;32:1335–1343.
  An extensive review of the definitions, causes, manifestations, pathophysiology, and treatment of DKA and HHS.

Magee MF, Bhatt BA. Management of decompensated diabetes. Diabetic ketoacidosis and hyperglycemic hyperosmolar syndrome. *Crit Care Clin.* 2001;17(1):75–106.
  Review of DKA and HHS.

Wolfsdorf J, Craig ME, Daneman D, et al. Diabetic ketoacidosis. *Pediatr Diabetes.* 2007;8:28–43.
  Consensus guidelines from the International Society for Pediatric and Adolescent Diabetes for the management of DKA.

30 Glucose Control in the ICU

David A. Rometo, Marin H. Kollef, and Garry S. Tobin

Hyperglycemia is a common finding in patients in the intensive care unit (ICU), occurring in both diabetic and nondiabetic patients. Factors contributing to hyperglycemia in critically ill patients include increased counterregulatory hormones (cortisol and glucagon), hepatic insulin resistance, decreased physical activity with resultant decrease in insulin-stimulated glucose uptake in heart and skeletal muscle, glucocorticoid therapy, dextrose-containing intravenous fluids, and dense caloric enteral and parenteral nutrition. Numerous observational studies have shown that hyperglycemia is an independent risk factor for morbidity and mortality in patients in the medical, surgical, neurology, and cardiac ICUs, including postoperative cardiac and general surgery patients, patients with acute myocardial infarction and stroke, and general medicine patients.

Until recently, it was less clear if hyperglycemia was a benign, physiologic marker of more severe critical illness, or a treatable cause of worse clinical outcomes. A few earlier single-center randomized trials have addressed this question, and they have suggested that treating hyperglycemia in critically ill patients could reduce morbidity and mortality. However, which patients benefit the most from treatment and the optimal glucose targets were unclear from those studies. More recent multicenter trials have demonstrated that hypoglycemia and intensive glycemic control were associated with adverse outcomes including increased hospital mortality. The following discussion addresses the current evidence, recommendations, and areas of uncertainty in regards to glucose control in the ICU.

TRIALS

The seminal randomized study treating hyperglycemia in critically ill patients was published by Van den Berghe et al. in 2001 and included 1548 intubated patients (13% with known diabetes) in a surgical ICU who were randomly assigned to intensive glycemic control with a target glucose between 80 and 110 mg/dL ($n = 765$), versus a standard care group that was treated with insulin when the blood glucose (BG) was >215 mg/dL, with a target glucose between 180 and 200 mg/dL ($n = 783$). The study found that the intensive care mortality rate was 42% lower (8% vs. 4.6%, $p < 0.04$) in the intensive treatment group, with the benefit reaching statistical significance in patients who remained in the ICU for more than 5 days. The major difference in mortality was attributed to a decrease in the development of multiorgan failure with sepsis.

Van den Berghe et al. addressed nonsurgical patients in 2006 with a follow-up trial limited to patients in a medical ICU, which randomized 1200 patients (16.9% with known diabetes) to intensive glucose control versus standard care utilizing the same protocol as in their 2001 trial. The study did not replicate the mortality benefit seen in the surgical ICU study. Overall, there was no significant difference in the in-hospital mortality rate (37.3% vs. 40%, $p = 0.33$). While the study did show decreased in-hospital mortality for the 767 patients who stayed in the ICU ≥ 3 days (43% vs. 52.5%, $p = 0.009$), there was increased mortality in the patients who stayed in the ICU <3 days (12.9% vs. 9.6%, $p = 0.41$ after correcting for baseline risk factors). This difference did not reach statistical significance. Despite no overall mortality benefit, there was reduced morbidity in the intensive treatment group, including less newly acquired kidney injury, reduced duration of mechanical ventilation, shorter ICU stay, and shorter hospital stays. There were no significant differences in bacteremia rates or duration of antibiotics.

In the two trials by Van ben Berghe et al., hypoglycemic episodes were increased in the intensive treatment group (5.2% vs. 0.7% in the surgical ICU, 18.7% vs. 3.1% in the medical ICU). Despite the high incidence of hypoglycemia, serious immediate side effects such as hemodynamic compromise and seizures were not reported. While hypoglycemia is more common in patients with renal and hepatic failure, which may partially explain the increased incidence of hypoglycemia in the medical ICU, hypo-glycemia was identified as an independent risk factor for death in the medical ICU population. However, the effect was not seen until at least 24 hours after the hypo-glycemic episode. The reason for this is unclear. The first Van den Berghe trial utilized arterial blood and arterial blood gas analyzers, not capillary glucose or point of care (POC) glucometers. The second trial utilized capillary BG normalized to whole blood and a Hemo Cue meter which has less variance than other POC techniques. Patients in these trials also consistently received early caloric intervention, often with total parental nutrition (TPN).

Brunkhorst et al., randomized patients to an intensive insulin treatment arm (mean morning BG level 112 mg/dL) and a conventional insulin treatment arm (mean morning BG level 151 mg/dL) in a multicenter randomized trial. No significant difference in 28-day mortality or mean organ failure score was observed between treatment groups. However, the intensive insulin treatment arm was associated with a statistically greater incidence of severe hypoglycemia, defined as ≤ 40 mg/dL, (17.0% vs. 4.1%; $p <0.001$) and serious adverse events (10.9% vs. 5.2%; $p = 0.01$) compared to the conventional insulin treatment arm.

More recently, the NICE-SUGAR study randomized critically ill patients expected to remain in the ICU >3 days to intensive glucose control (81–108 mg/dL) versus conventional glucose control (180 mg/dL or less) in a multinational random-ized trial. They found that severe hypoglycemia was more common in the intensive glucose control group (6.8% vs. 0.5%; $p <0.001$) and that 90-day all-cause mortality was increased (27.5% vs. 24.9%; $p = 0.02$). The treatment effect did not differ sig-nificantly between surgical patients and medical patients. Trauma patients and those on corticosteroids showed a trend for mortality benefit with intensive control. These authors concluded that a BG target of 180 mg/dL or less resulted in lower morbidity and mortality compared to a more aggressive glucose control target.

The Glucontrol study was another recent randomized control trial of intense versus intermediate glucose control in medico-surgical ICUs. The trial was stopped early due to a high rate of unintended protocol violations. They only studied one third of their intended number of patients, and the study was therefore underpowered.

The intense group did have significantly more hypoglycemia, and no difference in ICU mortality was seen. Twenty out of 111 hypoglycemic events were attributed to inappropriate continuation of insulin infusion, seen more in the intense therapy group. Other trials over the years have tried to determine benefits of intense glucose control in specific patient populations with conflicting results. What is consistent, however, is the increase in hypoglycemic events with more intense therapy, making hypoglycemia the limiting factor in lower target glucose protocols.

MANAGEMENT

The conclusions and current recommendations based on these studies are still somewhat controversial. Table 30.1 lists the most recent recommendations for glucose control in the ICU by the American Diabetes Association (Position Statement 2009) and the American College of Endocrinology, which includes patients in all ICUs and hospital wards. The authors of the Surviving Sepsis Campaign advocate blood sugar goals of <150 mg/dL in critically ill patients in large part to limit hypoglycemia and to simplify management. Overall, some studies support intensive glucose control in patients who are expected to stay in the ICU more than 3 to 5 days, and those on corticosteroids or suffering from recent trauma. The postulated reason for this is that preventing hyperglycemia prevents complications from hyperglycemia, and complications take time to develop. It seems reasonable to exclude medical ICU patients who are eating and who are expected to be in the ICU <3 days. However, it is not always possible to predict the length of ICU stays, and physician discretion is needed.

The benefits seen in the surgical ICU study by Van den Berghe were not replicated in later studies. Potential reasons for this include the strict use of blood gas analyzers on arterial blood (which would increase the accuracy of the readings compared to POC bedside analyzers on capillary blood), and the use of early parenteral nutrition, which may increase morbidity/mortality from blood stream infections in the conventional group.

In critically ill patients admitted to the ICU, all oral antihyperglycemic agents and subcutaneous insulin should be stopped. Insulin in critically ill patients should be given intravenously. The half-life of intravenous insulin is 5 to 9 minutes, which allows for rapid reversal of hypoglycemia when it occurs. Most ICUs now have standardized glucose algorithms, generally managed by nurses, which have been shown to be valid ways to manage glucose. The most effective glucose algorithms are dynamic and incorporate the rate of glucose change into the insulin dose adjustments.

TABLE 30.1	Recommended Target BG for Patients in the ICU

American Diabetes Association
  <180 mg/dL to 200 mg/dL

American College of Endocrinology
  <180 mg/dL

Surviving Sepsis Campaign
  <150 mg/dL

TABLE 30.2 | Insulin-Infusion Protocol

Initiating insulin infusion

Standard insulin infusion 100 U *regular human insulin* in 100 mL 0.9% normal saline.

Preferred administration IV ($t^1/_2$ 5–9 min) via an infusion pump.

Give initial bolus if BG >150 mg/dL;

    Divide initial BG by 70 and round to nearest 0.5 U (e.g., BG 250:250/70 = 3.57, rounded to 4, so IV bolus 4 U.)

After bolus, start infusion at same hourly rate as bolus (4 U/hr IV in above example).

If *BG less than 150 mg/dL,* divide by 70 for initial hourly rate with *NO bolus* (e.g., BG 150 would be 150/70 = 2.15, rounded to 2, so start at 2 U/hr IV).

Go to Algorithm 30.1 for instructions on changing the insulin-infusion rate.

BG Monitoring

Check BG q1h until stable (three consecutive values in target range).

Once stable can change BG monitoring to q2h.

If stable q2h for 12–24 hours can change to q3–4h if

    no significant change in nutrition or clinical status

Resume q1h BG monitoring for BG >70 md/dL with any of the following:

    Change in insulin-infusion rate.

    Initiation or cessation of corticosteroid or vasopressor therapy.

    Significant change in clinical status.

    Change in nutritional support (initiation, cessation, or rate change).

    Initiation or cessation of hemodialysis or CVVHD.

Hypoglycemia (BG ≤70 mg/dL)

If *BG <50 mg/dL,* stop infusion and give 25 g dextrose 50% (1 amp D50) IV. Recheck BG q10–15 min.

When BG >90 mg/dL, recheck in 1 hr. If still >90 mg/dL after 1 hr, resume insulin infusion at *50% most recent rate.*

If *BG 50–69 mg/dL,* stop infusion.

    If symptomatic or unable to assess, give 25 g dextrose 50% (1 amp D50) IV. Recheck BG q15 min.

    If asymptomatic, consider 12.5 g dextrose 50% (1/2 amp D50) or 8 oz. fruit juice PO.

        Recheck q15–30 min.

    When, BG >90 mg/dL, recheck in 1 hr. If still >90 mg/dL after 1 hr, resume insulin infusion at *75% most recent rate.*

BG, blood glucose; CVVHD, continuous venovenous hemodialysis; IV, intravenous; PO, by mouth. Modified from Goldberg PA, Siegel MD, Sherwin RS, et al. Implementation of a safe and effective insulin-infusion protocol in a medical intensive care unit. *Diabetes Care.* 2004;27:461–467, with permission.

Table 30.2 contains a validated insulin-infusion protocol outlining how to initiate an insulin infusion, monitor BG, and manage hypoglycemia. Algorithm 30.1 shows how to manage the insulin-infusion rate. It is important that one does not draw the wrong conclusions from trials examining intensive glucose control in the ICU. The standard of care in all of these studies is IV insulin to prevent hyperglycemia in critically ill,

ALGORITHM 30.1 — Changing the Insulin-Infusion Rate

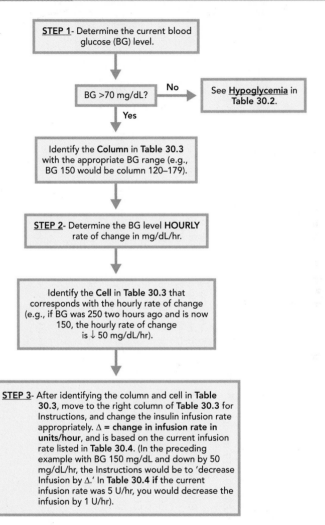

STEP 1- Determine the current blood glucose (BG) level.

BG >70 mg/dL? — **No** → See **Hypoglycemia** in Table 30.2.

Yes

Identify the **Column** in Table 30.3 with the appropriate BG range (e.g., BG 150 would be column 120–179).

STEP 2- Determine the BG level **HOURLY** rate of change in mg/dL/hr.

Identify the **Cell** in Table 30.3 that corresponds with the hourly rate of change (e.g., if BG was 250 two hours ago and is now 150, the hourly rate of change is ↓ 50 mg/dL/hr).

STEP 3- After identifying the column and cell in **Table 30.3**, move to the right column of **Table 30.3** for Instructions, and change the insulin infusion rate appropriately. Δ = **change in infusion rate in units/hour**, and is based on the current infusion rate listed in **Table 30.4**. (In the preceding example with BG 150 mg/dL and down by 50 mg/dL/hr, the Instructions would be to 'decrease Infusion by Δ.' In **Table 30.4** if the current infusion rate was 5 U/hr, you would decrease the infusion by 1 U/hr).

intubated patients. What is in dispute is the target BG range to achieve. NICE-SUGAR and other trials mentioned here should not be used to support the decision to use subcutaneous insulin over IV insulin, or to allow persistent hyperglycemia >180 mg/dL, in a critically ill patient.

In managing glucose, one must make insulin-infusion adjustments based on changes in carbohydrate intake. For example, a change in the dextrose 5% rate from 150 mL/hr (180 g carbohydrates normalized during a 24-hour period) to 75 mL/hr (90 g carbohydrates normalized during a 24-hour period) will require a decrease in

TABLE 30.3 Current Blood Glucose (BG) Level and Rate of Change[a]

BG 70–89 mg/dL	BG 90–119 mg/dL	BG 120–179 mg/dL	BG >180 mg/dL	Instructions (see Table 30.4 for Δ)
	BG ↑ by >20 mg/dL/hr	BG ↑ by >40 mg/dL/hr	BG ↑	*INCREASE INFUSION by 2Δ*
		BG ↑ by 1–40 mg/dL/hr OR BG UNCHANGED	*BG UNCHANGED OR* BG ↓ by 1–40 mg/dL/hr	*INCREASE INFUSION by Δ*
BG ↑	BG ↑ by 1–20 mg/dL/hr, *BG UNCHANGED, OR* BG ↓ by 1–20 mg/dL/hr	BG ↓ by 1–40 mg/dL/hr	BG ↓ by 41–80 mg/dL/hr	*NO INFUSION CHANGE*
BG UNCHANGED OR BG ↓ by 1–20 mg/dL/hr	BG ↓ by 21–40 mg/dL/hr	BG ↓ by 41–80 mg/dL/hr	BG ↓ by 81–120 mg/dL/hr	*DECREASE INFUSION by Δ*
BG ↓ by >20 mg/dL/hr See below[b]	BG ↓ by >40 mg/dL/hr	BG ↓ by >80 mg/dL/hr	BG ↓ by >120 mg/dL/hr	*HOLD INFUSION × 30 min then DECREASE by 2Δ*

[a]See Algorithm 30.1 for instructions.
[b]Hold insulin infusion; check BG q15–30 min; when >90 mg/dL, restart infusion at 75% most recent rate.

TABLE 30.4	Changes in Insulin-Infusion Rate (Δ) in U/hr	
Current-infusion rate (U/hr)	Δ = Rate change (U/hr)	2Δ = 2 × Rate change (U/hr)
<3	0.5	1
3–6	1	2
6.5–9.5	1.5	3
10–14.5	2	4
15–19.5	3[a]	6[a]
20–24.5[a]	4[a]	8[a]
>25[a]	5[a]	10[a]

[a]Infusions typically range 2–10 U/hr. Doses in excess of 20 U/hr are unusual and a physician should be notified to explore potential contributing factors such as errors in insulin dilution and administration.

the insulin-infusion rate in order to prevent hypoglycemia. In critically ill patients, multiple sources of carbohydrate need to be taken into consideration when calculating the insulin dose such as parenteral nutrition, enteral tube feeds, and glucose containing IV fluid. Nutrition, whether enteral or parenteral, should be given as a continuous infusion rather than intermittent boluses to prevent significant fluctuations in BG. It is often critical to reassess caloric intake every 12 to 24 hours. The patients most at risk for hypoglycemia are those with renal failure and hepatic failure. Close attention to details and a less aggressive upward titration schedule in patients with liver and renal failure should allow insulin drips to be safely used. Meticulous attention must also be paid to patients with impaired mental status who are unable to perceive and respond to low glucose levels.

The implementation of any protocol, whether taken from the literature or developed locally, especially one as complex as an IV insulin drip protocol, requires a significant amount of education and training. Even under controlled conditions, the protocol can be violated frequently, as seen in the Glucontrol study. The violations could be as simple as missed BG or as serious as a failure to adjust the insulin-infusion rate. Human error has to be taken into consideration when evaluating BG control. Computerized calculation of the drip rate has been shown to minimize mistakes and may improve outcome.

Once diabetic patients improve and are ready to be discharged from the ICU, intravenous insulin needs to be switched to subcutaneous insulin. Using an insulin sliding scale alone results in rebound hyperglycemia. The development of diabetic ketoacidosis and hyperglycemic hyperosmolar state in the hospital are considered "never events" by center for medicare and medicaid services. Using basal long-acting insulin (neutral protamine hagadorn, glargine, or detemir) combined with prandial and sliding scale short-acting insulin (aspart, lispro, glulisine) will lead to better glycemic control. When calculating the dosage, one needs to take into account the prior history of diabetes, type of diabetes, stress level, prior insulin dosage, steroid use, and general clinical status. Long-acting insulin needs to overlap with discontinuation of the drip to prevent hyperglycemia. We give short acting insulin at two times the drip rate plus long acting insulin (generally starting with 0.2–0.3 U/kg of body weight/day) and turn the drip off immediately. If short-acting insulin is not given, then the drip should overlap 2 to 3 hours to allow the long-acting insulin to be effective.

Attention should be paid to what glucose analyzer is used (blood gas, core laboratory, POC glucose oxidase, or POC glucose dehydrogenase), the source of patient sample (arterial, capillary, central venous), and what conditions the patient has (anemia, hypoxia, poor peripheral perfusion) or medications they are receiving (acetaminophen, ascorbic acid, intravenous immunoglobulin, peritoneal dialysis) that cause changes in glucose results.

Anemia (Hct <34%) has been shown to cause significant error, overestimating glucose with POC glucometers. Dosing insulin based on falsely elevated glucose values could contribute to hypoglycemia in intensively treated patients in ICU settings. The use of formulas correcting for the level of anemia have been shown to reduce hypoglycemic events in ICU patients.

Meters using glucose dehydrogenase strips are affected by maltose in IVIG, and Icodextrin from peritoneal dialysis, and therefore should not be used in healthcare facilities until these problems are corrected. New meters that automatically correct for hematocrit, hypoxia, and interfering reducing substances have been developed, but are not in regular use in hospitals. Even without an identified clinical interference, glucometers can have an error margin of up to 20%, where as laboratory analyzers must be below 10% to meet Food and Drug Administration (FDA) standards. Arterial blood measured by POC glucometers is more accurate than capillary glucose, and should be used when available in ICU patients on IV insulin.

In summary, although the current recommendations for glucose targets are still somewhat controversial, treating hyperglycemia in critically ill patients can lead to decreased morbidity and mortality. Available data suggest medical and postsurgical patients who are in the ICU more than 3 to 5 days are most likely to benefit from a lower target range, but mortality benefit is lessened or eliminated when hypoglycemic events increase. Insulin in critically ill patients should be given intravenously to allow rapid reversal of hypoglycemia if it occurs, with early data suggesting that critically ill medical and cardiac patients may be most sensitive to the effects of hypoglycemia. Insulin-infusion protocols implemented by well-trained staff can be effective ways to manage BG. Paying careful attention to changes in patients' clinical condition and nutritional status, as well as vigorous glycemic monitoring by hospital staff, will minimize hypoglycemic events. Standardizing the glucose monitoring methods and using more accurate technologies may reduce hypoglycemic events and allow for safer intense glucose management, resulting in better outcomes in future trials.

SUGGESTED READINGS

American Diabetes Association. Standards of medical care in diabetes-2009. *Diabetes Care.* 2009;32:S13–S61.
  ADA summary and recommendations for diagnosing and treating diabetes and hyperglycemia.
Brunkhorst FM, Engel C, Bloos F, et al. Intensive insulin therapy and pentastarch resuscitation in severe sepsis. *N Engl J Med.* 2008;358:125–139.
  Randomized trial demonstrating increased incidence of hypoglycemia and adverse events among patients receiving intensive glucose control.
Dellinger RP, Levy MM, Carlet JM, et al. Surviving Sepsis Campaign: international guidelines for management of severe sepsis and septic shock: 2008. *Crit Care Med.* 2008;36:296–327.
  Recommendations from the authors of the Surviving Sepsis Campaign for glucose control in critically ill septic patients.
Fahy BG, Sheehy AM, Coursin DB. Glucose control in the intensive care unit. *Crit Care Med.* 2009;37:1769–1776.
  A recent comprehensive review summarizing the recommendations for glucose control in critically ill patients and the evidence in support of these recommendations.

Garber AJ, Moghissi ES, Bransome ED Jr, et al. American College of Endocrinology position statement on inpatient diabetes and metabolic control. *Endocr Pract.* 2004;10:77–82.

Summary of the current evidence for glycemic control in hospitalized diabetic and non-diabetic patients, including current ACE recommendations.

Goldberg PA, Siegel MD, Sherwin RS, et al. Implementation of a safe and effective insulin infusion protocol in a medical intensive care unit. *Diabetes Care.* 2004;27:461–467.

Results of a nurse-implemented insulin infusion protocol which incorporated the velocity of glycemic change, showing it to be a safe and effective protocol for managing blood glucose in critically ill patients.

Inzucchi SV. Management of Hyperglycemia in the Hospital Setting. *N Engl J Med.* 2006;355: 1903–1911.

A review of glycemic control in hospitalized and critically ill patients, including evidence for treatment, strategies for glucose control, and current recommendations.

Krinsley JS. Association between hyperglycemia and increased hospital mortality in a heterogeneous population of critically ill patients. *Mayo Clin Proc.* 2003;78:1471–1478.

Retrospective analysis of blood glucose levels in intensive care unit patients showing the lowest hospital mortality (9.6%) among patients with mean glucose values between 80 and 99 mg/dL, with mortality increasing progressively as glucose values increased (42.5% in patients with mean glucose values above 300 mg/dL).

Malmburg K, Ryden L, Efendic S, et al. Randomized trial of insulin-glucose infusion followed by subcutaneous insulin treatment in diabetic patients with acute myocardial infarction (DIGAMI study): effects on mortality at 1 year. *J Am Coll Cardiol.* 1995;26:57–65.

Randomized trial of patients with acute MI showing a 29% reduction in 1 year mortality in patients assigned to intensive glucose control starting in-hospital and continuing for 3 months when compared with standard glucose control.

Malmberg K, Ryden L, Wedel H, et al. Intensive metabolic control by means of insulin in patients with diabetes mellitus and acute myocardial infarction (DIGAMI 2): effect on mortality and morbidity. *Eur Heart J.* 2005;26:650–651.

Randomized trial of patients with acute MI comparing intensive inpatient glucose control to intensive outpatient glucose control compared to standard care which showed no difference in 1-year mortality. However the study was underpowered and the difference in mean glucose values was small.

NICE-SUGAR Study Investigators, Finfer S, Chittock DR, Su SY, et al. Intensive versus conventional glucose control in critically ill patients. *N Engl J Med.* 2009;360:1283–1297.

A multinational study of intensive versus conventional glucose control in critically ill patients. Demonstrated increased incidences of hypoglycemia and mortality in the intensive glucose control group.

Pidcoke HF, Wade CE, Mann EA, et al. Anemia causes hypoglycemia in intensive care unit patients due to error in single-channel glucometers: methods of reducing patient risk. *Crit Care Med.* 2010;38(2):471–476.

Pinot DS, Skolnick AH, Kirtane AJ. U-Shaped relationship of blood glucose with adverse outcomes among patients with ST-segment Elevation Myocardial Infarction. *J Am Coll Cardiol.* 2005;46:178–180.

Report on pooled data from the TIMI 10-A/B, LIMIT-AMT, and OPUS studies showing significantly higher 30-day mortality in patients with acute STEMI who had hypoglycemia (BG <81 mg/dL), with only 8.7% of the hypoglycemic patients diagnosed with diabetes.

Preiser JC, Devos P, Ruiz-Santana S, et al. A prospective randomised multi-centre controlled trial on tight glucose control by intensive insulin therapy in adult intensive care units: the Glucontrol study. *Intensive Care Med.* 2009;35:1738–1748.

Randomized trial in a medico-surgical ICUs showed increased hypoglycemia but no change in mortality with intense (target BG 4.4–6.1 mmol/L) compared to intermediate (target BG 7.8–10.0 mmol/L) glucose control. Stopped early for protocol errors.

Scott MG, Bruns DE, Boyd JC, et al. Tight glucose control in the intensive care unit: are glucose meters up to the task? *Clin Chem.* 2009;55(1):18–20.

Van Den Berghe G, Wilmer A, Hermans G, et al. Intensive insulin therapy in the medical ICU. *N Eng J Med.* 2006;354:449–461.

Randomized trial in a medical ICU which showed significantly reduced morbidity but not in-hospital mortality in patients assigned to intensive glucose treatment (goal 80–110 mg/dL) compared with standard care (goal 180–200 mg/dL).

Van Den Berghe G, Wouters P, Weekers F, et al. Intensive insulin therapy in critically ill patients. *N Engl J Med.* 2001;345:1359–1367.

Randomized trial in a surgical ICU which showed decreased ICU mortality in hyperglycemic patients assigned to intensive glucose treatment (goal 80–110 mg/dL) compared with standard care (goal 180–200 mg/dL).

31

Oncologic Emergencies

Ryan Roop and Alex Denes

Cancers can cause metabolic, space occupying, and hematologic complications which require immediate recognition and treatment to prevent death or significant morbidity. This chapter will review the acute management of spinal cord compression, tumor lysis syndrome (TLS), superior vena cava (SVC) syndrome, and leukostasis, which can occur in patients with known malignancy or at initial presentation. Acute management of other serious complications of malignancy such as airway and gastrointestinal obstruction, cardiac tamponade, hypercalcemia, adrenal insufficiency, hematologic abnormalities, increased intracranial pressure, and febrile neutropenia is discussed in other chapters.

SPINAL CORD COMPRESSION

Back pain is the most frequent presenting symptom associated with spinal cord compression and commonly precedes neurologic impairment. The pain may be localized to the back, or radiate unilaterally or bilaterally in the distribution of spinal roots. Coughing or movement can often exacerbate the pain secondary to radiculopathy. Patients may also complain of sensory paresthesias such as burning, skin sensitivity, and numbness. Compression of the long sensory tracts in the cervical cord may cause paresthesias to appear in various lower dermatomes. Motor symptoms usually precede sensory symptoms but can be variable and can accompany or develop after sensory deficits. Common motor symptoms include weakness or heaviness of the affected limbs, flaccid paralysis, and loss of bladder and bowel control. Cord compression symptoms may present abruptly or progress gradually.

The most important aspect of the patient's evaluation is suspicion for the presence of cord compression by the examining health care provider. New-onset back pain in a patient at risk mandates a careful history and neurologic examination. In cases of gradual cord compression, patients may be unaware of sensory deficits, but they may be noted on neurologic exam. Regions distal to the cord compression may be weak and hyperreflexic with up-going (extensor plantar) reflexes in the toes, while reflexes at the level of a lesion are decreased. Patients with voiding symptoms may have urinary retention and should be evaluated by obtaining a post-void bladder residual or by ultrasound examination. Anal sphincter function is usually preserved until late in cord compression, but should be evaluated by digital rectal examination. Acute, severe cord compression can cause spinal shock, with hyporeflexia and flaccid paralysis in all regions below the lesion.

All patients with suspected cord compression should undergo urgent spine imaging. Magnetic resonance imaging (MRI) with contrast is the modality of choice when available. Contrast computed tomography (CT) or CT myelography is recommended if MRI is not available or cannot be performed. It is important to image the entire spine, as some patients may have compression or metastases at multiple levels. Plain films and bone scans have a limited role, since they may miss the soft tissue components of tumors. If the nature of the compressing mass is uncertain, surgical or image-guided biopsy for tissue diagnosis is essential. When cord compression is the initial presentation of cancer, further examination or imaging studies may reveal a lesion such as a lymph node, which may be more accessible for biopsy.

Treatment

The general approach to the evaluation and management of the patient with spinal cord compression is outlined in Algorithm 31.1. The importance of early recognition and intervention is to preserve or improve the patient's neurologic function. This is truly a medical urgency and should receive urgent evaluation and treatment.

Corticosteroids should be started if spinal cord compression is suspected and may be started in the absence of a tissue diagnosis. Steroids decrease edema associated with spinal cord compression and transiently improve symptoms. One common approach is dexamethasone given as a loading dose of 10 mg IV or PO followed by 4 mg IV or PO every 6 hours. Selected patients may benefit from prophylactic gastric acid suppression (with an H2 blocker or proton pump inhibitor) to prevent the development of stress ulcers. Dexamethasone should be continued during the initial evaluation and treatment period and then tapered over the subsequent 2 to 3 weeks regardless of symptom improvement. Longer duration of steroids may be beneficial in patients with cord compression due to multiple myeloma or lymphoproliferative disorders.

Because early studies of surgical decompression through posterior laminectomy followed by radiation therapy (XRT) seemed equivalent to XRT alone, external beam XRT became the treatment of choice. Commonly recommended radiation doses range from 2500 to 4000 cGy delivered in 10 to 20 fractions. Traditional indications for surgical intervention have included the need for a tissue diagnosis, resection of relatively "radioresistant" tumors, tumors primarily treated by surgery (such as sarcomas), spinal instability, and cord compression in a previously irradiated spine. A recent randomized study comparing surgical decompression followed by XRT to XRT alone has led to a major change in the approach to patients with spinal cord compression. The study was stopped after an interim analysis revealed significantly better outcomes for patients treated surgically, with more ambulatory patients remaining ambulatory (84% vs. 57%) and nonambulatory patients regaining the ability to walk (62% vs. 19%). For these reasons, surgery should be considered initially in all patients presenting with cord compression. Our approach at Washington University is to have all patients presenting with spinal cord compression evaluated by spine surgery, radiation oncology, and medical oncology to determine optimal therapy.

Sudden or very rapid onset of neurologic symptoms and back pain suggest the possibility of vertebral burst fracture causing bony impingement on the cord. This requires urgent surgical intervention to remove bone fragments from the spinal canal. Patients with extensive bony destruction by tumor and vertebral instability may be at risk for further compression fractures and symptom recurrence after completing XRT. These patients should be considered for vertebral stabilization. Surgical patients usually require 7 to 10 days for wound healing before beginning postoperative XRT. Systemic therapy using hormonal therapy or chemotherapeutic agents should be initiated when appropriate, especially in highly sensitive tumors such as prostate cancer, germ cell tumors, small cell lung cancer, multiple myeloma, and lymphoma.

ALGORITHM 31.1 Approach to the Evaluation and Management of Patients with Suspected or Documented Spinal Cord Compression from Cancer

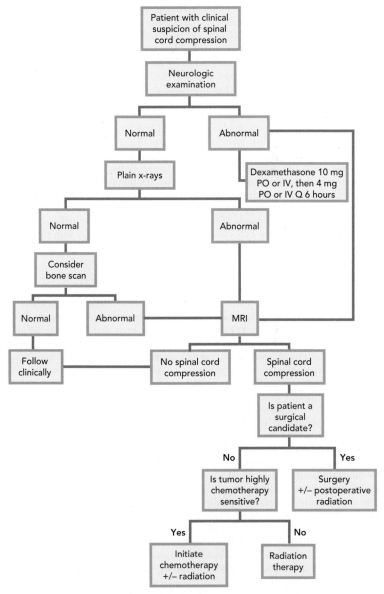

MRI, magnetic resonance imaging.

TUMOR LYSIS SYNDROME

The TLS refers to the metabolic consequences resulting from the sudden release of potassium, phosphates, and purine metabolites from tumor cells undergoing cell death. TLS is classically associated with malignancies such as acute lymphoblastic leukemia (ALL) or Burkitt's lymphoma, which are characterized by a high growth fraction, present with substantial systemic tumor burden, and which respond rapidly to cyto-toxic chemotherapy. Patients with other "treatment-sensitive" malignancies such as chronic lymphocytic leukemia (CLL) and small cell lung cancer and high tumor burden should also be considered at risk. However, TLS can occur in any situa-tion in which considerable tissue bulk is rapidly destroyed within the body, and may occur after cytotoxic chemotherapy, biologic treatments, corticosteroids, radiation, and chemoembolization. Clinical manifestations are variable and should not be used to monitor the course of TLS, but may include arrhythmias, mental status changes, tetany, stupor, renal failure, and even sudden death from hyperkalemic cardiac arrest. Ideally, the treating physician should anticipate TLS and intervene before the patient develops symptoms or serious metabolic complications.

TLS is diagnosed by analysis of venous blood and is characterized by acute renal failure and electrolyte derangements including hyperkalemia, hyperuricemia, hyper-phosphatemia, and hypocalcemia. Renal failure occurs from the precipitation of phos-phate and urate salts in the renal tubules. The resulting renal impairment leads to further accumulation of phosphorus and uric acid, creating an escalating destructive cycle. Patients with some degree of renal insufficiency prior to chemotherapy are at increased risk of developing TLS. Patients at highest risk include those with high grade or bulky lymphoid malignancies such as Burkitt's lymphoma and ALL.

Treatment

The general approach to the prevention and management of TLS is summarized in Algorithm 31.2. The best approach to TLS is prevention. Patients at high risk of TLS should be volume repleted before initiating chemotherapy, and isotonic fluids should be infused at 200 to 300 mL/hr to achieve a brisk diuresis during the first 2 to 3 days of treatment. The goal of hydration is to preserve renal function and to eliminate cellular breakdown products as they are released. Patients should have blood chemistries (especially potassium, phosphorous, calcium, creatinine, uric acid, and lactate dehydrogenase [LDH]) monitored every 8 to 12 hours during the first 2 to 3 days of treatment. Furosemide may be given to maintain urine output and may also increase excretion of potassium. The utility of urine alkalization is controversial, as evidence supporting its clinical benefit is lacking. In addition, urine alkalization has a theoretical risk of promoting soft tissue deposition of calcium phosphate. For this reason, we do not recommend the routine use of urine alkalization over hydration alone. In situations when urine alkalization is considered, we recommend administration of IV fluids containing 1 amp $NaHCO_3$ in 0.45% NaCl or 2 to 3 amps $NaHCO_3$ in D5W. Bicarbonate should be cautiously used in severe hyperphosphatemia, as this may cause calcium phosphate crystallization in the renal microvasculature and renal tubules, leading to worsening renal failure.

If the serum uric acid is <8 mg/dL, allopurinol should be given PO at 300 to 600 mg/day starting 24 to 48 hours before chemotherapy, as it requires 2 to 3 days to decrease uric acid levels. Allopurinol blocks xanthine oxidase, preventing the con-version of xanthine to uric acid, leaving xanthines, which are more soluble and easily

ALGORITHM 31.2 Prevention and Management of Tumor Lysis Syndrome (TLS) in Patients at High Risk

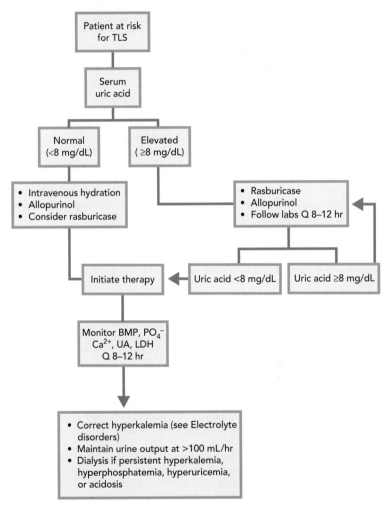

BMP, basic metabolic panel; UA, uric acid; LDH, lactate dehydrogenase.

excreted. The allopurinol dose should be decreased in patients with preexisting renal insufficiency and as tumor bulk decreases.

Urate oxidase (uricase) is a proteolytic enzyme absent in humans, which converts uric acid into allantoin, which is highly soluble and is readily excreted by the kidney. Recombinant urate oxidase, rasburicase, should be given to all patients with a serum uric acid level ≥8 mg/dL as well as to patients at high risk for TLS. Dosing is

0.15 to 0.2 mg/kg IV and can be repeated daily for a maximum of 7 days for uric acid levels above 8 mg/dL, but repeated dosing is rarely required. Rasburicase induces a rapid decline in serum uric acid levels often with normalization of uric acid levels within 4 hours and improvement in renal function. Rasburicase also causes phosphate reabsorption, and calcium phosphate deposition can be a persistent problem requiring aggressive hydration and diuresis even after uric acid levels are undetectable.

Hyperkalemia may develop rapidly and patients at risk should have serum electrolytes checked at least every 8 to 12 hours, and more frequently if TLS develops. Mild hyperkalemia (>5.5–6 mmol/L) may be managed with Kayexalate resin and hydration. More serious hyperkalemia (>6 mmol/L or with ECG changes) may be treated acutely with 2 amps of calcium gluconate IV rapidly to stabilize the cardiac membrane potentials, followed by 50 mL of 50% glucose solution IV with 10 units regular insulin IV, to transport extracellular potassium intracellularly. This should be followed by Kayexalate to decrease total body potassium as these treatments are only associated with transient improvement in hyperkalemia as potassium shifts intracellularly (see "Hyperkalemia" section of Chapter 24, Electrolyte Abnormalities, for more detailed treatment).

Hyperphosphatemia may be treated with noncalcium-based phosphate binders, and patients should be placed on a renal diet with restricted phosphorous and potassium intake.

Indications for hemodialysis include volume overload, serum uric acid >10 mg/dL despite multiple doses of rasburicase, or rapidly rising phosphorus and uncontrolled hyperkalemia. Renal failure caused by TLS is usually reversible, and even patients requiring hemodialysis often regain normal kidney function as the TLS resolves.

SUPERIOR VENA CAVA SYNDROME

Patients with SVC syndrome commonly present with dyspnea; cough; swelling of the face, neck, and upper extremities; headaches; and chest pain. Symptoms may develop acutely or gradually, and bending forward or lying flat may worsen symptoms. Even in the presence of severe symptoms, patients are rarely critically ill as a result of SVC syndrome alone. While SVC occlusion is usually not a life-threatening emergency, it can cause significant discomfort and morbidity and mandates immediate attention. Potentially life-threatening complications of SVC syndrome that warrant urgent intervention are cerebral edema causing coma and laryngeal edema causing central airway obstruction.

On physical examination, dilated neck veins are usually present, as is edema of the face, arms, neck, and supraclavicular region. Gradual occlusion of the SVC allows the development of collateral veins that may be easily visible over the upper chest. The chest radiograph often shows a right suprahilar mass or mediastinal widening but can be normal in some patients.

Contrast CT or MRI of the chest can provide information regarding the patency of the SVC, the presence of thrombus, the presence or absence of compressive mass lesions, and is useful in planning subsequent diagnostic or therapeutic interventions. A surgical or percutaneous biopsy of an accessible site should be performed in patients who present with SVC syndrome as the initial manifestation of malignancy, patients without a prior tissue diagnosis, or in patients in whom the diagnosis of the mass is uncertain (e.g., patients with multiple known malignancies). A tissue diagnosis is important in the management of SVC syndrome, as specific treatment may be

ALGORITHM 31.3 Evaluation and Management of Patients with Suspected or Confirmed Superior Vena Cava (SVC) Syndrome

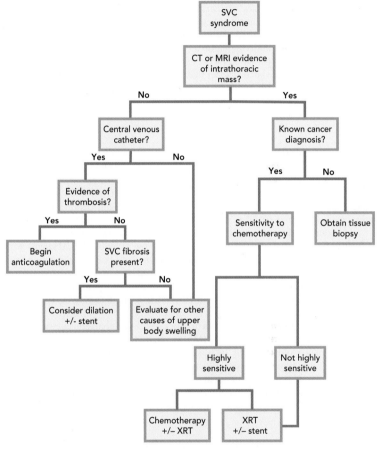

XRT, radiation therapy.

influenced by the tumor type. Only in very rare circumstance should therapy be initiated without confirming a histologic diagnosis.

Treatment

The general approach to the management of SVC syndrome is outlined in Algorithm 31.3. Radiotherapy is one of the mainstays of treatment for SVC syndrome. While success depends on the tumor type, 87% of patients respond when treated with regimens delivering 2000 cGy or more. Patients with "chemoresponsive" tumors, such as germ cell carcinoma, small cell lung cancer, and malignant lymphoma, can be treated with chemotherapy, followed by radiation if indicated. Expandable vena caval stents can be helpful in relieving SVC obstruction. Stenting can provide immediate relief to patients who are not expected to have a rapid response to radiation and to patients who have symptom recurrence after therapy.

A subset of patients develop SVC syndrome from benign causes, and stenting should be considered in these patients. Occlusive SVC thrombosis may occur as a complication of central venous catheters. At Washington University, we generally recommend leaving the central catheter in place to prevent dislodging of the clot and initiate therapeutic anticoagulation as with any DVT. Anticoagulation should be continued as long as the patient has active cancer, and for 6 months after the removal of the catheter in patients who are cancer free. Central venous catheters may also lead to stenosis of the SVC, which can be treated with fluoroscopy-guided balloon dilatation with or without stenting.

LEUKOSTASIS

Leukostasis is a syndrome usually associated with high numbers of immature leukocytes (blasts) in the peripheral circulation. Symptoms may include shortness of breath, headache, confusion, stupor, or focal neurologic deficits. Leukostasis is a clinical diagnosis as the symptoms are nonspecific and may be attributed to infection, heart failure, or vascular disease. However, without prompt recognition and treatment, mortality rates may be as high as 40% and can occur within hours of presentation.

Leukostasis is associated with high and rapidly rising blast counts, usually over 100,000/mL, but may occur with blast counts as low as 50,000/mL. Patients with leukostasis are usually hypoxemic, but spuriously low PaO_2 levels can result from the high metabolic rate of blasts in the arterial blood sample if the specimen is not processed in a timely fashion. A nonspecific diffuse infiltrate is often present on chest radiograph. There may be impairment of other end organs, including the eye, kidney, and liver. Lactic acidosis can occur as a late event.

Leukostasis is most commonly seen in patients with acute leukemias, especially the myelomonocytic (M4) and monocytic (M5) subtypes, though it has been described in other forms of myeloid leukemias, such as chronic myelogenous leukemia in blast crisis. It is not very common in ALL or CLL even in the presence of very high lymphocyte counts. The classic pathologic finding in leukostasis is occlusive intravascular aggregates of blasts blocking the microcirculation in multiple organs, especially the lungs and the brain.

Treatment

The general approach to the patient with hyperleukocytosis is outlined in Algorithm 31.4. Initiation of leukapheresis should not be delayed while a pathologic diagnosis is being determined. Initial management includes IV hydration, allopurinol and/or rasburicase, and hydroxyurea at a dose of 50 to 100 mg/kg/day in three divided doses as long as the blast count remains above 50,000/mL. Red blood cell transfusion should be resisted if possible, even in patients with significant anemia, as this increases whole blood viscosity and may exacerbate symptoms of leukostasis. Leukapheresis should be initiated, with a goal of rapidly reducing the blast count to <50,000/mL. Leukapheresis can attenuate or reverse the symptoms of leukostasis, and patients who undergo leukapheresis have a decreased incidence of central nervous system complications. Since blast counts may rebound rapidly after leukapheresis, a definitive treatment plan must be initiated as soon as possible.

ALGORITHM 31.4 **Evaluation and Management of Patients Presenting with Hyperleukocytosis**

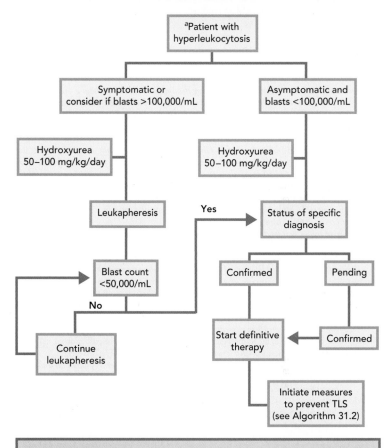

TLS, tumor lysis syndrome; IV, intravenously; ICU, intensive care unit.

Coexisting disorders should be sought and reversed. If present, disseminated intravascular coagulation or thrombocytopenia should be corrected to minimize the risk of central nervous system bleeding. Platelet counts should be monitored closely after leukapheresis, as the procedure often removes a significant number of platelets.

Patients suspected of having coexisting infection should have blood drawn for culture and be treated with broad-spectrum antibiotics, as local inflammatory processes may increase the expression of cellular adhesion molecules and contribute to leukostasis, even in the setting of moderate blast counts.

SUGGESTED READINGS

Ahmann FR. A reassessment of the clinical implications of the superior vena cava syndrome. *J Clin Oncol.* 1984;2(8):961–969.

Review of 1986 cases of SVC syndrome where therapy was initiated without a cancer diagnosis, which determined that treatment without a histologic diagnosis was not advised.

Patchell RA, Tibbs PA, Regine WF, et al. Direct decompressive surgical resection in the treatment of spinal cord compression caused by metastatic cancer: a randomized trial. *Lancet.* 2005;366:643–648.

Randomized, multi-institutional, non-blinded trial, which randomly assigned patients with spinal cord compression from metastatic cancer to surgery followed by radiotherapy (n = 50) or radiotherapy alone (n = 51), prematurely stopped after it was found that decompressive surgery with postoperative radiotherapy was superior to treatment with radiotherapy alone (as discussed in text).

Rampello E, Fricia T, Malaguarnera M. The management of tumor lysis syndrome. *Nat Clin Pract Oncol.* 2006;3(8):438–447.

Review of tumor lysis syndrome management.

Silverman P, Distelhorst CW. Metabolic emergencies in clinical oncology. *Semin Oncol.* 1989;16(6):504–515.

Review of metabolic complications of malignancy, including tumor lysis syndrome.

Tanigawa N, Sawada S, Mishima K, et al. Clinical outcome of stenting in superior vena cava syndrome associated with malignant tumors. *Acta Radiol.* 1998;39:669–674.

Small study of 33 patients with SVC syndrome with 23 receiving an expandable metallic stent and 10 receiving radiation therapy alone. The study showed no difference in survival, and similar improvements in clinical symptoms.

Wilson E, Lyn E, Lynn A, et al. Radiological stenting provides effective palliation in malignant central venous obstruction. *Clin Oncol (R Coll Radiol).* 2002;14(3):228–232.

Review of 18 patients presenting with SVC obstruction from tumor or thrombus, all undergoing stenting or thrombolysis, showing a mean duration of palliation of 87 days with no procedure related complications.

Zarkovic M, Kwaan HC. Correction of hyperviscosity by apheresis. *Semin Thromb Hemost.* 2003;29(5):535–542.

Review of apheresis principles, methods, indications for, and complications.

32

Temperature Alterations
Derek E. Byers

TEMPERATURE REGULATION

Temperature regulation involves a balance between heat production and dissipation. Basic metabolic processes generate heat, and various adaptive processes ranging from vasodilation and sweating to vasoconstriction and shivering help to maintain the normal body temperature at 37°C (98.6°F). Maintenance of euthermia is controlled by the hypothalamus, the brainstem's serotonergic system, and cellular mitochondrial oxidative phosphorylation. Interruption or changes in any of these processes can lead to temperature dysregulation.

FEVER AND HYPERTHERMIA

Fever is a preserved evolutionary response to infection, and involves an increase in the hypothalamic temperature set point with resulting increase in body temperature. Hyperthermia, in contrast, refers to an increase in body temperature associated with normal thermoregulatory center settings, and can be due to increased heat production or decreased heat loss. Studies have shown that immune activity is augmented at elevated temperatures, while bacterial growth is suppressed, and that blocking the body's normal increase in body temperature in response to infection (by forced cooling or antipyretic therapy) may prolong the duration of infectious symptoms. However, high fevers can have undesired consequences including seizures, disseminated intravascular coagulation, renal failure, and death.

A task force that includes societies in critical care medicine and infectious disease define *fever* as a temperature ≥38.3°C (≥101°F) measured from a reliable site (oral, rectal, auditory, or intravenous or bladder thermistor). Temperatures above 38.3°C warrant a thorough physical examination to determine if infection is the cause. At least two sets of blood cultures drawn from two different sterile sites, chest radiograph (especially for intubated patients), and further cultures and testing may be needed, as shown in Algorithm 32.1. The decision to begin antibiotic therapy is based on the patient's clinical stability, likelihood of infection, and immune status. Immunocompromised patients should be administered empiric broad-spectrum antibiotic coverage (see Chapter 3). Stable patients without an obvious infectious source may be monitored closely for fever recurrence and culture results prior to initiating therapy.

Table 32.1 lists infectious and noninfectious causes of fever and hyperthermia in the ICU. Most fevers are the result of infection, and appropriate antibiotic therapy should lead to improvement within a few days. However, a temperature ≥38.3°C

ALGORITHM 32.1 **Workup for Fever/Hyperthermia**

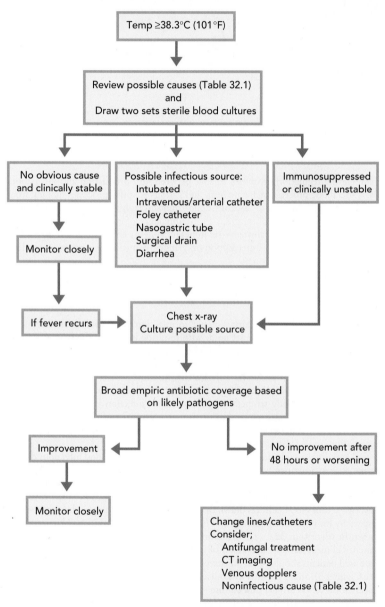

CT, computed tomography.

TABLE 32.1	**Causes of Fever and Hyperthermia**

Infectious causes
- Ventilator associated pneumonia
- *Clostridium difficile* colitis
- Intravenous catheter infection
- Urinary tract infection
- Nosocomial pathogen (Gram negative bacteria, *Candida* species)
- Sinusitis
- Abscess formation (intra-abdominal and elsewhere)
- Wound infection (decubitus ulcer)

Noninfectious causes
- Post-transfusion
- ARDS
- Deep vein thrombus
- Chemical thrombophlebitis
- Fat embolism
- Pancreatitis
- Acalculous cholecystitis
- Subarachnoid hemorrhage
- Alcohol/drug withdrawal
- Hyperthyroidism/thyroid storm
- Acute adrenal insufficiency
- Pheochromocytoma
- Transplant rejection
- Rhabdomyolysis/tetanus
- Connective tissue diseases
- Thrombotic thrombocytopenic purpura
- Malignancy ("B symptoms")
- Central/hypothalamic fever
- Drugs (antibiotics, chemotherapeutic agents, cytokines)
- Baclofen withdrawal
- Hyperthermic syndromes:
    - Malignant hyperthermia (halothane, isoflurane, succinylcholine)
    - Serotonin syndrome (SSRIs, mixed reuptake inhibitors)
    - Neuroleptic malignant syndrome (antipsychotic phenothiazines. haloperidol, metoclopramide, and prochlorperazine)
    - Anticholinergic toxicity (atropine, TCAs, antihistamines)
    - Sympathomimetic poisoning (MAOIs, cocaine, amphetamines, methamphetamines)

ARDS, acute respiratory distress syndrome; SSRI, selective serotonin reuptake inhibitors; TCAs, tricyclic antidepressants; MAOIs, monoamine oxidase inhibitors.

($\geq 101°F$) can be associated with several noninfectious sources and workup can lead to futile use of diagnostic testing, antibiotics, and time only to yield negative results. Temperatures $>38.9°C$ ($>102°F$) are uncommon for noninfectious causes, with the exception of drugs (including hyperthermic syndromes), blood transfusions, and hematologic malignancies.

Although numerous drugs can cause hyperthermia, certain drugs cause specific hyperthermic syndromes. Diagnosis of drug-induced hyperthermic syndromes can be made based on medication history and clinical signs.

Malignant hyperthermia occurs within minutes to hours of exposure to volatile anesthetics (i.e., halothane, isoflurane) or depolarizing muscle relaxants such as succinylcholine. Clinical signs include dramatic temperature elevation, tachycardia, muscle rigidity, and hypercarbia, and can progress to rhabdomyolysis, hemodynamic collapse, and death. Malignant hyperthermia is genetically inherited as a defect in calcium metabolism in skeletal muscle.

Serotonin syndrome typically develops within hours of combined treatment with medications that act on the serotonergic pathway, including selective serotonin-reuptake inhibitors and related antidepressants, tricyclic antidepressants, monoamine oxidase inhibitors, linezolid, dextromethorphan, and meperidine. Clinical diagnosis is based on a triad of cognitive problems (confusion, agitation), autonomic instability, and neuromuscular abnormalities (clonus, hyperreflexia, and tremor). Hyperthermia is found in approximately half of the cases and arises from increased muscle activity due to agitation and tremor.

Neuroleptic malignant syndrome usually occurs within several hours to days of starting a new neuroleptic medication (including phenothiazines, haloperidol, metoclopramide, and prochlorperazine), or acute withdrawal of dopamine agonists such as L-dopa. Clinical signs include hyperthermia, "lead-pipe" muscle rigidity (not clonus in contrast to serotonin syndrome), autonomic instability, and altered mental status (stupor, depression), and it occurs most often in young to middle-aged men. Hyperthermia is the result of muscle rigidity and central hypothalamic dysregulation.

Anticholinergic toxicity is rare and occurs after administration of drugs that block central and peripheral muscarinic receptors, such as antihistamines, atropine, and tricyclic antidepressants. Clinical findings include confusion, tremor, hallucinations, mydriasis, xerostomia, constipation, urinary retention, and coma (see also Chapter 33).

Sympathomimetic poisoning can follow ingestion of monoamine oxidase inhibitors and several drugs of abuse including cocaine, amphetamine, and methamphetamine and its derivatives (e.g., ecstasy). Clinical findings include hyperthermia, diaphoresis, tachycardia, ataxia, insomnia, rhabdomyolysis, and seizures. These drugs act largely through serotonergic pathways, but dopaminergic pathways are also involved (see also Chapter 33).

Damage to the hypothalamus from trauma, tumor, hemorrhage, or ischemia can raise the hypothalamic temperature set point, causing what is termed a *hypothalamic* or *central fever*. This is a true fever as opposed to a hyperthermic process. Clues to suggest a central fever include a plateau fever curve, poor response to antipyretics, lack of sweat, and suspected or confirmed hypothalamic injury. However, hypothalamic lesions are most commonly associated with hypothermia.

Treatment

The decision to treat fever is based on the cause, clinical situation, and severity of temperature elevation. Treatment options are listed in Table 32.2. There is no clear benefit to treating low-grade fevers, and treatment can mask characteristic disease-specific fever patterns (such as tertian and quartan fevers in plasmodium infections, or Pel-Ebstein fevers in patients with lymphoma). Treatment of fever is warranted in cases of mental status changes, seizures, and in critically ill patients with severe underlying pulmonary or cardiovascular disease. Hyperthermic syndromes require removal of the inciting agent and pharmacologic therapy as outlined in Table 32.2. In addition, they

TABLE 32.2 | **Therapeutic Options for Fever and Hyperthermia**

Antipyretics
  Acetaminophen (preferred if no contraindications)
  Nonsteroidal anti-inflammatory drugs

External cooling
  Cooling blankets
  Sponging
  Fans
  Ice baths

Internal cooling
  Gastric or peritoneal lavage
  Intravenous fluid replacement
  Hemodialysis
  Endovascular cooling catheter

Sedation with paralysis if necessary
Drug-induced hyperthermia
Remove inciting agent

Pharmacologic therapy[a]
  Dantrolene: MH and NMS
  Bromocriptine: NMS
  Cyproheptadine: SS
  Physostigmine: AS
  Procainamide should be considered prophylactically for NMS due to the high
    risk of ventricular fibrillation.

---

[a]See common drug dosages and side effects in Appendix.
MH, malignant hyperthermia; NMS, neuroleptic malignant syndrome; SS, serotonin syndrome;
AS, anticholinergic syndrome.

do not respond well to antipyretic therapy, and external cooling methods should be started immediately. In severe cases, internal cooling methods may be needed.

HYPOTHERMIA

Hypothermia is defined as core body temperature <35°C (<95°F). Table 32.3 lists possible causes. Excessive cold exposure is the most common cause in emergency department settings, but severe sepsis, intoxications, and endocrinopathies are frequent causes seen in the ICU. The majority of cases occur in elderly, debilitated, homeless, or intoxicated patients, and in those with underlying chronic illnesses.

Hypothermia can be divided into three grades based on a reliable core body temperature measurement: mild (32–35°C or 90–95°F), moderate (28–32°C or 82–90°F), and severe (<28°C or <82°F). Mild hypothermia is characterized by shivering, cool extremities, and pallor. Moderate and severe hypothermia are characterized by depressed mental status, ataxia, bradycardia or supraventricular arrhythmias, hyporeflexia, hypoventilation, impalpable pulses, and dilated pupils, and may lead to coma, pulmonary edema, and cardiac arrest. Shivering decreases as hypothermia worsens.

TABLE 32.3	Causes of Hypothermia

Cold exposure
Fulminant sepsis
Drugs (alcohol intoxication, sedatives, general anesthetics, antihypertensives)
Hypothyroidism/myxedema coma
Diabetic ketoacidosis
Multisystem trauma
Prolonged cardiac arrest
Kidney failure
Liver failure
Aggressive intravenous fluid replacement
Continuous or intermittent hemodialysis
Hypothalamic lesions (multiple sclerosis)

Laboratory studies may demonstrate acidosis, coagulopathy, and renal and liver abnormalities, but electrolyte changes are unpredictable. End-organ dysfunction is the result of decreased cardiac output and diminished metabolic clearance of toxins and drugs. Electrocardiographic abnormalities include J (Osborn) waves and prolonged PR, QRS, and QT intervals. J waves are positive deflections at the QRS-ST junction in the left ventricular leads, can be found in up to 80% of hypothermic patients, and may be mistaken for new right bundle branch block.

Patients with severe hypothermia are most at risk for developing cardiac arrest, and advanced cardiac life support management is modified for hypothermic cardiac arrest patients. It should be noted that hypothermia-induced bradycardia and peripheral vasoconstriction can make palpation of peripheral pulses difficult. Therefore, hypothermic patients without palpable pulses should be connected to a cardiac monitor quickly to determine the cardiac rhythm. Initial treatment follows the airway, breathing, and circulations of advanced cardiac life support, but also aims at aggressive active external and internal rewarming as outlined in Table 32.4. An initial defibrillation attempt is appropriate for ventricular fibrillation and ventricular tachycardia if the core temperature is <30°C, but further attempts should be withheld until the core temperature is increased to >30°C. In addition, cardiovascular drug metabolism is decreased and the effects reduced in hypothermic patients. Thus cardioactive medications are often not administered at body temperatures <30°C. If >30°C, the interval between drug administration should be increased to avoid toxic buildup. Induced hypothermia following cardiac arrest is discussed in Chapter 19.

Treatment

Management of hypothermia begins with removal of wet clothing, protection from heat loss, and avoidance of excessive movement to prevent cardiac dysrhythmias. Passive rewarming is usually sufficient for mild hypothermia, but additional active rewarming therapy may be required for moderate and severe cases (Table 32.4). External rewarming can cause temperature "afterdrop" as cold peripheral blood is mobilized to the interior. This can be avoided by the concomitant use of active internal rewarming. Hypotension can also occur during the rewarming process from peripheral vasodilation. Thus, patients should be treated with intravenous fluids and the blood pressure should be monitored frequently. Continuous core body temperature monitoring helps to ensure

TABLE 32.4	Therapies for Hypothermia and Expected Change in Core Body Temperature
Warming Method	**°C/hr**

Passive external
    Blankets
    Warmed ambient environment
    Humidified inspired air
	0.5–4

Active external
    Blankets (prewarmed or heated with forced air or fluid)
    Warm water immersion
    Warm water packs
	1–4

Active internal
    Warmed (42°C) humidified air
    Warmed (42°C) intravenous fluids
    Body cavity lavage with warm saline (GI, bladder,
      peritoneal, pleural)
	Variable

Extracorporeal
    Hemodialysis/hemofiltration
    Continuous arteriovenous rewarming
    Cardiopulmonary bypass
	2–3
	3–4
	7–10

GI, gastrointestinal.
Modified from Aslam AF, Aslam AK, Vasavada BC, et al. Hypothermia: evaluation, electrocardiographic manifestations, and management. *Am J Med*. 2006;119:297–301, with permission.

the goal increase of 1°C to 2°C (2–4°F) per hour, and continuous cardiac monitoring and frequent serum electrolyte tests with prompt correction help to minimize the risk of arrhythmias. More rapid rewarming is used for patients with severe hypothermia and cardiac arrest. Prognosis depends on cause, comorbidities, and complications. Mortality rates up to 100% are reported in the most severe cases, but, in practice, death should not be proclaimed with certainty until the patient has been successfully rewarmed.

In frostbite, affected body parts should be manipulated as little as possible. Affected areas should be thawed by warm water immersion (40–42°C), as hotter water can cause further damage. Blisters may form during the rewarming process. Clear blisters can be debrided to avoid continued tissue damage, but hemorrhagic blisters should be left intact to avoid infection. Thawed body parts should be kept on sterile sheets and evaluated by a surgeon to assess tissue viability. Urgent amputation is rarely indicated, but patients should be monitored for the development of compartment syndrome.

INDUCED HYPOTHERMIA AS THERAPY

Hypothermia can help to minimize the deleterious effects of ischemia-reperfusion injury. The American Heart Association recommends induced hypothermia for comatose patients following cardiac arrest, and induced hypothermia has become a standard of care in some medical centers for cerebral edema in cases of traumatic brain injury, acute liver failure, and following neonatal asphyxiation. In cardiac arrest, therapeutic hypothermia should be considered for all patients who are non-responsive and have a return of spontaneous circulation (ROSC). Exceptions include patients with ROSC >8 hours, imminent cardiovascular collapse, life-threatening bleeding or infection, or an underlying terminal condition. Treatment protocols vary, but generally include initiation of hypothermia as soon as possible by active external and/or intravascular cooling, sedation and paralysis, and mechanical ventilation with a goal core temperature of 32 to 34°C. Maintenance of hypothermia is continued with close ICU monitoring for up to 24 hours, and slow rewarming (or "decooling") at a rate of 0.2 to 0.33°C per hour may minimize hemodynamic complications that can develop. Fluid boluses, inotropes, and vasopressors may be required to maintain adequate cerebral perfusion, and combinations of sedatives, analgesics, and neuromuscular blockade can help to control shivering. For these reasons, therapeutic hypothermia should be reserved for centers equipped to closely monitor and treat hemodynamic and neurologic side effects that can occur.

SUGGESTED READINGS

Aslam AF, Aslam AK, Vasavada BC, et al. Hypothermia: evaluation, electrocardiographic manifestations, and management. *Am J Med*. 2006;119:297–301.
  A review of the causes, diagnostic signs, and management of patients with hypothermia.
Hadad E, Weinbroum AA, Ben-Abraham R. Drug-induced hyperthermia and muscle rigidity: a practical approach. *Eur J Emerg Med*. 2003;10:149–154.
  A review of the drug-induced hyperthermic syndromes, help in differential diagnosis, and therapeutic options.
Marik PE. Fever in the ICU. *Chest*. 2000;117:855–869.
  A review of the causes of fever in the ICU and rational approach to management.
O'Grady NP, Barie PS, Bartlett J, et al. Practice parameters for evaluating new fever in critically ill adult patients. *Crit Care Med*. 1998;26:392–408.
  Consensus statement from a panel of 13 experts from the Society of Critical Care Medicine and Infectious Disease Society of America that provides a rational and cost-effective approach to diagnosis and management of patients with fevers in the ICU.
Peberdy MA, Callaway CW, Neumar RW, et al. Part 9: Post cardiac arrest care: 2010 American Heart Association Guidelines for Cardiopulmonary Resuscitation and Emergency Cardiovascular Care. *Circulation*. 2010;122(18 Suppl 3):S768–S786.
  Current AHA guidelines for modifications of ACLS in hypothermic patients.
Seder DB, Van der Kloot TE. Methods of cooling: Practical aspects of therapeutic temperature management. *Crit Care Med*. 2009;37(Suppl):S211–S222.
  From a supplemental publication that focuses on the clinical and biological aspects of therapeutic hypothermia and temperature management.

33 Toxicology

Nicholas M. Mohr, Devin P. Sherman, and
Steven L. Brody

More than 2.5 million cases of accidental or intentional poisoning were recorded by U.S. poison control centers in 2008, resulting in 1315 deaths and over 93,000 intensive care unit admissions. Among fatalities, 91% were 20 years of age or older. Deaths were most common following ingestion of sedatives/hypnotics/antipsychotics (14.8%), opioids (12.7%), acetaminophen alone or in combination (12.7%), antidepressants (7.8%), cardiovascular drugs (7.5%), ethanol (6.7%), and stimulant street drugs (5.8%). Although much of the initial management is provided in the emergency department (ED), critical care physicians may subsequently manage the poisoned patient.

KEY STEPS IN THE MANAGEMENT OF THE POISONED PATIENT

Algorithm 33.1 presents an outline for managing the poisoned patient.

1. Before all else, address the "ABCs" (airway, breathing, and circulation):
   - Intubate and mechanically ventilate for airway protection or respiratory failure
   - Obtain intravenous access and give crystalloid for hypotension. Obtain electrocardiogram (EKG) and routine labs. Obtain extra tubes of blood for serum drug and toxin levels.
2. Treat potentially reversible causes of altered mental status or coma with:
   - Rapid glucose assessment and treatment, if indicated (prior to intubation if possible)
   - Thiamine 100 mg IV
   - Naloxone 0.4 to 2 mg IV or IM if possible opioid toxicity
3. Assess for and treat toxidrome and give specific antidotes when indicated (see Tables 33.1 and 33.2). Call the regional Poison Control Center at 1-800-222-1222 for management advice.
4. Block absorption of toxins when appropriate (see "Gastric Decontamination").
5. Enhance elimination of toxins when appropriate (see "Enhancing Drug Elimination").

EMERGENCY EVALUATION

The initial assessment of the poisoned patient should begin with an assessment of the ABCs: airway, breathing, and circulation. Respiratory depression, loss of airway protective reflexes, and aspiration are common consequences of ingestion. Awake patients may need close monitoring for delayed drug effects, and lethargic or obtunded patients,

ALGORITHM 33.1 Key Steps in the Initial Management of the Poisoned Patient

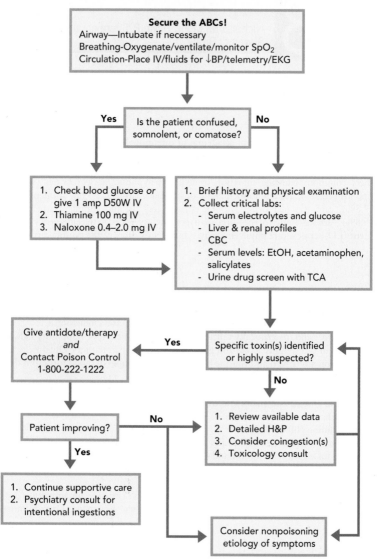

IV, intravenous; D50W, dextrose 50% in water; CBC, complete blood count; EtOH, ethanol; TCA, tricyclic antidepressant; H&P, history and physical examination.

TABLE 33.1	Clinical Toxidromes	
	Possible features	Offending agents
Sympathomimetic	Hypertension, tachycardia, tachypnea, hyperthermia, mydriasis, agitation, hallucinations, diaphoresis	Cocaine Amphetamines Ephedrine Pseudoephedrine Theophylline Caffeine
Anticholinergic "Hot as a hare, dry as a bone, red as a beet, mad as a hatter."	Hypertension, tachycardia, tachypnea, hyperthermia, mydriasis, agitation, delirium, hallucinations, dry skin, dry mouth, ileus, urinary retention	Tricyclic antidepressants Antihistamines Atropine Phenothiazines Scopolamine Belladonna alkaloids
Cholinergic "SLUDGE"	Salivation, lacrimation, urination, diarrhea, gastrointestinal distress, emesis; also bradycardia, miosis, confusion, coma, bronchoconstriction	Organophosphates Physostigmine Pyridostigmine Edrophonium
Opioid	Hypotension, bradycardia, hypopnea, bradypnea, hypothermia, miosis, CNS depression/coma, decreased bowel sounds, pulmonary edema	Heroin Oxycodone Morphine Meperidine Fentanyl Codeine Methadone
Sedative-hypnotic	Hypotension, bradycardia, hypopnea, bradypnea, CNS depression, coma	Benzodiazepines Barbiturates Alcohols
Extrapyramidal	Rigidity, torticollis, opisthotonos, trismus, oculogyric crisis, dysphoria	Prochlorperazine Haloperidol Chlorpromazine Other antipsychotics

or those with recurrent seizures may require immediate endotracheal intubation. When in doubt, the airway should be secured by intubation. Care should be taken to clear the airway of secretions or obstruction.

Ventilatory failure in the poisoned patient may be a consequence of respiratory depression (e.g., from sedatives) or muscle paralysis/weakness (e.g., from botulism). Arterial blood gas (ABG) measurement will reveal an elevated $PaCO_2$. Somnolence or obtundation in the setting of a rising $PaCO_2$ is an indication for intubation and assisted ventilation. Bronchospasm may be observed in cases of inhalational injury and other toxins, and bronchodilators may be useful.

TABLE 33.2	Selected Causes of an Elevated Anion Gap
Toxic ingestions	Other causes
Salicylate	Lactic acidosis
Ethylene glycol	Ketoacidosis
Methanol	Diabetic
Paraldehyde	Starvation
Isoniazid	Alcoholic
Iron	Uremic acidosis
Selected causes of a low anion gap	
Lithium	Hypoalbuminemia
	Elevated IgG (e.g., myeloma)

IgG, immunoglobulin G.

Hypoxemia can result as a consequence of toxin-associated hypoventilation, aspiration, or pulmonary edema. Oxygen should be administered in all lethargic patients during initial workup. Treatment of significant hypoxemia may require mechanical ventilation or high fractions of inspired oxygen (FiO_2).

Arrhythmias, hypotension, and circulatory failure/shock can occur with poisonings. Venous access should be obtained and IV fluids given for hypotension. Continuous electrocardiogram monitoring should be initiated and an EKG obtained. Pulseless or hemodynamically unstable patients should receive standard advanced cardiac life support therapies. However, toxin-induced cardiac arrest may at times require specific therapies. For example, wide QRS pulseless rhythms due to tricyclic antidepressant (TCA) toxicity should be rapidly treated with sodium bicarbonate, as should hyperkalemic arrests due to salicylate toxicity. Furthermore, some common therapies should be avoided with certain intoxications (e.g., beta-blockers in cocaine intoxication).

All patients (especially the poisoned patient) with altered mental status should be screened for hypoglycemia or treated empirically with IV dextrose (25 g, or one ampule of D50W). Thiamine (100 mg IV) and naloxone (0.4 to 2 mg IV) should also be given to these patients for possible Wernicke encephalopathy and opiate intoxication, respectively. Patients receiving thiamine should also receive IV dextrose.

DIAGNOSTIC STRATEGIES

Important Principles

• All overdoses are considered to be polysubstance overdoses until proven otherwise. Ethanol and opiates are common components of polysubstance overdose.
• The following lethal ingestions with specific therapies should always be ruled out:
   Acetaminophen (serum level)
   TCAs (qualitative urine screen, EKG)
   Salicylates (serum level)
• Pre-existing illnesses and coingestions can confound a "classic" poisoning presentation.
• Toxins screened on "drug screens" vary among institutions, and are often insensitive and non-specific. Avoid over reliance on drug screens in the face of a clinical toxidrome.

- History, physical examination, and laboratory testing should be directed at identifying or confirming exposure to specific toxins if these are not already known.

Toxidromes

A *toxidrome* is a constellation of signs and symptoms that may be seen after exposure to a specific class of intoxicant (Table 33.1). The physical examination should be performed with particular attention to vital signs, mental status, pupillary size, and psychomotor state that may suggest a specific toxidrome.

Ingestion History

An accurate accounting of the ingestion should be obtained. Specific details including type and quantity of ingestion should be sought, and an outpatient medication profile should be established. Relevant details may come from initial responders (e.g., emergency medical services) or patient contacts. Be aware that the history obtained may be unreliable or incomplete, mandating a rigorous evaluation for possible polysubstance ingestions.

The Optimal Use of Laboratory Tests

Basic tests should include a comprehensive metabolic panel and complete blood cell count. Arterial blood should be analyzed by co-oximetry in the presence of respiratory distress, altered mental status, somnolence, coma, or cyanosis. Serum levels of ethanol, acetaminophen, and salicylate, and urine screen for common drugs of abuse and TCAs should be sent. Serum levels of digoxin, lithium, theophylline, phenytoin, and iron may be useful if the patient is known to take or have immediate access to these medicines. Do not delay treatment awaiting test results if an ingestion is suspected.

One should be cautious about the use and interpretation of toxicology screening tests. Qualitative urine or serum screening assays may reveal "exposure" to various classes of drugs, but cannot discern whether an exposure is responsible for the presentation. Many substances are not included on screens for drugs of abuse. Further, depending on the timing of the ingestion, coingestions, and the sensitivity of the test used, results may be falsely negative even in the presence of intoxication. Some tests evaluate for metabolites of a drug, and others may test for only some drugs in a particular drug class (e.g., some opiate screens are negative in the presence of methadone or fentanyl). Thus, toxicology screening tests can be used to support clinical suspicion, but management should be guided by a careful history and identification of a toxidrome, and therapy driven by clinical findings.

Clues to specific poisonings may be found by attention to the "three gaps": the anion gap, the osmolal gap, and the oxygen saturation gap.

Anion gap elevations may indicate the ingestion of toxins such as ethylene glycol, methanol or salicylates. The formula for calculating the serum anion gap follows, and causes of an elevated or low anion gap are included in Table 33.3.

$$\text{Anion gap} = [\text{Na}^+] - ([\text{Cl}_2^-] + [\text{HCO}_3^-])$$

The normal range is 7 to 13 mEq/L, but vary among laboratories.

Osmolal gap elevations may be present following toxic ingestions of alcohols. The serum osmolal gap is the difference between the measured and calculated serum osmolality. Thus, an elevated osmolal gap reflects the presence of an osmotically active substance in the blood that is not accounted for by routine calculation of osmolality. Formulas necessary for calculating the osmolal gap follow, and a list of causes of an elevated osmolal gap are included in Table 33.4.

TABLE 33.3	Selected Causes of an Elevated Osmolal Gap	
With normal anion gap	**With elevated anion gap**
Isopropanol	Methanol
Acetone	Ethylene glycol
Mannitol	Formaldehyde
Diethyl ether	Paraldehyde

$$\mathrm{Osm_{calculated}} = 2[\mathrm{Na^+}] + [\mathrm{urea}]/2.8 + [\mathrm{glucose}]/18 + [\mathrm{ethanol}]/4.6$$

where $[\mathrm{Na^+}]$ is in mmol/L and [urea], [glucose] and [ethanol] are in mg/dL.

$$\mathrm{Osmolal\ gap} = \mathrm{Osm_{measured}} - \mathrm{Osm_{calculated}} (\mathrm{normal} < 10)$$

Oxygen saturation gap describes differences between oxyhemoglobin percentage as measured by pulse oximetry ($\mathrm{SpO_2}$) or as estimated from arterial oxygen tension

TABLE 33.4	Specific Antidotes for Selected Toxins
Toxin	**Antidotes**
Acetaminophen	*N*-acetylcysteine
Carbon monoxide	100% O_2, hyperbaric O_2 in some cases
Cholinesterase inhibitors (e.g., organophosphates)	Atropine 1–5 mg IV, repeat q5–10 min for ongoing wheezing or bronchorrhea Pralidoxime 1–2 g IV over 30 min, repeat after 1 hr if ongoing weakness or fasciculations
Cyanide	Sodium nitrite 300 mg IV over 2–5 min
Digoxin	Digoxin-specific antibody fragments (Fab) Acute: 10–20 vials Chronic: 3–6 vials
Ethylene glycol	Fomepizole 15 mg/kg IV over 30 min (first dose), then 10 mg/kg q12h × 4 doses, then 15 mg/kg q12h as needed
Iron	Deferoxamine start at 5 mg/kg/hr, titrate as tolerated to 15 mg/kg/hr, max daily dose 6–8 g/day
Isoniazid	Pyridoxine 1 g for each gram of isoniazid ingested up to 70 mg/kg or 5 g max infused IV at 0.5 g/min until seizures stop, then the remainder infused during 4–6 hr
Methanol	Fomepizole 15 mg/kg IV over 30 min (first dose), then 10 mg/kg q12h × 4 doses, then 15 mg/kg q12h as needed
Methemoglobinemia	Methylene Blue 1–2 mg/kg IV over 5 min followed by 30 mL saline flush
Opioids	Naloxone 0.4–2 mg IV (IM, SC, or endotracheally)
Sulfonylureas	Octreotide 50 mcg SC q6h

IV, intravenously; IM, intramuscularly; SC, subcutaneously.

(PaO_2) when compared with the oxyhemoglobin percentage (SaO_2) as measured by co-oximetry. An oxygen saturation gap may indicate poisoning from carbon monoxide, cyanide or hydrogen sulfide, or the presence of an acquired hemoglobinopathy, as occurs with methemoglobinemia. If these toxins are suspected, arterial blood must be analyzed by a co-oximeter, which is capable of measuring the concentrations of oxyhemoglobin, deoxyhemoglobin, methemoglobin, and carboxyhemoglobin in the specimen.

TREATMENT STRATEGIES

Antidotes

Specific antidotes are available for relatively few toxins. Although potentially life-saving, many of these antidotes have adverse effects and can be harmful if used inappropriately. Consultation with a poison control center or a medical toxicologist is advised when prescribing an antidote with which one is unfamiliar. A select list of antidotes is included in Table 33.2.

Gastric Decontamination

Among methods for blocking the absorption of drugs in the gastrointestinal (GI) tract, activated charcoal and whole-bowel irrigation (WBI) are recommended for use in limited circumstances. The routine use of gastric lavage, induced emesis (e.g., with syrup of ipecac), and cathartics are not recommended.

Activated charcoal, given orally or through a nasogastric tube, readily adsorbs most toxins, thereby preventing systemic absorption and toxicity. Substances that are not well adsorbed by activated charcoal are alcohols, iron, and lithium. The efficacy of activated charcoal is greatest when given within 1 hour of ingestion. A single dose of activated charcoal (1 g/kg) is recommended in adolescents and adults. Multiple-dose activated charcoal (MDAC) may be used as means of drug elimination in the management of certain poisonings (see below). Contraindications to the use of activated charcoal include an unprotected airway and the ingestion of a hydrocarbon. Caution should be taken in the setting of significant GI pathology or recent GI surgery.

WBI involves the enteral administration of large volumes of an osmotically balanced polyethylene glycol electrolyte solution to induce diarrhea with rapid expulsion of unabsorbed toxins from the GI tract. No controlled studies have been published, but WBI may be considered in the management of certain ingestions (Table 33.5). WBI is best performed using a nasogastric tube, and a recommended regimen is 1500 to

---

TABLE 33.5 Potential Indications for Whole-Bowel Irrigation

Iron poisoning
Lithium poisoning
Sustained-release or enteric coated medication toxicity
Retained illicit drug packets (i.e., from "body packing")

Contraindications

Bowel obstruction	Ileus	Bowel perforation
Unprotected airway	Uncontrolled vomiting	
Hemodynamic instability	Toxic colitis	

TABLE 33.6	Potential Indications for Urine Alkalinization (with Selected Comments)

Salicylates: Severe cases not meeting criteria for hemodialysis
Methotrexate: Consider hemoperfusion instead
2,4-Dichlorophenoxyacetic acid: Goal urine pH >8 and urine output >600 mL/hr
Chlorpropamide: Dextrose infusion alone usually adequate
Phenobarbital: Multiple dose activated charcoal may be more effective
Diflunisal
Fluoride

Contraindications
Renal failure

2000 mL/hr of enterally administered WBI fluid continued at least until a clear rectal effluent is noted. Contraindications include an unprotected airway, bowel perforation or obstruction, ileus, significant GI hemorrhage, toxic colitis, uncontrolled vomiting, and hemodynamic instability.

Induced emesis and cathartics are not recommended because of the lack of proven efficacy and interference with enterally administered specific antidotes.

Enhancing Drug Elimination

Urine alkalinization is a method of enhancing the renal elimination of certain poisons by increasing urine pH to levels ≥7.5 through the administration of IV sodium bicarbonate (e.g., 1 to 2 mEq/kg IV during 3 to 4 hours). The strongest indication is moderately severe salicylate toxicity not meeting criteria for hemodialysis. Other possible indications are included in Table 33.6. Potassium supplementation may be required in the setting of hypokalemia to ensure effective urine alkalinization. Urine pH should be monitored frequently (every 1 hour initially) to ensure that the target pH ≥7.5 is reached. Serum electrolytes should be monitored every 2 to 4 hours as well. Complications of therapy include alkalemia and hypokalemia. Renal failure is a contraindication.

MDAC refers to the repeated enteral administration of activated charcoal, which may enhance the elimination of certain toxins (Table 33.7). Dosing regimens vary, but

TABLE 33.7	Potential Indications for MDAC (Severe Poisoning)

Carbamazepine
Dapsone
Phenobarbital
Quinine
Theophylline

Contraindications
Unprotected airway
Coadministration of cathartic with MDAC

MDAC, multiple-dose activated charcoal.

TABLE 33.8	Selected Toxins Removable by Hemodialysis or Hemoperfusion with Potential Indications
Hemodialysis	
Salicylates	Significant neurologic symptoms, CV instability, renal failure, level >100 mg/dL
Lithium	Renal failure, coma, seizures, CV instability, myoclonus
Methanol	New visual deficit, severe acidosis, level >50 mg/dL
Ethylene glycol	Severe acidosis, renal failure, level >50 mg/dL
Isopropanol	Hypotension, clinical worsening, level >400 mg/dL; rarely needed
Calcium channel blockers	Nicardipine, nifedipine, and nimodipine with severe cardiotoxicity, heart block requiring pacing, refractory hypotension
Beta-blockers	Limited to acebutolol, atenolol, and especially sotalol with CV instability, renal failure
Hemoperfusion	
Barbiturates	Clinical deterioration or renal failure
Carbamazepine	Life-threatening ingestion or clinical deterioration; consider MDAC
Theophylline	Seizures, arrhythmias, persistent hypotension
Valproic acid	Rapid deterioration, hepatic dysfunction, level >1,000 mg/L

CV, cardiovascular; MDAC, multiple-dose activated charcoal.

a typical regimen would include a 1 g/kg loading dose, followed by 0.5 g/kg every 2 to 4 hours for at least three doses. Drug elimination occurs by adsorption of toxins that have diffused from the blood into the gut lumen or that have undergone enterohepatic recirculation. Drugs with low volumes of distribution, low protein binding, and long elimination half-lives are the best candidates for MDAC. An unprotected airway is a contraindication to use of MDAC. Cathartics should not be coadministered with MDAC.

Hemodialysis and hemoperfusion are extracorporeal methods of toxin removal that may be required to treat life-threatening toxicity (Table 33.8). General indications for use include clinical deterioration despite intensive alternative therapy, impairment of normal toxin elimination capacity (e.g., liver or renal failure), and severe toxicity from drugs that can be removed faster by extracorporeal methods than by other means. Prompt nephrology and medical toxicology consultation should be obtained when hemodialysis or hemoperfusion are being considered.

Emerging evidence suggests a therapeutic role for intravenous lipid emulsion (e.g., lipid parenteral nutrition) in overdoses with lipophilic drugs (e.g., bupivacaine, verapamil, chlorpromazine, clomipramine). It is theorized that the intravenous lipid sequesters toxins from physiologic binding sites. Optimal dosing has not yet been defined, but a 1.5 mL/kg bolus of 20% lipid (as used for parenteral nutrition) followed by a 0.25 mL/kg/min infusion has been used. Evidence does not support routine use of lipid emulsion therapy except as a rescue therapy in consultation with a medical toxicologist.

SPECIFIC INTOXICATIONS AND MANAGEMENT STRATEGIES

Opioids

- Sx: Sedation, hypercarbic respiratory failure, miosis
- Dx: Clinical diagnosis
- Tx: Naloxone, mechanical ventilation

Opioid-intoxicated patients present with a syndrome that typically includes sedation, respiratory depression, miosis, and decreased GI motility. Life-threatening manifestations of opioid intoxication include respiratory depression, which may range from decreases in tidal volume and respiratory rate to complete apnea. ABG analysis will typically reveal an elevated $PaCO_2$, and hypoxemia may be present in severe intoxication. Hypotension (resulting from histamine release) is more common with certain agents (e.g., meperidine). Noncardiogenic pulmonary edema may occur. Seizures may occur as a result of the accumulation of the neurotoxic metabolites of certain opioids (specifically meperidine, propoxyphene, and tramadol). Acetaminophen or aspirin toxicity may complicate the patient presentation when combination analgesics have been ingested. Drug screens may not detect some opiate medications (e.g., fentanyl, methadone). As such, patients with a toxidrome consistent with opioid toxicity should be treated regardless of toxicology screening tests.

Management of opioid intoxication is primarily directed at ensuring adequate airway control and ventilation and the early use of the opioid antagonist naloxone. Naloxone is given initially at doses of 0.4 to 2 mg IV every 2 minutes until effect to a maximum of 10 mg. Naloxone should be viewed as an agent to prevent intubation, not for use after mechanical ventilation is initiated. The duration of naloxone action is 1 to 2 hours, which may be shorter than the activity of the opioid intoxicant, mandating a several-hour monitoring period after response. Intoxication with long acting opioids may require repeated doses of naloxone. Continuous naloxone infusions can be used at a dose of two-thirds the original response dose per hour (dosing assistance from a pharmacist or toxicologist is recommended). Opioid-dependent patients may suffer opioid withdrawal with naloxone treatment. Pregnant patients may develop uterine contractions and induction of labor with naloxone administration. Oral opiate overdose may be treated with a single dose of activated charcoal if started within the first hour of ingestion, while body packers should be treated with activated charcoal, WBI, and naloxone infusion if symptomatic.

Dextromethorphan

- Sx: Agitation, mydriasis, dizziness and hallucinations
- Dx: Clinical history and symptoms.
- Tx: Naloxone for respiratory depression

Dextromethorphan is an opioid used as an antitussive in some over-the-counter cough and cold preparations (e.g., Robitussin DM, NyQuil Nighttime Cold Medicine). Dextromethorphan-containing products are often intentionally abused for their psychoactive properties. Intoxicated patients may present with restlessness, mydriasis, ataxia, dizziness, and hallucinations. Stupor, coma, and seizure can occur in more severe cases. Mixed ingestions must be ruled out as over-the-counter cold remedies often contain other ingredients (e.g., acetaminophen, aspirin). Dysphoria associated with dextromethorphan intoxication may be treated with benzodiazepines, and naloxone is partially effective for reversal of respiratory depression. A serotonin syndrome of hyperthermia, hypertension, and muscle rigidity may occur in dextromethorphan-intoxicated patients also taking monoamine oxidase inhibitors.

Acetaminophen

- Sx: Asymptomatic early, nausea and vomiting, liver failure
- Dx: Serum acetaminophen level
- Tx: *N*-acetylcysteine (NAC)

The majority of acetaminophen ingestions cause no significant clinical toxicity, but life-threatening liver injury and even death can occur with overdose. Acute ingestions of 150 mg/kg (or 10 g), or the chronic ingestion in excess of 4 g/day may result in clinical toxicity. The generation of a toxic metabolite, *N*-acetyl-p-benzoquinoneimine (NAPQI), by the cytochrome P-450 mixed-function oxidase system (specifically the CYP2E1 enzyme) in the setting of overwhelmed hepatic glutathione results in hepatic and renal injury. Induction of CYP2E1 (e.g., by ethanol, rifampin, isoniazid, or carbamazepine) or decreased glutathione stores, as occurs with chronic malnutrition from alcoholism, increases the risk for acetaminophen toxicity.

The clinical presentation of acetaminophen overdose depends on the time of presentation and amount of acetaminophen taken. Patients may be entirely asymptomatic, but early symptoms include anorexia, nausea, and vomiting. Liver injury usually occurs within 24 to 36 hours of ingestion as evidenced by elevations in blood levels of aspartate aminotransferase (AST) and alanine aminotransferase (ALT). Maximal hepatotoxicity is usually seen 72 to 96 hours after ingestion and may result in encephalopathy, coagulopathy, renal failure, hypoglycemia, and shock. Elevations in pancreatic enzymes and acute myocardial injury have also been described.

In all cases of known or potential acetaminophen overdose, the serum level of acetaminophen should be measured 4 hours after ingestion or as soon as possible thereafter and plotted against time using the Rumack–Matthew nomogram (Fig. 33.1). Plasma concentrations above the lower line ("possible risk") are an indication for treatment with NAC. Administration of NAC should not be delayed while awaiting the serum level in cases of witnessed ingestions, hepatotoxicity or pregnancy. Repeating the serum acetaminophen level should be considered in cases of ingestion of extended-release products if the initial value is below the treatment line. Although the nomogram assesses risk of toxicity with levels obtained from 4 to 24 hours post-ingestion, patients who present after 24 hours with detectable acetaminophen levels or elevated liver enzymes should receive NAC therapy while awaiting further data or input from poison control.

NAC enhances both the synthesis of glutathione (which acts as an antioxidant) as well as the conversion of acetaminophen to (nontoxic) acetaminophen sulfate, rather than NAPQI. Several different NAC protocols have been used and are of similar efficacy (Table 33.9).

A specific pitfall of acetaminophen overdose management arises in patients with chronic ingestions or an unknown time of ingestion, because they cannot be plotted on the Rumack–Matthews nomogram. Considering the relatively safe profile of NAC therapy and the disastrous consequences of failing to treat acetaminophen toxicity, early NAC treatment is recommended. Any patient with a clinically suspected toxic acetaminophen ingestion with unknown time of ingestion should be treated if either: (i) the presenting acetaminophen level is detectable (even if below the Rumack–Matthews treatment line), or (ii) the serum hepatic transaminases (e.g., AST) are

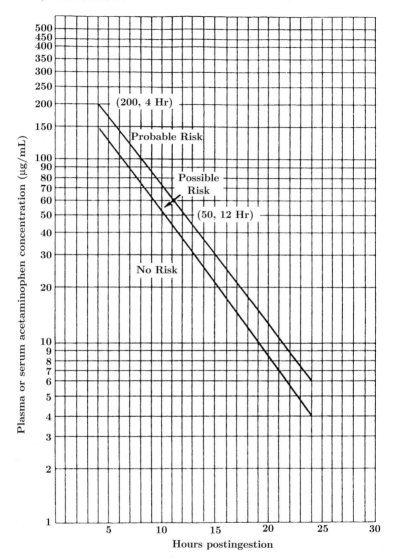

Figure 33.1. Rumack-Matthew acetaminophen toxicity nomogram.

elevated above baseline. In general, discontinuation of NAC therapy is appropriate in communication with a medical toxicologist either after a complete treatment course, normalization of serum transaminases, or clarification of the patient's ingestion history.

NAC therapy is available in both IV and oral formulations. Although neither seems to have superior efficacy, many centers now use the IV formulation for simplicity of administration. In general, NAC therapy is continued for the duration of

TABLE 33.9	Acceptable *N*-Acetylcysteine Protocols for the Treatment of Acetaminophen Toxicity
20-hr IV regimen (continuous infusion)	150 mg/kg IV given over 15 min, then 50 mg/kg IV given over 4 hr, then 100 mg/kg IV given over 20 hr
72-hr PO regimen	140 mg/kg PO once, then 70 mg/kg PO q4h × 17 doses
52-hr IV regimen	140 mg/kg given over 60 min, then 70 mg/kg IV q 4 hr × 12 doses

IV, intravenously; PO, orally.

therapy (20 hours for IV, 72 hours for oral) except in cases of hepatic failure, when longer treatment is usually recommended. Severe acetaminophen toxicity resulting in fulminant hepatic failure should be managed with early hepatology consultation or transfer to a tertiary center for evaluation for liver transplantation. A suspected suicide attempt and drug or ethanol abuse alone may not preclude transplantation, but formal psychiatric assessment may be required. The most often used predictor of the need for liver transplantation after acetaminophen overdose are the King's College Hospital criteria: (a) pH <7.25 in spite of adequate fluid resuscitation or (b) the combination of grade III-IV hepatic encephalopathy, serum creatinine >3.4 mg/dL and prothrombin time >100 seconds. Acute renal failure is common in the setting of acetaminophen-induced fulminant hepatic failure and is likely multifactorial in nature. Hemodynamic monitoring may be needed to assess intravascular volume status.

Salicylates

- Sx: Abdominal pain, nausea and vomiting, respiratory alkalosis, anion gap acidosis
- Dx: Salicylate level
- Tx: Alkalinization of the urine, hemodialysis

Salicylate toxicity results from both direct corrosive injury to the GI tract and multiple metabolic effects (e.g., respiratory stimulation, uncoupling of mitochondrial oxidative phosphorylation, inhibition of the tricarboxylic acid cycle, enhanced lipolysis with ketone generation). Patients may present with GI symptoms (e.g., abdominal pain, nausea and vomiting, and GI bleeding), diaphoresis, respiratory alkalosis with anion gap metabolic acidosis, deranged glucose regulation, tachycardia, ventricular arrhythmias, pulmonary edema/acute lung injury, prolonged prothrombin times, central nervous system (CNS) effects (e.g., agitation, confusion, seizures, and coma), tinnitus, rhabdomyolysis, and renal failure. The clinical course may be dynamic; for example, with GI symptoms prominent early but metabolic derangements, such as acidosis and renal failure seen later. The finding of coincident CNS changes with tachycardia and diaphoresis suggests severe toxicity and warrants immediate and aggressive action. Many salicylate overdoses are accidental, so laboratory screening should be performed on any patient with nonspecific symptoms, no clear diagnosis, and a significant anion gap metabolic acidemia.

The diagnosis of salicylate exposure can be confirmed by obtaining a serum salicylate level. Activated charcoal may be administered within an hour of suspected or

TABLE 33.10 Indications for Hemodialysis in Acute Salicylate Poisoning

Progressive hemodynamic deterioration
Persistent CNS derangement
Severe acid-base or electrolyte disturbances despite appropriate therapy
Renal failure
Acute lung injury
Serum salicylate level >100 mg/dL for acute ingestions

confirmed salicylate poisoning unless a contraindication exists. Serum glucose should
be measured or dextrose given empirically if confusion or seizures occur. Benzodiazepines should be administered for recurrent seizures. Fluid deficits may be substantial because of vomiting and insensible losses and should be treated with IV fluid.
In addition, sodium bicarbonate should be given intravenously to a target serum pH
of approximately 7.50 (to limit tissue redistribution of salicylate) and urine pH of
approximately eight (to enhance renal elimination of salicylate). Effective alkaluria
will require correction of hypokalemia and potassium supplementation in the setting
normokalemia should be considered. ABG analysis, urine pH, and serum chemistries
should be followed serially (every 1 to 4 hours) to guide therapy in the most ill
patients. Hemodialysis is indicated in severe intoxication (see Table 33.10). Delays
in initiating hemodialysis when indicated may result in unnecessary morbidity and
mortality.

Tricyclic Antidepressants
• Sx: Anticholinergic toxidrome, (especially, tachycardia, confusion)
• Dx: Prolonged QT interval, TCA use history
• Tx: IV sodium bicarbonate

TCA overdose can result in life threatening cardiovascular and CNS effects due
to the narrow therapeutic window for these agents. Toxicity may vary with the class of
TCA, but amitriptyline is particularly toxic. Symptoms from TCA toxicity are a result
of anticholinergic effects, alpha-adrenergic blockade, inhibition of norepinephrine
and serotonin reuptake, and blockade of the fast sodium channels in myocardium,
resulting in a quinidine-like effect. Cardiotoxicity may manifest with tachycardia,
prolongation of the PR, QRS, or QT intervals, atrioventricular block, arrhythmias,
depressed myocardial contractility, or hypotension. Seizures are a common consequence of TCA overdose, and when coupled with impaired sweating, can lead to
life-threatening hyperthermia.

TCA overdose should be considered in any patient with an anticholinergic toxidrome or with confusion or coma, especially if accompanied by tachycardia, QRS
prolongation, rightward axis deviation of the terminal 40 ms of the QRS complex,
or QT interval prolongation. Specific drug levels are neither valuable nor required
to make the diagnosis of acute intoxication. Qualitative urine and serum screens can
retrospectively support the diagnosis of intoxication.

Initial management of TCA overdose is directed at emergent management of airway, hemodynamic instability, and treatment of ongoing seizures. Sodium bicarbonate
infusion should be given as an antidote for cardiotoxicity in the setting of ventricular
arrhythmias or QRS prolongation >100 msec, or in the presence of hypotension with

acidosis (pH <7.20). A typical regimen would be an initial bolus of 1 to 2 mEq/kg, followed by an infusion of 150 mEq of sodium bicarbonate in 1 L of D5W given at 2 to 3 mL/kg/hr IV, adjusted to a target arterial pH of 7.45 to 7.50. The benefits of sodium bicarbonate therapy are multifactorial, related in part to the effect of sodium on myocardial channels. Hypertonic saline has been used in refractory cases. Combination therapy with bicarbonate infusion and hyperventilation should be avoided because of the risk of induction of a life-threatening alkalosis and hypokalemia. Type 1a and 1c antiarrhythmics (e.g., procainamide and flecainide) should be avoided in the management of arrhythmias and lidocaine has not been shown to have efficacy. Although the evidence is limited, magnesium sulfate has been shown to be effective for TCA-induced wide complex tachycardia unresponsive to other agents. Benzodiazepines should be used to treat TCA-induced seizures, with phenytoin, barbiturates, and propofol used for refractory cases. Activated charcoal should be given if no contraindication exists. Hemodialysis and hemoperfusion are not shown to be beneficial in TCA overdose. Physostigmine is not recommended in the management of TCA overdose because of significant toxicity associated with use.

Beta-Blockers

- Sx: Bradycardia, hypotension, AV blockade, confusion, hypoglycemia, hyperkalemia
- Dx: Clinical diagnosis
- Tx: Atropine, intravenous glucagon, cardiac pacing, cardiopulmonary bypass

Beta-adrenergic blockers can result in life-threatening toxicity when taken in doses even two to three times the therapeutic range. Potential cardiovascular manifestations of toxicity include bradycardia and hypotension, heart block of any degree, and cardiogenic shock. CNS toxicity including confusion, seizures, and coma may occur, particularly with lipid-soluble medications (e.g., propranolol, metoprolol, timolol). Bronchospasm can be life-threatening in patients with underlying chronic obstructive pulmonary disease or asthma. Metabolic derangements such as hypoglycemia and hyperkalemia may also occur. Many beta-blockers have long half-lives, potentially resulting in prolonged effects. Toxicity may even be seen with ocular preparations.

Diagnosis is made based on the clinical presentation and suspected or known history of ingestion. Exposure may be confirmed with qualitative urine screen.

Treatment is directed at the specific clinical manifestation and may include atropine, isoproterenol, or cardiac pacing for bradycardia or heart block, and nebulized bronchodilators for bronchospasm. Refractory bradycardia or hypotension may be treated with glucagon, starting with a 5- to 10-mg IV bolus, followed by continuous infusion at 1 to 10 mg/hr. Nausea, vomiting, hyperglycemia, and hypocalcemia may be seen with glucagon use. Adrenergic agents such as dobutamine, dopamine, epinephrine and norepinephrine may be ineffective at usual therapeutic doses. External or transvenous pacing should instead be considered early in the management of significant toxicity or large ingestions. Phosphodiesterase inhibitors such as milrinone may be useful in cases of cardiogenic shock. Refractory cases may require hemodynamic support by cardiopulmonary bypass.

Activated charcoal may be useful to block absorption in early presentations. Most beta-blockers have very large volumes of distribution, making them less susceptible to clearance by extracorporeal techniques. Acebutolol, atenolol, and sotalol are exceptions that are amenable to extracorporeal removal in cases of severe toxicity, particularly in the patient with renal failure.

Calcium Channel Blockers

- Sx: Hypotension, bradycardia, AV nodal blockade, hypoglycemia, seizures
- Dx: Clinical diagnosis
- Tx: IV calcium

Calcium channel blockers can result in significant toxicity, particularly in patients with underlying cardiovascular disease or when coingested with other cardiovascular medicines (e.g., beta-blockers). Clinical manifestations of calcium channel blocker toxicity are primarily cardiovascular. Hypotension is common. Bradycardia and cardiac conduction disturbances may occur, typically with nondihydropyridines (e.g. verapamil). By contrast, dihydropyridines may result in hypotension with reflex tachycardia due to a lack of activity on the sinoatrial and atrioventricular nodes. Noncardiovascular effects include nausea and vomiting, mental status changes, noncardiogenic pulmonary edema, hyperglycemia, and seizures. Sustained-release preparations may result in prolonged or delayed toxicity.

Diagnosis is made based on a typical presentation with a history of ingestion. Comprehensive urine toxicology screening may detect diltiazem and verapamil.

Treatment is directed at the particular manifestation of toxicity. IV fluid should be given initially for hypotension. IV calcium is given for hypotension or cardiac conduction disturbances. A typical dose is 10 mL of 10% $CaCl_2$ given over 2 to 3 minutes, with additional doses every 5 to 10 minutes for ongoing instability, followed by continuous infusion of 10% $CaCl_2$ at 10 mL/hour. IV dopamine, norepinephrine or epinephrine may be needed for refractory hypotension.

Glucagon and phosphodiesterase inhibitors should also be considered in these cases. Insulin-glucose infusions (to a target serum glucose between 100 and 200 mg/dL) may be useful in cases refractory to these measures. Invasive hemodynamic monitoring is encouraged in patients not responding to initial resuscitative measures. Severely poisoned patients may require support using ventricular pacing, ventricular assist devices, and even cardiopulmonary bypass, depending on the scenario.

Activated charcoal may be given to block absorption in early presentations or with sustained release preparations. Most calcium channel blockers have large volumes of distribution and are highly protein-bound, making them poor candidates for removal by hemodialysis, although lipid emulsion therapy has been described. Nicardipine, nifedipine, and nimodipine have lower volumes of distributions and are potentially removable by hemoperfusion in cases of severe toxicity (Table 33.8).

Digoxin

- Sx: Nausea, vomiting, and altered mental status
- Dx: Serum digoxin level
- Tx: Digoxin specific antibody (Fab) fragments

Digoxin toxicity may occur from acute or chronic ingestion owing to a narrow therapeutic window. Cardiac glycosides reversibly inhibit the sodium-potassium-ATPase, causing an increase in intracellular sodium and a decrease in intracellular potassium. Changes in volume of distribution, diminished protein binding from hypoalbuminemia, and renal impairment can result in decreased elimination and increased risk for toxicity. Clinical features of toxicity include anorexia, nausea, vomiting and abdominal pain, and if severe, lethargy and delirium. Chronic toxicity tends to more insidious and commonly includes the classic visual changes of blurred vision and alterations in color vision. Cardiac toxicity, predisposing to arrhythmias, is the most concerning effect. Digoxin toxicity may induce almost any cardiac arrhythmia (except for atrial fibrillation, atrial flutter, or Mobitz II heart block). Hypokalemia is more common with chronic ingestion while hyperkalemia often occurs with acute toxicity and is correlated with the increased mortality.

When digoxin toxicity is suspected, initial management includes acute stabilization, obtaining an EKG with continuous monitoring, measuring serum electrolytes, and a digoxin level. The normal therapeutic range for digoxin is 0.8 to 2 ng/mL; however, "toxic" levels have been described in asymptomatic patients while toxicity has also been described in the setting of "normal" levels. Symptoms of severe intoxication (life-threatening arrhythmia, acute renal failure, altered mental status, or hyperkalemia >5.5 mEq/L), are indications for treatment with digoxin-specific antibody (Fab). Evidence to support the administration of Fab in patients without these symptoms is lacking, although some advocate use when digoxin levels are > 10 ng/L in acute ingestions and >4 ng/mL in chronic ingestions based on the potential to develop symptoms. Hyperkalemia should be treated conservatively since hypokalemia can propagate lethal arrhythmias in the setting of high digoxin levels. Thus primary treatment with bicarbonate, insulin and glucose, or ion exchange resins is seldom warranted. Maintenance of normal serum levels of magnesium is also important. There is no proven beneficial role for GI decontamination with activated charcoal and or hemodialysis.

Cocaine

- Sx: Sympathomimetic toxidrome
- Dx: Clinical history, urine drug screen
- Tx: Benzodiazepines and anti-hypertensives (except beta-blockers)

Cocaine intoxication can result in life-threatening cardiovascular, pulmonary, and CNS complications. Mechanisms of toxicity include inhibited monoamine reuptake and enhanced catecholamine release (together resulting in increased levels of catecholamines), as well as blockade of Na^+ channel activity. In addition, cocaine promotes thrombogenesis and vasoconstriction. Many features of cocaine intoxication are shared with amphetamine toxicity, and management is similar. Both substances are commonly coingested with alcohol, which may complicate management.

The clinical presentations of cocaine intoxication can be quite varied. Hyperthermia, hypertension, and tachycardia are common. Neuropsychiatric presentations may include agitation and confusion ("agitated delirium"), dystonic reactions, acute cerebrovascular accidents, and seizures. Cardiovascular complications include acute myocardial infarction and arrhythmias. Pulmonary complications include pulmonary edema (cardiogenic or noncardiogenic), alveolar hemorrhage, inhalational heat or burn injury to the aerodigestive tract mucosa, and barotrauma (e.g., pneumothorax, pneumomediastinum) from coughing or intranasally inhaling cocaine. Vasoconstriction can cause intestinal or renal ischemia. Rhabdomyolysis is common in those with agitated delirium. Use of cocaine during pregnancy may result in fetal toxicity, abruptio placentae, spontaneous abortion, and premature labor.

Urine drug of abuse screens may be positive for cocaine for 2 to 3 days after use and false-negative test results can occur. Markers for cardiac injury and creatine phosphokinase levels as well as urinalysis should be obtained in patients with significant intoxication.

Management of cocaine toxicity depends on the presentation. Benzodiazepines (e.g., diazepam 5 to 10 mg every 5 minutes as needed) function as first-line therapy for agitation and most manifestations of toxicity. Treatment of hyperthermia includes

TABLE 33.11	Medications Contraindicated in the Setting of Cocaine Use

Beta-blockers (absolute contraindication)
　　Unopposed alpha adrenergic activity may cause HTN or coronary vasospasm

Phenothiazines and butyrophenone antipsychotics (absolute contraindication)
　　Increase seizure risk, prolong QT interval, promote dystonic reactions

Succinylcholine
　　May exacerbate rhabdomyolysis-induced hyperkalemia

Class Ia antiarrhythmics (e.g., procainamide)
　　May worsen QRS and QT prolongation and potentiate cocaine effects

HTN, hypertension.

adequate sedation and, if necessary, external cooling. Hypertension is best treated with sedation, and if necessary, calcium channel blockers, sodium nitroprusside, or phentolamine. Pure beta-blockers are contraindicated. Other contraindicated medications are listed in Table 33.11.

Chest pain should be thoroughly evaluated. Possible causes include acute coronary events, aortic dissection, and pneumothorax. Cocaine may impair the coronary artery perfusion by vasoconstriction via alpha-adrenergic stimulation, pro-thrombotic effects via thromboxane, and promotion of atherosclerosis in chronic use. Cardiac ischemia occurs in 5% to 6% of those with cocaine use presenting to the ED, so a high index of suspicion should prompt the use of oxygen, aspirin, nitroglycerin, and benzodiazepines. An EKG and serial troponin measurements should be obtained. Further diagnostic evaluation for cardiac ischemia, (e.g., stress testing, cardiac catheterization), is pursued when there is active infarction (ST-elevations) or significant clinical suspicion of fixed coronary lesions that may benefit from intervention.

Supraventricular arrhythmias are treated with calcium channel blockers and pure beta-blockers are contraindicated. Ventricular arrhythmias should be treated with benzodiazepines, oxygen, control of ischemia, correction of electrolytes, and if necessary, lidocaine. Class Ia antiarrhythmics (e.g., procainamide) should be avoided. Management of body packing by drug smugglers may include activated charcoal and WBI if asymptomatic, but immediate surgical removal is required in patients with any signs of cocaine intoxication, suggesting packet rupture. Attempts to retrieve packets by endoscopy risk drug spillage and are not recommended, particularly in the asymptomatic patient.

Alcohols

- Sx: All alcohols present similarly–ataxia, dysarthria, somnolence, respiratory depression, odor on breath
- Dx: Elevated osmolar gap, elevated anion gap (methanol, ethylene glycol), serum levels
- Tx: Fomepizole

Ethanol is widely abused and is a common component of mixed ingestions, particularly in suicide attempts. Toxicity may present with ataxia, dysarthria, CNS depression, and respiratory depression. The diagnosis should be suspected based on presence of symptoms with characteristic ethanol odor and can be confirmed by measuring the blood ethanol level. Treatment is largely supportive and is directed at ensuring adequate airway control and ventilation. Three non-ethanol toxic alcohol ingestions are important to diagnose quickly in critically ill patients: isopropanol, methanol, and ethylene glycol. The key to diagnosis for these ingestions is maintaining a high index of suspicion and measuring the anion and osmolar gaps.

Isopropanol is a component of rubbing alcohol and some other household compounds that may be intentionally ingested as an alternative to ethanol. Clinical manifestations include GI irritation, upper GI bleeding, CNS depression, respiratory depression, and ketosis. Diagnosis should be considered in patients with these symptoms, particularly when presenting with fruity breath (due to acetone production), unexplained ketosis, or an elevated serum osmolal gap. The diagnosis can be confirmed by measuring the serum level. As with ethanol intoxication, treatment is largely supportive. Confused or comatose patients should be screened for hypoglycemia and treated with thiamine 100 mg IV followed by 25 g dextrose. Isopropanol may be removed by hemodialysis, but this is rarely necessary. Upper GI bleeding should be managed with adequate volume resuscitation, correction of coagulopathies, and usual therapies for GI mucosal injury (proton pump inhibitors, endoscopic interventions as needed).

Methanol is found in many household solvents and may be ingested as a substitute for ethanol. Patients may present initially with inebriation. After a characteristic latent period of 12 or more hours, severe manifestations of toxicity including anion gap acidosis, visual disturbance, blindness, respiratory failure, seizures, and coma may occur. Physical examination should include assessment of the pupillary light reflex and funduscopic exam. Methanol ingestion should be considered in all cases of elevated anion gap. The screening test of choice is the osmolar gap. Definitive diagnosis may be made by measuring the serum methanol level, although later presentations may reveal undetectable methanol levels (but elevated formate levels). Toxicity results when methanol is converted to formaldehyde and then to formate by alcohol dehydrogenase. Fomepizole (or ethanol) should be given as a competitive inhibitor of alcohol dehydrogenase in cases of methanol levels >20 mg/dL, acidemia, or an elevated osmolal gap. Fomepizole is dosed at 15 mg/kg IV over 30 minutes, followed by 10 mg/kg IV every 12 hours for four doses, followed by 15 mg/kg IV every 12 hours as needed until the serum methanol level is <20 mg/dL. Folic acid (e.g., 50 mg IV every 6 hours) should be given to promote conversion of formate to CO_2 and water. Hemodialysis should be implemented in cases of visual disturbances, serum methanol levels >50 mg/dL, or severe acidosis. Treatment should be initiated rapidly in cases of an anion gap acidosis with elevation in the osmolar gap and clinical suspicion, not waiting for definitive measurement of a methanol level.

Ethylene glycol is found in antifreeze and may be ingested during suicide attempts or as a substitute for ethanol. Early toxicity manifests with CNS depression. As with methanol, delayed toxic manifestations (after 4 to 12 hours) are often more severe and may include metabolic acidosis, renal failure, seizures, coma, and death. Toxicity arises from the formation of toxic metabolites (e.g., glycolaldehyde and oxalate) under the action of alcohol dehydrogenase. Ethylene glycol should be considered in all cases of elevated anion gap and elevated osmolal gap. The patient's urine may fluoresce under a Wood's lamp or reveal oxalate crystals under microscopy. Diagnosis can be confirmed by measuring the serum level, but treatment should not be delayed if clinical suspicion of ingestion is high. Therapy with fomepizole should be used in a manner similar to that described for methanol poisoning in patients with serum ethylene glycol levels >20 mg/dL, the presence of acidosis, or an elevated osmolal gap. Hemodialysis should be instituted in the setting of renal failure, serum level >50 mg/dL, or severe acidosis. Seizures should be treated with benzodiazepines and correction of hypocalcemia, if present.

Carbon Monoxide

- Sx: Nausea and vomiting, headache, lethargy, confusion.
- Dx: Exposure history, oxygen saturation gap, elevated carboxyhemoglobin.
- Tx: 100% oxygen, hyperbaric oxygen when indicated.

Carbon monoxide (CO) competes with O_2 for hemoglobin-binding sites (forming carboxyhemoglobin, COHb) and has an affinity for hemoglobin that is >200 times that of O_2. Consequently, COHb dissociates extremely slowly, resulting in inadequate oxygen delivery to peripheral tissues.

Neurologic symptoms of toxicity include headache, altered mental status, vision changes, and coma. Nausea and vomiting are common. Cardiac manifestations include arrhythmias and myocardial ischemia or infarction. Less commonly, rhabdomyolysis, pancreatitis, and hepatic injury may be seen. Pulmonary edema may be seen as a consequence of primary cardiac disturbance or from smoke inhalation. Delayed neurologic manifestations (e.g., impaired concentration, amnesia, and depression) are common.

Carbon monoxide poisoning should be suspected after certain exposures (e.g., smoke or poorly ventilated car exhaust, gas stoves, and space heaters). The diagnosis can be confirmed by analyzing arterial blood by co-oximetry, which will allow measurement of COHb. Symptoms and signs of CO toxicity may correlate poorly with the measured COHb levels. Oxyhemoglobin assessments by pulse oximetry (SpO_2) or by estimates made from the partial pressure of oxygen (as reported by some ABG analyzers) can be misleading in CO poisoning. A device for measuring carboxyhemoglobin non-invasively using light transmitted through a capillary bed (similar to pulse oximetry) is now available, but several reports have questioned its accuracy, and laboratory confirmation is recommended.

The treatment of CO toxicity is 100% oxygen. The half-life of COHb varies inversely with the inspired partial pressure of O_2. For this reason, hyperbaric oxygen (HBO_2) therapy has been used to treat CO toxicity since the 1960s. The threshold indications to institute HBO_2 therapy are not well defined, but most experts recommend this therapy for patients who have had loss of consciousness, neurologic abnormalities, cardiac ischemia, or pregnancy. There is a lower threshold for treatment of pregnant patients due to increased affinity of CO by fetal hemoglobin. The benefits of HBO_2 therapy are thought to be greatest when administered promptly (e.g., within 6 hours of exposure) and has benefit in improving delayed neurologic sequelae.

Iron

- Sx: Vomiting, diarrhea, GI bleeding
- Dx: Serum iron level
- Tx: Deferoxamine

Iron toxicity results from both direct corrosive effects to the GI mucosa and from impairment of cellular respiration with resultant lactic acidosis. Doses of >60 mg/kg of elemental iron are potentially lethal. Patients may initially be asymptomatic or present with GI symptoms, or hypovolemia. Later manifestations may include shock and multiorgan failure. Diagnosis of iron poisoning can be made based on an ingestion history with an appropriate clinical presentation.

Abdominal radiographs should be obtained to evaluate for radiopaque tablets. The serum iron level should be measured on presentation (and followed serially up to 12 hours after ingestion), with toxicity likely if ≥450 μg/dL. WBI is indicated (in the absence of bowel perforation or obstruction) as the first-line method of gastric decontamination as activated charcoal will not adsorb iron. Patients presenting with altered mental status, shock, metabolic acidosis, or serum iron levels ≥500 μg/dL at 4 to 6 hours after ingestion should be treated with the iron chelator deferoxamine. Deferoxamine is given at 10 to 15 mg/kg/hr by continuous infusion with a recommended maximum daily dose of 6 to 8 g, and therapy should not be delayed while awaiting iron levels in the setting of clinical toxicity. Deferoxamine may cause infusion rate-related hypotension, and adequate IV fluid replacement is needed as prophylaxis against acute renal failure. Deferoxamine therapy may be stopped when the serum iron level normalizes (as measured by atomic absorption spectroscopy, as deferoxamine interferes with most routine assays), when systemic toxicity and acidosis resolve, or when the urine is no longer reddish-brown (an indication of the presence of chelated deferoxamine-iron complex). GI or surgical consultation is warranted in cases of tablet concretion/bezoar, continued GI bleeding, or bowel perforation.

SUGGESTED READINGS

Brent J, Wallace KL, Burkhart KK, et al., eds. Critical care toxicology: diagnosis and management of the critically poisoned patient. Philadelphia: Elsevier Mosby, 2005.
   A comprehensive and well-referenced toxicology textbook with a critical care focus.
Chyka PA, Seger D, Krenzelok EP, et al; American Academy of Clinical Toxicology; European Association of Poisons Centres and Clinical Toxicologists. Position paper: single-dose activated charcoal. Clin Toxicol (Phila). 2005;43:61–87.
   Discusses dosages, complications and indications for the use of activated charcoal.
Fertel BS, Nelson LS, Goldfarb DS, et al. Extracorporeal removal techniques for the poisoned patient: a review for the intensivist. J Intensive Care Med. 2010;25:139–148.
   A review of indications for extracorporeal removal of toxins.
Flomenbaum NE, Goldfrank LR, Hoffman RS, et al. eds. Goldfrank's toxicologic emergencies. 9th ed. New York: McGraw-Hill, 2010.
   This is a classic reference toxicology textbook.
Heard KJ. Acetylcysteine for acetaminophen poisoning. New Engl J Med. 2008;359:285–292.
   Recent perspectives regarding the management of acetaminophen overdose.
McCord J, Jneid H, Hollander JE, et al. Management of cocaine-associated chest pain and myocardial infarction: a scientific statement from the American Heart Association Acute Cardiac Care Committee of the Council on Clinical Cardiology. Circulation. 2008;117:1897–1907.
   Review article on the management of cardiac complications of cocaine use.
Mokhles B, Leiken JB, Murray P, et al. Adult toxicology in critical care, Parts I: General approach to the intoxicated patient. Chest. 2003;123:577–592.
Mokhles B, Leiken JB, Murray P, et al. Adult toxicology in critical care, Parts II: Specific poisonings. Chest. 2003;123:897–922.
   Review of critical care management of various poisonings.
Woolf AD, Erdman AR, Nelson LS, et al. Tricyclic antidepressant poisoning: an evidence-based consensus guideline for out-of-hospital management. Clin Toxicol. 2007;45:203–233.
   Consensus guidelines for management of TCA poisoning.

34 Central Nervous System Infections

Hitoshi Honda and Keith F. Woeltje

Meningitis and encephalitis cause significant morbidity and mortality, often requiring intensive care unit–level care. Approximately 50% of patients with bacterial meningitis require mechanical intubation, usually because of altered mental status. Physiologically, *meningitis* is characterized by the inflammation of the meninges surrounding the brain and spinal cord, while *encephalitis* refers to the inflammation within the brain parenchyma. Clinically, patients with encephalitis are more likely to have altered level of consciousness or confusion, although the clinical presentations of encephalitis and meningitis overlap considerably. The distinction between meningitis and encephalitis has important implications in the etiology, treatment, and prognosis of the illness. Table 34.1 identifies the most common etiologies of meningitis and encephalitis.

TABLE 34.1	Common Etiologies of Meningitis and Encephalitis
Type	Etiology
Bacterial meningitis	*Streptococcus pneumoniae*
	Neisseria meningitidis
	Haemophilus influenzae
	Listeria monocytogenes[a]
Viral meningitis	Enteroviruses[b]
	HSV
	Lymphocytic choriomeningitis virus
Encephalitis	Enteroviruses[b]
	HSV
	Arboviruses[b]
	West Nile virus
	St. Louis encephalitis virus
	Eastern equine virus
	Western equine virus

[a]More common in patients >50 years of age and immunocompromised individuals.
[b]Seasonal predominance in summer and fall.
HSV, herpes simplex virus.

The initial evaluation of patients with any type of suspected central nervous system (CNS) infection usually takes place outside the intensive care unit, but a thorough understanding of the workup is essential. An approach to the initial evaluation of CNS infections is presented in Algorithm 34.1. The sensitivity of the classic triad of fever, stiff neck, and altered mental status in predicting bacterial meningitis is <50%, but the absence of all three symptoms makes CNS infection unlikely. Retrospective studies have shown that almost all patients with bacterial meningitis have at least two of four critical symptoms, including fever, neck stiffness, headache, and altered mental status. Until the diagnosis of CNS infection is confirmed or rejected, antimicrobials should be administered empirically.

There is little evidence to suggest that imaging prior to lumbar puncture impacts management or outcomes in patients with CNS infection. Clinical and historical features suggestive of possible abnormalities on computed tomography include history of CNS disease, history of recent seizure, altered level of consciousness, new focal neurologic deficits on examination, or neurologic findings in the setting of immunosuppression. Many physicians will perform imaging in the presence of these findings. The presence of an abnormality on imaging is not predictive of brain herniation, a life-threatening complication of lumbar puncture, and the decision to obtain imaging should never delay the initiation of empirical antimicrobial treatment.

Because clinical history and physical examination can be unreliable in diagnosing CNS infection, analysis of cerebrospinal fluid (CSF) is crucial. CSF findings are essential in distinguishing bacterial from viral causes of infection. When performed by an experienced technician, Gram stain of the CSF is positive in approximately 50% to 75% of cases of bacterial meningitis. Sensitivity of the test varies by organism; it is positive in 90% of untreated cases of *Streptococcus pneumoniae* versus 30% to 35% of cases of *Listeria* meningitis. Although receipt of antibiotics prior to lumbar puncture will decrease the sensitivity of the cultures, antibiotic treatment should not be delayed to increase culture yield.

In addition to routine Gram stain and culture, CSF should be examined for glucose and protein quantitation, and cell count should be examined from the last tube of fluid obtained. Although rarely seen, cryptococcal meningitis may present as acute meningitis even in immunocompetent individuals. A cryptococcal antigen assay should be ordered on all patients. Fungal, viral, and acid-fast bacilli cultures are very low yield in the setting of acute meningitis or encephalitis and should not be routinely ordered. The laboratory can hold a quantity of CSF for additional testing if indicated from the initial CSF findings. Typical CSF findings for viral and bacterial meningitis as well as encephalitis are presented in Table 34.2.

Encephalitis caused by herpes simplex virus is most often seen in young children and individuals older than 50 years. Patients may present with altered level of consciousness, focal cranial nerve findings, or focal seizures and may have abnormal temporal lobe findings on imaging. Because herpes simplex virus encephalitis is associated with high morbidity and mortality when treatment is delayed, patients aged 50 years and older with symptoms of encephalitis should be given acyclovir empirically until the results of CSF polymerase chain reaction for herpes virus are obtained. Table 34.3 outlines specific recommendations for empirical and specific treatment regimens of CNS infection.

The use of adjuvant steroids in the treatment of bacterial meningitis remains controversial. Improvements in morbidity and mortality have been shown in a subgroup of patients with bacterial meningitis caused by *S. pneumoniae*. However, the benefit of improvement in clinical outcome using steroid for patients with bacterial meningitis

ALGORITHM 34.1 Initial Evaluation for Possible Central Nervous System (CNS) Infection

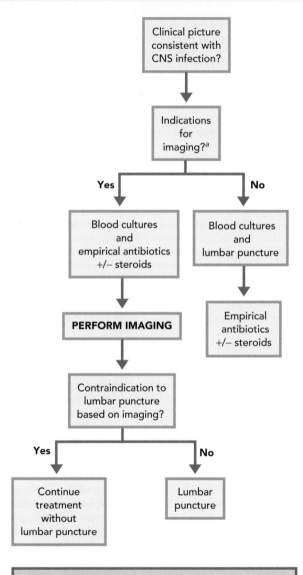

Clinical picture consistent with CNS infection?

↓

Indications for imaging?[a]

Yes ←→ **No**

Blood cultures and empirical antibiotics +/− steroids

Blood cultures and lumbar puncture

↓

PERFORM IMAGING

Empirical antibiotics +/− steroids

↓

Contraindication to lumbar puncture based on imaging?

Yes ←→ **No**

Continue treatment without lumbar puncture

Lumbar puncture

[a]History of CNS disease, history of recent seizure, altered level of consciousness, new focal neurologic deficits, or neurologic deficits in the setting of immunosuppression

TABLE 34.2	CSF Findings in Meningitis and Encephalitis		
CSF finding	Bacterial meningitis	Viral meningitis	Encephalitis
WBC/mm^3	≥1,000	100–10,000	<250
Differential	PMN predominance (≥80%)	Lymphocyte predominance[a] (≥50%)	Lymphocyte predominance[a]
Protein	>250	50–250	<150
CSF to serum glucose ratio	≤0.4	Normal to decreased	>0.5
Opening pressure (mm Hg)	>200	Usually normal	Normal to slightly increased

[a]May have neutrophilic predominance initially.
CSF, cerebrospinal fluid; WBC, white blood cell; PMN, polymorphonuclear cells.

TABLE 34.3	Treatment Recommendations for CNS Infection
Etiology	Suggested therapy
Empirical	Vancomycin 10–15 mg/kg IV q8h[a] PLUS Ceftriaxone 2 g IV q12h Addition of steroids if indicated[b] If ≥50 years, addition of ampicillin 2 g IV q4h[a] If suspicion for HSV, addition of acyclovir 10 mg/kg q8h[a]
Streptococcus pneumoniae	If PCN MIC ≤1 μg/mL, ceftriaxone 2 g IV q12h
	If PCN MIC ≥2 μg/mL OR ceftriaxone MIC ≥1 μg/mL, vancomycin 10–15 mg/kg IV q8h[a] AND Ceftriaxone 2 g IV q12h
Neisseria meningitidis	If PCN MIC <0.1 μg/mL, ampicillin 2 g IV q4h[a] If PCN MIC ≥0.1 μg/mL, ceftriaxone 2 g IV q12h
Listeria monocytogenes	Ampicillin 2 g IV q4h[a] If PCN allergy, use trimethoprim/sulfamethoxazole 5 mg/kg q8h[c]
Viral meningitis	Supportive measures
Herpes encephalitis	Acyclovir 10 mg/kg IV q8h[a]
Other viral encephalitis	Supportive measures

[a]Dose adjustment required for impaired renal function.
[b]Dexamethasone 0.15 mg/kg every 6 hr × 4 days.
[c]Dosing based on trimethoprim component.
IV, intravenous; HSV, herpes simplex virus; PCN, penicillin; MIC, mean inhibitory concentration.
Adapted from Infectious Diseases Society of America Guidelines.

TABLE 34.4	Suggested Length of Therapy for CNS Infection by Etiology
Etiology	Length of treatment (days)
Listeria monocytogenes	≥21
Gram-negative bacilli	21
Group B *Streptococcus*	14–21
HSV encephalitis	14[a]
Streptococcus pneumoniae	14
Haemophilus influenzae	7
Neisseria meningitidis	7

[a]Extend therapy to 21 days if there is immunosuppression.
HSV, herpes simplex virus.
Adapted from Infectious Diseases Society of America Guidelines

due to other pathogens (e.g., *Neisseria meningitidis, Haemophilus influenzae*) is not completely clear. Although in patients with suspected or proven *S. pneumoniae* meningitis, steroids prior to, or concurrent with, the initial dose of antibiotics should be considered, timely diagnosis of definite bacterial meningitis and prompt pathogen identification is a challenge. The benefit of steroids started after antibiotics is less ceratin, although one study suggests that it may be beneficial in patients with microbiologically proven diseases.

Nosocomial meningitis accounts for only 0.4% of all hospital infections and almost always occurs in the setting of neurosurgical intervention. In contrast to community-acquired bacterial meningitis, nosocomial meningitis is typically caused by Gram-negative organisms, coagulase-negative staphylococcal species, or *Staphylococcus aureus.* Empirical treatment should include vancomycin for Gram-positive organisms plus cefepime, ceftazidime, or meropenem to cover the possibility of aerobic Gram-negative bacilli including *Pseudomonas aeruginosa.* Recommendations regarding length of treatment are often based on historical practices rather than specific evidence from clinical trials. Given the variable absorption of certain oral antimicrobials, treatment should be given intravenously for the duration of therapy. The choice of intravenous antimicrobial therapy for bacterial meningitis is also influenced by its penetration to CSF. Suggested lengths of treatment for various CNS infections are shown in Table 34.4.

There is often confusion about the need for isolation in patients diagnosed with meningitis. Two common causes of bacterial meningitis, *H. influenzae* and *N. meningitidis,* are spread via large particle droplets >5 μm in size. Infection with either of these organisms warrants droplet precautions for the first 24 hours of treatment. Healthcare workers, who examine (i.e., funduscopic exam) or perform procedures (intubation, bronchoscopy, suctioning endotracheal secretes) on patients with suspected bacterial meningitis, should wear surgical mask to prevent potential exposure to droplet particles. Individuals entering the room should wear standard masks when working within 3 feet of the patient as well. Patient movement should be limited if possible; however, if transport is required, the patient should wear a mask to minimize potential spread of infection. Because the etiology of bacterial meningitis is typically unknown at the time of presentation, all patients with suspected meningitis should initially be placed on droplet precautions in addition to standard precautions.

SUGGESTED READINGS

deGans J, van de Beek D. Dexamethasone in adults with bacterial meningitis. *N Engl J Med.* 2002;347:1549–1556.

> *A recent randomized, placebo-controlled trial of adjuvant steroid therapy in bacterial meningitis concluding that early steroid therapy decreases mortality and morbidity in patients with bacterial meningitis.*

Flores-Cordero JM, Amaya-Villar R, Rincón-Ferrari MD, et al. Acute community-acquired bacterial meningitis in adults admitted to the intensive care unit: clinical manifestations, management and prognostic factors. *Intensive Care Med.* 2003;29:1967–1973.

> *A focused look at patients with bacterial meningitis requiring admission to the intensive care unit suggesting that clinical course of disease over the first 24 hours of hospitalization is a major predictor of morbidity and mortality.*

Hasbun R, Abrahams J, Jekel J, et al. Computed tomography of the head before lumbar puncture in adults with suspected meningitis. *N Engl J Med.* 2001;345:1727–1733.

> *Large prospective study of CT scan prior to lumbar puncture in patients with clinical suspicion of meningitis that shows certain clinical features are predictive of normal head CT in patients with suspected meningitis.*

Korinek AM, Baugnon T, Golmard JL, et al. Risk factors for adult nosocomial meningitis after craniotomy: role of antibiotic prophylaxis. *Neurosurgery.* 2006;59:126–133.

> *Brief review of nosocomial meningitis with evaluation of peri-operative antibiotic prophylaxis. Findings demonstrate antibiotic prophylaxis at the time of neurosurgery improves surgical site infection rates but does not have significant impact on rates of post-operative meningitis.*

Nguyen TH, Tran TH, Thwaites G, et al. Dexamethasone in Vietnamese adolescents and adults with bacterial meningitis. *N Engl J Med.* 2007;357(24):2431–2440.

> *A recent, randomized controlled trial for dexamethasone use in patients with bacterial meningitis concluded the dexamethasone does not improve outcome for patients with suspected bacterial meningitis although the benefit of dexamethasone use was observed for patients with microbiologically proven bacterial meningitis even those who received the prior antibiotic treatment.*

Palabiyikoglu I, Tekeli E, Cokca F, et al. Nosocomial meningitis in a university hospital between 1993 and 2002. *J Hosp Infect Control.* 2006;62:94–97.

> *Retrospective evaluation of 51 cases of nosocomial meningitis which showed the major risk factor for hospital-acquired meningitis was neurosurgical procedure. The most common causative organisms were gram-negative bacilli and Staphylococcus species.*

Rotbart HA. Viral meningitis. *Semin Neurol.* 2000;20:277–292.

> *Complete review of all aspects of viral meningitis including epidemiology, pathogenesis, clinical presentations, diagnosis, and treatment options.*

Sejvar JJ. The evolving epidemiology of viral encephalitis. *Curr Opin Neurol.* 2006;19:350–357.

> *A current look at emerging causes of viral encephalitis which shows ongoing transmission of West Nile Virus in the United States and explores transfusions and transplants as potential sources of transmission for viral encephalitis.*

Tunkel AR, Hartman BJ, Kaplan SL, et al. Practice guidelines for the management of bacterial meningitis. *Clin Infect Dis.* 2004;39:1267–1283.

> *A thorough review of evidence-based treatments for bacterial meningitis with evaluation and treatment guidelines endorsed by the Infectious Diseases Society of America.*

van de Beek D, deGans J, Tunkel AR, et al. Community-acquired bacterial meningitis in adults. *N Engl J Med.* 2006;354:44–53.

> *An up-to-date review of recent studies and advances in bacterial meningitis including management of complications.*

van de Beek D, Drake JM, Tunkel AR. Nosocomial meningitis. *N Engl J Med.* 2010;362(2):146–154.

> *A thorough review of current evidence of nosocomial meningitis.*

35 Community-Acquired Pneumonia

Bernard C. Camins

Community-acquired pneumonia (CAP) affects about 2 to 3 million patients each year. Although mortality is relatively low (<1%) for nonhospitalized patients, mortality among hospitalized patients can be as high as 30%, with the majority of deaths occurring in patients admitted to the intensive care unit (ICU). One of the most important decisions to make is to determine if the patient truly has CAP as opposed to healthcare-associated pneumonia (HCAP). CAP patients are those patients from whom the first positive bacterial culture is obtained within 48 hours of hospital admission and lack risk factors for HCAP. Please see Chapter 36 for the HCAP criteria.

Direct admission to the ICU is recommended for patients on vasopressors or those requiring intubation and mechanical ventilation. The American Thoracic Society and the Infectious Diseases Society of America (ATS/IDSA) guidelines recommend that patients who meet at least three minor criteria should also be admitted to the ICU (see Table 35.1). The decision to admit a patient to the ICU can have significant implications since studies have shown that patients who are admitted to a hospital ward but later require admission to the ICU have a higher morbidity and mortality than patients directly admitted to the ICU.

While not recommended for all patients with CAP, routine testing to determine the etiology of CAP is recommended for all patients admitted to the ICU. These tests should at least include blood and sputum cultures, Legionella and Pneumococcal urinary antigen testing, and endotracheal aspirate if the patient is intubated or even possibly bronchoscopy or nonbronchoscopic bronchoalveolar lavage (BAL). Patients with cavitary infiltrates should have fungal or mycobacterial cultures performed. Antibiotic therapy should not be delayed in favor of collecting samples for laboratory testing. Sputum culture results are particularly helpful when an organism that is not part of the normal flora is recovered.

Blood cultures should preferably be obtained prior to the administration of antibiotics. Obtaining blood cultures within 24 hours of admission has been shown to reduce mortality simply because resistant pathogens are identified earlier with the availability of culture results. A *Legionella* urine antigen test is recommended for all immunocompromised patients with CAP or any patient with severe CAP admitted to the ICU. This diagnostic test only detects *Legionella pneumophila* serogroup 1, so a negative result does not rule out *Legionella* pneumonia. A pneumococcal urinary antigen assay may also help in the diagnosis of pneumococcal pneumonia. However, this test is not as reliable as the *Legionella* urine antigen assay because it only has a sensitivity of 50% to 80%.

TABLE 35.1	**Criteria for Severe Community-Acquired Pneumonia and admission to the ICU[a]**

Major criteria
    Invasive mechanical ventilation
    Septic shock with the need for vasopressors
Minor criteria
    Respiratory rate $\geq$30 breaths/min[b]
    PaO_2/FIO_2 ratio $\leq$250[b]
    Multilobar infiltrates
    Confusion/disorientation
    Uremia (BUN level $\geq$20 mg/dL)
    Leukopenia from infection (WBC count <4000 cells/mm^3)
    Thrombocytopenia (platelet count <100,000 cells/mm^3)
    Hypothermia (core temperature <36°C)
    Hypotension requiring aggressive fluid resuscitation

[a]Patients who meet one major criterion or at least three minor criteria are recommended to be admitted to the ICU.
[b]Noninvasive ventilation can be substituted for respiratory rate $\geq$30 breaths/min or PaO_2/FIO_2 ratio $\leq$250.
Adapted from Mandell LA, Wunderink RG, Anzueto A, et al. Infectious Diseases Society of America/American Thoracic Society consensus guidelines on the management of community-acquired pneumonia in adults. *Clin Infect Dis.* 2007;44:S27–72.

Finally, during influenza season, rapid antigen or polymerase chain reaction assay testing for presence of influenza A or B virus is recommended for both treatment and epidemiologic purposes. Before any empiric antibiotic regimen is selected, a determination needs to be made if the patient truly has CAP or HCAP. Table 35.2 presents information for the treatment of patients admitted to the ICU with severe CAP. Combination therapy for bacteremic pneumococcal pneumonia is recommended at least during the first 48 hours of treatment. Recently, experts have recommended shorter courses of therapy for CAP. Even in patients with pneumococcal bacteremia from CAP, a 5-day course of therapy may be adequate. A recent randomized controlled trial showed that levofloxacin, 750 mg by mouth daily for 5 days, was equivalent to a 10-day course of the 500-mg dose. However, this study included all hospitalized patients, not only patients with severe CAP. Patients with severe CAP may require at least 10 days of antibiotic therapy. Patients with *Legionella* pneumonia should always be treated with a 14-day course of therapy unless azithromycin is prescribed.

The patient should be clinically stable within 72 hours of initiation of therapy. If there is clinical deterioration after 24 hours of therapy, several possibilities should be considered. First, a resistant pathogen may be the etiologic agent and the initial empiric therapy may be inadequate. Some patients may have *drug-resistant Streptococcus pneumoniae* or *Pseudomonas aeruginosa* despite the lack of risk factors. Alternatively, unusual bacterial pathogens may be the cause of severe CAP. Recent reports of severe necrotizing pneumonia in young patients without any risk factors should alert the clinician to the possibility of severe CAP caused by community-associated methicillin-resistant *Staphylococcus aureus* (CA-MRSA). These patients may have a viral prodrome that is followed by acute onset of shortness of breath, sepsis, and hemoptysis. There should

TABLE 35.2	**Antibiotic Recommendations for the Intensive Care Unit Patient with Community-Acquired Pneumonia**
No risk factors for *Pseudomonas* infection	Recommended antibiotics

Streptococcus pneumoniae including DRSP
Haemophilus influenza
Legionella streptococcus
Staphylococcus aureus
Streptococcus pyogenes
Less common pathogens
  Klebsiella pneumoniae and other Gram negatives
  Mycoplasma pneumoniae
  Respiratory viruses
  Miscellaneous
    Chlamydophila pneumoniae
    Mycobacterium tuberculosis
    Endemic fungi
	β-Lactam[a] + azithromycin OR respiratory fluoroquinolone[b] OR respiratory fluoroquinolone,[b] with aztreonam if patient has β-lactam allergy

Risk factors for *Pseudomonas* infection present[c]	Recommended antibiotics
All the above agents and *Pseudomonas aeruginosa*	Antipseudomonal β-lactam[d] with gram positive coverage + ciprofloxacin OR levofloxacin (750 mg dose) OR Antipseudomonal β-lactam with Gram positive coverage[d] + an aminoglycoside + a respiratory fluroquinolone[b] OR azithromycin OR Aztreonam + levofloxacin OR Aztreonam + moxifloxacin with an aminoglycoside if patient has β-lactam allergy

[a]Cefotaxime, ceftriaxone, ampicillin-sulbactam, or ertapenem.
[b]Levofloxacin or moxifloxacin.
[c]Severe structural lung disease (e.g., bronchiectasis, severe COPD), recent antibiotic therapy, recent stay in the hospital, malnutrition, chronic corticosteroid therapy (e.g., prednisone >10 mg/day).
[d]Cefepime, piperacillin, piperacillin-tazobactam, imipenem, or meropenem.
DRSP, drug-resistant *Streptococcus pneumoniae*.

also be a low threshold in screening for human immunodeficiency virus infection and *Pneumocystis jiroveci* pneumonia. Nocardiosis, tuberculosis, or endemic fungi should also be considered in patients who test positive for human immunodeficiency infection. The patient's history should be reviewed again for certain exposures: cattle, sheep, or goat for *Coxiella burnetii,* birds for *Chlamydophila psittaci,* and rabbits for tularemia.

Respiratory tract viruses are common causes of pneumonia. Viral pneumonia may be severe in the elderly, immunocompromised, or patients with chronic obstructive lung disease and other comorbid illnesses. Although the results were varied, previous studies have shown that 4% to 39% of patients hospitalized for CAP had evidence of a viral infection. Severe pneumonia from influenza warrants treatment with an antiviral agent in most situations.

Complications of CAP should also be suspected in patients who fail to respond to initial therapy. About 10% of patients with pneumococcal pneumonia have metastatic disease such as meningitis, arthritis, endocarditis, and peritonitis. A parapneumonic effusion or empyema may require drainage with a chest tube. A repeat chest x-ray or a computed tomography scan may be warranted in patients who fail to respond to therapy. Finally, noninfectious causes such as pulmonary embolus, lung malignancy, hypersensitivity pneumonitis, Wegener's granulomatosis, or eosinophilic pneumonia can be misdiagnosed as CAP.

SUGGESTED READINGS

Arbo MD, Snydman DR. Influence of blood culture results on antibiotic choice in the treatment of bacteremia. *Arch Intern Med.* 1994;154:2641–2645.

A randomized controlled trial showing that blood cultures immediately prior to initiation of therapy for CAP leads to improved survival.

Bartlett JG, Breiman RF, Mandell LA, et al. Community-acquired pneumonia in adults: guidelines for management. The Infectious Diseases Society of America. *Clin Infect Dis.* 1998;26:811–838.

An evidence-based guidelines from the IDSA for the management of CAP in immunocompetent adults.

Dunbar LM, Wunderink RG, Habib MP, et al. High-dose, short-course levofloxacin for community-acquired pneumonia: a new treatment paradigm. *Clin Infect Dis.* 2003;37: 752–760.

A randomized controlled trial showing that a short course of levofloxacin at higher doses was as efficacious as the longer course treatment for CAP.

Mandell LA, Bartlett JG, Dowell SF, et al. Update of practice guidelines for the management of community-acquired pneumonia in immunocompetent adults. *Clin Infect Dis.* 2003;37:1405–1433.

An update of the evidence-based guidelines from the IDSA for the management of CAP in immunocompetent adults.

Mandell LA, File TM Jr. Short-course treatment of community-acquired pneumonia. *Clin Infect Dis.* 2003;37:761–763.

A review article advocating shorter courses to avoid the emergence of antibiotic resistance.

Mandell LA, Wunderink RG, Anzueto A, et al. Infectious Diseases Society of America/American Thoracic Society consensus guidelines on the management of community-acquired pneumonia in adults. *Clin Infect Dis.* 2007;44:S27–S72.

The latest evidence based recommendations from the IDSA and ATS for the treatment of immunocompetent adults.

36

Nosocomial Pneumonia

Michael J. Durkin and Marin H. Kollef

Hospital-acquired pneumonia (HAP) is defined as a nosocomial pneumonia (NP) that occurs 48 hours or more after hospital admission, which was not incubating at the time of hospital admission (Table 36.1). Ventilator-associated pneumonia (VAP) refers to NP that develops more than 48 to 72 hours after endotracheal intubation. Prevention strategies for HAP and VAP should be routinely employed to minimize the occurrence of this nosocomial infection (Table 36.2). It is important to thoroughly evaluate patients with suspected NP in order to exclude other conditions that can mimic

TABLE 36.1	Definitions of Pneumonia[a] (with Focus on Bacterial Pathogens)
Pneumonia category	Definition
Community-acquired pneumonia	Patients with a first positive bacterial culture obtained within 48 hours of hospital admission lacking risk factors for health care–associated pneumonia
Health care–associated pneumonia	Patients with a first positive bacterial culture within 48 hours of admission and any of the following: admission source indicates a transfer from another health care facility (e.g., hospital, nursing home); receiving hemodialysis, wound, or infusion therapy as an outpatient; prior hospitalization for at least 3 days within 90 days; immunocompromised state due to underlying disease or therapy (human immunodeficiency virus, chemotherapy)
Hospital-acquired pneumonia	Patients with a first positive bacterial culture >48 hours after hospital admission
Ventilator-associated pneumonia	Mechanically ventilated patients with a first positive bacterial culture >48 hours after hospital admission or tracheal intubation, whichever occurred first

[a]Criteria for pneumonia include new or progressive lung infiltrate and at least two of the following clinical criteria: hyperthermia or hypothermia, elevated white blood cell count, purulent tracheal secretions or sputum, and worsening oxygenation.

TABLE 36.2	Strategies for the Prevention of Nosocomial Pneumonia	
Strategy	Recommendation	Evidence level
Topical iseganan	No	1
Orodigestive decontamination[a] (Topical/topical plus intravenous antibiotics)	No	1
Oral chlorhexidine	Yes	1
Aerosolized antibiotics[a]	No	1
Intravenous antibiotics[a]	No	1
Specific stress ulcer prophylaxis regimen	No	1
Short-course antibiotic therapy (when clinically applicable)	Yes	1
Routine antibiotic cycling/rotation/heterogeneity[b]	No	2
Restricted (conservative) blood transfusion	Yes	2
Use of noninvasive mask ventilation	Yes	1
Avoid reintubation	Yes	2
Avoid patient transports	Yes	2
Orotracheal intubation preferred for airways	Yes	1
Orogastric intubation preferred for feeding tubes	Yes	2
Routine ventilator circuit changes	No	1
Use of heat–moisture exchanger	Yes	1
Closed endotracheal suctioning	Yes	1
Subglottic secretion drainage	Yes	1
Shortening the duration of mechanical ventilation	Yes	1
Adequate intensive care unit staffing	Yes	2
Silver-coated endotracheal tube	Yes	1
Polyurethane endotracheal tube cuff	Yes	1
Semierect positioning	Yes	1
Rotational beds	Yes	1
Chest physiotherapy	No	1
Early tracheostomy	No	1
Use of protocols/bundles incorporating multiple prevention elements	Yes	2

[a]Routine antibiotic prophylaxis not recommended due to potential emergence of antibiotic-resistant bacteria.
[b]May be useful in specific clinical circumstances (as an adjunct to controlling an outbreak of a multidrug-resistant bacterial infection).
Evidence levels: 1, supported by randomized trials; 2, supported by prospective or retrospective cohort studies; 3, supported by case series.

the presentation of NP (Table 36.3). HAP is the second most common nosocomial infection in the United States after urinary tract infection, but is the leading cause of mortality attributed to nosocomial infections. The incidence of NP is between 5 and 10 cases per 1,000 hospital admissions and, although the incidence of VAP is difficult to determine because of differences in the case definition, it is estimated that 9% to 27% of patients undergoing mechanical ventilation for >48 hours are affected. "Attributable mortality" from NP is estimated to be between 33% and 50%, with the

TABLE 36.3	Noninfectious Causes of Fever and Pulmonary Infiltrates Mimicking Nosocomial Pneumonia

Chemical aspiration without infection
Atelectasis
Pulmonary embolism
Acute respiratory distress syndrome
Pulmonary hemorrhage
Lung contusion
Infiltrative tumor
Radiation pneumonitis
Drug reaction
Bronchiolitis obliterans organizing pneumonia

higher mortality occurring in patients with bacteremia or infections with *Pseudomonas aeruginosa* or *Acinetobacter* species (Table 36.4).

The American Thoracic Society and the Infectious Diseases Society of America published guidelines for the management of adults with HAP, VAP, and health care-associated pneumonia in early 2005. These guidelines provide recommendations for the antibiotic management of NP as summarized in Table 36.5 and Algorithm 36.1. It is important for clinicians treating patients with suspected NP to prescribe initial antimicrobial regimens that are likely to be active against the offending pathogen in order to optimize outcome. Clinicians should be aware of the prevailing bacterial pathogens associated with NP, and their antimicrobial susceptibility, in order to optimize antimicrobial treatment. Once the pathogens and antimicrobial susceptibilities are known, narrowing or de-escalation of the antimicrobial regimen can occur.

TABLE 36.4	Most Common Pathogens Associated with Various Pneumonia Categories
Infection site	**Pathogens**
I. Pneumonia (immunocompetent) **1.** Community-acquired pneumonia (nonimmuno-compromised host)	*Streptococcus pneumoniae* *Haemophilus influenzae* *Moraxella catarrhalis* *Mycoplasma pneumoniae* *Legionella pneumophila* *Chlamydia pneumoniae* Methicillin-resistant *Staphylococcus aureus* (MRSA) Influenza virus

(continued)

TABLE 36.4	Most Common Pathogens Associated with Various Pneumonia Categories (*Continued*)
Infection site	**Pathogens**
2. Health care-associated pneumonia	Methicillin-resistant *S. aureus* *Pseudomonas aeruginosa* *Klebsiella pneumoniae* *Acinetobacter* species *Stenotrophomonas* species *L. pneumophila*
3. Pneumonia (immunocompromised host)	
a. Neutropenia	Any pathogen listed above *Aspergillus* species *Candida* species
b. Human immunodeficiency virus	Any pathogen listed above *Pneumocystis carinii* *Mycobacterium tuberculosis* *Histoplasma capsulatum* Other fungi Cytomegalovirus
c. Solid-organ transplant or bone marrow transplant	Any pathogen listed above (Can vary depending on timing of infection to transplant)
d. Cystic fibrosis	*H. influenzae* (early) *S. aureus* *Pseudomonas aeruginosa* *Burkholderia cepacia*
4. Lung abscess	*Bacteroides* species *Peptostreptococci* *Fusobacterium* species *Nocardia* (in immunocompromised patients) Amebic (when suggestive by exposure)
5. Empyema	*S. aureus* *S. pneumoniae* Group A Streptococci *H. influenzae* } Usually acute Anaerobic bacteria *Enterobacteriaceae* *M. tuberculosis* } Usually subacute or chronic

TABLE 36.5 Antibiotic Recommendations for Nosocomial Pneumonia[a]

Category of pneumonia	Organisms	Empiric therapy	Additional information
HCAP/HAP/VAP Not at risk for MDR pathogens and hospitalized for <5 days	Multidrug-resistant (MDR) potential pathogens unlikely: *Streptococcus pneumoniae* *Haemophilus influenzae* Methicillin-sensitive *Staphylococcus aureus* *Escherichia coli* *Klebsiella pneumoniae* *Enterobacter* species *Proteus* species *Serratia marcescens*	Third-generation cephalosporin (ceftriaxone) Or Ampicillin–sulbactam Or Respiratory fluoroquinolone (Levofloxacin or moxifloxacin) Or Nonantipseudomonal carbapenem (ertapenem)	Azithromycin should be considered for atypical coverage in very ill patients or ones with a high suspicion for atypical organisms or *Legionella* who are not on a respiratory fluoroquinolone.
HCAP/HAP/VAP At risk for MDR pathogens or hospitalized for ≥5 days	Potential MDR pathogens likely: *Pseudomonas aeruginosa* *Klebsiella pneumoniae* (extended-spectrum β-lactamase+) *Acinetobacter* species *Legionella pneumophila* Methicillin-resistant *S. aureus*	Antipseudomonal cephalosporin (cefepime, ceftazidime) Or Antipseudomonal carbapenem (imipenem or meropenem) Or Antipseudomonal penicillin with beta-lactamase inhibitor (piperacillin-tazobactam) Plus Antipseudomonal fluoroquinolone (ciprofloxacin or levofloxacin) Or Aminoglycoside (gentamicin, tobramycin, or amikacin) Plus Anti MRSA agent (linezolid or vancomycin)	Carbapenems are often effective against ESBL organisms (*E. coli, Klebsiella*) or *Acinetobacter.* For patients with penicillin allergy consider substituting β-lactam with: • Aztreonam • Meropenem (<1% cross reactivity to penicillin allergy) Inhaled antibiotics (colistin and aminoglycosides) have been used in selected populations and should be used only after consultation with a subspecialist.

[a]Clinicians should be aware of the prevailing bacterial pathogens associated with nosocomial pneumonia and the antibiotic susceptibility patterns of these pathogens locally in order to optimize clinical outcomes.

ALGORITHM 36.1 A Step-by-Step Approach to the Management of Nosocomial Pneumonia

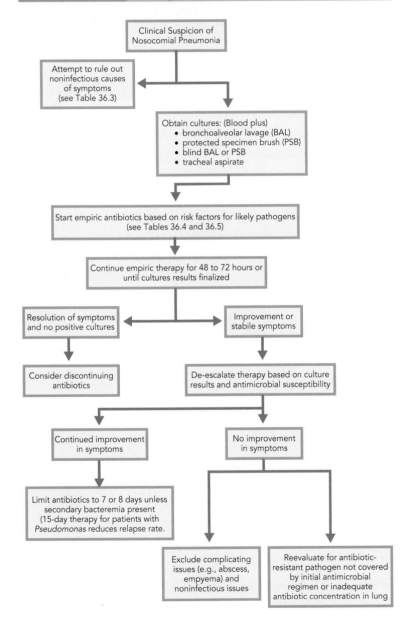

SUGGESTED READINGS

American Thoracic Society; Infectious Diseases Society of America. Guidelines for the management of adults with hospital-acquired, ventilator-associated, and healthcare-associated pneumonia. *Am J Respir Crit Care Med.* 2005;171:388–416.
  Management guidelines for nosocomial pneumonia.
Chastre J, Fagon JY. Ventilator-associated pneumonia. *Am J Respir Crit Care Med.* 2002;165:867–903.
  State-of-the-art review of nosocomial pneumonia.
Morrow LE, Kollef MH. Recognition and prevention of nosocomial pneumonia in the ICU and infection control in mechanical ventilation. *Crit Care Med.* 2010;38:s352–s362.
  Concise review on the prevention and diagnosis of nosocomial pneumonia.

37 Cellulitis/Fasciitis/ Myositis

Kevin W. McConnell, John P. Kirby
and John E. Mazuski

Skin and soft tissue infections can occur anywhere in the body. They may be characterized either on the basis of anatomic criteria, or whether a necrotizing infection is present.

ANATOMIC CLASSIFICATION

Although infections have traditionally been stratified by the depth of tissue involvement, this classification has limited prognostic value. Nonetheless, terminology based on anatomic depth continues to be widely used and therefore retains relevance in clinical practice (Fig. 37.1). Patients with superficial infections involving only the epidermis and dermis, such as pyoderma, impetigo, erysipelas, folliculitis, furuncles, and carbuncles, rarely need admission to the intensive care unit. In contrast, deeper soft tissue infections, including cellulitis, fasciitis, and myositis, are associated with significant morbidity and mortality, depending on the clinical situation.

Cellulitis is an acute bacterial infection involving the skin and subcutaneous tissue, including the superficial fascia. The disease most commonly involves the lower extremities; other areas that may be affected include the periorbital regions, areas near body piercings, incisions, puncture wounds ("skin-popping"/illicit drugs), bites, and areas with any preexisting skin condition such as venous stasis, ischemia, or decubitus ulcers. Critically ill patients may have increased susceptibility to these infections because of their impaired immune status and altered skin flora. The most common causative organisms are *Streptococcus pyogenes* and *Staphylococcus aureus*. Less common causes of cellulitis may be suspected based on the patient's history or comorbidities (Table 37.1).

Fasciitis involves the subcutaneous tissue and deep fascia. The clinical presentation may be masked, as changes in the overlying skin may only be observed later in the disease process. Trauma is the most common cause; however, approximately 20% of cases of necrotizing fasciitis occur in healthy patients with no known injury, source, or predisposition.

Myositis involves infection down to muscle and is generally differentiated into myonecrosis or pyomyositis. Myonecrosis is associated with gas gangrene and clostridial infections, and pyomyositis is usually the result of a puncture wound with abscess formation. The distinction is vital, as myonecrosis necessitates immediate operative

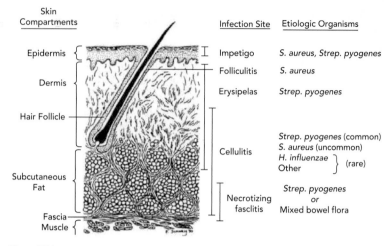

Figure 37.1. Anatomic classification of soft tissue infections.

debridement, whereas pyomyositis may be amenable to antibiotics and percutaneous drainage.

NECROTIZING INFECTIONS

Although anatomic location may be used to name a process, the more important clinical distinction is between necrotizing and nonnecrotizing skin and soft tissue infections. Regardless of depth of infection, nonnecrotizing infections usually respond to antibiotics or simple drainage procedures. However, necrotizing infections require immediate surgical debridement. Early diagnosis and intervention represent the most important factors in determining patient outcomes from necrotizing soft tissue infections.

TABLE 37.1	Less Common Sources of Soft Tissue Infections
History	**Source**
Freshwater swim with laceration or abrasion	*Aeromonas hydrophila*
Saltwater swim or seafood contamination of wound	*Vibrio* species (especially *Vibrio vulnificus*)
Cat/dog bite	*Pasteurella multocida,* polymicrobial anaerobes
Human bite	*Bacteroides fragilis, Eikenella* spp., polymicrobial anaerobes
HIV	*Haemophilus influenzae,* fungus, infected Kaposi's sarcoma
Diabetes, pregnancy, cirrhosis	Group B *Streptococcus*

HIV, human immunodeficiency virus.

TABLE 37.2	Characteristics of Necrotizing Infections

Signs/symptoms associated with increased likelihood that a necrotizing infection is present

Pain out of proportion to examination
Bullae
Systemic toxicity
Serum sodium <135 mmol/L
WBC >15,400 cell/mm^3
Tenderness beyond the area of erythema
Crepitus
Cutaneous anesthesia
Cellulitis refractory to antibiotic therapy

WBC, white blood count.

Determining whether or not a necrotizing infection is present can be challenging, because physical examination is often unreliable (Table 37.2). Patients with these infections frequently have normal overlying skin. Overt signs of necrotic tissue, such as crepitus, occur in only 30% of patients. Laboratory abnormalities, including C-reactive protein hemoglobin, sodium, creatinine, glucose levels and white blood cell counts, have been used to construct risk scores, but these are not yet in widespread use.

Radiographic imaging may assist in the diagnosis of necrotizing soft tissue infections. However, plain radiography shows soft tissue gas in only 15% to 30% of necrotizing infections. Computed tomography and ultrasound are sometimes helpful ancillary studies to identify soft tissue gas or necrotic tissue. Magnetic resonance imaging (MRI) may delineate the extent of the infection and has a high sensitivity for detection of necrotizing soft tissue infections; however, specificity is somewhat low, and logistic difficulties in obtaining this study limit its utility in critically ill patients. In equivocal cases, biopsy with frozen section has been recommended for definitive diagnosis, but again is associated with significant logistical difficulties when needed urgently. An alternative means of establishing the severity of the infection is to make a bedside incision under local anesthesia and digitally examine the tissue planes; facile separation of the subcutaneous tissue from the fascia is a characteristic sign of a necrotizing soft tissue infection. A management algorithm for distinguishing necrotizing from nonnecrotizing infections is presented in Algorithm 37.1.

Antibiotic therapy directed against Gram-positive cocci, particularly *Streptococcus* and *Staphylococcus,* has generally been used for initial therapy of nonnecrotizing soft tissue infections. However, one-third of isolates from patients with soft tissue infections are Gram-negative organisms, so additional antibiotic therapy directed against common Gram-negative organisms may be needed, particularly with infections involving the axillae or perineum. Antimicrobial management of nonnecrotizing infections is complicated by the increased prevalence of resistant organisms such as methicillin-resistant *S. aureus,* including those positive for the Panton–Valentine leukocidin. Methicillin-resistant *S. aureus* was responsible for 59% of the skin/soft tissue infections of patients presenting to emergency departments at 11 facilities across the country. Therefore, it is generally appropriate to include an antimicrobial agent that has activity against this organism. Vancomycin has traditionally been used for this, but linezolid and daptomycin may be alternatives in the critically ill patient.

ALGORITHM 37.1 Algorithm for Managing Soft Tissue Infections

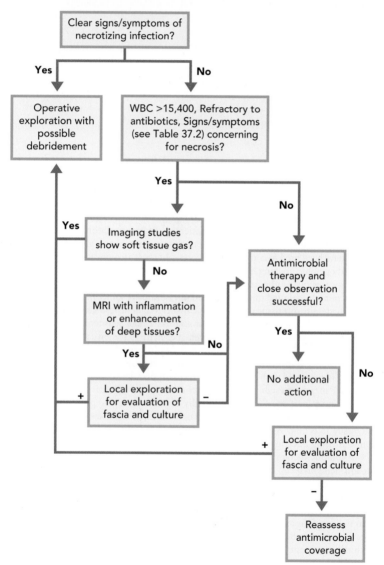

WBC, white blood cells; MRI, magnetic resonance imaging.

Necrotizing soft tissue infections are lethal disorders, associated with a 20% to 30% mortality. Patients with these infections should undergo immediate surgical debridement and antibiotic therapy. These antimicrobial therapies should be broad based, including coverage of Gram-positive cocci, Gram-negative bacilli, and anaerobes. For patients with monomicrobial infections due to streptococci or clostridia, penicillin is still advocated. Agents that can decrease toxin production, such as clindamycin or linezolid, may also be useful in selected patients with necrotizing soft tissue infections.

Hyperbaric oxygen is sometimes used as an adjunct to surgical debridement and antibiotics, but may not be applicable unless a hyperbaric chamber is immediately available. Potential benefits include a reduction in alpha-toxin production, improved tissue demarcation, and diminished tissue loss. Other adjunctive therapies include extracorporeal plasma treatment and intravenous immunoglobulin. Data are inadequate for any of these adjuncts to be recommended as standard therapy. Current guidelines continue to emphasize timely diagnosis, effective surgical debridement, and appropriate initial antibiotic coverage as proven ways to optimize outcome in patients with necrotizing skin and soft tissue infections.

SUGGESTED READINGS

Feldmeier J. Hyperbaric oxygen: indications and results. The hyperbaric oxygen therapy committee report. Undersea and hyperbaric Medicine Society. New York, NY: Kensington MD Publishing, 2003.
Evidenced-based review on hyperbaric oxygen usage includes indications for usage in soft tissue infection.

Lopez FA, Lartchenko S. Skin and soft tissue infections. *Infect Dis Clin North Am.* 2006;20; 759–772.
A review article which emphasizes microbiology and emergence of MRSA in soft tissue infection.

Malangoni MA, McHenry R. Approach to the patient with soft tissue infection. In: Wilmore DW, Fink MP, Jurkovich GJ, et al., eds. ACS surgery: principles and practice. 6th ed. BC Decker, 2007.
This is a comprehensive review with emphasis on identification of necrotizing infections.

May AK, Stafford RE, Bulger EM, et al. Treatment of skin and soft tissue infections. *Surg Infect.* 2009;10:467–499.
These are the guidelines of the Surgical Infection Society, a comprehensive evidence-based review of the literature on this topic.

Moran GJ, Krishnadasan A, Gorwitz RJ, et al. Methicillin-resistant *S. aureus* infections among patients in the emergency department. *N Engl J Med.* 2006;355:666–674.
Multicenter trial showing the emergence of MRSA in soft tissue infections.

Turecki MB, Taljanovic MS, Stubbs AY, et al. Imaging of musculoskeletal soft tissue infections. *Skeletal Radiol.* 2010;39:957–971.
This is an updated, comprehensive review of radiologic modalities used to image soft tissue infections.

Wall DB, Klein SR, Black S, et al. A simple model to help distinguish necrotizing fasciitis from nonnecrotizing soft tissue infection. *J Am Coll Surg.* 2000;191:227–231.
This article describes the use of serum sodium and white blood cell count to identify patients with necrotizing infections.

Weigelt J, Itani K, Stevens D, et al. Linezolid vs. vancomycin in treatment of complicated skin and soft tissue infections. *Antimicrob Agents Chemother.* 2005;49:2260–2266.

Wong CH, Khin LW, Heng KS, et al. The LRINEC (Laboratory Risk Indicator for Necrotizing Fasciitis) score: a tool for distinguishing necrotizing fasciitis from other soft tissue infections. *Crit Care Med.* 2004;32:1535–1541.
This article describes the use of common laboratory values in predicting the presence of a necrotizing infection.

38 Bacteremia and Catheter-Related Bloodstream Infections

David K. Warren

Bacteremia is a common complication in the critically ill. Bloodstream infections can be secondary to a recognized infection site, or primary infections either without an obvious source, or from the intravascular devices commonly used in critical care. Central venous catheters (CVCs) are the most common source of primary bloodstream infection in critically ill patients, and provide a unique opportunity for pathogens to enter the bloodstream. CVCs become infected through multiple mechanisms. The intra- and extraluminal portions of the catheter or the catheter hub(s) become colonized by bacteria that then enter the bloodstream. Rarely, contaminated intravenous solutions can create outbreaks of bacteremia with uncommon pathogens. Potentially, hematogenous seeding from bacteremia originating at another source can occur. Successful treatment of catheter-associated bloodstream infection is more difficult than simple bacteremia, as organisms on intravascular catheters exist within a slime-like biofilm, reducing their susceptibility to antimicrobial therapy and host defenses.

Local infection of the catheter insertion site presents as inflammation and purulent drainage from the entry site. However, local signs of infection are typically absent in catheter-associated bacteremia. Embolic phenomena distal to the catheter (e.g., septic pulmonary emboli) are also highly suggestive of a catheter-associated infection, although not commonly seen. More often, the clinician is faced with a critically ill patient who is febrile without an obvious source and has a CVC in place.

Determining if a CVC is the source of a new fever presents a diagnostic and management challenge. A conservative strategy of removing all catheters and replacing them at new sites at the first sign of fever would benefit some patients, but also leads to the removal of many uninfected CVCs, unnecessarily exposing patients to the risks of line replacement. A reasonable approach would be to draw blood cultures, and then immediately remove the catheter if there are obvious signs of infection at the insertion site (especially in the case of nontunneled catheters) or the patient is in septic shock. If a thorough evaluation does not reveal a source of infection and the patient is stable, it is reasonable to leave the catheter in place, follow the blood cultures, and start empirical antibiotics at the clinician's discretion. If the cultures become positive, the catheter can be removed and a new catheter placed at a different site, if still indicated.

Because the sensitivity and specificity of blood cultures are imperfect, multiple strategies have been studied in an attempt to improve the diagnosis of

ALGORITHM 38.1 Evaluation of Suspected Catheter-Associated Bacteremia

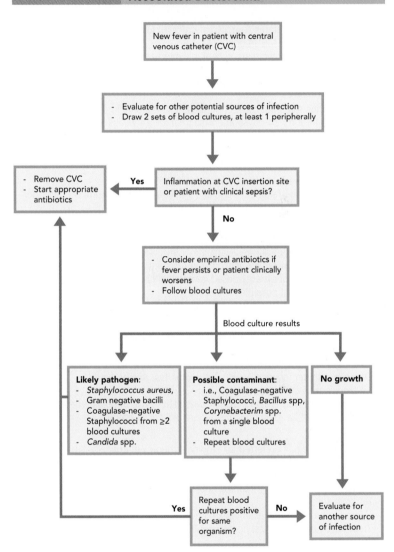

New fever in patient with central venous catheter (CVC)

- Evaluate for other potential sources of infection
- Draw 2 sets of blood cultures, at least 1 peripherally

Inflammation at CVC insertion site or patient with clinical sepsis?

Yes →
- Remove CVC
- Start appropriate antibiotics

No

- Consider empirical antibiotics if fever persists or patient clinically worsens
- Follow blood cultures

Blood culture results

Likely pathogen:
- *Staphylococcus aureus*,
- Gram negative bacilli
- Coagulase-negative Staphylococci from ≥2 blood cultures
- *Candida* spp.

Possible contaminant:
- i.e., Coagulase-negative Staphylococci, *Bacillus* spp, *Corynebacterim* spp. from a single blood culture
- Repeat blood cultures

No growth

Repeat blood cultures positive for same organism?

Yes / **No**

Evaluate for another source of infection

catheter-associated bloodstream infection. Currently, two methods are practical for widespread application. The first takes advantage of the continuous monitoring system for blood cultures used in most modern microbiology laboratories. Blot et al. found that, in cases of catheter-associated bloodstream infection, a blood culture drawn from a catheter became positive for growth faster than a paired sample from a peripheral

TABLE 38.1	Management of Bloodstream Infections by Common Pathogens

Staphylococcus aureus

Use parenteral β-lactams (oxacillin or nafcillin) for susceptible strains

Use vancomycin for MRSA only

Linezolid and daptomycin are acceptable alternatives for MRSA if unable to tolerate vancomycin

TEE recommended, if possible, evaluating for endocarditis

Remove catheters

If endocarditis ruled out by TEE, no prosthetic material in place and catheter removed, treat for 14 days; otherwise treat for ≥4 weeks

Treat complicated infections (endocarditis, septic thrombophlebitis, prolonged bacteremia) for 4–6 weeks (6–8 weeks for osteomyelitis)

Coagulase-negative Staphylococci

If catheter removed, treat with vancomycin for 5–7 days after removal

If catheter must be retained, treat for 10–14 days with vancomycin, consider antibiotic lock, and repeat blood cultures if signs/symptoms recur

Enterococci

Ampicillin for susceptible isolates

Vancomycin for ampicillin-resistant, vancomycin-sensitive isolates

Linezolid or daptomycin for vancomycin-resistant, ampicillin-resistant isolates

Consider addition of synergy-dosed gentamicin (1 mg/kg IV q8h)

Remove catheters if possible

Treat for 7–14 days of systemic antibiotic therapy for uncomplicated infection

Gram-negative bacilli

Empiric therapy should include agents active against *Pseudomonas aeruginosa*

Tailor antibiotics to sensitivity results

Remove catheter, especially with *Pseudomonas, Acinetobacter, Stenotrophomonas* spp.

If catheter removed, treat for 10–14 days of systemic antibiotic therapy; if catheter must be retained, consider antibiotic lock therapy

Candida species

An echinocandin is preferred for empirical therapy in critically ill patients; liposomal amphotericin B is an alternative therapy

Antifungal susceptibility can be inferred from the species identification

Repeat blood cultures on therapy until negative

Remove catheters

Dilated ophthalmologic examination on treatment to exclude endophthalmitis

Treat for 14 days after first negative culture in uncomplicated infections

---

MRSA, methicillin-resistant *Staphylococcus aureus;* IV, intravenous; TEE, transesophageal echocardiogram.

venipuncture. If a catheter-drawn blood culture becomes positive for growth at least 2 hours earlier than a peripherally drawn culture obtained at the same time, this strongly suggests the catheter as the source of the bacteremia. The other common method is culturing segments of catheters after their removal. A variety of techniques have been studied, but the semiquantitative roll plate technique described by Maki et al. remains the most common. Documenting significant colonization of a catheter with the same organism isolated from blood cultures provides strong evidence that the catheter is the source of infection. An approach to suspected catheter-associated bloodstream infection in the intensive care unit is presented in Algorithm 38.1.

Management strategies for specific pathogens can be found in Table 38.1. Special care should be taken in the case of *Candida* species (discussed in Chapter 39) and *Staphylococcus aureus,* given their ability to establish metastatic foci of infection. *S. aureus* bacteremia should prompt a thorough examination for metastatic sites of infection. High rates of endocarditis have been reported in catheter-associated *S. aureus* bacteremia, and transesophageal echocardiography should be considered in all cases, if not contraindicated.

The decision to remove a tunneled catheter or implanted port in the face of bacteremia is more difficult, given the expense and risk involved. In general, these devices should be removed when there is a soft tissue infection of the tunnel or the port reservoir, when there are systemic complications (i.e., septic shock, septic thromboembolic disease, endocarditis, osteomyelitis, or other metastatic foci of infection), when infection is due to *S. aureus* or *Candida* spp., and prolonged bacteremia not responding to appropriate antibiotic therapy. If salvage of the catheter is deemed necessary, there is evidence that use of high-concentration antibiotic lock therapy may improve success rates. Consultation with an infectious diseases specialist is recommended for complicated cases.

SUGGESTED READINGS

Beutz M, Sherman G, Mayfield J, et al. Clinical utility of blood cultures drawn from central vein catheters and peripheral venipuncture in critically ill medical patients. *Chest.* 2003;123:854–861.
  Blood cultures drawn from central venous catheters or from peripheral venipuncture had similar positive and negative predictive values for detected bloodstream infection.
Blot F, Schmidt E, Nitenberg G, et al. Earlier positivity of central-venous- versus peripheral-blood cultures is highly predictive of catheter-related sepsis. *J Clin Microbiol.* 1998;36:105–109.
  Paired sets of blood cultures from a catheter and peripheral venipuncture can be used to diagnose catheter-related bacteremia.
Fowler VG Jr, Li J, Corey GR, et al. Role of echocardiography in evaluation of patients with Staphylococcus aureus bacteremia: experience in 103 patients. *J Am Coll Cardiol.* 1997;30:1072–1078.
  Transesophageal echocardiography found a surprisingly high rate of endocarditis in patients with S. aureus bacteremia who had negative transthoracic echocardiograms.
Maki DG, Weise CE, Sarafin HW. A semiquantitative culture method for identifying intravenous-catheter-related infection. *N Engl J Med.* 1977;296:1305–1309.
  The original paper describing the commonly used roll plate culture technique.
Mermel LA, Allon M, Bouza E, et al. Clinical practice guidelines for the diagnosis and management of intravascular catheter-related infection: 2009 Update by the Infectious Diseases Society of America. *Clin Infect Dis.* 2009;49:1–45.
  The most recent evidence-based guidelines for managing catheter-associated bacteremia.

Stewart PS, William Costerton J. Antibiotic resistance of bacteria in biofilms. *Lancet.* 2001; 358:135–138.

A review of possible mechanisms of bacterial resistance within biofilms.

Weinstein MP, Towns ML, Quartey SM, et al. The clinical significance of positive blood cultures in the 1990s: a prospective comprehensive evaluation of the microbiology, epidemiology, and outcome of bacteremia and fungemia in adults. *Clin Infect Dis.* 1997;24: 584–602.

A prospective study of bacteremia from three large medical centers; appropriate antibiotic therapy was associated with lower mortality.

39 Invasive Fungal Infection

Toshibumi Taniguchi and Keith F. Woeltje

Invasive fungal infections are a significant cause of morbidity and mortality worldwide. The incidence of these infections is steadily increasing. In addition, strains resistant to many commonly used antifungal agents are becoming more prevalent.

Candida species are by far the most common fungal pathogens encountered in the intensive care unit. *Candida* is now the fourth most common cause of nosocomial bloodstream infection. The term *invasive candidiasis* comprises several conditions including candidemia, endocarditis, meningitis, and other forms of deep organ involvement (e.g., endophthalmitis and hepatosplenic candidiasis). The attributable mortality for an episode of invasive candidiasis has been reported to be as high as 40% to 50%.

Perhaps the strongest risk factor for invasive candidiasis is length of intensive care unit stay, with most studies revealing peak incidence at approximately day 10. Colonization with *Candida* (e.g., rectal, sputum, urine, or superficial wound colonization) is also considered a risk factor for the development of invasive disease. The importance of multifocal colonization remains an area of debate. Multiple single-center studies have suggested that multifocal colonization carries higher predictive value for development of invasive disease; however, one of the largest multicenter prospective trials done to date did not show a significant relationship between the number of colonized sites and the development of invasive disease. Other risk factors are listed in Table 39.1.

Candida albicans remains the most common species isolated from patients, accounting for 44% to 71% of disease. However, an epidemiologic shift toward non-*albicans* species is occurring, with the most common non-*albicans* isolates being *Candida glabrata, Candida parapsilosis, Candida tropicalis,* and *Candida krusei.* Recent data from the Prospective Antifungal Therapy Alliance (PATH) database from 2004 to 2008 showed the incidence of candidemia caused by the non-*albicans Candida species* was higher (54.4%) than the *C. albicans* (45.6%). This shift has particularly important implications for therapy because of intrinsic fluconazole resistance carried by *C. glabrata* and *C. krusei.*

The presence of *Candida* in a blood culture should never be perceived simply as a contaminant and should always prompt further investigation for possible sources. Although *Candida* grows readily in current blood culture bottles, blood cultures are positive in only 50% to 70% of patients with invasive candidiasis. However, a positive culture from a nonsterile site often provides little evidence to distinguish between infection and colonization. Biopsy of a specific lesion (from a normally sterile site) demonstrating characteristic histopathology can be considered definitive, but this is

TABLE 39.1 Risk Factors for Invasive Candidiasis

Prolonged ICU stay
Candida colonization
Central venous catheterization
Broad-spectrum antimicrobials
Renal failure
Hemodialysis
Diabetes
Parenteral nutrition
Malignancy
Chemotherapy/immunosuppressive medications
Surgery (particularly abdominal)
Transplantation
APACHE II score ≥20
Acute pancreatitis

ICU, intensive care unit; APACHE, acute physiology and chronic health evaluation.

often not feasible in critically ill patients. Because of these limitations, a reliable, nonculture-based method has been vigorously sought. 1,3-β-D-glucan, which is a major component of fungal cell wall, can be detected and its assay is recently approved by the Food and Drug Administration (FDA). This test has sensitivity of 75% to 100% and a specificity of 88% to 100%. However, it is a broad-spectrum assay that detects *Aspergillus, Candida, Fusarium, Acremonium,* and *Saccharomyces* species, thus careful interpretation is needed. None of the currently available tests have adequate sensitivity and specificity for reliable diagnosis. For this reason, empiric therapy for invasive candidiasis is often appropriate for the critically ill patient with risk factors who is not improving with appropriate antibacterial agents. Furthermore, recent evidence suggests a decrease in mortality when antifungal therapy is started early in high-risk hosts showing clinical signs of disease rather than holding therapy until definitive diagnosis (i.e., *Candida* growth in blood culture). Although no major conclusions can be drawn from this limited analysis, we believe that early empiric therapy in high-risk patients pending culture results is justifiable.

Evidence-based guidelines regarding general management and treatment of candidiasis were published by the Infectious Diseases Society of America in 2009. Fluconazole is an appropriate choice for nonneutropenic, hemodynamically stable patients unless there is high suspicion for a fluconazole-resistant species (e.g., previous colonization with *C. glabrata, C. krusei,* or history of recent azole exposure). If fluconazole is used for empiric therapy, a relatively high dose (e.g., 800 mg intravenously daily and adjusted for renal function) should be used until species identification is made. In patients who are neutropenic, hemodynamically unstable, or who are being treated in units with high rates of infection with fluconazole-resistant species (regardless of immune function or hemodynamic status), treatment with an echinocandin is preferred until species identification of the *Candida* isolate is made (Algorithm 39.1); amphotericin B formulation may be used as an alternative if there is intolerance to or limited availability of other antifungals. Voriconazole is another alternative, however, if offers little advantage over fluconazole and is recommended as step-down oral therapy for selected cases of candidiasis due to *C. krusei* or voriconazole-susceptible *C. glabrata.*

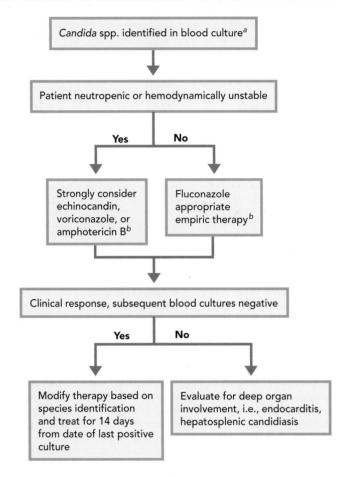

ALGORITHM 39.1   **Empiric Treatment of Candidemia**

Candida spp. identified in blood culture[a]

↓

Patient neutropenic or hemodynamically unstable

Yes / **No**

Strongly consider echinocandin, voriconazole, or amphotericin B[b]

Fluconazole appropriate empiric therapy[b]

↓

Clinical response, subsequent blood cultures negative

Yes / **No**

Modify therapy based on species identification and treat for 14 days from date of last positive culture

Evaluate for deep organ involvement, i.e., endocarditis, hepatosplenic candidiasis

[a]Removal of central lines and ophthalmologic exam recommended with diagnosis of candidemia when clinically stable.
[b]Also consider echinocandin, voriconazole, or amphotericin B for patients colonized with *Candida glabrata* or *Candida krusei,* those residing in units with high rates of infection with these organisms, and recipients of previous fluconazole prophylaxis or therapy.

For infection due to *C. parapsilosis,* treatment with fluconazole is recommended since they are less susceptible to echinocandins. In the case of candidemia, the standard duration of therapy is 14 days from the last positive blood culture. Recommended treatment may be considerably longer, depending on the site of involvement. Early removal of the central venous catheter is recommended, but not all studies have shown that early removal is associated with clinical benefit; thus, timing of removal of central venous

TABLE 39.2	Risk Factors for Invasive Aspergillosis

Prolonged neutropenia (>10 days)
Hematopoietic stem cell transplantation
Solid organ transplantation
Corticosteroid/other immunosuppressive therapy
Advanced HIV
Chronic granulomatous disease

HIV, human immunodeficiency virus.

catheter should be carefully individualized for each patient. Additional components of management include ophthalmologic examination to exclude endophthalmitis.

Because fungal pathogens represent a growing proportion of nosocomial infections, prophylaxis with antifungal agents in high-risk patients has been implemented at several centers. The few trials performed to date have shown a nonsignificant risk reduction with the use of either fluconazole or ketoconazole as prophylaxis; however, these studies were limited by relatively small numbers. Although these results are encouraging, they have not led to definitive recommendations for antifungal prophylaxis. Antifungal prophylaxis may be a reasonable approach in selected high-risk patients such as transplant recipients or patients with chemotherapy-induced neutropenia.

Although a much less common cause of invasive disease, *Aspergillus* species remain an important consideration in a certain subset of patients, particularly those who are immunosuppressed (Table 39.2). Sinopulmonary involvement is the most common manifestation of invasive disease; however, dissemination can occur virtually anywhere, including the skin, central nervous system, eyes, and abdominal viscera. Computed tomography may suggest the diagnosis with findings such as the "halo sign," a haziness surrounding a nodular pulmonary infiltrate. However, this feature can be seen with other angioinvasive infections, so it is far from diagnostic. The organism will grow on culture; however, its presence in samples from nonsterile sites may indicate colonization rather than true infection. The sensitivity of the serum galactomannan assay varies widely in the literature between 29% and 100% and the specificity is typically greater than 85%. False-positive results may also occur in patients receiving piperacillin–tazobactam. β-D-glucan may be also useful to support the diagnosis of *Aspergillus* infection. These assays potentially can be used as a diagnostic adjunct but should not be used as sole criterion for diagnosis. Demonstration of the organism on biopsy is considered the gold standard for diagnosis.

According to an international, multicenter, randomized open-label trial comparing amphotericin B and voriconazole as initial therapy for invasive aspergillosis, voriconazole was associated with improved survival (71% vs. 58%, respectively). Based on this trial, use of voriconazole is recommended as first-line therapy. The echinocandins are alternative therapy for *Aspergillus* and therefore used in patients who cannot tolerate or who are refractory to standard therapy (Table 39.3). Combination therapy is often used in these patients; however, because of conflicting results from clinical trials, no definitive recommendation can be given.

Mucormycosis is a life-threatening mold infection caused by fungi of the order *Mucorales*. The term *zygomycosis* was used in the past but with recent reclassification, the order *Zygomycetes* was abolished and placed the order *Mucorales* in the subphylum *Mucormycotina*. There are multiple organisms within this general classification, and

TABLE 39.3	Activity of Antifungal Agents			
Fungus	Fluconazole	Voriconazole	Echinocandin[a]	Amphotericin B
Candida albicans	+	+	+	+
Candida parapsilosis	+	+	+/−	+
Candida tropicalis	+	+	+	+
Candida glabrata	DD/−	+/−	+	+
Candida krusei	−	+	+	+
Aspergillus spp.[b]	−	+	+	+
Cryptococcus spp.[c]	+	+	−	+
Mucorales (Zygomycetes)	−	−	−	+
Fusarium spp.	−	+	−	+/−

[a]Only caspofungin and anidulafungin approved for candidemia.
[b]Aspergillus terreus often resistant to amphotericin B.
[c]In vitro data suggest susceptibility to voriconazole, although no clinical trials have been performed to demonstrate efficacy.
+, susceptibility; −, resistance; DD, dose-dependent susceptibility.

those most commonly isolated include *Rhizopus, Rhizomucor, Absidia,* and *Mucor.* These organisms are known for their predilection of immunocompromised hosts and typically present with relatively rapid-onset angioinvasive disease. Predisposing factors include diabetes, acidosis, solid organ and bone marrow transplantation recipients, iron overload, deferoxamine treatment, and other forms of immunosuppression.

The most common presentation is that seen in the diabetic, acidotic patient manifesting as rhinocerebral disease. Pulmonary involvement is the more typical presentation in the posttransplant immunosuppressed host. Although the incidence of *mucormycosis* remains relatively low, it has shown a definite increase in recent years because of the increasing population with immunosuppression. Furthermore, there has been an association between *mucormycosis* and those high-risk patients receiving long-term voriconazole as posttransplant prophylaxis, although a direct causal link has not been established. The organism can be difficult to grow on standard laboratory media; thus, diagnosis is often made based on biopsy demonstrating characteristic histopathology.

The typical broad-spectrum antifungal classes, echinocandins and azoles (including voriconazole), are not effective against the agents of *mucormycosis.* High-dose amphotericin B is considered standard first-line therapy (e.g., amphotericin B deoxycholate 1 to 1.5 mg/kg/day or amphotericin B lipid formulations at doses of at least 5 mg/kg/day [Table 39.4]). Higher doses are often used (e.g., 7.5 to 10 mg/kg/day), although the efficacy of this approach has not been validated. Because of the angioinvasive nature and propensity to rapidly progress, urgent surgical intervention is always required for rhinocerebral disease and often for pulmonary disease. Initiation of amphotericin B-based therapy within 5 days after diagnosis of *mucormycosis* was associated with improvement in survival compared with initiation of treatment at ≥6 days

TABLE 39.4 Indications/Dosing of Commonly Used Antifungal Agents

Agent	Dose	Dosing adjustment necessary
	Invasive candidiasis	
Fluconazole	400–800 mg/day, IV or PO	Renal insufficiency
Voriconazole	IV: 6 mg/kg every 12 hr for 2 doses followed by 3–4 mg/kg every 12 hr	Hepatic dysfunction IV vehicle may accumulate in renal insufficiency
	PO: <40 kg–100 mg every 12 hr ≥40 kg–200 mg every 12 hr	
Caspofungin	70 mg loading dose followed by 50 mg/day, IV	Hepatic dysfunction
Anidulafungin	200 mg loading dose followed by 100 mg/day, IV	None
Amphotericin B deoxycholate[a]	0.6–1 mg/day, IV	None, careful monitoring renal and liver function
Amphotericin B lipid formulations[a] • Colloidal dispersion (Amphotec) • Lipid complex (Abelcet) • Liposomal (AmBisome)	3–5 mg/kg/day, IV	None, careful monitoring renal and liver function
	Invasive aspergillosis	
Itraconazole	IV: 200 mg every 12 hr for 4 doses followed by 200 mg/day PO: 200–400 mg/day	Multiple drug interactions IV not recommended for CrCl <30 mL/min
Voriconazole	As listed above	As listed above
Amphotericin B deoxycholate[a]	1–1.5 mg/kg/day	As listed above
Amphotericin B lipid formulations[a]	5 mg/kg/day, IV	As listed above Higher doses sometimes used
Caspofungin	As listed above	As listed above
	Mucormycosis	
Amphotericin B deoxycholate[a]	1–1.5 mg/kg/day	As listed above
Amphotericin B lipid formulations[a]	≥5 mg/kg/day, IV[b]	As listed above Higher doses sometimes used

[a]Bolus infusion of normal saline with dose recommended to decrease incidence of nephrotoxicity. Premedication with acetaminophen and diphenhydramine may decrease infusion-related reactions. In severe cases, hydrocortisone 50–100 mg IV may also be administered.
[b]Recommended start dose. Higher doses of 7.5–10 mg/kg/day are sometimes used, although there are no prospective trials of efficacy in zygomycosis.
IV, intravenous; PO, by mouth; CrCl, creatine clearance.

after diagnosis (83% vs. 49% survival). Establishing an early diagnosis of *mucormycosis* is critical to commence early antifungal treatment. Posaconazole, recently approved for fungal prophylaxis in the severely immunosuppressed patient, has shown activity against *mucormycosis* as salvage therapy in case reports. However, pharmacokinetic and pharmacodynamic data raise concerns about reliability of achieving adequate levels of oral posaconazole *in vivo*. Therefore, therapeutic drug monitoring may be warranted. Posaconazole is not currently approved by the FDA as standard treatment.

SUGGESTED READINGS

Herbrecht R, Denning DW, Patterson TF, et al. Voriconazole versus amphotericin B for primary therapy of invasive aspergillosis. *N Engl J Med.* 2002;347:408–415.
  Randomized, unblinded trial showing improved outcomes with voriconazole compared to amphotericin B as primary therapy for invasive aspergillosis.
Horn DL, Neofytos D, Anaissie EJ, et al. Epidemiology and outcomes of candidemia in 2019 patients: data from the prospective antifungal therapy alliance registry. *Clin Infect Dis.* 2009;48:1695–1703.
  Multicenter prospective cohort study assessing risk factors for developments of candidemia.
Marr KA, Boeckh M, Carter RA, et al. Combination antifungal therapy for invasive aspergillosis. *Clin Infect Dis.* 2004;39:797–802.
  Retrospective analysis showing improved 3-month survival with combination of voriconazole and caspofungin when used as salvage therapy.
Mennink-Kersten MA, Donnelly JP, Verweij PE. Detection of circulating galactomannan for the diagnosis and management of invasive aspergillosis. *Lancet Infect Dis.* 2004;4(6):349–357.
  Review of utility of aspergillus galactomannan assay.
Morrell M, Fraser VJ, Kollef MH. Delaying the empiric treatment of *Candida* bloodstream infection until positive blood culture results are obtained: a potential risk factor for hospital mortality. *Antimicrob Agents Chemother.* 2005;49:3640–3645.
  Retrospective cohort analysis showing higher mortality with delay in antifungal therapy.
Odabasi Z, Mattiuzzi G, Estey E, et al. Beta-D-glucan as a diagnostic adjunct for invasive fungal infections: validation, cutoff development, and performance in patients with acute myelogenous leukemia and myelodysplastic syndrome. *Clin Infect Dis.* 2004;39:199–205.
  Diagnostic utility of β-D-Glucan among patients with hematologic malignancies.
Ostrosky-Zeichner L, Pappas PG. Invasive candidiasis in the intensive care unit. *Crit Care Med.* 2006;34:857–863.
  Review of current epidemiologic trends and management strategies for invasive candidiasis in the ICU.
Pappas PG, Kauffman CA, Andes D, et al. Clinical practice guidelines for the management of candidiasis: 2009 update by the Infectious Diseases Society of America. *Clin Infect Dis.* 2009;48:503–535.
  Evidence-based review and treatment recommendations.
Playford EG, Webster AC, Sorrell TC, et al. Antifungal agents for preventing fungal infections in non-neutropenic critically ill and surgical patients: systematic review and meta-analysis of randomized clinical trials. *J Antimicrob Chemother.* 2006;57:628–638.
  Meta-analysis of 12 studies evaluating efficacy of antifungal prophylaxis in high-risk patients.
Spellberg B, Walsh TJ, Kontoyiannis DP, et al. Recent advances in the management of mucormycosis: from bench to bedside. *Clin Infect Dis.* 2009;48:1743–1751.
  Review of recent strategies for treatment of mucormycosis.
Walsh TJ, Anaissie EJ, Denning DW, et al. Treatment of aspergillosis: clinical practice guidelines of the Infectious Diseases Society of America. *Clin Infect Dis.* 2008;46:327–360.
  Evidence-based review and treatment recommendations of aspergillosis.

40 Infections in the Immunocompromised Host

Stephen Y. Liang and Steven J. Lawrence

Infections in the critically ill immunocompromised patient carry significant morbidity and mortality. While empiric antimicrobial therapy is universally indicated in the early stages of care, definitive diagnosis and therapy requires knowledge of the patient's level of immunosuppression, inherent or iatrogenic, upon which a broad differential of suspect pathogens can then be assembled. Immunocompromised patients are at risk for community-acquired infections as well as a myriad of opportunistic and nosocomial infections. Clinical signs and symptoms of infection are frequently atypical and nonspecific. Muted inflammatory responses arising from neutropenia, corticosteroids, and other forms of immunosuppressive therapy may render identification of an infectious focus difficult. Multiple prior hospitalizations for infection and the outpatient use of prophylactic antimicrobials to prevent opportunistic infection may place patients at risk for acquiring multidrug-resistant organisms. The management of infections in an immunocompromised patient can be challenging and is often best accomplished in consultation with an infectious disease specialist.

NEUTROPENIC FEVER

Neutropenia is a common complication in patients receiving chemotherapy or with a primary hematologic malignancy. Prolonged duration and severity of neutropenia translate into a heightened risk of bloodstream and other serious infections. Neutropenic fever is defined as an absolute neutrophil count (ANC) of <500 cells/mm³ or <1000 cells/mm³ with an anticipated decline below 500 cells/mm³ over the next 48 hours coupled with the presence of a single temperature of ≥38.3°C (101°F) or a persistent temperature of ≥38.0°C (100.4°F) for more than an hour. Considered a medical emergency, neutropenic fever should always be assumed infectious in etiology until proven otherwise through a comprehensive evaluation. More than half of all patients with neutropenic fever are ultimately found to have either an established or occult infection.

Mucositis secondary to chemotherapy places the neutropenic patient at high risk for infections of the sinuses, oropharynx, and the gastrointestinal tract. Invasive fungal sinusitis (mucormycosis) caused by Zygomycetes can progress to severe rhino-orbital-cerebral infections requiring extensive surgical debridement. Neutropenic enterocolitis (typhlitis) manifesting as a necrotizing infection of the cecum can extend to the terminal ileum and ascending colon, leading to bowel perforation, peritonitis, hemorrhage, and sepsis. *Clostridium difficile* infection (CDI) may present as abdominal pain with diarrhea. Translocation of intestinal bacteria across damaged mucosal membranes can precipitate serious bloodstream infections with *Enterococcus* species and Gram-negative organisms. Pneumonia and urinary tract infections are common. Cutaneous and mucosal infections caused by herpesviruses and fungi increase the risk of bacterial superinfection. Long-term vascular access sites present avenues of infection for skin flora. Catheter-related infections associated with severe sepsis, suppurative thrombophlebitis, endocarditis, septic emboli, and bacteremia with *Staphylococcus aureus,* Gram-negative organisms, mycobacteria, and fungi usually require catheter removal in order to clear the infection.

In the last two decades, the continuum of pathogens implicated in neutropenic fever has shifted from Gram-negative bacilli (*Pseudomonas aeruginosa, Escherichia coli,* and *Klebsiella* species) toward Gram-positive organisms (*S. aureus, Staphylococcus epidermidis, Streptococcus* species, and *Enterococcus* species) and fungi, though Gram-negative infections still abound. Patients with a prior history of tuberculosis are at heightened risk for reactivation of their disease. With protracted chemotherapy and neutropenia, *Nocardia* and fungal infections with *Aspergillus* (invasive pneumonia, sinusitis), *Fusarium, Cryptococcus neoformans,* and endemic mycoses (*Histoplasma capsulatum, Blastomyces dermatitidis,* and *Coccidioides immitis*) may be encountered. Disseminated candidiasis with hepatic and splenic abscess formation may present with fever, abdominal pain, and an elevated alkaline phosphatase. Patients with acute lymphocytic leukemia (ALL) or other malignancies receiving high-dose corticosteroids without adequate antimicrobial prophylaxis may develop *Pneumocystis jiroveci* pneumonia. Viral infections secondary to herpes simplex virus (HSV), cytomegalovirus (CMV), Epstein–Barr virus (EBV), varicella zoster virus (VZV), and human herpesvirus-6 (HHV-6) may assume a wide range of clinical manifestations including meningitis, encephalitis, esophagitis, hepatitis, and skin disease.

Early empiric antimicrobial therapy in neutropenic fever decreases mortality and takes precedence once adequate blood cultures have been obtained. Based on local antimicrobial resistance patterns, monotherapy with an antipseudomonal cephalosporin, beta-lactam, or carbapenem for broad Gram-negative coverage is initially recommended with or without vancomycin for Gram-positive coverage (Algorithm 40.1). If blood cultures remain negative and a fever persists for more than 5 days, empiric antifungal therapy is usually warranted to cover mold infections. Empiric antiviral therapy is generally not recommended unless characteristic skin or cutaneous lesions suggestive of HSV or VZV are identified or active influenza has been identified in the community.

SOLID ORGAN TRANSPLANTATION

The spectrum of infectious diseases encountered in patients who have undergone solid organ transplantation varies over time and with the degree of immunosuppression used to ensure graft survival (Table 40.1). The majority of infections in the first month following a solid organ transplant represent complications of surgery and prolonged hospitalization. Wound dehiscence, leaking surgical anastomoses, infected fluid collections (blood, urine, and bile), and other infectious complications may be encountered depending on the type of graft (Table 40.2). The importance of early surgical debridement and drainage of infected fluid collections cannot be overemphasized in addition to antimicrobial therapy. Health care–associated

ALGORITHM 40.1   **Management of Neutropenic Fever**

Fever ≥38.3°C or persistently ≥38.0°C for at least 1hr **AND** ANC ≤500/mm^3 or ANC ≥500/mm^3 with expected decline to ≤500/mm^3

↓

- Blood cultures × 2, urinalysis and urine culture, chest radiograph, other testing as indicated (*e.g.* nasopharyngeal swab for influenza and other respiratory viruses; *Clostridium difficile* toxin)
- Empiric Gram negative antibiotics*
- Vancomycin 1 g q12hr × 72 hr (target troughs of 15–20 mcg/mL) if indicated**

← If suspected *intra-abdominal source* or *Clostridium difficile infection*, consider adding Metronidazole 500 mg po/IV q8hr

↓

New temp after afebrile ≥48 hr **OR** persistently febrile ≥72 hr and cultures negative

← If *clinically unstable* consider adding double Gram negative coverage with aminoglycoside × 72 hr

Discontinue aminoglycoside if cultures negative after 72 hr

↓

Clinically stable
- Culture negative: continue same regimen
- Culture positive: per culture and sensitivities

← **Clinically unstable**
- Change Gram negative coverage
- Consider addition of Vancomycin **

↓

Persistently febrile ≥5 days and cultures negative
- Consider infectious disease consult
- Consider addition of antifungal agent (voriconazole vs. liposomal amphotericin B)

(**) Indications for Vancomycin
- Severe mucositis
- Clinical evidence of catheter-related infection
- Known colonization with resistant streptococci or staphylococci
- Sudden temperature spike of >40°C
- Hypotension

Discontinue Vancomycin after 72 hr if cultures negative for coagulase negative staphylococci, methicillin-resistant *Staphylococcus aureus*, or cephalosporin-resistant streptococci

(*) Gram-negative coverage (including *Pseudomonas aeruginosa*)

Cefepime 1 g IV q8hr **OR** Meropenem 500 mg IV q6hr **OR** Piperacillin-tazobactam 4.5 g IV q6hr

Penicillin allergy
Ciprofloxacin 400 mg IV q8hr **OR** Aztreonam 2 g IV q8hr

All drug doses provided assume normal venal function. Dose adjusements may be necessary in the setting of renal impairment.

TABLE 40.1 Timeline of Infections in the Solid Organ Transplant Patient

≤1 month	1–6 months	≥6 months
Postoperative complication and nosocomial infection • Surgical site infection • Graft ischemia/superinfection • Anastomotic leak • Abscess/infected fluid collection • Pneumonia • Urinary tract infection • Catheter-associated infection • *Clostridium difficile* infection **Donor-derived infection** • *Aspergillus* spp, *Cryptococcus neoformans*, endemic fungi (*Histoplasma capsulatum, Coccidioides immitis*) • Herpesviruses (CMV, EBV, HSV, VZV, HHV-6), HIV, HBV, HCV, WNV, LCMV, rhabdovirus (rabies) • *Toxoplasma gondii, Trypanosoma cruzi* (Chagas) • *Balamuthia mandrillaris, Strongyloides stercoralis* **Recipient-derived infection** • *Mycobacterium tuberculosis* • *Cryptococcus neoformans*, endemic fungi • Herpesviruses, HIV, HBV, HCV • *Toxoplasma gondii, Strongyloides stercoralis* (hyperinfection)	**Postoperative complication (less common)** **Nosocomial infection** **Opportunistic infection** (Depending on antimicrobial prophylaxis) • *Listeria monocytogenes* • *Nocardia* spp • *Mycobacterium tuberculosis* • Nontuberculous mycobacteria • *Pneumocystis jiroveci* • *Aspergillus* spp • *Cryptococcus neoformans* • Endemic fungi • Herpesviruses (CMV, EBV, HSV, VZV, HHV-6/7/8) • HBV, HCV • Adenovirus • Influenza, RSV • Parvovirus B19 • BK polyomavirus (nephropathy) • *Toxoplasma gondii* (myocarditis) • *Leishmania* • *Trypanosoma cruzi* • Cryptosporidium • Microsporidium • *Strongyloides stercoralis* (hyperinfection)	**Low-level immunosuppression** • Community-acquired infection (pneumonia, UTI) • *Nocardia* spp • *Rhodococcus* • *Mycobacterium tuberculosis* • Nontuberculous mycobacteria • *Aspergillus* spp • *Mucor* spp • *Cryptococcus neoformans* • Endemic fungi • Herpesviruses (CMV, EBV, HSV, VZV), EBV-related PTLD • HBV, HCV • JC polyomavirus (PML) • BK polyomavirus **High-level immunosuppression** See *Opportunistic Infection* (1–6 months)

CMV, cytomegalovirus; EBV, Epstein–Barr virus; HBV, hepatitis B virus; HCV, hepatitis C virus; HHV, human herpesvirus; HIV, human immunodeficiency virus; HSV, herpes simplex virus; LCMV, lymphocytic choriomeningitis virus; PML, progressive multifocal leukoencephalopathy; PTLD, posttransplant lymphoproliferative disorder; WNV, West Nile virus; VZV, varicella zoster virus.
Adapted from Fishman JA. Infection in solid-organ transplant recipients. *N Engl J Med*. 2007;357:2601–2614.

TABLE 40.2	Graft Site-Specific Infections
Heart	Myocarditis (*Toxoplasma gondii* seropositive donor to seronegative recipient) Mediastinitis/sternal wound infection (*Staphylococcus aureus, Staphylococcus epidermidis*)
Lung	Pneumonia (*Pseudomonas aeruginosa, Escherichia coli, Klebsiella pneumoniae, Stenotrophomonas maltophilia, Staphylococcus aureus, Burkholderia cepacia, Mycobacterium tuberculosis,* CMV, *Candida* species, *Aspergillus* species) Mediastinitis (*Pseudomonas aeruginosa, Escherichia coli, Klebsiella pneumoniae, Staphylococcus epidermidis*)
Liver	Biloma/hepatic abscess/peritonitis (*Enterococcus, Klebsiella pneumoniae, Enterobacter cloacae, Candida* species)
Kidney	Urinary tract infection (*Escherichia coli, Enterobacter cloacae, Klebsiella* species, *Proteus mirabilis, Enterococcus* species) Nephropathy (BK polyomavirus)

pneumonia, urinary tract infection, and infections of vascular catheters, surgical drains, and other foreign objects are also common during the postoperative period. Reactivation of latent infections (HBV, HCV, HIV, tuberculosis, strongyloidiasis) and infection by colonizing or nosocomial bacteria and fungi are possible. Infection with multidrug-resistant organisms (MRSA, VRE, extended spectrum beta-lactamase Gram-negative organisms, azole-resistant *Candida* species) must be considered. Although rare, infections transmitted to a transplant recipient through an infected donor organ can be devastating and must be considered in the setting of clinical deterioration during the first week after transplant if no other obvious explanations are plausible.

Following the first month after transplant, immunosuppression to prevent acute rejection substantially increases the risk of opportunistic infection. In particular, patients receiving high-dose corticosteroids and T-lymphocyte depleting agents (antithymocyte globulins, OKT3, alemtuzumab) may be especially vulnerable to severe viral (HHV) infections. CMV infection and reactivation are common in patients not on prophylactic antiviral therapy. CMV donor–recipient mismatch leading to primary CMV infection carries the highest risk of invasive disease (pneumonitis, hepatitis, colitis). Coinfection with immunomodulating viruses (CMV, EBV, HHV-6, HBV, HCV) may further predispose a patient to serious bacterial and fungal infections. Information concerning a patient's antimicrobial prophylaxis regimen, geographic location, and epidemiologic exposures may lend further insight into the types of opportunistic infections possible. In heart transplant recipients, infection with *Toxoplasma gondii* may lead to myocarditis.

As the risk of acute graft rejection declines over time, the requirement for immunosuppression generally stabilizes and decreases. At 6 months posttransplant, most patients are more likely to suffer from community-acquired infections (e.g., pneumonia) than opportunistic ones. However, patients still on significant doses of immunosuppressive regimens remain prone to the latter.

HEMATOPOIETIC STEM CELL TRANSPLANTATION

The risk of infection after allogeneic hematopoietic stem cell transplant bears a resemblance to that of the neutropenic patient and can be separated into three general phases (Table 40.3). Patients undergoing autologous transplant share the same risks of infection during the first phase but largely recover immune function thereafter. Usually comprising the first 3 weeks after transplant, the pre-engraftment phase represents the period of greatest bone marrow suppression and is defined by neutropenia following conditioning chemotherapy. Recipients are at high risk for Gram-negative infections as a result of chemotherapy-related mucositis and translocation of gut flora as described above. Gram-positive infections from skin and oropharyngeal flora are also common. Infection with *Streptococcus viridans* can lead to a rapidly fatal shock

TABLE 40.3	**Timeline of Infections in the Hematopoietic Stem Cell Transplant Patient**	
Pre-engraftment (<3 weeks)	Early postengraftment (3 weeks–3 months)	Late postengraftment (>3 months)
• Gram-negative bacteria (*Pseudomonas aeruginosa,* Enterobacteriaceae, *Stenotrophomonas maltophilia*) • Gram-positive bacteria (*Staphylococcus aureus,* coagulase-negative staphylococcus, *Streptococcus* spp, *Enterococcus*) • *Clostridium difficile* • *Candida* spp • *Aspergillus* spp • *Fusarium* spp • Zygomycetes • HSV (seropositive) • Respiratory viruses (RSV, parainfluenza, rhinovirus, influenza, adenovirus, human metapneumovirus)	• *Legionella pneumophila* • *Listeria monocytogenes* • *Nocardia* spp • *Mycobacterium tuberculosis* • Nontuberculous mycobacteria • *Candida* spp • *Aspergillus* spp • *Fusarium* spp • Zygomycetes • *Pneumocystis jiroveci* • CMV (seropositive) • EBV • HHV-6, -7 • VZV (seropositive) • Respiratory viruses • BK polyomavirus • *Toxoplasma gondii* • *Strongyloides stercoralis* • *Cryptosporidium*	• Encapsulated bacteria (*Streptococcus pneumoniae,* Haemophilus influenzae, Neisseria meningitidis*) • *Nocardia* spp • Endemic mycoses • CMV • EBV • VZV (seropositive) • BK/JC polyomavirus • Parvovirus B19 • If chronic GVHD, then consider pre-engraftment and early postengraftment organisms as well

CMV, cytomegalovirus; EBV, Epstein–Barr virus; GVHD, graft versus host disease; HBV, hepatitis B virus; HCV, hepatitis C virus; HHV, human herpesvirus; HIV, human immunodeficiency virus; HSV, herpes simplex virus; RSV, respiratory syncytial virus; VZV, varicella zoster virus.

Adapted from Hiemenz JW. Management of infections complicating allogeneic hematopoietic stem cell transplantation. *Semin Hematol.* 2009;46:289–312.

syndrome. Bacteremia, pneumonia, and CDI figure prominently during this phase. Localized and disseminated azole-resistant candidiasis as well as invasive mold infections (*Aspergillus, Fusarium, Zygomycetes*) presenting as pneumonia, sinusitis, central nervous system infection, or skin lesions are also encountered. Seropositive recipients not taking antiviral prophylaxis are highly vulnerable to reactivation of HSV, which can involve the skin, liver, and gastrointestinal tract.

Bone marrow recovery marks the beginning of the immediate postengraftment phase that typically lasts from 3 weeks to 3 months after transplant. Cell-mediated and humoral deficiencies predominate. Acute graft versus host disease (GVHD) and its treatment with high-dose immunosuppression can further increase the risk of infection. Many of the same fungal infections seen in the pre-engraftment phase persist. *P. jiroveci* pneumonia is less common now as a result of effective antimicrobial prophylaxis. Reactivation of immunomodulating HHVs, most importantly CMV, can result in life-threatening pneumonia, encephalitis, colitis, and marrow suppression. Reactivation of toxoplasmosis may also be seen during this phase.

Six months after transplantation, the recipient enters the late postengraftment phase. If a recipient has not developed GVHD, immune function may be largely restored within 1 to 2 years. Conversely, recipients who have chronic GVHD and receive additional immunosuppression remain at high risk for severe infection, particularly with encapsulated bacteria (*Streptococcus pneumoniae, Haemophilus influenzae, Neisseria meningitidis*), *Nocardia* spp, fungi, and viruses (CMV, EBV, VZV).

HUMAN IMMUNODEFICIENCY VIRUS

The advent of antiretroviral therapy (ART) has revolutionized the care of patients with human immunodeficiency virus (HIV). ART-adherent patients are more likely to be admitted to the intensive care unit with medical problems unrelated to their HIV infection or directly related to the antiretroviral regimens themselves. However, underdiagnosis of HIV in the community coupled with barriers to access and adherence with effective ART and antimicrobial prophylaxis mean that a significant number of patients with HIV/AIDS will continue to present to the intensive care unit with severe, life-threatening opportunistic infections. The $CD4^+$ lymphocyte cell count remains an accurate gauge of susceptibility to opportunistic infection in HIV patients.

Community-acquired pneumonia (*S. pneumoniae, H. influenzae,* and increasingly *S. aureus*) remains a common cause of pulmonary infection in this population, irrespective of $CD4^+$ cell count. *Mycobacterium tuberculosis* may present with pulmonary or extrapulmonary manifestations in HIV. The prevalence of *P. jiroveci* pneumonia increases dramatically once the $CD4^+$ cell count drops below 200 cells/mm^3. Other fungal pneumonias caused by *C. neoformans* and *H. capsulatum* may also be seen below this threshold. Bacteremia associated with pneumonia and disseminated mycobacterial and fungal disease are more common at lower $CD4^+$ cell counts. Below a $CD4^+$ cell count of 50 cells/mm^3, pneumonia secondary to *Mycobacterium avium complex* (MAC), CMV, and VZV becomes possible.

Central nervous system infections are more common when the CD4+ cell count is severely depressed (Table 40.4). Generally seen when the $CD4^+$ cell count falls below 100 cells/mm^3, *Toxoplasma encephalitis* may manifest with fever, headache, altered mental status, neurologic deficits, and seizure. In most cases, ring-enhancing lesions are seen on CT and MRI. Less common infections associated with ring-enhancing lesions may include bacterial brain abscess, cryptoccomas, and syphilitic gummas. Below a $CD4^+$ cell count of 50 cells/mm^3, meningoencephalitis secondary to

TABLE 40.4	**Common and Important Pathogens in the Immunocompromised Host**
I. Neutropenia	
A. Pneumonia	Bacteria, *Aspergillus* spp, CMV, respiratory viruses
B. CNS infection	Bacteria, *Listeria monocytogenes, Aspergillus* spp, *Cryptococcus neoformans,* HSV, CMV, HHV-6
II. Transplant	
A. Pneumonia	Bacteria, *Nocardia* spp, *Mycobacterium tuberculosis,* nontuberculous mycobacteria, *Pneumocystis jiroveci, Aspergillus* spp, CMV, respiratory viruses, *Strongyloides stercoralis*
B. CNS infection	*Nocardia* spp, *Listeria monocytogenes, Aspergillus* spp, *Cryptococcus neoformans,* endemic fungi, CMV, HHV-6, HSV, VZV, *Toxoplasma gondii*
III. HIV	
A. Pneumonia	
Any CD4$^+$	Bacteria, *Mycobacterium tuberculosis*
CD4$^+$ <200	Above + *Pneumocystis jiroveci,* endemic mycoses, *Toxoplasma gondii*
CD4$^+$ <50	Above + *Mycobacterium avium complex,* CMV, VZV
B. CNS infection	
Any CD4$^+$	Bacteria, *Listeria monocytogenes,* HSV
CD4$^+$ <100	*Toxoplasma gondii*
CD4$^+$ <50	*Cryptococcus neoformans,* CMV, EBV-associated lymphoma, VZV, JC polyomavirus (PML)

CMV, cytomegalovirus; EBV, Epstein–Barr virus; HHV, human herpesvirus; HSV, herpes simplex virus; VZV, varicella zoster virus.

C. neoformans may present with severe headache, photophobia, and even coma in the face of elevated intracranial pressures. Herpesvirus encephalitis (HSV, CMV, VZV), primary CNS lymphoma (EBV), and progressive multifocal leukoencephalopathy (JC polyomavirus) must be considered in the patient with rapid neurologic deterioration and abnormalities on brain imaging.

Immune reconstitution inflammatory syndrome (IRIS) is a life-threatening complication of ART that can be indistinguishable from an acute opportunistic infection. Usually apparent within days to weeks of initiating ART, improvements in immune function can lead to an exuberant inflammatory response against infectious agents that may previously have been clinically silent. *M. tuberculosis,* MAC, *P. jiroveci,* endemic fungi, and CMV infections are most commonly seen and may occur at previously known sites of infection or at new sites altogether. Corticosteroids may attenuate the inflammatory response and their use should be weighed against the risk of further immunosuppression.

ASPLENIA

Patients who have undergone splenectomy or who are functionally asplenic secondary to underlying disease (sickle cell disease, splenic artery thrombosis, malaria, infiltrative disease) are at increased risk for severe sepsis by encapsulated organisms including *S. pneumoniae, H. influenzae,* and *N. meningitidis.* It is important to inquire about prior immunizations as effective vaccines exist against each of these organisms.

BIOLOGIC AGENTS

Tumor necrosis factor (TNF) antagonists (etanercept, infliximab, adalimumab) have found increased use in the treatment of rheumatoid arthritis, Crohn's disease, and other inflammatory autoimmune disorders. Patients with untreated latent *M. tuberculosis* infection are susceptible to developing active disease after initiation of a TNF antagonist. Infections with opportunistic organisms (*T. gondii,* endemic fungi) as well as nontuberculous mycobacteria, *Legionella pneumophila,* and *Listeria monocytogenes* have been reported.

SUGGESTED READINGS

Corona A, Raimondi F. Caring for HIV-infected patients in the ICU in the highly active antiretroviral therapy era. *Curr HIV Res.* 2009;7:569–579.

Fishman JA. Infection in solid-organ transplant recipients. *N Engl J Med.* 2007;357:2601–2614.

Hiemenz JW. Management of infections complicating allogeneic hematopoietic stem cell transplantation. *Semin Hematol.* 2009;46:289–312.

Linden PK. Approach to the immunocompromised host with infection in the intensive care unit. *Infect Dis Clin North Am.* 2009;23:535–556.

41

Prevention of Infection in the Intensive Care Unit

Amy M. Richmond

Infections acquired in the intensive care unit (ICU) are a significant contributor to morbidity and mortality in hospitalized patients. ICU-acquired infections increase patient length of stay and can lead to excess costs well beyond $50,000 per occurrence. Multiple measures to prevent the transmission of organisms within the ICU are necessary. Transmission-based precautions including contact, droplet, and airborne should be instituted when necessary, and health care worker compliance should be monitored. Contact precautions (gowns and gloves) should be instituted for those with antibiotic-resistant organisms such as methicillin-resistant *Staphylococcus aureus,* vancomycin-resistant *Enterococcus,* multiple-drug resistant Gram-negative bacterium, and *Clostridium difficile.* Droplet precautions (donning a surgical mask) are necessary for large droplet infectious agents such as influenza and the meningococcus. Airborne precautions (N95 respirator and negative-pressure ventilation) are used for airborne infectious agents such as *Mycobacterium tuberculosis* and varicella. To prevent health care worker and patient exposure, transmission-based precautions must be instituted on first clinical suspicion. Infection prevention should be consulted in cases in which a patient or health care worker exposure may have taken place.

Foremost in prevention of infections is adequate hand hygiene prior to placing and/or handling an invasive device or examining a patient. Alcohol-based hand rubs placed at the bedside have been shown to increase compliance as well as maintain the skin integrity of health care workers' hands and should be encouraged. Alcohol hand rubs can be used whenever hands are not visibly soiled. Antimicrobial soaps should also be available in the ICU setting for use when hands are soiled or following a body substance exposure. Effective cleaning and disinfection of the ICU environment also plays a key role in transmission of microorganisms.

Hospital-acquired infections that are device-associated, such as ventilator-associated pneumonia (VAP) and central line-associated bloodstream infections (CLABSI), pose the greatest risk to hospitalized patients. VAP is reported by the Centers for Disease Control (CDC) as the second most common hospital-acquired infection after Foley catheter-associated urinary tract infections. Central venous catheter-related BSIs are also a concern and can lead to other infectious complications such as endocarditis, septic thrombophlebitis, and osteomyelitis. The CDC, the Institute for Healthcare Quality Improvement (IHI) and the Society for Healthcare Epidemiology

TABLE 41.1	Summary of Recommendations for the Prevention of Ventilator-Associated Pneumonia

Education and training

Educate health care workers regarding the epidemiology of, and infection control procedures for, preventing health care-associated bacterial pneumonia in such manner as to ensure worker competency according to the worker's level of responsibility in the health care setting.

Hand hygiene and aseptic technique

Decontaminate hands with soap and water or with a waterless antiseptic agent after contact with mucous membranes, respiratory secretions, or objects contaminated with respiratory secretions, before and after contact with a patient who has an endotracheal or tracheostomy tube in place, before and after contact with any respiratory device that is used on patients, between contacts with different patients, after handling respiratory secretions or objects contaminated with secretions from one patient and before contact with another patient, object, or environmental surface; and between contacts with a contaminated body site and the respiratory tract of, or respiratory device on, the same patient.

When soiling with respiratory secretions from a patient is anticipated, wear a gown and change it after soiling occurs and before providing care to another patient. Use only sterile or pasteurized fluid to remove secretions from the suction catheter if the catheter is to be used for re-entry into the patient's lower respiratory tract. If the closed-system suction is used, change the in-line suction catheter when it malfunctions or becomes visibly soiled.

Prevention of aspiration

Remove devices such as endotracheal, tracheostomy, and/or enteral (i.e., oro- or nasogastric, or jejunal) tubes from patients and discontinue enteral-tube feeding as soon as the clinical indications for these are resolved.

As much as possible, avoid subjecting patients who have received mechanically assisted ventilation to repeat endotracheal intubations.

Maintain an endotracheal cuff pressure of at least 20 cm H_2O.

Unless contraindicated by the patient's condition, perform orotracheal rather than nasotracheal intubation.

If there is no medical contraindication, elevate at an angle of 30 to 45 degrees the head of the bed of a patient at high risk for aspiration pneumonia, e.g., a person receiving mechanically assisted ventilation and/or who has an enteral tube in place.

Routinely assess the patient's intestinal motility (e.g., by auscultating for bowel sounds and measuring residual gastric volume or abdominal girth) and adjust the rate and volume of enteral feeding to avoid regurgitation.

Routinely verify appropriate placement of the feeding tube.

Perform regular antiseptic oral care in accordance with product guidelines.

Ventilator circuits

Do not change routinely, on the basis of duration of use, the ventilator circuit (i.e., ventilator tubing, exhalation valve, and the attached humidifier) that is in use on an individual patient. Rather, change the circuit when it is visibly soiled or mechanically malfunctioning.

(continued)

TABLE 41.1	Summary of Recommendations for the Prevention of Ventilator-Associated Pneumonia (*Continued*)

Periodically drain and discard any condensate that collects in the tubing of a mechanical ventilator, taking precautions not to allow condensate to drain toward the patient.

Use an endotracheal tube with a dorsal lumen above the endotracheal cuff to allow drainage (by continuous suctioning) of tracheal secretions that accumulate in the patient's subglottic area.

Before deflating the cuff of an endotracheal tube in preparation for tube removal, or before moving the tube, ensure that secretions are cleared from above the tube cuff.

Use sterile water to rinse reusable respiratory equipment.

Store and disinfect respiratory therapy equipment properly.

Adapted from Tablan OC, Anderson LJ, Besser R, et al. Guidelines for preventing health-care-associated pneumonia, 2003. *MMWR Recomm Rep.* 2004;53(RR03):1–36 and Coffin SE, Klompas M, Classen D, et al. Strategies to prevent ventilator-associated pneumonia in acute care hospitals. *Infect Control Hosp Epidemiol.* 2008;29:S31–S40.

(SHEA) have published evidence-based guidelines for the prevention of device-associated infections and are summarized in Tables 41.1 and 41.2.

Invasive devices allow organisms a portal of entry during a time when the patient is particularly susceptible to infection. Therefore, general prevention measures should include a daily review of the necessity of all invasive devices and removing them as soon as they are no longer clinically necessary. Clinician-driven ventilator-weaning protocols have been shown to be effective in decreasing VAP rates and are reviewed in Chapter 17.

Additional prevention measures are aimed at the placement and maintenance of the device. Recommendations to prevent VAP are aimed at preventing aspiration of secretions, colonization of the aerodigestive tract, and contamination of the ventilator circuit. Maintaining the head of the patient's bed at a minimum of 30 degrees assists with prevention of aspiration of gastric contents. In addition, the ventilator circuit should remain closed as much as possible and in-line suctioning devices should be collected after use.

The use of sucralfate, H_2-antagonists, or proton pump inhibitors (PPI) for peptic ulcer disease prophylaxis in ventilated patients has come into question in recent years. While the IHI ventilator bundle promotes peptic ulcer disease prophylaxis, the SHEA and CDC documents consider this to be an unresolved issue. The SHEA guidelines state this in an unresolved issue stating that acid-suppressive therapy may increase colonization of the aerodigestive tract.

The risk for CLABSI in the ICU is high due to the prolonged use of multiple catheters that are frequently accessed. Recommendations to prevent BSI include placing the central venous catheter (CVC) while observing aseptic technique and using maximal sterile barriers including sterile gown, sterile gloves, mask, and a full drape. A chlorhexidine and alcohol tincture is the preferred agent for skin antisepsis prior to CVC placement, as well as preparation during dressing changes. When selecting a site for insertion, the femoral vain should be avoided. The subclavian vein has the least instance of infection; however, the risk and benefits of infections and noninfectious

TABLE 41.2	Summary of Recommendations for the Prevention of Bloodstream Infection

Education and training

Educate health care workers regarding the indications for intravascular catheter use, proper procedures for the insertion and maintenance of intravascular catheters, and appropriate infection control measures to prevent intravascular catheter related infections.

Assess knowledge of and adherence to guidelines periodically for all persons who insert and manage intravascular catheters.

Designate trained personnel for the insertion and maintenance of intravascular catheters and designate personnel who have been trained and exhibit competency in the insertion of catheters to supervise trainees.

Hand hygiene and aseptic technique

Observe proper hand-hygiene procedures either by washing hands with conventional antiseptic-containing soap and water or with alcohol-based hand rubs (ABHR). Observe hand hygiene before and after inserting, replacing, accessing, repairing, or dressing an intravascular catheter. Use of gloves does not obviate the need for hand hygiene.

Use aseptic technique including the use of a cap, mask, sterile gown, sterile gloves, and a large sterile sheet, for the insertion of CVCs (including peripherally inserted CVCs) or guidewire exchange.

Wear clean or sterile gloves when changing the dressing on intravascular catheters.

Disinfect clean skin with an appropriate antiseptic before catheter insertion and during dressing changes. Although a 0.5% chlorhexidine-based preparation is preferred, tincture of iodine, or 70% alcohol, can be used.

Allow the antiseptic to remain on the insertion site and to air dry before catheter insertion. Allow povidone iodine to remain on the skin for at least 2 minutes, or longer if it is not yet dry before insertion.

Use either sterile gauze or sterile, transparent, semipermeable dressing to cover the catheter site. Replace catheter-site dressing at least every sevendays, and if the dressing becomes damp, loosened, or visibly soiled.

Do not use topical antibiotic ointment or creams on insertion sites (except when using dialysis catheters) because of their potential to promote fungal infections and antimicrobial resistance.

Clean catheter hubs, caps, or injection ports prior to access with an alcoholic chlorhexidine preparation or 70% alcohol to reduce contamination.

Site and catheter selection

Select the catheter, insertion technique, and insertion site with the lowest risk for complications (infectious and noninfectious) for the anticipated type and duration of IV therapy. Use a subclavian site (rather than a jugular or a femoral site) in adult patients to minimize infection risk for nontunneled CVC placement when not contraindicated.

Use a CVC with the minimum number of ports or lumens essential for the management of the patient.

Do not routinely replace central venous or arterial catheters solely for the purposes of reducing the incidence of infection.

(continued)

TABLE 41.2	Summary of Recommendations for the Prevention of Bloodstream Infection (*Continued*)

Catheter discontinuation and replacement

Promptly remove any intravascular catheter that is no longer essential.

Replace any short-term CVC if purulence is observed at the insertion site.

Do not use guidewire exchanges to replace catheters in patients suspected of having catheter-related infection or routinely to prevent infection.

Pressure monitoring

Use disposable, rather than reusable, transducer assemblies when possible.

Replace disposable or reusable transducers at 96-hour intervals. Replace other components of the system (including the tubing, continuous-flush device, and flush solution) at the time the transducer is replaced.

When the pressure monitoring system is accessed through a diaphragm rather than a stopcock, wipe the diaphragm with an appropriate antiseptic before accessing the system.

CVC, central venous catheter; IV, intravenous.

Adapted from O'Grady NP, Alexander M, Dellinger EP, et al. Guidelines for the prevention of intravascular catheter-related infections. *MMWR*. 2002;51(RR10):1–29 and Marschall J, Mermel LA, Classen D, et al. Strategies to prevent central line-associated bloodstream infections in acute care hospitals. *Infect Control Hosp Epidemiol*. 2008;29;S22–S30.

complications should be weighed out on an individual basis. The use of a catheter insertion checklist and a standardized insertion kit to promote best practices is also recommended. The decision to use antimicrobial or antiseptic impregnated catheters, devices, dressings, or sponges should be made by the critical care and infection prevention team and based on an evaluation of current infection rates and compliance with evidence-based practices. A summary of CDC and SHEA guidelines for CVC placement and maintenance can be viewed in Table 41.2. Clinical management of catheter-related BSIs is described in Chapter 37.

Finally, surveillance for ICU-acquired infections using standardized definitions should take place on a routine basis in order to monitor patient outcomes of care. Infection rates should be provided to ICU medical and nursing staff for review, and immediate action taken in times of increased rates. Additionally, prevention measures should be monitored regularly for consistency of application. For optimal reduction in the transmission of infections, all evidence-based prevention methods for each infection must be applied together. Such a concept is the basis for the IHI prevention of infection "bundles."

SUGGESTED READINGS

Coffin SE, Klompas M, Classen D, et al. Strategies to prevent ventilator-associated pneumonia in acute care hospitals. *Infect Control Hosp Epidemiol*. 2008;29:S31–S40.

Ely EW, Meade MO, Haponik EF, et al. Mechanical ventilator weaning protocols driven by nonphysician health-care professionals: evidence-based clinical practice guidelines. *Chest*. 2001;120(6, suppl):454S–463S.
  Recommendations based on 4 randomized controlled trials and 11 nonrandomized control trials for the protocol-driven weaning of patients from mechanical ventilation.

Marschall J, Mermel LA, Classen D, et al. Strategies to prevent central line-associated bloodstream infections in acute care hospitals. *Infect Control Hosp Epidemiol.* 2008;29:S22–S30.

O'Grady NP, Alexander M, Dellinger EP, et al. Guidelines for the prevention of intravascular catheter-related infections. *MMWR Recomm Rep.* 2002;51(RR10):1–29.

CDC guidelines discussing the microbiology, pathogenesis, and prevention of intravascular catheter-related infections.

Tablan OC, Anderson LJ, Besser R, et al. Guidelines for preventing health-care-associated pneumonia, 2003. *MMWR Recomm Rep.* 2004;53(RR03):1–36.

CDC update discussing the prevention of HCAP, including prevention of transmission of bacterial, viral, and fungal pathogens.

The Hospital Infection Control Practices Advisory Committee. Guideline for isolation precautions in hospitals. Part II. Recommendations for isolation precautions in hospitals. *Am J Infect Control.* 1996;24:24–52.

The Centers for Disease Control and Prevention and the Hospital Infection Control Practices Advisory Committee's revised recommendations for isolation policies/procedures regarding hospital infection control.

42

Clostridium difficile and Other Infectious Causes of Diarrhea

Linda D. Bobo and Erik R. Dubberke

The most commonly encountered etiologies of infectious diarrhea in hospitalized adults in industrialized countries are *Clostridium difficile*, with *Salmonella spp.*, norovirus, and rotavirus, and *Cryptosporidium* in the immunocompromised host being less common.

INFECTIOUS ETIOLOGIES

Diarrhea adversely impacts critically ill patients by contributing to dehydration, electrolyte imbalances, hemodynamic instability, malnutrition, and skin breakdown. Most diarrhea in hospitalized patients is noninfectious. However, it is essential to consider an infectious etiology in an ICU patient with diarrhea, especially if the patient has ≥3 watery bowel movements per day, blood or mucus in the stool, vomiting, severe abdominal pain, and/or fever. A modified "3-day rule" was proposed to aid in when to culture stool for enteropathogenic bacteria other than *C. difficile*. This rule is a safe and cost-effective cut-off for rejecting stool samples of adult patients. Non-*C. difficile* enteric pathogenic bacteria and parasites are detected in <1% of patients hospitalized for >3 days with diarrhea. Proposed exceptions to the "3-day rule" are the presence of neutropenia ($<0.5 \times 10^6$ cells/mL), human immunodeficiency virus (HIV) infection, suspected nondiarrheal manifestation of enteric infection (erythema nodosum, mesenteric lymphadenitis, polyarthritis, fever of unknown origin), patient older than 65 years with comorbidities causing end-organ damage, or a suspected hospital-acquired outbreak.

Establishing the etiology if an infectious cause of diarrhea is suspected is important so pathogen-specific treatment can by initiated (if available), and the appropriate precautions can be taken to prevent transmission to other patients. It is important to obtain history of recent antibiotic use, type of food consumed, ingestion of untreated water, recent travel, contact with animals and ill family members, immunosuppression due to HIV or chemotherapy, asplenia, sickle cell disease, and residence in a nursing home in the past 30 days. It is also important to be cognizant that some etiologies of infectious diarrhea occur seasonally, such as norovirus because hospital outbreaks can be coincident with those in the community. The fecal-oral route is the usual mode of infection, and person-to-person spread is the most common form of transmission. It is important to work with Infectious Diseases and Infection Prevention and

Control personnel to implement appropriate measures to halt the spread of the causative organism to other patients and staff in the ICU.

Clostridium difficile Infection

C. difficile is the leading cause of hospital-associated infectious diarrhea. It has also surpassed methicillin-resistant *Staphylococcus aureus* as the leading cause of hospital-associated infections. In the past 10 years, there has been a dramatic increase in incidence and severity of *C. difficile* infection (CDI). These increases are associated in part with the emergence of a new prevalent strain of *C. difficile*, the BI/NAP1/027 strain. This strain is highly fluoroquinolone resistant, produces more toxin A and B *in vitro* than typical strains that cause disease in humans, and produces a third toxin, binary toxin.

C. difficile is a spore-forming anaerobic bacillus that produces two exotoxins, A and B, which cause intestinal pathology. Most patients who acquire *C. difficile* remain asymptomatic. When *C. difficile* does cause symptomatic infection, this is referred to as CDI. Most strains produce both toxin A and B. A low percentage of strains produce only toxin B. These strains can cause the same spectrum of illness as strains that produce both toxins, and have caused hospital-associated outbreaks. Nontoxigenic strains are nonpathogenic. The differences in ability to produce toxin are important from a diagnostic standpoint, as some diagnostics detect *C. difficile* whether or not it produces toxin, and some detect only toxin A. This is discussed in more detail below.

Antimicrobial exposure is the most common and potentially modifiable risk factor for CDI, especially in the ICU where patients are frequently on several antibiotic classes concurrently. Historically, the most common antibiotics associated with CDI have been clindamycin, broad-spectrum cephalosporins, and ampicillin/amoxicillin, but most all antibacterial agents can predispose to CDI. In addition, the fluoroquinolones have been increasingly associated with CDI due in part to the emerging epidemic NAP1/027 strain that is highly fluoroquinolone resistant. Patients can become symptomatic during treatment or several weeks after antibiotics have been stopped. Other risk factors include increasing age and severity of underlying illness. Although the mechanism is unclear, gastric acid suppressants such as H_2 antagonists and proton pump inhibitors are also associated with increased CDI. Recently CDI pressure, or the number of other patients with CDI in the same patient care area as the patient at risk, was found to be one of the factors most strongly associated with CDI. This provides additional evidence CDI is caused from acquisition of *C. difficile* within the hospital setting, and stresses the importance of preventing transmission of *C. difficile* from patients with CDI.

Assessment

Symptoms of CDI range from mild, self-limited diarrhea to life-threatening colitis. Fatal ileitis has also been recently recognized, but is uncommon. Common symptoms of CDI include a watery, distinctive-smelling diarrhea (barn-like odor), nausea, and mild abdominal pain or cramping. About 30% of patients with CDI are febrile and 50% have a leukocytosis. A white blood count (WBC) >20,000 may herald a patient at risk for rapid progression to fulminate colitis with the systemic inflammatory response syndrome and shock. Although diarrhea is the hallmark for symptomatic CDI, severe abdominal pain and lack of diarrhea could indicate the patient has ileus with toxic megacolon. There are no validated methods to identify patients at risk for poor outcomes due to CDI, but factors associated with poor outcomes due to CDI include advanced age, acute renal insufficiency, WBC >20,000, immunosuppression, and hypoalbuminemia.

Diagnosis

C. difficile should be suspected in adults and children ≥1 year old with unexplained diarrhea or if ileus is present in association with recent antibiotic use. Patients with pseudomembranes at endoscopy should be presumed to have CDI, but pseudomembranes are present in only 50% of patients with CDI. Diagnosis of CDI is most commonly established with detection of *C. difficile* and/or its toxins in patients with diarrhea. The most commonly used method is a toxin A/B enzyme immunoassay (EIA). Although results can be obtained in several hours and most clinical laboratories can perform the test, it has variable sensitivity and specificity. It is important to note that some toxin EIAs detect only toxin A, and these assays will miss strains that produce only toxin B. The cell culture cytotoxicity assay is often referred to as the "gold standard" of *C. difficile* diagnostics, but it is not as sensitive or specific as toxigenic culture. In addition, this test requires a tissue culture facility, is labor intensive, is operator dependent, and takes 24 to 48 hours, or longer, for results.

An EIA for *C. difficile* glutamate dehydrogenase (GDH) is advocated by some in an algorithmic approach as a screening test. The GDH EIA is highly sensitive in general but it isn't specific for toxigenic *C. difficile*. It will detect nontoxigenic *C. difficile* and some non-*C. difficile* strains that also produce GDH. In the algorithmic approach, stools submitted for *C. difficile* testing are first screened with the GDH EIA. GDH-negative results are reported out as negative. GDH-positive specimens are tested with a confirmatory assay, typically an assay that is more sensitive than a toxin EIA but may be prohibitive to use from a cost or labor stand point on every specimen, such as the cell culture cytotoxicity assay, polymerase chain reaction (PCR), or toxigenic culture. A caveat to the algorithmic approach is the GDH assay has not always been found to be 100% sensitive. If the initial screen is not 100% sensitive, any benefit of this approach to avoid false negative results versus toxin EIAs is quickly lost. A positive GDH test would need to be followed with confirmatory cell culture cytotoxicity test. The most sensitive and specific testing is anaerobic culture of stool with confirmation that the isolate produces neutralizable toxin by tissue culture cytotoxicity testing.

The most sensitive and specific method to detect toxigenic *C. difficile*, when performed correctly, is toxigenic culture. Anaerobic culture of stool using selective methods is used to isolate *C. difficile*, and toxin production is confirmed *in vitro*. However, this method is not typically clinically feasible due to cost, labor, and minimal 72 to 96 hour turnaround time. PCR assays that detect the *C. difficile* toxin B gene are also available. These tests are rapid, and have increased sensitivity but are expensive. Common practices that are discouraged include automatic repeat testing (e.g., *C. difficile* × 3), test of cure, and testing asymptomatic patients, as all of these can lead to misleading results.

Treatment

Supportive therapy with fluid and electrolytes repletion should be provided. In addition, it is recommended to discontinue the offending antibiotic if possible as this may reduce the risk of CDI recurrence. Recently published guidelines recommend specific anti-*C. difficile* treatment should be based on CDI severity and whether the infection is recurrent (Table 42.1). Metronidazole at 500 mg three times a day orally is used for mild or moderate CDI, and oral vancomycin at 125 mg four times a day is recommended for severe or multiply recurrent CDI. In a prospective, randomized blinded placebo

TABLE 42.1	Treatment Guidelines Based on Clinical Severity and Number of Recurrences
Presentation	Treatment and cautions
Initial infection with mild or moderate infection	Metronidazole 500 mg PO q8h, 10–14 days; multiple and prolonged courses can cause irreversible peripheral neuropathy
Severe infection without complications	Vancomycin 125 mg PO q6h, 10–14 days
Severe infection with complications	Vancomycin 500 mg q6h PO or by NG tube plus metronidazole 500 mg IV q8h Vancomycin 250 mg q6h per rectal retention enema for ileus Surgical consult for possible subtotal colectomy
First recurrence	Same as initial infection based on disease severity
After a second relapse within 30–90 days or if the patient's condition significantly worsens after treatment cessation	Vancomycin taper or pulse dosing Taper: Week 1: 125 mg PO q6h; Week 2: 125 mg q12h; Week 3: 125 mg daily; Week 4: 125 mg every other day; Week 5–6: 125 mg every 3 days. Pulse dosing: up to 125–500 mg PO every 2–3 days for 3 weeks

controlled trial, there was no difference between metronidazole and vancomycin for clinical cure of mild CDI, but vancomycin was associated with increased cure in severe disease. There was no difference for either drug for preventing recurrent CDI. The caveat, as previously stated, is there are no validated methods to reliably detect which patients are most likely to benefit from oral vancomycin based on CDI severity.

It is recommended to administer both intravenous metronidazole and a higher dose of oral vancomycin for patients with CDI who are hemodynamically unstable. There are no data to indicate there is synergy between metronidazole and vancomycin, or data to suggest a higher dose of vancomycin is better than the standard 125 mg dose (which achieves levels of vancomycin 500 to 1000 times the MIC_{90} of *C. difficile* in stool). Rather, the rationale behind this recommendation is an attempt to get therapeutic antibiotics to the colon as quickly as possible in these acutely ill patients. It is also recommended that a surgical consult be obtained for these patients as they may require a therapeutic colectomy. Vancomycin retention enemas of 250 mg in 250 mL of normal saline four times daily should be considered if the patient has an ileus. Intravenous immunoglobulin (IVIG) at 500 mg/kg for 1 to 3 doses has been used as well in patients with fulminate colitis. A retrospective, propensity score matched case-control study failed to demonstrate benefit of IVIG for severe CDI; however, time from symptom onset to administration of IVIG was not controlled for.

In general, about 20% of patients with an initial episode of CDI will have a recurrence, 45% of patients with one recurrence will have another recurrence, and at >60% with at least two recurrences will recur again. The recommended treatment of multiply recurrent CDI (defined as at least third episode of CDI) is tapered oral vancomycin. Vancomycin is initially administered four times a day for 10 to 14 days, and then a dose per day is removed a week at a time until the patient is taking one dose every 2 to 3 days. The rationale for this regimen is as the doses are spaced out it allows the colonic flora to regenerate.

There are numerous adjunctive treatments of CDI in the literature with poor quality of data to support their use. Anion-binding resins, such as cholestyramine and colestipol, are often administered for recurrent CDI. These agents have been found to be inferior to vancomycin and no better than placebo for the treatment of CDI. These agents do bind vancomycin, so it is advisable to not administer them concomitantly if the patient requires oral vancomycin for severe CDI. Probiotics have not been found to be of benefit when treating an acute episode of CDI or for preventing recurrent CDI when studied in randomized trials. In addition, patients in ICUs are at increased risk for infections due to probiotic organisms. IVIG has also been used to treat relapsing CDI. Many of patients who develop recurrent CDI individuals have a poor immunoglobulin G response to *C. difficile* toxins. In a small unmatched study of relapsing CDI cases, IVIG along with 500 mg of oral vancomycin three times per day was used, and a durable response was reached at 3 months in most of the patients.

There are several investigational agents that show some promise. Fidaxomicin (also known as OPT-80 and PAR-101) is a new narrow spectrum macrocyclic antibiotic that is not absorbed systemically. Fidaxomicin achieves very high levels in the stool, and it does not disrupt the normal intestinal microflora to the extent of metronidazole and vancomycin. These properties may contribute to its increased efficacy in phase 3 trials as compared with vancomycin for global cure of CDI by decreasing the relapse rate. It was also shown to be noninferior to oral vancomycin for clinical cure of CDI. Fully humanized monoclonal antibodies to toxins A and B (Medarex/Merck CDA1+CDB1) are in trials for treating relapsing infection. The Medarex/Merck antibodies were designed to be given with anti-*C. difficile* antibiotics, as it does not cure the infection. Vaccine research aimed at prevention of infection is underway.

Infection Control

The approaches for preventing acquisition of CDI in the hospital are to decrease risk of CDI if exposure occurs, and to prevent transmission to other patients. Decreasing the risk of CDI if transmission occurs involves antimicrobial stewardship. The first line of defense against CDI is healthy intestinal flora. By decreasing the numbers of patients on antimicrobials and/or decreasing high-risk antimicrobial exposures, the number of patients at risk for CDI is decreased if *C. difficile* exposure occurs. Up to 25% of antibiotic usage is not needed and this is true even in the ICU setting.

C. difficile transmission is through fecal-oral route. Infected patients can excrete large numbers of spores in feces. The resistant spore serves as a vehicle for transmission by contaminating hands of health care workers, bedding, and other structures in the patient's room and unit. Hand contamination can occur even when the patient is not touched. Strategies to interrupt transmission involve using contact precautions, signage, and environmental cleaning. Quaternary detergents used to clean patient rooms are not sporicidal, so using sporicidal hypochlorite-based disinfectants on surfaces (1000 to 5000 ppm) is recommended in outbreak settings. Routine use of sporicidal agents to clean the environment is not routinely recommended in nonoutbreak settings, as they do not appear to be associated with reductions in CDI. Despite the fact that alcohol does not kill *C. difficile* spores and alcohol-based hand hygiene products are less effective than hand washing at removing spores from hands of volunteers, it is not recommended to preferentially perform hand hygiene after caring for a patient with CDI in non-outbreak settings. Numerous studies have failed to demonstrate an increase in CDI with the use of alcohol-based hand hygiene products, and no studies have demonstrated decrease in CDI with use of soap and water. Potential explanations for these findings are extremely poor adherence to hand hygiene when soap and water is the preferred method, gloves are effective at preventing contamination of hands, and potential for contamination of hands after removing gloves if the sink used to wash hands is the same sink used by the patient.

Other Infectious Agents

Many bacteria, viruses, and parasites have similar clinical presentations. The most commonly encountered in industrialized countries are *Salmonella spp.*, norovirus, rotavirus, and *Cryptosporidium* (Table 42.2). Excluding *C. difficile*, these four organisms have a higher reported incidence of infection in the health care setting than other bacterial, viral, or parasitic pathogens. They may occur concurrently with community or institutional outbreaks. When associated with large institutional outbreaks, these organisms have caused substantial economic loss due to unit closures, furloughing or cohorting staff, with need for extensive disinfection.

Recognition of *Salmonella* outbreaks can be difficult due to longer incubation period and because this organism can cause extraintestinal infection. Antibiotics are usually not used because the gastroenteritis is usually self-limited, and antibiotics will prolong shedding in the stool after symptoms resolve. The exceptions are moderate or severe disease, bacteremia, sickle cell disease or prosthetic grafts, extraintestinal disease, and disease in immunocompromised hosts. Stool cultures are the main stay of diagnosis, and blood cultures are indicated if persistent fever or signs of sepsis are present. *Salmonella* is a reportable disease, and local reporting requirements should be followed. It is frequently associated with contaminated food, and one case should prompt an investigation of whether it is health care associated. Because the hospital case/outbreak could be part of a larger epidemic, it is important that the ICU works closely with infectious diseases specialists, infection prevention and control personnel, and public health officials. Standard disinfectants and alcohol-based hand hygiene products are effective against *Salmonella spp.* Contact precautions are reserved for incontinent or diapered patients to control institutional spread.

Norovirus is disseminated by transfer of infective feces and/or vomitus. Specific diagnosis requires laboratory confirmation because the signs and symptoms of norovirus are not specific. Testing is not routinely done in clinical laboratories in the United States and may require collaboration with the local department of public health. Serology can be useful because diarrhea is generally short lived and limits the time available to collect samples for characterizing outbreaks. Norovirus has been associated with pseudo-outbreaks of *C. difficile* due to more frequent testing for *C. difficile* and detection of asymptomatic *C. difficile* colonization in patients with diarrhea due to norovirus. Treatment is supportive in nature. Early recognition of norovirus is important because it has a short incubation period of 24 hour and can disseminate rapidly in the hospital causing large economic loss and morbidity. All patients with norovirus injection should remain in contact precautions for the duration of their illness. Special attention to environmental cleaning is needed even if surfaces do not appear to be soiled. It may be necessary to use bleach (500 ppm available chlorine) to clean the environment during an outbreak. Aerosolization as a mode of infection may occur, so those engaged in cleaning heavily infected areas should wear masks. Although norovirus is relatively resistant to alcohol, there is no evidence that alcohol-based hand hygiene products are not effective for hand decontamination.

TABLE 42.2 Other Common Causes of Bacterial, Viral, and Parasitic Diarrhea Found in the Hospital

Organism	Transmission	Incubation period	Symptom duration	Laboratory diagnosis	Treatment	Control measures
Salmonella spp.	Food, water, fecal contact	6–48 hr	3–7 days	Culture	Non-typhi: supportive; ciprofloxacin 500 mg PO daily 5–7 days; bacteremia-ciprofloxacin 400 mg IV q12h ×14 days (switching to 750 mg bid when possible) or ceftriaxone 2 gm IV q24h × 14 days (switch to PO cipro)	Review food handling; contact precautions
Norovirus	Fecal, vomitus contact	24 hr	2–3 days	If needed EIA, RT-PCR	Supportive	Contact precautions; consistent environmental cleaning, disinfection; hypochlorite if continued transmission; consider cohorting affected patients to separate airspaces, toilet facilities
Rotavirus	Fecal contact	24–72 hr	1–4 days	RT-PCR, EIA, EM	Supportive	Contact precautions; consistent environmental cleaning, disinfection, frequent diapering
Cryptosporidium	Fecal contact, food, water	1–30 days	5–10 days or chronic	Smear, EIA, PCR	Supportive: immunocompetent-no HIV: nitazoxanide 500 mg PO bid × 3 days; HIV-effective antiretrovirals; nitazoxanide not licensed for immunodeficient patients	Contact precautions

Laboratory diagnosis – EIA, enzyme immunoassay; RT-PCR, reverse transcriptase polymerase chain reaction.

Rotavirus is spread by fecal-oral route. Infection is more prevalent in children but has caused severe infection with associated mortality in hospitalized adults. Profuse watery diarrhea with dehydration and electrolyte abnormalities is generally more severe in infants and children than diarrhea with other common enteric pathogens. In immunocompromised children, rotavirus can be associated with chronic diarrhea, prolonged shedding, and extraintestinal infection. Confirmation of rotavirus is important in complicated cases, in immunocompromised patients, and for epidemiologic infection control purposes. Rotavirus can be detected by EIA for VP2 and VP6 viral proteins in stool, but reverse transcriptase PCR is now the major diagnostic test. Treatment is primarily supportive. All patients with rotavirus infection should be placed on contact precautions for the duration of their illness. Rotavirus is generally a hardy virus and resists inactivation by chlorination in sewage effluents and drinking water. It can be inactivated by antiseptics with >40% alcohol, free chlorine >20,000 ppm, and phenol-based compounds.

Cryptosporidium is a protozoan parasite that is infectious by way of feces contaminated with the oocyst. Symptoms vary from mild, self-limited to extremely severe. Relapses can occur following a diarrhea-free period of days to weeks. It can also cause chronic diarrhea, especially in HIV patients with low CD4 counts who have had inadequate highly active retroviral therapy (HAART). Chronic diarrhea is characterized by frequent, foul-smelling bulky stools with development of malabsorption, or less frequently, voluminous watery diarrhea. In HIV-AIDS patients, *Cryptosporidium* can also cause extraintestinal infection. For laboratory diagnosis, sensitivity and specificity for the acid-fast stain of the oocyst is poor, and antigen EIA gives variable sensitivity and specificity. PCR has the best sensitivity and specificity for detection in stool of the diagnostic tests. Treatment of immunocompetent patients is primarily supportive. For HIV patients, HAART is their best option, and nitazoxanide has had variable results. Large community outbreaks have occurred due to contamination of surface water. Hospital-associated infections are uncommon, and this organism has been shown to have low infection transmission in the hospital setting. Patients with bowel incontinence or who are diapered should be placed in contact precautions for the duration of their illness. The oocyst is relatively resistant to a variety of environmental cleaners, but a 1000-fold decrease in infectivity occurs with a 4-minute exposure to 6% to 7% hydrogen peroxide. Despite the resistance of *Cryptosporidium* oocysts to multiple agents, standard hospital disinfectants can be used in the absence of an institutional outbreak.

SUGGESTED READINGS

Bauer TM, Lalvani A, Fehrenbach J, et al. Derivation and validation of guidelines for stool cultures for enteropathogenic bacteria other than Clostridium difficile in hospitalized patients. *JAMA*. 2001;285:313–319.

Bobo LD, Dubberke ER. Recognition and prevention of hospital-associated enteric infections in the intensive care unit. *Crit Care Med*. 2010;38(suppl):S324–S334.

Cohen SH, Gerding DN, Johnson S, et al. Clinical Practice Guidelines for *Clostridium difficile* Clinical Practice Guidelines *for Clostridium difficile* Infection in Adults: 2010 Update by the Society for Healthcare Epidemiology of America (SHEA) and the Infectious Diseases Society of America (IDSA). *Infect Control Hosp Epidemiol*. 2010;31:431–455.

Fan K, Morris AJ, Reller LB. Application of rejection criteria for stool cultures for bacterial enteric pathogens. *J Clin Microbiol*. 1993;31:2233–2235.

Valenstein P, Pfaller M, Yungbluth M. The use and abuse of routine stool microbiology: a College of American Pathologists Q-probes study of 601 institutions. *Arch Pathol Lab Med*. 1996;120:206–211.

43 Acute Kidney Injury

Tingting Li and Anitha Vijayan

Acute kidney injury (AKI) is the term proposed by the Acute Kidney Injury Network (AKIN) to represent the entire spectrum of acute renal dysfunction. It is a common clinical problem encountered in critically ill patients, frequently in the setting of multiorgan failure, and is an independent risk factor for increased in-hospital and long-term mortality.

DEFINITION

The lack of consensus definition for AKI confounds the comparisons between studies of prevention, therapy, and outcome. The RIFLE (risk, injury, failure, loss of kidney function, and end-stage kidney disease) criteria (Table 43.1) and the AKIN criteria (Tables 43.2 and 43.3) are two currently accepted definitions developed in an effort to standardize the definition of AKI.

RIFLE is a multilevel classification system of AKI, consisting of three graded levels of injury (risk, injury, and failure), and two clinical outcome categories (loss and ESKD). The RIFLE criteria seem to correlate with prognosis, with a progressive increase in mortality as the level of injury increases.

The AKIN criterion is a modification of the RIFLE criteria. It consists of both diagnostic criteria for AKI and a staging system. The staging system corresponds to risk, injury, and failure of the RIFLE criteria.

Patients with AKI are frequently classified as being nonoliguric (urine output >400 mL/day), oliguric (urine output <400 mL/day), or anuric (urine output <100 mL/day). Lower urine output suggests more severe renal injury, and is associated with a worse outcome. Prognosis is also worse in patients who require renal replacement therapy. Therefore, a timely diagnosis is critical, as identification and prompt treatment of the cause of renal injury may hasten recovery and avoid the need for dialysis.

DIAGNOSTIC APPROACH TO THE PATIENT WITH AKI

AKI is a syndrome of multiple etiologies. In using an algorithmic approach in the evaluation of AKI, a key step early in the process is to delineate whether the insult is prerenal, intrinsic, or postrenal (Algorithm 43.1). In many cases, the patient's history, physical examination, laboratory/radiographic data, and meticulous review of medical records will provide the necessary information in making such a determination.

The history should focus on recent events that might have led to renal hypoperfusion, or recent exposure to nephrotoxins, both endogenous and exogenous. Causes

TABLE 43.1 — RIFLE Classification

Category	GFR and serum creatinine criteria	Urine output
Risk	GFR decrease ≥25% OR Creatinine up 1.5 times baseline	<0.5 mL/kg/hr for 6 hr
Injury	GFR decrease ≥50% OR Creatinine up 2 times baseline	<0.5 mL/kg/hr for 12 hr
Failure	GFR decrease ≥75% OR Creatinine up 3 times baseline OR Creatinine ≥4.0 mg/dL Acute rise >0.5 mg/dL	<0.3 mL/kg/hr for 24 hr or anuria for 12 hr
End stage	End-stage kidney disease (>3 mo)	

GFR, glomerular filtration rate; RIFLE, risk, injury, failure, loss, and end stage.

TABLE 43.2 — AKIN Criteria for AKI

Diagnostic criteria

An abrupt (within 48 hours) reduction in kidney function defined as an absolute increase in serum creatinine of ≥0.3 mg/dL, a percentage increase in serum creatinine of ≥50%, or a reduction in urine output (oliguria of <0.5 mL/kg per hour for more than 6 hours).

AKIN, Acute Kidney Injury Network.

TABLE 43.3 — AKIN Criteria for AKI

	Staging system[a]	
Stage	Serum creatinine criteria	Urine output criteria
1	Increase in serum creatinine of ≥0.3 mg/dL or increase to ≥150%–200% (1.5- to 2-fold) from baseline	<0.5 mL/kg/hr for >6 hr
2	Increase in serum creatinine to >200%–300% (>2- to 3-fold) from baseline	<0.5 mL/kg/hr for >12 hr
3[b]	Increase in serum creatinine to >300% (>3-fold) from baseline (or serum creatinine of ≥4.0 mg/dL with an acute increase of at least 0.5 mg/dL)	<0.3 mL/kg/hr for 24 hr or anuria for 12 hr

[a]Only one criterion (creatinine or urine output) has to be fulfilled to qualify for a stage.
[b]Individuals who receive RRT are considered to have met the criteria for stage 3 irrespective of the stage they are in at the time of RRT.
AKIN, Acute Kidney Injury Network.

ALGORITHM 43.1 Features to Distinguish Among the Three Categories of Acute Kidney Injury

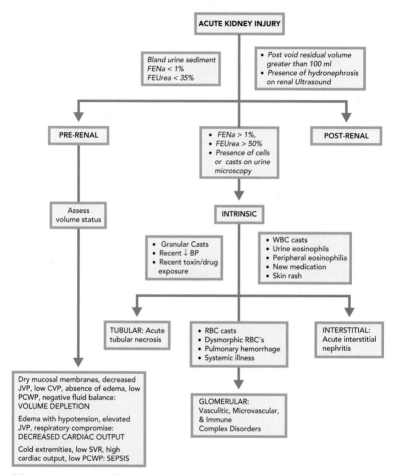

CVP, central venous pressure; FENa, fractional excretion of sodium; FEUrea, fractional excretion of urea; JVP, jugular venous pressure; PCWP, pulmonary capillary wedge pressure; SVR, systemic vascular resistance; BP, blood pressure; RBC, red blood cell; WBC, white blood cell.

of renal hypoperfusion must be investigated (e.g., intravascular volume depletion, decreased cardiac output, shock, cirrhosis, and renal vasoconstriction of various causes). Recent trauma should raise the suspicion for myoglobin-induced acute tubular necrosis (ATN). Pulmonary manifestations such as dyspnea and hemoptysis may raise the possibility of a pulmonary-renal syndrome such as Goodpasture's disease and Wegener's granulomatosis. A history of fever, rash, and arthralgia may suggest vasculitides or an infectious etiology (e.g., endocarditis). Flank pain can be seen in nephrolithiasis, urinary obstruction, renal vein thrombosis, or renal infarct. The presence or absence of anuria and hematuria are important clues as well. A detailed examination of medical history and of recent medications (e.g., antibiotics, nonsteroidal anti-inflammatory drugs (NSAIDs), diuretics, and chemotherapeutic agents), including over-the-counter drugs and radiocontrast agents, should be conducted. In the setting of postoperative AKI, careful review of intraoperative records may reveal episodes of hypotension or use of nephrotoxic drugs. In the in-patient setting, an ischemic or nephrotoxic event should be sought. In patients with mental status changes, obtaining history from a family member or friend is crucial as it can provide clues regarding overdose (e.g., acetaminophen or other medications) or accidental or deliberate ingestion (e.g., ethylene glycol and methanol).

On examination, a careful assessment of the patient's volume status often yields valuable clues as to the nature and degree of renal dysfunction. Systemic signs such as arthritis, rash, and mental status changes also give valuable clues as these can be associated with systemic illnesses such as infection, vasculitides, atheroembolic disease, or thrombotic microangiopathy. The finding of lower abdominal distention makes bladder outlet obstruction highly likely as the cause of AKI. A very tense and distended abdomen in the setting of ascites or recent abdominal surgery raises the suspicion for abdominal compartment syndrome.

Objective laboratory and radiologic tests that are essential include complete blood count, renal function panel, urinalysis, microscopy of the fresh spun urine sediment, calculated fractional excretion of sodium (FENa) and urea (FEUrea), and, when obstruction is suspected, a renal ultrasound. Physician examination of the urinary sediment is essential as abnormal urinary sediment is strongly suggestive of an intrarenal process. Based on the initial suspicion, additional diagnostic tests such as serologic studies or renal ultrasound with Doppler can be obtained. Renal biopsy is necessary to make a diagnosis when glomerulonephritis is suspected and is also used to make a definitive diagnosis of interstitial nephritis. The diagnosis of ATN should be based on clinical findings and supporting laboratory data.

ETIOLOGY OF AKI

Prerenal AKI

Etiology
In the prerenal process, the integrity of renal parenchyma is preserved. The decreased glomerular filtration rate is a physiological response to renal hypoperfusion that is due to either true or "effective" volume depletion. Examples include true hypovolemia of various causes, decreased cardiac output, liver failure, anaphylaxis, and sepsis. Renal vasoconstriction (e.g., hypercalcemia, sepsis, liver failure, calcineurin inhibitors, and norepinephrine) and impairment of renal autoregulation (e.g., NSAIDs, angiotensin-converting enzyme inhibitor [ACEI], and angiotensin II receptor blockers [ARBs]) are common scenarios leading to prerenal azotemia. Hypoperfusion may also result from sustained intraabdominal pressure >20 mm Hg, leading to abdominal compartment syndrome. This syndrome can be seen in intraabdominal hemorrhage, massive ascites, bowel distension, abdominal surgery, and post-liver transplantation.

Diagnosis
The diagnosis is suspected from the history and physical examination. In prerenal AKI, the urine sediment is typically bland, lacking cells, crystals, and cellular casts. The urine chemistry reflects the appropriate tubular response to hypoperfusion, with avid sodium reabsorption. The calculated FENa is <1% and the urine sodium is usually

<10 mmol/L. The urine is markedly concentrated and urine osmolality is usually >500 mOsm/kg. FENa is the most sensitive index and is most useful for oliguric patients not exposed to loop diuretics. For patients taking diuretics, the FEUrea has been demonstrated to be superior, with a specificity and sensitivity >95%. A FEUrea of <35% would suggest renal hypoperfusion. It is important to appreciate that a FENa of <1% can be seen in several other renal conditions, including acute glomerulonephritis, contrast nephropathy, pigment-induced ATN, and in early urinary obstruction. In patients with impaired urinary concentrating ability (CKD or elderly patients), FENa can be >1% in the prerenal state. Other useful parameters in differentiating prerenal problems from tubular dysfunction include the blood urea nitrogen to creatinine ratio (>20:1).

Management

Rapid reversal of the cause of renal hypoperfusion is critical because prolonged renal ischemia leads to renal tubular injury (Algorithm 43.2). All offending drugs/agents should be discontinued immediately. In cases of hypovolemia, depending on the source of fluid loss, volume resuscitation with normal saline or blood products should be administered without delay. In conditions associated with overfill situations, such as congestive heart failure or cardiogenic shock, treatment is directed at maximizing cardiac function, particularly with diuretics, positive inotropes, afterload reduction, and possibly cardiac-assist devices. Invasive hemodynamic monitoring of central venous pressure can be an important tool to guide management when intravascular volume status is difficult to determine based on noninvasive assessment.

Management of hepatorenal syndrome (HRS) remains a clinical challenge. HRS is a serious but potentially reversible complication of end-stage liver disease as well as fulminant hepatic failure of any cause (e.g., tumor infiltration and acetaminophen toxicity). It is a result of severe intrarenal vasoconstriction in the setting of splanchnic vasodilatation and effective hypovolemia. It can occur spontaneously in advanced liver disease, or develop after a precipitating event such as infection (e.g., spontaneous bacterial peritonitis), gastrointestinal bleeding, or large-volume paracentesis without albumin. In patients with spontaneous bacterial peritonitis, albumin infusion may prevent development of HRS.

HRS is a diagnosis of exclusion (see Table 43.4 for diagnostic criteria of HRS). The prognosis of HRS is very poor (type 1 worse than type 2) as there are very few therapeutic strategies in HRS and liver transplantation is the only definitive treatment (Table 43.5). Resolution of HRS can occur with improvement in hepatic function in the cases of acute liver injury and alcoholic hepatitis.

POSTRENAL AKI

A postrenal process occurs when the glomerular filtration rate is decreased secondarily by an impediment to urine outflow as a result of structural or functional changes in the urinary tract. The increased pressure in the urinary tract is conveyed proximally from the obstruction, resulting in a rise in tubular pressure and an eventual decrease in the hydraulic pressure gradient across the glomerular capillaries, leading to a decline in glomerular filtration rate as well as changes in tubular function (decreased concentrating ability, distal renal tubular acidosis).

Urinary obstruction can be unilateral or bilateral, acute or chronic, partial or complete, intrarenal (tubular obstruction from crystals, casts) or extrarenal. Clinical symptoms vary according to duration, degree, and site of obstruction. Unilateral

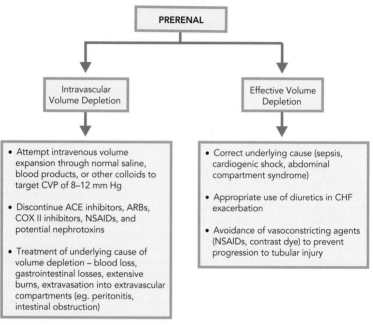

ALGORITHM 43.2 Management of Prerenal Causes of Acute Kidney Injury

PRERENAL

Intravascular Volume Depletion

- Attempt intravenous volume expansion through normal saline, blood products, or other colloids to target CVP of 8–12 mm Hg

- Discontinue ACE inhibitors, ARBs, COX II inhibitors, NSAIDs, and potential nephrotoxins

- Treatment of underlying cause of volume depletion – blood loss, gastrointestinal losses, extensive burns, extravasation into extravascular compartments (eg. peritonitis, intestinal obstruction)

Effective Volume Depletion

- Correct underlying cause (sepsis, cardiogenic shock, abdominal compartment syndrome)

- Appropriate use of diuretics in CHF exacerbation

- Avoidance of vasoconstricting agents (NSAIDs, contrast dye) to prevent progression to tubular injury

ACE, angiotensin-converting enzyme; ARBs, angiotensin II receptor blockers; CHF, congestive heart failure; COX, cyclo-oxygenase; CVP, central venous pressure; NSAIDs, nonsteroidal anti-inflammatory drugs.

TABLE 43.4 Diagnostic Criteria of Hepatorenal Syndrome

- Cirrhosis with presence of ascites
- Worsening renal function over days to weeks with serum creatinine at least 1.5 mg/dl
- Absence of intrinsic renal disease as indicated by proteinuria (>500 mg/day), microscopic hematuria (>50 red blood cells per high power field), and/or structural abnormalities detected by imaging studies.
- Absence of shock
- Absence of concurrent or recent use of nephrotoxic medications
- No improvement of renal function after diuretic withdrawal and volume expansion with albumin for at least two days. Albumin should be dosed one gram/kg of body weight per day up to a maximum of 100 grams/day.

SUBTYPES	**Type 1:** Rapidly progressive form, with doubling of serum creatinine to a level >2.5 mg/dL in <2 wk
	Type 2: moderate renal failure, with a slowly progressive course. Serum creatinine 1.5–2.5 mg/dl. Typically associated with refractory ascites

Diagnostic criteria of hepatorenal syndrome are adapted from: Salerno F, et al. Diagnosis, prevention, and treatment of hepatorenal syndrome in cirrhosis. Gut 2007;56:1310–1318.

TABLE 43.5	Treatment of Type 1 Hepatorenal Syndrome

Vasoconstrictors and albumin
- Terlipressin: not available in the United States
- Midodrine (systemic vasoconstrictor) + octreotide (inhibitor of endogenous vasodilator release)
  - Midodrine 5–15 mg orally three times a day
  - Octreotide 100–200 μg subcutaneously three times a day
- Norepinephrine: limited data

Transjugular intrahepatic portosystemic shunt
- Treatment of refractory ascites
- May provide gradual improvement in renal function
- Data very limited
- Effect on survival unclear

Hemodialysis
- Bridge to liver transplantation OR
- Awaiting recovery of hepatic function
- May be difficult to perform due to hemodynamic instability (CVVHD)

Liver transplantation

obstruction does not typically lead to renal failure. UOP is nondiagnostic except in the case of anuria that suggests complete obstruction.

The diagnosis is initially suspected based on the history and physical examination, and confirmed by findings of hydronephrosis on renal ultrasound or CT. Absence of hydronephrosis on radiologic testing does not completely exclude obstruction. In the setting of severe volume depletion, retroperitoneal fibrosis, and in the very early phase of obstruction, dilatation of the calyces may not occur and ultrasound may be falsely negative. A simple method to evaluate for distal obstruction is to measure the postvoid residual that, if more than 100 mL, is consistent with bladder outlet obstruction. Obstruction of the Foley catheter with clots should also be considered, and this is ruled out either by flushing the catheter or replacing it with a new one. In the intensive care setting, unless there is high index of suspicion based on the clinical picture (e.g., recent abdominal surgery, history of malignancy, and anticholinergic medications), the yield from renal ultrasound is low.

Once the diagnosis of urinary obstruction/obstructive nephropathy is made, prompt intervention is necessary to minimize long-term renal impairment. The method of intervention is dictated by the location and cause of the obstruction. Postobstructive diuresis with marked polyuria is often seen after relief of complete obstruction. Although this is considered an appropriate response in many cases, volume depletion and electrolyte imbalances can occur and require close monitoring and intervention.

INTRINSIC AKI

Intrinsic renal disease is present when the injury is at the level of the kidney parenchyma. Further classification depends on the area of involvement: glomeruli, vasculature, tubules, or interstitium. Such differentiation can frequently be achieved by careful analysis of the urine sediment. "Muddy" granular casts and tubular epithelial cell casts are most often seen in ATN. Red blood cell casts and dysmorphic red blood cells suggest a glomerular origin, and white blood cell casts are found when inflammation is present in the interstitium as in acute interstitial nephritis (AIN) and pyelonephritis. It is important to note that red and white blood cell casts are fragile and that their absence alone does not necessarily eliminate their associated disorders from the differential diagnosis. In the critical care setting, ischemic and nephrotoxic ATN account for up to 90% of intrinsic AKI.

Acute Tubular Necrosis

Etiology

ATN can result from prolonged prerenal states (e.g., volume depletion and hypotension) or toxins (e.g., intravenous contrast, aminoglycosides, antiviral and antifungal medications, and myoglobin). In the critical care setting, the insults are usually simultaneous or sequential and no single precipitating factor can be identified (Table 43.6 contains a list of common causes of ATN). In severe cases, renal hypoperfusion can result in bilateral cortical necrosis and irreversible renal damage.

Diagnosis

With severe or prolonged injury, the renal tubules lose their ability to retain sodium and concentrate urine. The FENa is usually above 1% and the FEUrea is >50% with a serum blood urea nitrogen to creatinine <20:1. Examination of the urine sediment can reveal muddy brown granular casts in majority of the patients. Because the glomeruli and interstitium are typically spared, other urinary findings such as heavy proteinuria and hematuria are absent.

Although the FENa is a useful indicator to differentiate between prerenal states and ATN, as noted before, there are some exceptions to the rule. Certain conditions that result in ATN can demonstrate a low FENa. Contrast-induced nephropathy (CIN) typically manifests as nonoliguric AKI, occurring 3 to 5 days after radiocontrast exposure. Early in the course of the renal injury, the FENa is low (<1%) despite the absence of systemic volume depletion. This is a result of the profound renal vasoconstriction caused by release of endothelin induced by intravenous contrast. Rhabdomyolysis and severe hemolysis release pigments (myoglobin and hemoglobin, respectively) that are toxic to the tubules, but may also present early in the course with a low FENa secondary to renal vasoconstriction.

Prevention

Close monitoring of intravascular volume status and cautious use of nephrotoxic agents can dramatically reduce the incidence of AKI secondary to ATN. The majority of the preventive techniques have been studied in the area of CIN. Various intravenous hydration regimens have been shown to reduce the risk of renal injury in patients undergoing radiocontrast procedures, with regimens consisting of normal saline or sodium bicarbonate-based intravenous fluids being most effective. "Renal-dose" dopamine infusions have *not* shown to be beneficial in prevention nor aid in recovery from renal injury. In fact, some studies have suggested increased risk for AKI, and thus there is *no* role for this agent in the prevention or treatment of AKI. *N*-acetylcysteine has been studied in small randomized trials, and its combination with intravenous hydration may result in a lower incidence of CIN. Although this advantage has not been clearly defined, *N*-acetylcysteine can be considered for use in high-risk patients undergoing contrast administration, given its low cost, safety, and potential benefit.

TABLE 43.6	Common Causes of Acute Tubular Necrosis
Cause	Description
Ischemia	Results from prolonged prerenal state (hypovolemia, sepsis, cardiogenic shock) Treat by addressing underlying cause and maximizing renal perfusion
Intravascular iodinated contrast	Characterized by both renal vasoconstriction and tubular injury Risk factors: preexisting renal dysfunction, heart failure, diabetes, volume depletion, multiple myeloma, large volume of contrast, and high-osmolarity contrast FENa <1% Hydration with intravenous sodium chloride or sodium bicarbonate shown to be beneficial N-acetylcysteine orally or intravenously may help in prevention Most patients recover renal function
Rhabdomyolysis	May result from crush injury, prolonged immobilization, status epilepticus, hyperthermia, statin medication, cocaine use, hypophosphatemia, hypokalemia, snake venom, or inherited metabolic disorders Degree of muscle enzyme elevation does not always correlate with severity of renal injury Mechanisms of AKI: renal vasoconstriction, proximal tubular injury, and tubular obstruction by pigment casts Hyperkalemia, hyperphosphatemia, hypocalcemia, hyperuricemia Urine dipstick may show heme pigment in absence of RBCs on urine sediment Urine supernatant red to brown in color FENa <1% Treat with vigorous hydration (may require up to 10 L of normal saline during 24 hr) to replete volume and increase urinary flow rate
Hemoglobinuria	Result from intravascular hemolytic processes Urine dipstick may show heme pigment in absence of RBCs on urine sediment FENa <1% Lactate dehydrogenase elevated, haptoglobin decreased, and unconjugated bilirubin elevated Treatment similar to rhabdomyolysis and focus on underlying cause
Cast nephropathy	Casts composed of light chain (myeloma) and Tamm–Horsfall protein can lead to direct tubular injury and intratubular obstruction Risk factors: volume depletion, loop diuretics, hypercalcemia, IV contrast Role of plasmapheresis unclear

(continued)

TABLE 43.6	Common Causes of Acute Tubular Necrosis (*Continued*)
Cause	Description
Aminoglycosides	Typically presents 5–7 days after initiating drug Length of treatment correlates with increased incidence of nephrotoxicity FENa >1% in most cases Usually nonoliguric Significant urinary loss of magnesium, potassium, and calcium Recovery may take several weeks, even if drug is promptly discontinued
Amphotericin B	Effect is cumulative Causes intense renal vasoconstriction as well as direct toxicity to tubules by disrupting cell membrane Liposomal preparations have lower incidence of nephrotoxicity
Intravenous acyclovir	Insoluble precipitation in renal tubules resulting in obstruction Needle-shaped crystals may be seen on urine sediment Discontinuation of medicine usually reverses renal injury
Cisplatin	Dose-related and cumulative effect Profound renal magnesium wasting; hypokalemia can be seen Vigorous fluid hydration should be given prior to medication to increase urine flow
Ethylene glycol/ methanol	Toxicity can result from ingestion of wood alcohol (methanol) or antifreeze radiator fluid (ethylene glycol) Elevated osmol gap Anion gap metabolic acidosis presents later in course Oxalate crystals (envelope-shaped) are present in the urine sediment with ethylene glycol but not with methanol intoxication Fomepizole antidote is loaded as 15 mg/kg over 30 minutes, then 15 mg/kg every 12 hr Hemodialysis may be required to treat refractory metabolic acidosis/AKI
Tumor lysis syndrome	Results after large numbers of neoplastic cells are rapidly killed after cancer treatment or tumor autolysis Intracellular contents are released into the circulation, including potassium, phosphate, and uric acid Most often seen 48–72 hr after cancer treatment Renal injury is through uric acid precipitation in the acidic environment of the tubules Hyperphosphatemia can lead to calcium–phosphate crystal formation and nephrocalcinosis Patients are typically oliguric; may require temporary dialysis, although usually reversible if addressed early Treatment is with aggressive hydration, allopurinol, and rasburicase

FENa, fractional excretion of sodium; RBCs, red blood cells.

Management and Prognosis

There is no specific treatment of ATN once it has occurred. Therapy is generally supportive and includes the use of renal replacement therapy if necessary. Attempts to reverse the initial insult should be made. Management should also focus on avoiding additional nephrotoxic insults and adjusting drug doses appropriately for the level of renal function. Depending on the cause and severity, as well as the baseline renal function, renal recovery takes days, weeks, or even months, if at all. Generally, renal recovery can be expected in >90% of patients who previously had normal baseline function.

Glomerular and Microvascular Processes

Glomerular causes of renal injury are much less common in an acute intensive care setting (Table 43.7). However, the pulmonary-renal syndromes of Wegener's granulomatosis and Goodpasture's disease should be considered in anyone presenting with simultaneous respiratory and renal dysfunction, as they are universally fatal if not recognized and treated in a timely manner. The presence of red blood cell casts specifically suggests a glomerular origin. In the appropriate clinical setting, such findings should trigger a search for vasculitic and nephritic disorders. Serologic tests are helpful in these cases, although kidney biopsy may ultimately be necessary for a definitive diagnosis.

The antiglomerular basement membrane antibody is a highly sensitive (95%) and specific test (99%) for Goodpasture's disease. In Wegener's granulomatosis, the serine proteinase 3 antibody (c-ANCA, cytoplasmic antineutrophil cytoplasmic antibody) is elevated in >75% of cases; approximately 20% have an elevated myeloperoxidase antibody (p-ANCA) and <5% are ANCA-negative. Treatment of these syndromes is with immediate intravenous corticosteroids (methylprednisolone at 7 mg/kg/day for 3 days followed by oral prednisone at 1 mg/kg/day up to 60 mg) and with cytotoxic immunosuppressants (cyclophosphamide at 2 to 3 mg/kg/day). Therapeutic plasma exchange is also employed in the treatment of Goodpasture's disease. In ANCA-positive vasculitis with advanced renal failure, one study demonstrated that the single predictive factor associated with long-term independence from dialysis was the use of therapeutic plasma exchange. Therapeutic plasma exchange is also recommended for the management of pulmonary hemorrhage associated with ANCA-positive vasculitis. The differential diagnoses of pulmonary-renal syndromes include community-acquired pneumonia with sepsis and ATN, systemic lupus erythematosus with lung involvement and lupus nephritis, sarcoidosis, infections such as leptospirosis, legionella, ehrlichiosis (pneumonia with AIN or ATN), and pancreatitis with pneumonia and ATN.

Hemolytic-uremic syndrome (HUS) and thrombotic thrombocytopenic purpura (TTP) are two distinct thrombotic microangiopathies that can result in renal injury. Although distinct clinical entities, they share several common precipitating factors such as human immunodeficiency virus infection, malignancy, calcineurin inhibitors, pregnancy, and chemotherapeutic agents. Ticlopidine and, less commonly, clopidogrel are more closely associated with TTP. In the diarrheal form of HUS, a Shiga-like toxin enters the circulation through compromised colonic epithelium and results in inflammation, endothelial injury, and thrombosis in the renal microvasculature. Therapy is supportive for HUS, with no proven efficacy of antibiotics, anticoagulation, immunoglobulin, or plasmapheresis. In the case of TTP, daily plasma volume exchange is a life-saving therapy and thus must not be delayed. In resistant cases, immunosuppression with high-dose prednisone and rituximab can be used. Splenectomy has been attempted in refractory cases, but is of unproven benefit.

TABLE 43.7	Selected Glomerular and Microvascular Disorders in the ICU	
Cause	Characteristics	Treatment
Immune complex	Hypocomplementemia seen with postinfectious GN, MPGN, SLE, endocarditis, and cryoglobulinemia	Treat the underlying cause
Pauci-immune and anti-GBM disease	Pulmonary hemorrhage syndromes may have positive serum c-ANCA or p-ANCA or anti-GBM antibody (Goodpasture's) Dysmorphic RBCs in urine suggest glomerular origin	Supportive therapy for pulmonary compromise, mechanical ventilation if necessary Corticosteroids and cytotoxic agents Plasma exchange for Goodpasture's or vasculitis with pulmonary hemorrhage or advanced renal failure
Microvascular	HUS and TTP with low platelets, hemolytic anemia, and schistocytes on peripheral smear	TTP requires emergent plasma exchange Supportive care for HUS Refractory TTP may benefit from immunosuppression with prednisone and/or rituximab
	Atheroembolic disease Subacute renal failure, days to weeks after invasive vascular procedure, with livedo reticularis and transient peripheral eosinophilia	Avoid anticoagulation and further vascular procedures

GN, glomerulonephritis; MPGN, membranoproliferative glomerulonephritis; SLE, systemic lupus erythematosus; c-ANCA, cytoplasmic antineutrophilic cytoplasmic antibody; p-ANCA, perinuclear antineutrophilic cytoplasmic antibody; GBM, glomerular basement membrane; RBCs, red blood cells; HUS, hemolytic-uremic syndrome; TTP, thrombotic thrombocytopenic purpura.

Another microvascular process affecting the kidneys is atheroembolic disease. As hospitalized patients frequently undergo invasive vascular procedures, a high index of suspicion for atheroembolic disease should be maintained in the appropriate clinical setting. These patients demonstrate renal dysfunction days to weeks after manipulation of aorta or other large arteries, and follow a slowly progressive course. Transient peripheral eosinophilia may be present in >65% of cases. Hypocomplementemia can be seen in the initial phase of the disease. Skin findings are highly variable and may include livedo reticularis of the extremities or digital necrosis with gangrene (blue toe syndrome). Distal pulses are typically present as the occlusion is at the level of smaller arteries and arterioles. The general rule from the renal standpoint is a slow decline in renal function during months, with a third of the patients requiring dialysis. In multivisceral atheroembolic disease, manifested by intestinal ischemia, pancreatitis,

TABLE 43.8 Selected Causes of Acute Interstitial Nephritis

Agent	Diagnosis	Course
Methicillin	Hypersensitivity symptoms predominate with fever in 85% Urinary findings also very common, as >80% of patients with hematuria, pyuria, eosinophiluria, or non-nephrotic proteinuria	Most patients recover renal function within 2 months, although nearly one-fifth require temporary dialysis CKD remains in only 10%
Rifampin	Gastrointestinal symptoms (nausea, vomiting, abdominal pain) Oliganuria in nearly all patients Eosinophilia uncommon, although other hematologic abnormalities such as hemolysis (25%) and thrombocytopenia (50%) may occur Elevation of liver enzymes seen in one-quarter of patients Anti-rifampin antibodies in almost all patients Renal biopsy rarely shows immune complex deposition at tubular basement membrane	Occurs 24 hr following dose with prior exposure (up to 1 year prior) Temporary dialysis required in almost all cases CKD remains in only 3%
Other antibiotics (sulfonamides, fluoroquinolones, beta-lactams)	Fever less common than with methicillin (45%), but with rash and flank pain in almost 50%; oliguria in 40% Urinary findings less common than with methicillin	Mean exposure to antibiotic is 10 days CKD remains in approximately 40%
NSAIDs	Hypersensitivity symptoms uncommon More than one-third with nephrotic range proteinuria Renal biopsy may show minimal change disease	Exposure is frequently months before presentation CKD remains in half of patients
Allopurinol	Hypersensitivity symptoms very common and robust with accumulation of metabolite oxypurinol Eosinophilia and hepatitis are common Renal biopsy may show immune complex deposition at tubular basement membrane	Mortality may be as high as 25%

(continued)

TABLE 43.8 Selected Causes of Acute Interstitial Nephritis (*Continued*)

Agent	Diagnosis	Course
Proton-pump inhibitors	Class effect Initial signs and symptoms are nonspecific Requires high level of clinical suspicion	Can occur many months after initiation of PPIs Prognosis generally good once PPIs discontinued Steroids may be tried
Leptospiral nephropathy	Fever and jaundice are very common Other findings may include hepatomegaly, gingival and gastrointestinal bleeding, macroscopic hematuria, conjunctival suffusion, altered mental status; oligoanuria in nearly all patients Rhabdomyolysis, cholestatic hepatitis, hemolytic anemia, and thrombocytopenia are common findings Confirm with positive blood/urine culture or serology Renal biopsy shows inflammation predominantly at proximal tubules, and may also show interstitial hemorrhage	Nephropathy occurs in 40% of leptospirosis Mortality is approximately 25% CKD remains in only 10%
Sarcoidosis	Extrarenal symptoms predominate, most commonly affecting lungs, eyes, and skin Eosinophilia seen in one-quarter of patients Hypercalcemia common despite advanced renal failure Hilar adenopathy on chest radiograph ACE levels not reliable with renal involvement Renal biopsy can show noncaseating granulomas and giant cells	Often remitting and relapsing course CKD remains in 90%

CKD, chronic kidney disease; NSAIDs, nonsteroidal anti-inflammatory drugs; ACE, angiotensin-converting enzyme.

and other systemic manifestations, 1-year mortality can be as high as 70%. There is no effective medical treatment. Avoidance of further vascular procedures along with judicious control of blood pressure, use of ACEIs, and nutritional support have also been associated with better prognosis. A case series has noted a possible benefit from statin therapy in improving the long-term renal outcome.

Interstitial Processes

AIN is an inflammatory process caused by medications or by infections. The classic triad of rash, eosinophilia, and fever is not commonly seen. Urinary findings suggestive of AIN include white blood cells, white blood cell casts, and eosinophils. Occasionally, the urine sediment can be bland. Detection of eosinophiluria should be done with the Hansel's stain. However, eosinophiluria is a nonspecific finding and has a relatively low sensitivity and specificity. Renal biopsy may be necessary to establish a definitive diagnosis. Beta-lactam antibiotics are common culprits, although nearly every antibiotic and many nonantibiotic medications have been implicated. Table 43.8 lists some of the more common causes of AIN in the ICU.

Removal of the offending agent or treatment of the underlying infectious disease is the mainstay of therapy. Recovery of renal function may not occur for days to weeks, and sometimes several months. The role of corticosteroid therapy remains controversial. Some studies suggest a better outcome in patients who are treated with steroids. Cyclophosphamide, mycophenolate mofetil, or other immunosuppressants have also been used in corticosteroid nonresponders after 2 to 3 weeks of therapy.

SUMMARY

An algorithmic approach to AKI can help uncover the etiology and devise a treatment plan. Early in the investigation, it is important to determine if the insult is prerenal, intrinsic, or postrenal in nature, using the history, physical examination, laboratory data, and imaging studies. Microscopic examination of the urine sediment is of high value in identifying the underlying renal disorder and may help in further classifying some disorders. Once a specific diagnosis is made, one can initiate specific treatment and, in many cases, achieve successful reversal of kidney injury.

SUGGESTED READINGS

Bellomo R, Ronco C, Kellum JA, et al. Acute renal failure. Definition, outcome measures, animal models, fluid therapy, and information technology needs: the second international consensus conference of the Acute Dialysis Quality Initiative (ADQI) Group. *Crit Care.* 2004;8:204–212.
  Consensus committee report for defining and managing renal injury.
Keyserling HF, Fielding JR, Mittelstaedt CA. Renal sonography in the intensive care unit: when is it necessary? *J Ultrasound Med.* 2002;21:517–520.
  Retrospective study of the efficacy of renal sonography in making a diagnosis.
Marenzi G, Assanelli E, Marana I, et al. N-acetylcysteine and contrast-induced nephropathy in primary angioplasty. *N Engl J Med.* 2006;354:2773–2782.
  Randomized controlled trial comparing high and low doses of N-acetylcysteine in preventing contrast-induced nephropathy.
Markowitz GS, Perazella MA. Drug-induced renal failure: a focus on tubulointerstitial disease. *Clin Chim Acta.* 2005;351:31–47.
  Review of pattern of drug-induced renal injury.

Mehta RL, Kellum JA, Shah SV, et al. Acute Kidney Injury Network: report of an initiative to improve outcomes in acute kidney injury. *Crit Care.* 2007;11:R31.

Merten GJ, Burgess WP, Gray LV, et al. Prevention of contrast-induced nephropathy with sodium bicarbonate: a randomized controlled trial. *JAMA.* 2004;291:2328–2334.
Randomized study evaluating efficacy of sodium bicarbonate in preventing renal injury.

Mueller C, Buerkle G, Buettner HJ, et al. Prevention of contrast media-associated nephropathy: randomized comparison of 2 hydration regimens in 1620 patients undergoing coronary angioplasty. *Arch Intern Med.* 2002;162:329–336.
Randomized study comparing different intravenous fluids in preventing renal injury.

Praga M, González E. Acute interstitial nephritis. *Kidney Int.* 2010;77:956–961.

Ruggenenti P, Noris M, Remuzzi G. Thrombotic microangiopathy, hemolytic uremic syndrome, and thrombotic thrombocytopenic purpura. *Kidney Int.* 2001;60:831–846.
Review of TTP and HUS.

Salerno F, Gerbes A, Ginès P, et al. Diagnosis, prevention and treatment of hepatorenal syndrome in cirrhosis. *Gut.* 2007;56:1310–1318.

Tsai JJ, Yeun JY, Kumar VA, et al. Comparison and interpretation of urinalysis performed by a nephrologists versus a hospital-based clinical laboratory. *Am J Kidney Dis.* 2005;46:820–829.
Blinded study comparing ability of different examiners in evaluating urinalyses.

Tublin ME, Murphy ME, Tessler FN. Current concepts in contrast media-induced nephropathy. *Am J Roentgenol.* 1998;171:933–939.
Review of contrast-induced renal injury.

44 Renal Replacement Therapy

Tingting Li and Anitha Vijayan

The principal strategy regarding acute kidney injury (AKI), particularly in the intensive care setting, is prevention. Once AKI occurs, the presentation and course are variable and treatment is generally supportive. The optimal time to initiate renal replacement therapy (RRT) remains unknown.

INDICATIONS

Conventional indications for RRT include metabolic acidosis, hyperkalemia, volume overload, and severe uremic symptoms refractory to medical management. Other indications include certain intoxications of certain substances (ethylene glycol, methanol, lithium, etc.), where either the substance or the toxic metabolite will be cleared with dialysis.

Acidosis

Refractory metabolic acidosis is an acute indication for dialytic therapy in the severely ill patient. Progressive acidemia can develop as the kidneys lose their ability to reclaim bicarbonate and excrete organic acids. More commonly in the intensive care setting, tissue hypoperfusion with multiorgan system failure results in severe lactic acidosis. Aggressive alkali therapy can encounter problems with volume overload, metabolic alkalosis, and hypocalcemia. Initiation of RRT would obviate the concern over volume overload and could restore the blood pH to its physiologic range.

Hyperkalemia

Hyperkalemia can be rapidly fatal and need to be addressed promptly. Temporizing measures include intravenous calcium to stabilize the myocardial cell membrane, as well as insulin (with dextrose 50% in water), sodium bicarbonate, and inhaled beta-agonists to promote an intracellular shift in potassium. Elimination of potassium from the body can be achieved with ion-exchange resins, but this effect is unpredictable and inefficient. In the volume-depleted patient, aggressive fluid resuscitation can enhance sodium delivery to the distal nephron. The reabsorption of sodium makes the lumen electronegative, promoting secretion of potassium via the potassium channel (see Chapter 24 for further discussion).

When these efforts are unsuccessful, urgent RRT becomes necessary. Intermittent hemodialysis (IHD) with higher blood flow and dialysate flow rates is very effective in lowering potassium rapidly and is the preferred modality of choice. The patients are dialyzed using a 0 or 1 mEq/L potassium concentration in the dialysate. However, in a critically ill hypotensive patient with or without pressors, continuous renal replacement therapy (CRRT) with high flow rates (>35 mL/kg/hr) of replacement fluid and dialysate with 0 potassium concentration can also be utilized to lower potassium levels.

Volume Overload

Volume overload is another frequently encountered problem in the critical care setting. There is evidence that in patients with AKI, fluid overload is an independent risk factor for mortality. Although randomized trials studying the use of diuretics in AKI have not demonstrated any survival advantage, improvement in renal recovery, or avoidance of dialytic therapy, it is not unreasonable to offer a trial of high-dose loop diuretic (160 to 200 mg of furosemide) in the setting of fluid overload. Respiratory compromise with pulmonary edema and/or significant soft tissue edema that impairs the barrier defense of the skin is the most common subjective criteria for initiating renal replacement in the oliguric patient.

Uremia

With progressive renal dysfunction, there is an impaired ability to excrete nitrogenous wastes and glycosylated end products. Blood urea nitrogen (BUN) level is generally used as a surrogate marker for uremic toxin accumulation. Unfortunately, many signs and symptoms commonly found in the uremic syndrome do not always correlate with BUN levels, and therefore there is no established objective cutoff beyond which dialytic therapy is recommended. Rather, acute indications for initiating urgent RRT center on the presence of specific clinical findings, namely uremic encephalopathy and uremic pericarditis. The latter possesses a high risk of converting into hemorrhagic pericarditis with cardiac tamponade.

TIMING OF INITIATION OF RRT

The optimal timing for initiation of RRT is undefined at this time. A few studies have shown a survival advantage with early initiation (definition varies greatly among studies; most used BUN <60 vs. >60). However, all the studies have significant design flaws and no definitive conclusions can be drawn.

MODALITIES

Once the decision has been made to initiate RRT, one needs to select a modality. The available modalities are IHD, CRRT, sustained low-efficiency dialysis (SLED), or peritoneal dialysis. The choice depends on the availability of therapies at the institution, physician preference, the patient's hemodynamic status, and the presence of comorbid conditions. Intermittent modalities generally cause greater fluctuations in blood pressure and produce greater fluid shifts in a short amount of time. Continuous modalities allow for the same solute clearance and fluid removal, but spread out during a 24-hour period, and thus are favored in hemodynamically unstable patients such as those with sepsis or fulminant hepatic failure.

In the United States, CRRT is performed in approximately 30% of adult patients with AKI and has almost completely replaced peritoneal dialysis in the intensive care unit (ICU) setting. However, although CRRT has some potential benefits over IHD, as seen in randomized trials, CRRT has not shown improved survival over IHD in critically ill patients. Likewise, randomized trials have not shown a difference in time to renal recovery or length of ICU or hospital stay between groups treated with IHD versus CRRT.

In the recent years, the use of SLED or extended daily dialysis (EDD) has risen and is mainly driven by its convenience, safety, excellent control of electrolytes and volume status, and lower cost compared to CRRT. Treatments are intermittent but with longer duration (8 to 10 hours/session), lower blood and dialysate flow rate, lower small solute, and fluid removal than IHD (and higher blood and dialysate flow rate, small solute and fluid removal than CRRT). SLED is often performed 5 to 6 times per week, usually during the night. It is an excellent modality for those patients who are prone to hemodynamic instability, provides "down time" for procedures, and at the same time does not compromise the dialysis dose. SLED usually requires little or no anticoagulation, demands less nursing care, and is a good alternative to CRRT in the ICU. Randomized, controlled studies have suggested similar safety and effectiveness compared to CRRT and IHD.

Table 44.1 lists the advantages and disadvantages of the different modalities of dialysis.

TABLE 44.1	Renal Replacement Modalities	
Modality	Advantages	Disadvantages
IHD	High-efficiency transport of solutes when rapid clearance of toxins or electrolytes is required Allows time for off-unit testing	Hemodynamic intolerance secondary to fluid shifts "Saw-tooth" pattern of metabolic control between sessions
CRRT	Gentler hemodynamic shifts than IHD Steady solute control	Continuous need for specialized nursing Requires continuous anticoagulation (heparin vs. citrate)
SLED	All of the advantages of CRRT Provides "down time" for off-unit testing Less nursing care than CRRT Less expensive than CRRT Anticoagulation generally not necessary	Requires almost daily treatments Less "middle molecule" removal than CRRT
Peritoneal dialysis	Gentler hemodynamic shifts than IHD	Requires invasion of peritoneal cavity, which may not be possible in postoperative patients Less predictable fluid removal rates

CRRT, continuous renal replacement therapy; IHD, intermittent hemodialysis; SLED, sustained low-efficiency dialysis.

DIALYSIS DOSE

The ideal dose of dialytic therapy in critically ill patients has not yet been conclusively determined. Evidence from end-stage, dialysis-dependent patients suggests that a thrice-weekly regimen should be performed with a urea reduction of approximately 70% per session. However, in the acutely ill intensive care population, these calculations are not always equivalent. The actual urea clearances are approximately 25% lower than what would be expected in a stable chronic dialysis patient, and thus it has been proposed that additional benefit may be derived from higher treatment doses, more frequent treatments, or greater hemofiltration.

In IHD, a few small studies had shown a survival advantage in critically ill patients who receive either a higher delivered dialysis dose three times per week or undergo daily dialysis. In contrast, the VA/NIH Acute Renal Failure Trial Network (ATN) study, a large multicenter, prospective, randomized trial, did not find a decrease in mortality or increase in renal recovery with more frequent dialysis (six times per week vs. three times). We recommend IHD be provided three time a week, targeting the urea reduction ratio of >70%, or Kt/V of 1.2 to 1.4 per treatment.

Similarly, in CRRT, small randomized controlled trials had shown a survival benefit with high intensity dialysis. Subsequent trials have shown conflicting results. The largest trials to date, the ATN study (effluent rate of 35 mL/kg/hr vs. 20 mL/kg/hr) and the study from the RENAL Replacement Therapy Study Investigators (effluent rate of 40 mL/kg/hr vs. 25 mL/kg/hr), did not demonstrate a survival advantage with higher intensity dialysis at day 60. In the ATN study, higher intensity dialysis did not improve recovery of renal function or reduce the rate of nonrenal organ failure. Subsequent meta-analysis showed similar results. We recommend using flow rates of 20 mL/kg/hr, divided equally between the replacement flow rate and dialysate flow rate, using the continuous venovenous hemodiafiltration (CVVHDF) modality. With this dosing we recommend that patients remain on therapy for a minimum of 20 hours per day. If the patient is not receiving at least 18 to 20 hours of CRRT in a 24-hour period, then flow rates may have to be increased to 25 mL/kg/hr. Also, in patients who need higher clearances for severe acidosis or hyperkalemia, then higher flow rates should be used.

DRUG DOSING IN CRRT

Various factors affect the dosing of medications in the setting of CRRT. The pharmacokinetics of drug removal during CRRT can be highly complex, depending on the drug's molecular size, protein-binding, volume of distribution, dialyzer membrane permeability, the dose of dialysis, and the modality of CRRT (continuous venovenous hemodialysis [CVVHD] vs. continuous venovenous hemofiltration [CVVH] vs. CVVHDF). The clearance of a drug can also be affected by its elimination by nonrenal routes or by the degree of residual renal function. Generally, the nonrenal clearance is taken to be constant, although in critically ill patients with multiorgan system failure, this component may be less than predicted. In sepsis, certain variables such as volume of distribution and protein binding can be altered. There is a paucity of data about drug dosing during CRRT in critically ill patients. One important principle to remember is that elimination is continuous; therefore, most drugs will need to given twice or thrice daily. Drug levels, when available, should be measured daily. The recommended doses for some of the more commonly prescribed antibiotics are listed in Table 44.2. These recommendations should not replace clinical judgment as clinical situations vary greatly.

TABLE 44.2	Dosing of Common Antimicrobial Agents During Continuous Renal Replacement Therapy (CRRT)	
Drug	Dosing in CVVH	Dosing in CVVHD or CVVHDF
Vancomycin	LD 15–20 mg/kg, then 1 g q48h	LD 15–20 mg/kg, then 1 g q24h
Cefepime	1–2 g q12h	2 g q12h
Ceftazidime	1–2 g q12h	2 g q12h
Cefotaxime	1–2 g q12h	2 g q12h
Ceftriaxone	2 g q12–24h	2 g q12–24h
Imipenem–cilastatin	250 mg q6h or 500 mg q8h	250 mg q6h, 500 mg q6h, or 500 mg q8h
Meropenem	1 g q12h	1 g q12h
Ciprofloxacin	200 mg q12h	200–400 mg q12h
Metronidazole	500 mg q8h	500 mg q8h
Piperacillin–tazobactam	2.25 g q6h	3.375 g q6h
Amikacin	LD 10 mg/kg, then 7.5 mg/kg q24–48h	LD 10 mg/kg, then 7.5 mg/kg q24–48h
Tobramycin	LD 3 mg/kg, then 2 mg/kg q24–48h	LD 3 mg/kg, then 2 mg/kg q24–48h
Gentamicin	LD 3 mg/kg, then 2 mg/kg q24–48h	LD 3 mg/kg, then 2 mg/kg q24–48h
Daptomycin	4 or 6 mg/kg q48h	4 or 6 mg/kg q48h
Linezolid	600 mg q12h	600 mg q12h
Fluconazole	200–400 mg q24h	400–800 mg q24h
Acyclovir	5–7.5 mg/kg q24h	5–7.5 mg/kg q24h

LD, loading dose.

DRUG DOSING IN SLED

There is limited data on drug clearance and appropriate drug dosing in patients undergoing SLED. The same factors affecting drug dosing in CRRT are applied here. However, drug clearance is more unpredictable due to the intermittent nature of SLED. It is also difficult to make general dosing recommendations for a particular drug as the half-life can be quite variable due to lack of uniformity in dialyzer membrane, blood, and dialysate flow rates (machine and center dependent). For once a day medications, the dose should be given post-SLED. For twice a day medications, the first dose should be given post-SLED and the second dose 12 hours later. Serum levels of antibiotics should be measured immediately postdialysis and supplemental dose given if necessary. The SLED machine should be set up around the same time everyday if possible. Close communication between the nephrology team and the ICU team is essential to ensure adequate drug dosing.

COMPLICATIONS OF RENAL REPLACEMENT THERAPY

As with any procedure, there are certain complications and adverse events that can be associated with renal replacement therapies. Vigilance for such complications and their immediate rectification are essential to prevent life-threatening situations, especially in the vulnerable population of the ICU. In addition, the necessity for a central venous catheter places the patient at risk for infectious complications.

Hypotension

Intradialytic hypotension can occur in all clinical settings with all modalities, although it is more commonly seen with IHD. Volume-depleted and septic patients are at heightened risk, and careful attention to the physical examination and invasive hemodynamic monitoring when indicated can help ensure adequate volume resuscitation prior to initiating the dialysis session. A target central venous pressure of 8 to 12 mm Hg can be used in these settings and may dictate a reduction or stoppage of fluid ultrafiltration. Other factors can also result in intradialytic hypotension. The rapid clearance of uremic solutes can lower the serum osmolality and lead to a fluid shift toward the intracellular space, depleting the intravascular volume. A normal saline bolus of 250 mL or administration of 25% albumin in 100 mL can be used as initial management steps in the treatment of intradialytic hypotension, and ultrafiltration may need to be turned off. The dialysate temperature can be decreased to promote vasoconstriction. Patients who are persistently hypotensive may need to switch to a continuous modality. Air embolism is a very rare complication of dialysis that can lead to hemodynamic instability. Other differential diagnoses to consider include internal hemorrhage, pericardial tamponade, and myocardial infarction.

Arrhythmias

Cardiac arrhythmias can occur in the setting of rapid electrolyte shifts in acute hemodialysis. The removal of certain anti-arrhythmic drugs during dialysis is also a risk factor. In chronic dialysis, a bath with a potassium concentration of 2 to 3 mEq/L is frequently used. However, when hyperkalemia necessitates a dialysate with a potassium concentration of 0 to 1 mEq/L, it is important to monitor hourly potassium levels. A low-potassium dialysate should not be used longer than 1 hour unless the serum potassium remains critically elevated. Patients on digitalis are especially sensitive to hypokalemia. Supraventricular arrhythmias can also be triggered during the placement of the dialysis catheter, by a malpositioned dialysis catheter, and sometimes during dialysis. If the arrhythmia is resulting in hemodynamic compromise, then therapy is discontinued immediately and cardioversion should be attempted.

Dialyzer Reactions

Dialyzer reactions are rare during hemodialysis. Type A, or anaphylactic, reactions are estimated to occur in 4 of every 100,000 sessions and present in the first few minutes once the blood in the circuit returns to the patient. Symptoms are varied and may include urticaria, flushing, chest pain, back pain, dyspnea, vomiting, and chills. Severe cases can progress to hypotension, cardiac arrest, and death. The cause for this reaction is believed to be related to residual amounts of ethylene oxide, which is used to sterilize dialyzers. Type A reactions are treated by immediately discontinuing the dialysis session and discarding the blood in the circuit. Further therapy with epinephrine or bronchodilators depends on the severity of the reaction.

Type B reactions are more common, and are distinguished from Type A reactions in that they are usually less severe and present later, usually after the first 15 minutes of dialysis. They are thought to be due to the use of unsubstituted cellulose dialyzer membranes and complement activation. They occur in 3% to 4% of sessions and also present with chest pain, back pain, dyspnea, or gastrointestinal symptoms. If the symptoms are not severe, then dialysis is continued and the symptoms slowly resolve. Treatment is supportive, with appropriate use of intravenous saline, analgesics, and antiemetics.

Dialysis Catheter-Related Problems

The dialysis catheter itself can also pose problems. When needed acutely, a nontunneled catheter can be inserted into a central vein at the bedside. When infection and bacteremia occur, prompt catheter removal is generally recommended unless vascular access is especially difficult. Thrombus or fibrin sheaths can form around or inside the catheters causing inadequate blood flows for dialysis. Even though heparin is usually instilled into the hub of the catheter after each dialysis, this does not necessary prevent the clot formation. An attempt at clot lysis can be made by instilling 2 mg of alteplase into each catheter lumen. The catheter is then capped for 2 to 3 hours and the medication is aspirated before dialysis is again attempted. Alteplase should not be administered systemically for this purpose. If the catheter continues to malfunction, it may be changed over a guidewire or replaced completely.

In patients with chronic kidney disease, subclavian veins are not used for dialysis catheters, as there is a high risk of subclavian venous stenosis, which can prevent the future placement of an arteriovenous fistula or graft in that extremity for dialysis. There are no data to suggest that tunneled catheters are more beneficial regarding infection rates or adequacy of dialysis in intensive care patients with AKI. Tunneled catheters are typically used in patients with multiple malfunctioning temporary catheters, poor chance for early renal recovery, or for those being transferred out of the ICU to a different facility. For clotted tunneled catheters, interventional radiology consultation is required to perform endoluminal brushing to dislodge thrombi and fibrin sheaths.

Problems Associated with CRRT

One of the advantages of CRRT over IHD is that the slower blood flow rates place a gentler hemodynamic burden on unstable patients. However, hypotension can still occur in this group, especially when high ultrafiltration rates are attempted. Some adverse events are specific to continuous modalities, mostly related to electrolyte abnormalities. Uninterrupted high-flow CRRT can cause dramatic hypophosphatemia, hypokalemia, and hypomagnesemia. Serum electrolytes need to be monitored at least twice daily. Hypokalemia can be corrected by increasing the potassium concentration in the replacement fluid and dialysate. Hypophosphatemia and hypomagnesemia can be corrected by supplementation.

Given its lower flow rates, CRRT usually requires some form of anticoagulation to prevent clotting in the extracorporeal circuit. Heparin is the preferred anticoagulant at many institutions. In cases of heparin-induced thrombocytopenia, the direct thrombin inhibitor argatroban can be used. When systemic anticoagulation is contraindicated, citrate can be used regionally in the dialysis circuit. Citrate chelates calcium in the serum and inhibits activation of the coagulation cascade. Citrate is quickly metabolized to bicarbonate in the liver and thus does not result in systemic anticoagulation. Calcium is replaced through a separate central venous line and this process requires close monitoring of serum ionized calcium levels. With the breakdown of citrate to bicarbonate, the development of a metabolic alkalosis is another concern with this form of anticoagulation. Metabolic alkalosis can be treated by changing the replacement fluid to normal saline from a bicarbonate-based product.

Hypothermia is a well-known complication of CRRT and is common at high flow rates. Significant amounts of heat are lost from the slow-flowing extracorporeal circuit and can cause drops in body temperature of 2°C to 5°C. This can be addressed by warming the replacement fluid being infused or by rewarming the blood returning to the patient through specialized devices that can be attached to the machine. However, this poses a problem regarding the detection of fever. Unpublished reports have shown no advantage to checking routine cultures; therefore, reliance on the other clinical signs of infection is needed.

SUMMARY

RRT is initiated when more conservative medical management has failed to control the fluid, electrolyte, and metabolic complications of AKI. Several modalities are available to the clinician, and selection between intermittent and continuous forms depends on the availability at the institution, the patient's hemodynamic stability, and comorbid illnesses. Despite the overall safety of these procedures, complications and adverse events can occur, requiring meticulous attention and, in some cases, frequent laboratory monitoring to anticipate and prevent their occurrence.

SUGGESTED READINGS

Bagshaw SM, Berthiaume LR, Delaney A, et al. Continuous versus intermittent renal replacement therapy for critically ill patients with acute kidney injury: a meta-analysis. *Crit Care Med.* 2008;36:610.

Brause M, Nuemann A, Schumacher T, et al. Effect of filtration volume of continuous venovenous hemofiltration in the treatment of patients with acute renal failure in intensive care units. *Crit Care Med.* 2003;31:841–846.
  Prospective pilot study comparing patients dialyzed with different target Kt/V.

Cho KC, Himmelfarb J, Paganini E, et al. Survival by dialysis modality in critically ill patients with acute kidney injury. *J Am Soc Nephrol.* 2006;17:3132–3138.
  Multicenter observational study comparing continuous and intermittent dialysis.

Jun M, Heerspink HJ, Ninomiya T, et al. Intensities of renal replacement therapy in acute kidney injury: a systemic review and meta-analysis. *Clin J Am Soc Nephrol.* 2010;5:956–963.

Kroh UF, Holl TJ, Steinhauber W. Management of drug dosing in continuous renal replacement therapy. *Semin Dial.* 1996;9:161–165.
  Review of factors determining drug dosing in CRRT.

Mushatt DM, Mihm LB, Dreisbach AW, et al. Antibiotic dosing in slow extended daily dialysis. *Clin Infect Dis.* 2009;49:433–437.

O'Reilly P, Tolwani A. Renal replacement therapy III: IHD, CRRT, SLED. *Crit Care Clin.* 2005;21:367–378.
  Review of replacement options.

Palevsky PM. Renal replacement therapy I: indications and timing. *Crit Care Clin.* 2005;21:347–356.
  Review of dialytic indications.

Ricci Z, Ronco C. Renal replacement therapy II: dialysis dose. *Crit Care Clin.* 2005;21:357–366.
  Review of dialysis dosing.

Ronco C, Bellomo R, Homel P, et al. Effects of different doses in continuous veno-venous haemofiltration on outcomes of acute renal failure: a prospective randomised trial. *Lancet.* 2000;356:26–30.
  Randomized study comparing patients assigned to different ultrafiltration doses.

Schiffl H, Lang SM, Fischer R. Daily hemodialysis and the outcome of acute renal failure. *N Engl J Med.* 2002;346:305–310.
  Randomized study comparing daily and intermittent conventional dialysis.

The RENAL Replacement Therapy Study Investigators. Intensity of continuous renal-replacement therapy in critically ill patients. *N Engl J Med.* 2009;361:1627–1638.

The VA/NIH Acute Renal Failure Trial Network. Intensity of renal support in critically ill patients with acute kidney injury. *N Engl J Med.* 2008;359:7–20.

Trotman RL, Williamson JC, Shoemaker DM, et al. Antibiotic dosing in critically ill adult patients receiving continuous renal replacement therapy. *Clin Infect Dis.* 2005;41:1159–1166.

Vinsonneau C, Camus C, Combes A, et al. Continuous venovenous haemodiafiltration versus intermittent haemodialysis for acute renal failure in patients with multiple-organ dysfunction syndrome: a multicentre randomised trial. *Lancet.* 2006;368:379–385.
Multicenter randomized study comparing continuous and intermittent dialysis.

45

Fulminant Hepatic Failure

Anupam Aditi and Jeffrey S. Crippin

Fulminant hepatic failure (FHF) is a rare entity characterized by coagulopathy, encephalopathy, and acute hepatic failure in the absence of preexisting cirrhosis (Table 45.1). Exceptions to the absence of preexisting liver disease include autoimmune hepatitis and Wilson's disease, if the disease has only been recognized within the last 26 weeks. Approximately 2000 cases of FHF are reported per year, with a high morbidity and mortality rate noted in patients who do not receive hepatic transplantation.

CAUSES AND DIAGNOSIS

In patients with FHF, it is imperative to ascertain the etiology of the liver failure, as this can dictate treatment. A prospective multicenter review of 308 patients enrolled between 1998 and 2001 by the Acute Liver Failure Study Group found the following distribution of causes: acetaminophen overdose (39%), indeterminate etiology (17%), idiosyncratic drug reactions (13%), and viral hepatitis (hepatitis A virus or hepatitis B) (12%). Table 45.1 outlines the possible causes of FHF, as well as the diagnostic evaluation needed for each etiology. On presentation, initial laboratory analysis should include a complete blood cell count, basic metabolic panel, liver chemistries, magnesium, phosphate, lactic acid, arterial blood gas, acetaminophen level, acute viral hepatitis panel, toxicology screen, ceruloplasmin level, antinuclear antibodies, anti-smooth muscle antibodies, HIV status, and a pregnancy test.

MANAGEMENT OF ETIOLOGY-SPECIfiC FHF (SEE ALGORITHM 45.1)

The benefit of N-acetylcysteine (NAC) in acetaminophen toxicity has been demonstrated for decades; however, its role in nonacetaminophen-related acute liver failure (ALF) has only recently been established. In a prospective, double-blind trial with 173 patients with ALF without clinical or historical evidence of acetaminophen overdose, a transplant-free survival benefit was demonstrated in patients who received NAC therapy. Patients with grade 1 to 2 encephalopathy treated with NAC were 2.46 times more likely to survive to 21 days without a transplant than patients with grade 1 to 2 encephalopathy receiving a placebo. The data also demonstrated a statistically significant transplant-free survival at 1 year in the NAC group. Given its minimal adverse reaction profile, NAC therapy should be initiated for all patients with ALF presenting

TABLE 45.1   Diagnosis and Causes of Acute Liver Failure

1. Acute hepatic disease <26 weeks without evidence of preexisting cirrhosis
2. Encephalopathy
3. Coagulopathy (INR >1.5)

Etiology	History and physical examination	Diagnostic evaluation and biopsy
Acetaminophen	History of ingestion	Acetaminophen level, suspect ingestion even with low level, use nomogram
Drug toxicity	New medications, antibiotics, NSAIDS, anticonvulsants, psychiatric history, herbals, unlikely if >1 yr on medication	Serum osmolality, drug levels
Substance abuse	Mushroom poisoning, cocaine use	Urine drug screen, serum osmolality
Viral	Viral syndrome, pregnancy, recent travel, skin lesions, immunocompromised state	HBsAg, IgM anti-HBc, IgM anti-HAV, IgM anti-HEV, anti-HCV, HCV-RNA by PCR, HIV, HSV, parvovirus B19, adenovirus, CMV, EBV
Shock liver	History of heart failure, cardiac arrest, volume depletion, or substance abuse	BNP, lactate, urine drug screen, serum osmolality, 2D echocardiogram
Malignancy	Budd–Chiari syndrome, infiltrating disease, lymphadenopathy, venous thromboembolism	Abdominal ultrasound with Doppler, abdominal computed tomography, tumor markers
Wilson's disease	Patient <18 yr old, Kayser–Fleischer rings Coombs-negative hemolytic anemia	Ceruloplasmin (<20 mg/dL), 24-hr urinary Cu (>100 μg), nonceruloplasmin Cu >25 μg/dL (serum Cu-[3 × ceruloplasmin]), subnormal alkaline phospatase/bilirubin ratio <2, uric acid, hemolytic anemia *Bx: Hepatic copper >250 μg/g dry weight*
Acute fatty liver of pregnancy, HELLP	Pregnancy	β-HCG, low platelets, hemolytic anemia, proteinuria *Bx: Oil Red O staining*
Autoimmune	Erythroderma, history of autoimmune disease (e.g., thyroiditis, arthritis)	Autoimmune serologies: antinuclear antibody, anti–smooth muscle antibody, anti-LKM1 *Bx: interface hepatitis and portal plasma cell infiltrate*

INR, international normalized ratio.

ALGORITHM 45.1 Treatment Algorithm for Acute Liver Failure

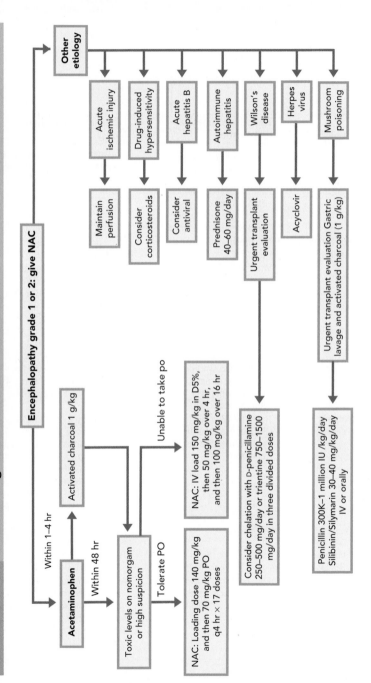

with grade 1 to 2 encephalopathy. Treatment with NAC should not delay transfer to a transplant facility.

Acetaminophen Toxicity

Acetaminophen toxicity is the leading cause of FHF, and clinicians should have a low threshold for starting NAC therapy. Indications for empiric treatment with NAC include known ingestion of >10 g/day, a high suspicion of acetaminophen overdose, inadequate knowledge of circumstances surrounding admission, and any elevated acetaminophen level (Fig. 45.1). A single dose of acetaminophen at 150 mg/kg or more carries a risk of liver damage, but much smaller doses over several days can also be damaging as well. If ingestion is known to have occurred within 4 hours of presentation, activated charcoal (1 g/kg) is more effective in lowering the plasma acetaminophen level than gastric lavage, ipecac, or supportive treatment. Administration of activated charcoal prior to treatment with NAC does not reduce the efficacy of either agent. NAC should be administered as early as possible, although its effect is seen even 48 hours after ingestion. A Cochrane database review reported that NAC reduces mortality (odds ratio, 0.26) in patients with FHF. Refer to Algorithm 45.1 for PO and IV NAC dosing. In a review of transplantation for acetaminophen overdose, there was no difference in survival rate between the use of oral and various intravenous protocols of NAC administration.

Viral Hepatitis

Hepatitis B, with or without hepatitis D, accounts for >50% of viral causes of FHF. Treatment with lamivudine (100 mg/day) has been used anecdotally for acute hepatitis B, and case reports have shown clinical benefits; however, the only randomized controlled trial (RCT) with lamivudine did not show significant clinical and biochemical improvement compared to placebo. One study did demonstrate a mortality benefit of lamivudine therapy in patients with reactivation of hepatitis B during immunosuppressive therapy. Hepatitis E is a more common cause of FHF in immigrants from endemic countries such as Russia, India, Pakistan, and Mexico. Treatment of acute hepatitis A and E is supportive. Hepatitis C alone rarely causes ALF; however, other viruses such as HSV, EBV, adenovirus, and parvovirus B19 have been noted in the literature.

MANAGEMENT OF SYSTEMIC COMPLICATIONS

Central Nervous System

Cerebral edema and increased intracranial pressure (ICP) are serious complications of FHF, seen in up to 80% of patients who die in the setting of FHF. The risk of cerebral edema increases with progression of encephalopathy, with a >75% incidence in patients with grade 4 encephalopathy. Advanced cerebral edema can lead to uncal herniation and death.

Management of neurologic complications is outlined in Algorithm 45.2. Patients with grade 1 or 2 encephalopathy should be transferred to a liver transplant center. Patients with grade 3 to 4 encephalopathy should be intubated for airway protection. Endotracheal lidocaine should be used before suctioning to decrease choking/Valsalva. Frequent neurologic examinations are imperative, and clinical clues such as systemic hypertension, bradycardia, posturing, and decreased pupillary reflexes can suggest impending herniation.

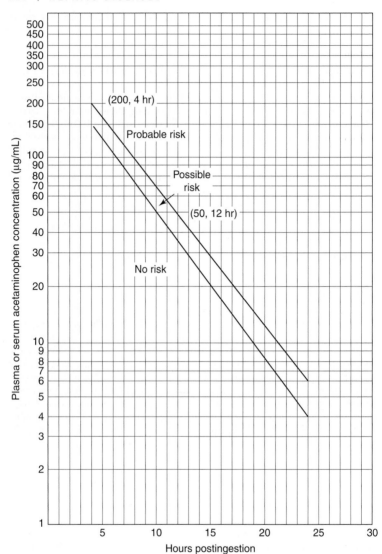

Figure 45.1. Nomogram for acetaminophen hepatotoxicity. (Adapted from Rumack BH, Peterson RC, Koch GG, et al. Acetaminophen overdose: 662 cases with evaluation of oral acetylcysteine treatment. *Arch Intern Med.* 1981;141:380.)

ALGORITHM 45.2 CNS Complications of Fulminant Hepatic Failure

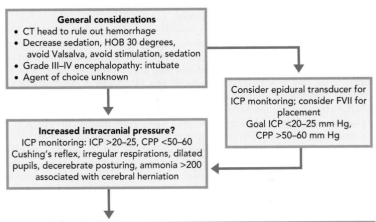

General considerations
- CT head to rule out hemorrhage
- Decrease sedation, HOB 30 degrees, avoid Valsalva, avoid stimulation, sedation
- Grade III–IV encephalopathy: intubate
- Agent of choice unknown

Consider epidural transducer for ICP monitoring; consider FVII for placement
Goal ICP <20–25 mm Hg, CPP >50–60 mm Hg

Increased intracranial pressure?
ICP monitoring: ICP >20–25, CPP <50–60
Cushing's reflex, irregular respirations, dilated pupils, decerebrate posturing, ammonia >200 associated with cerebral herniation

Intervention	Administration	Comments
Mannitol	Bolus 0.5–1 g/kg. Can repeat twice.	No role in prophylaxis Keep serum osmolality <320 mOsm/kg; monitor for hyperosmolality Side effects: hyper/hyponatremia, volume overload
Hyperventilation	Titrate to pCO₂ 25–30 mm Hg	No role in prophylaxis Temporary measure to prevent acute decompensation
Hypertonic saline	145–155 mmol/L	Prophylactic level 145–155 mmol/L can prevent rise in ICP without survival benefit
Barbiturates	Thiopental 185–500 mg/15 min Or pentobarbital bolus 3–5 mg/kg followed by continuous infusion of 0.2–1 mg/kg/hr	Can decrease ICP in failed cases Side effects: Severe hypotension
Steroids	10 mg IV q 6° dexamethasone	Only indicated for CNS infection or brain tumor Does not increase survival in acute liver failure
Hypothermia	Goal 32–34°C	Uncontrolled trials suggest benefit Side effects: arrhythmias, infection, and coagulopathy

CNS, central nervous system; FVII, factor VII; HOB, head of bed.

ICP monitoring should be considered for patients with rapidly progressive encephalopathy and those listed for liver transplantation. It is currently used by approximately 50% of liver transplant programs; however, no RCT has been performed to demonstrate a mortality benefit. Three types of catheters are used for monitoring ICP: epidural, subdural, and parenchymal. A review of 262 patients showed a complication rate of 4% with epidural transducers and approximately 20% with subdural and parenchymal monitors; however, epidural catheters are less reliable in comparison. The most common complications include bleeding in the setting of coagulopathy, infection, and volume overload resulting from correction of coagulopathy. Recombinant factor VII has been used in a small trial to aid with placement of ICP transducers with favorable results. ICP should be maintained at a level <20 mm Hg, with a cerebral perfusion pressure (mean arterial pressure [MAP] minus ICP) >50 mm Hg.

Once increased ICP or cerebral edema is present, aggressive measures should be undertaken to prevent herniation. Minimal sedation, avoidance of sensory stimulation, and raising the head of the bed can be helpful. Therapies focused on decreasing cerebral edema include osmotic agents (mannitol or hypertonic saline) or decreasing cerebral blood flow (hyperventilation or hypothermia).

Mannitol is administered as a bolus dose (0.5 to 1 g/kg of a 20% solution). The dose can be repeated twice; however, administration is limited by maintaining a serum osmolality <320 mOsm/kg. If patients have concomitant renal failure, hemofiltration should be considered. Hyperventilation has only a short-term benefit but can be used with the goal of reducing $PaCO_2$ to 25 mm Hg. An RCT demonstrated no benefit of prophylactic continuous hyperventilation in ALF. A study of 30 patients with ICP monitoring randomized to 3% hypertonic saline with a goal serum sodium concentration of 145 to 155 mmol/L showed a significant decrease in average ICP and episodes of increased ICP, but no survival benefit. Hypothermia (32°C to 34°C) has been associated with a beneficial effect in uncontrolled trials. Patients with FHF may have seizure activity, but prophylactic phenytoin has not proven to be effective in improving survival. Despite an association between an arterial ammonia level of >200 μmol/L and herniation, no benefit of gut decontamination or lactulose has been demonstrated in ALF. Barbiturate coma can be attempted for refractory increased ICP, but requires close monitoring of MAP due to its association with hypotension. Dexamethasone is not effective at prolonging survival.

Coagulopathy

The management of coagulopathy is outlined in Algorithm 45.3. Synthesis of coagulation factors I, II, V, VII, IX, and X is depressed in patients with FHF. Sources of bleeding include procedure sites, stress ulcers, lungs, and the oropharynx. Proton pump inhibitors should be used for stress ulcer prophylaxis. Platelets should only be transfused for counts <10,000/μL or in the face of active bleeding. Vitamin K is routinely given, but fresh-frozen plasma should not be transfused unless there is active bleeding or a planned procedure. Packed red blood cells can be transfused for symptomatic anemia or to replace blood loss secondary to hemorrhage.

The role of recombinant factor VII has been evaluated during the placement of ICP monitors. In an unblinded study comparing patients with FHF given recombinant factor VII with a cohort of historic controls, patients receiving recombinant factor VII all had successful placement (7/7 vs. 3/8). Patients receiving recombinant factor VII also had a significant decrease in mortality and anasarca from fluid overload.

Hypotension

Hypotension is multifactorial in patients with FHF, resulting from volume depletion, third spacing, infection, gastrointestinal bleeding, or as a result of overall low systemic vascular resistance and a hyperkinetic cardiovascular state. Fluid resuscitation should be balanced with avoidance of volume overload and the theoretical risk of increasing ICP. Maintenance fluid should be glucose based because of hypoglycemia associated with liver failure. Although not compared directly in trials, dopamine or norepinephrine can be used for vasopressor support. In a small study, dopamine led to a significant increase in cardiac output, systemic oxygen delivery, and hepatic and splanchnic blood flow when used to increase MAP by 10 mm Hg. Although systemic oxygen consumption was increased, splanchnic oxygen consumption was decreased. A small trial evaluating the role of norepinephrine in FHF noted an increase in MAP, although it was not associated with an increase in cardiac index and actually resulted in a decrease in

ALGORITHM 45.3   Management of the Complication of Fulminant Hepatic Failure

SC, subcutaneously; FFP, fresh-frozen plasma; Cx, chest x-ray; MAP, mean arterial pressure; inh, inhibitors; plts, platelets; PMN, polymorphonuclear leukocyte; CVVHD, continuous venovenous hemodialysis; HD, hemodialysis; D5%, 5% dextrose; CRRT, continuous renal replacement therapy; IHD, intermittent hemodialysis; FVII, factor VII.

383

systemic oxygen consumption. Terlipressin has also been studied in ALF, and two research studies have found conflicting data on whether terlipressin causes detrimental elevations in ICP. Resuscitation with colloid is theoretically better than crystalloid, given that albumin induces a more effective expansion of the central blood volume, but no mortality benefit has been shown.

Infection

Infections are found in 80% of patients with FHF, with 25% of patients developing documented bacteremia and 33% developing systemic fungal infections. Periodic surveillance cultures should be obtained to detect infections as early as possible. Although prophylactic antibiotics do not provide a survival advantage, a low threshold for initiation of broad-spectrum coverage should be maintained. Infections and hyperthermia increase the risk of hepatic encephalopathy; therefore, a theoretical benefit of empiric antibiotic therapy exists for patients with worsening encephalopathy.

Renal Failure

Renal failure is multifactorial in patients with FHF because of the direct toxic effect of ingested substances, volume depletion, hypotension, acute tubular necrosis, and/or the hepatorenal syndrome. In contrast to acute tubular necrosis, renal failure due to the hepatorenal syndrome is characterized by a low urinary sodium (<10 mEq/L), progressive hyponatremia, and a lack of improvement with volume expansion. Nephrotoxic agents such as aminoglycosides and nonsteroidal anti-inflammatory drugs should be avoided and NAC should be used prior to intravenous contrast studies. When dialysis is needed, continuous renal replacement therapy should be used over daily intermittent hemodialysis, due to its association with improved cardiovascular dynamics.

Metabolic Complications

Metabolic complications include hypoglycemia resulting from diminished glucose synthesis and lactic acidosis due to anaerobic glucose metabolism. Patients benefit from glucose monitoring and treatment of hypoglycemia with dextrose-based solutions. Electrolytes such as phosphorus, potassium, and magnesium are usually abnormal and should be repleted as indicated. Enteral or parenteral nutrition should be initiated early, and protein should not be restricted. A recent Cochrane database review did not find convincing evidence of a beneficial role of branched chain amino acids in the treatment of patients with hepatic encephalopathy.

PROGNOSTIC INDICATORS

The most important prognostic indicator in FHF is the etiology of hepatic damage. Acetaminophen toxicity, hepatitis A, ischemic liver injury, and pregnancy-related liver failure portend a transplant-free survival of >50%, whereas idiosyncratic drug reactions, hepatitis B, autoimmune hepatitis, Wilson's disease, and Budd–Chiari syndrome carry a survival rate of <25% without transplantation. The timing of the presentation is also important; however, these data may be confounded by the etiology of FHF. An illness of <1 week in duration suggests ischemic hepatopathy or acetaminophen overdose and is associated with improved survival, whereas an illness >4 weeks in duration suggests an indeterminate or viral etiology and indicates a poor transplant-free survival. The degree of encephalopathy is another strong

TABLE 45.2	West Haven Criteria for Semiquantitative Grading of Mental State
Grade 1	Trivial lack of awareness Euphoria or anxiety Shortened attention span Impaired performance of addition
Grade 2	Lethargy or apathy Minimal disorientation for time or place Subtle personality change Inappropriate behavior Impaired performance of subtraction
Grade 3	Somnolence to semistupor, but responsive to verbal stimuli Confusion Gross disorientation
Grade 4	Coma (unresponsive to verbal or noxious stimuli)

Atterbury et al. *Am J Dig Dis.* 1978;23:398–406.

predictor of outcome (Table 45.2). Patients with grade 2 encephalopathy have a 65% to 70% chance of survival, whereas patients with grades 3 and 4 have a 30% to 50% and a 20% chance of survival, respectively. The King's College Criteria (Table 45.3) are important indicators of outcome. In patients with nonacetaminophen-associated FHF, the presence of a single factor is associated with a mortality rate

TABLE 45.3	King's College Hospital Criteria for Liver Transplantation in Fulminant Hepatic Failure
Acetaminophen-induced disease	Arterial pH <7.30 OR Prothrombin time >100 sec AND Creatinine > 3.4 mg/dL AND Grade III or IV encephalopathy
Nonacetaminophen-induced disease	Prothrombin time >100 sec (regardless of encephalopathy grade) OR Any 3 of the following (regardless of encephalopathy grade): Age <10 or >40 yr Etiology: non-A, non-B hepatitis, halothane hepatitis, or idiosyncratic drug reaction Duration of jaundice before onset of encephalopathy >7 days Prothrombin time >50 sec Serum bilirubin >18 mg/dL

O'Grady et al. *Gastroenterology.* 1989;97:439–445.

of 80% whereas the presence of any three factors is associated with a 95% mortality rate. In patients with acetaminophen hepatotoxicity and FHF, a single risk factor is associated with a mortality of 55% and the presence of severe acidosis confers a 95% mortality.

LIVER TRANSPLANTATION

Liver transplantation is a proven treatment of FHF, although limited by the prompt availability of donors. Posttransplant survival rates are as high as 80% to 90%. The decision to pursue transplantation versus continuing medical therapy (such as NAC) is difficult. Factors to consider include the possibility of spontaneous recovery, the feasibility of transplantation, and assessment of contraindications to transplantation. Prognostic models such as the King's College Criteria (Table 45.3) and the Acute Physiology and Chronic Health Evaluation (APACHE) II score help in determining the need for liver transplantation. For patients with acetaminophen-associated FHF, a recent meta-analysis reported that the King's College Criteria had a sensitivity of 0.59 and specificity of 0.92 in determining the need for transplantation. An APACHE II score of >15 was associated with a specificity of 0.81 and sensitivity of 0.92 in determining the need for transplantation. The APACHE II score had a higher positive likelihood ratio of 16.4 and negative likelihood ratio of 0.19 (one study) versus the King's College Criteria with a positive and negative likelihood ratio of 12.33 and 0.29, respectively, based on six pooled studies.

SUGGESTED READINGS

Brok J, Buckley N, Gluud C. Interventions for paracetamol (acetaminophen) overdose. *Cochrane Database Syst Rev.* 2006;CD003328.
> *This meta-analysis provides a comprehensive review of proven and unproven therapies for the leading cause of fulminant hepatic failure.*

Hoofnagle JH, Carithers RL, Shapiro C, et al. Fulminant hepatic failure: summary of a workshop. *Hepatology.* 1995;21:240–252.
> *This paper summarizes issues in the management of fulminant hepatic failure.*

Kulkarni S, Cronin DC. Fulminant hepatic failure. In: Hall JB, Schidt GA, Wood LD, eds. Principles of critical care. 3rd ed. New York, NY: McGraw-Hill Professional, 2005:1279–1288.
> *This chapter provides an excellent overview of the pathophysiology and management issues in fulminant hepatic failure.*

Polson J, Lee WM. AASLD position paper: the management of acute liver failure. *Hepatology.* 2005;41:1179–1197.
> *This paper provides guidelines by the American Association for the Study of Liver Diseases on the management of fulminant hepatic failure.*

Raghavan M, Marik PE. Therapy of intracranial hypertension in patients with fulminant hepatic failure. *Neurocrit Care.* 2006;4:179–189.
> *This paper provides an excellent overview of treatment for intracranial hypertension and reviews the current understanding of the mechanisms leading to this life-threatening complication.*

Yee HF Jr, Lidofsky SD. Acute liver failure. In: Feldman M, Scharschmidt BF, Sleisenger MH, eds. Sleisenger & Fordtran's gastrointestinal and liver disease. 7th ed. Philadelphia, PA: Saunders, 2002:1567–1576.
> *This chapter provides an excellent overview of the pathophysiology and management issues in fulminant hepatic failure.*

46 Hyperbilirubinemia

Anupam Aditi and Jeffrey S. Crippin

PHYSIOLOGY

Heme is a breakdown constituent of senescent erythrocytes. It is converted to biliverdin by heme oxygenase and further reduced by biliverdin reductase to bilirubin in the reticuloendothelial system. Bilirubin, unconjugated and water insoluble at this point, is tightly bound to albumin and delivered to the liver. It is transported into the hepatocytes by carrier-mediated mechanisms, transferred to the endoplasmic reticulum bound by cytosolic proteins, and converted to a water-soluble form with the addition of uridine diphosphate (UDP) glucuronic acid. An ATP-dependent export pump, the rate-limiting step in bilirubin transport, transfers conjugated bilirubin into the biliary canaliculi, where it is added to bile. Bile eventually drains into the small intestine and is subsequently metabolized by ileal and colonic bacteria to urobilinogen. Eighty percent of urobilinogen is excreted in stool, whereas approximately 20% is reabsorbed in the small intestine and enters the portal circulation. The reabsorbed urobilinogen is subsequently excreted in stool and urine.

On the basis of the aforementioned physiology, the bilirubin pathway can be divided into four steps: (1) bilirubin production, (2) hepatic bilirubin uptake, (3) bilirubin conjugation, and (4) bilirubin excretion. Hyperbilirubinemia is classically divided into unconjugated and conjugated forms, with pathology at steps 1, 2, and 3 leading to unconjugated hyperbilirubinemia and pathology at step 4 causing conjugated hyperbilirubinemia. However, this division is rarely absolute and clinicians may encounter a mixed picture.

Indirect Hyperbilirubinemia

Unconjugated hyperbilirubinemia occurs when the indirect bilirubin is >80% of the total bilirubin. This may be caused by increased bilirubin production or decreased hepatocyte uptake and conjugation. Hemolysis, resorption of internal bleeding or hematoma, and dyserythropoiesis are frequent causes of unconjugated hyperbilirubinemia. Hemolysis is characterized by an elevated reticulocyte count, schistocytes or spherocytes on peripheral smear, a positive Coombs test, an increased lactate dehydrogenase, and a decreased haptoglobin level. A decrease in hepatocyte uptake and conjugation is the result of inhibition of uptake mechanisms, inhibition of glucuronidation, or defects in conjugation. Competitive inhibition of bilirubin uptake may be caused by medications such as rifampin and probenecid, whereas inhibition of glucuronidation can occur with hyperthyroidism and estradiol therapy. A common enzymatic defect, that is, decreased activity of bilirubin UDP-glucuronyl transferase, results in asymptomatic unconjugated hyperbilirubinemia, better known as Gilbert's syndrome. A more severe quantitative defect in UDP-glucuronyl transferase leads to Crigler–Najjar types I and II.

Direct Hyperbilirubinemia

Conjugated or direct hyperbilirubinemia is usually secondary to hepatocellular dysfunction, biliary obstruction, or biliary injury. Hepatocellular dysfunction, whether acute or chronic, can cause reflux of conjugated bilirubin into the circulation. This is dependent largely on the fact that active canalicular excretion of conjugated bilirubin is the rate-limiting step in the bilirubin pathway and extremely sensitive to liver dysfunction. Acute hepatocellular dysfunction is suggested by an elevated bilirubin level in association with elevated aminotransferase levels. Chronic dysfunction results in lower aminotransferase levels, and common causes include chronic viral hepatitis and alcoholic liver disease. Both acute and chronic liver dysfunction may give rise to a mixed hyperbilirubinemia if a disease process causing unconjugated hyperbilirubinemia is superimposed on hepatic dysfunction.

Biliary dysfunction results from obstruction of the extrahepatic biliary ducts or nonobstructive injury of the intra- or extrahepatic ducts. A direct bilirubin fraction >50% of the total bilirubin suggests a hepatobiliary etiology and, if accompanied by an elevated alkaline phosphatase and γ-glutamyl transpeptidase (GGTP) level, favors biliary obstruction. Causes of intrinsic obstruction include choledocholithiasis, biliary strictures, cholangiocarcinoma, primary sclerosing cholangitis, AIDS cholangiopathy, and parasitic infection. Extrinsic compression can be secondary to pancreatic masses (tumor, fibrosis, pseudocyst, or abscess), or lymphadenopathy. Nonobstructive biliary disease also presents with an elevated alkaline phosphatase level, an elevated GGTP level, and direct hyperbilirubinemia but without imaging evidence of obstruction. Potential etiologies include acute viral hepatitis, primary biliary cirrhosis, infiltrative diseases such as amyloidosis and sarcoidosis, drug toxicity, sepsis, total parenteral nutrition, and paraneoplastic syndrome secondary to renal cell carcinoma.

Diagnosis and Therapy

Imaging is required for diagnosis and guides therapy. Imaging modalities include ultrasonography, computed tomography (CT), endoscopic retrograde cholangiopancreatography (ERCP), percutaneous transhepatic cholangiography (PTC), and magnetic resonance cholangiopancreatography (MRCP) (Algorithm 46.1). An abdominal ultrasonography or CT, both with high specificity, can confirm an obstructive process. Ultrasonography is a more sensitive technique for detecting stones within the gallbladder, whereas both techniques are less apt to identify choledocholithiasis. An ultrasonography is less helpful in obese patients and when overlying bowel gas is present. If these studies fail to reveal a cause of biliary obstruction, an MRCP gives better visualization of the intrahepatic ducts. If an obstructive process is confirmed, cholangiography can provide direct access to the biliary tree. An ERCP gains access to the proximal biliary tree, whereas PTC, starting at the peripheral bile ducts, allows visualization of the biliary tree. Either study allows decompression of obstructive processes via sphincterotomy and stone retrieval, stricture dilation, or stent placement. Superimposed infection of an obstructed biliary tract must promptly be treated with broad-spectrum antibiotics and prompt decompression of the biliary tree. If no obstruction is found and a cholestatic pattern still persists, cholangiography may be useful to delineate biliary

ALGORITHM 46.1 Evaluation and Management of Hyperbilirubinemia

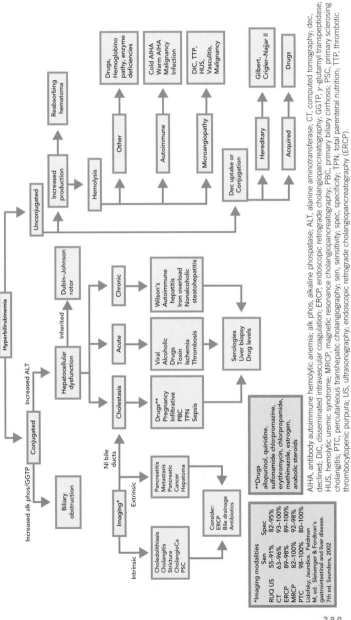

AIHA, antibody autoimmune hemolytic anemia; alk phos, alkaline phospatase; ALT, alanine aminotransferase; CT, computed tomography; dec, declined; DIC, disseminated intravascular coagulation; ERCP, endoscopic retrograde cholangiopancreatography; GGTP, γ-glutamyl transpeptidase; HUS, hemolytic uremic syndrome; MRCP, magnetic resonance cholangiopancreatography; PBC, primary biliary cirrhosis; PSC, primary sclerosing cholangitis; PTC, percutaneous transhepatic cholangiography; sen, sensitivity; spec, specificity; TPN, total parenteral nutrition; TTP, thrombotic thrombocytopenic purpura; US, ultrasonography; endoscopic retrograde cholangiopancreatography (ERCP).

*Imaging modalities

	Sen	Spec
RUQ US	55–91%	82–95%
CT	63–96%	93–100%
ERCP	89–98%	89–100%
MRCP	82–100%	92–98%
PTC	98–100%	80–100%

Lidofsky: Jaundice. Feldman
M, ed. Sleisenger & Fordtran's
gastrointestinal and liver disease.
7th ed. Saunders, 2002

**Drugs
allopurinol, quinidine,
sulfonamide chlorpromazine,
erythromycin, chlorpropamide,
methimazole, estrogen,
anabolic steroids

389

anatomy. CT imaging can reveal infiltrative disease, and a liver biopsy is often required to further define the extent and type of liver injury.

SUGGESTED READINGS

Greenberger NJ, Paumgartner G. Diseases of the gallbladder and bile ducts. In: Kasper D, et al., eds. Harrison's principles of internal medicine. 16th ed. New York, NY: McGraw-Hill, 2005:1880–1891.

This chapter discusses common causes of biliary dysfunction and provides an approach to diagnosing biliary disease.

Lidofsky S. Jaundice. In: Feldman M, ed. Sleisenger & Fordtran's gastrointestinal and liver disease. 7th ed. Philadelphia, PA: Saunders, 2002:249–261.

This chapter provides a systematic approach to evaluating a patient with jaundice and compares the various imaging modalities to evaluate biliary disease.

Pratt DS, Kaplan MM. Jaundice. In: Kasper D, et al., ed. Harrison's principles of internal medicine. 16th ed. New York, NY: McGraw-Hill, 2005:238–243.

This chapter also provides a systematic approach to evaluating a patient with jaundice.

Summerfield JA. Diseases of the gallbladder and biliary tree. In: Warrell D, et al., ed. Oxford textbook of medicine. 4th ed. Oxford: Oxford University Press, 2003:700–708.

This source provides an excellent overview of investigations in biliary disease.

Wolkoff A. The hyperbilirubinemias. In: Kasper D, et al., ed. Harrison's principles of internal medicine. 16th ed. New York, NY: McGraw-Hill, 2005:1817–1822.

This chapter provides a great review of the pathophysiology and disorders of the biliary system.

47 End-Stage Liver Disease

Mrudula V. Kumar and Kevin M. Korenblat

The shared outcome of most untreated, chronic liver diseases is the development of cirrhosis. The resulting clinically evident liver disease is commonly referred to as decompensated cirrhosis and is characterized by both portal hypertension and hepatic synthetic dysfunction. These complications typically coexist in patients with cirrhosis and are the major cause of liver disease–related morbidity and mortality. Common complications of portal hypertension are ascites, portal hypertensive-related bleeding, hepatic encephalopathy, and thrombocytopenia. ICU admissions for these complications are a frequent occurrence, and successful management depends on prompt diagnosis and treatment.

ASCITES

Ascites describes the pathologic accumulation of a serous fluid in the peritoneal cavity. It is the most frequent manifestation of decompensated cirrhosis and is associated with a 2-year mortality rate of 50%. Cirrhotic ascites is identified by its low albumin content and a >1.1 g/dL difference between serum and ascites albumin concentrations (serum–ascites albumin gradient).

Paracentesis for the sampling of the ascites is required in all patients with new-onset ascites or in those with a change in their clinical condition, such as confusion, renal dysfunction, or gastrointestinal bleeding. Paracentesis (Fig. 47.1) is a safe procedure that can be done even in patients with coagulopathy and thrombocytopenia. The right and left lower quadrants are the preferred site for paracentesis, and complications are unusual and mostly limited to abdominal wall hematomas. The ascites should be analyzed for albumin, cell count, and differential and the fluid inoculated directly into blood culture media.

Although ascites is best managed with oral furosemide and spironolactone, diuretics may need to be withheld in ICU patients who frequently have renal dysfunction or hypovolemia. Intravenous (IV) diuretics should be avoided in patients with cirrhosis, as they can precipitate renal failure. Repeated large-volume paracentesis is a valid strategy for the management of ascites refractory to medical therapy. The administration of albumin at the time of paracentesis has been advocated to ameliorate the risk of postparacentesis circulatory dysfunction. In practice, 12.5 g of 25% albumin can be infused for every 2 L of ascites removed. The timing of administration has not been rigorously studied, but owing to the long half-life of albumin in the circulation, its administration after completion of the paracentesis is likely to be sufficient.

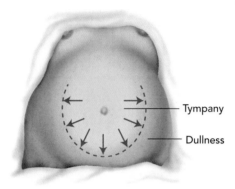

Figure 47.1. Areas of dullness in both right and left lower abdominal quadrants are ideal sites for diagnostic paracentesis.

The benefits of albumin notwithstanding, there are no compelling data that albumin administered with paracentesis improves patient survival; however, the sample size of the studies available may make detection of a survival advantage difficult. The principal benefit of large-volume paracentesis is relief of symptoms; there is no evidence that those with large-volume cirrhotic ascites are at risk for the abdominal compartment syndrome and thus large-volume paracentesis to decrease peritoneal ascites volume should not be expected to improve renal function.

Hepatic hydrothorax occurs in as many as 13% of patients with ascites, is typically right sided, and occurs as a result of defects in the diaphragm that permit passage of ascites into the pleural space. This complication can be managed by thoracentesis, diuretics, and, when refractory to medical therapy, transjugular intrahepatic portosystemic shunt (TIPS) placement. Tube thoracostomy should be avoided because volume losses can be substantial and precipitate renal dysfunction.

SPONTANEOUS BACTERIAL PERITONITIS

The most important complication of ascites is the development of spontaneous bacterial peritonitis (SBP). Between 10% and 27% of patients with cirrhotic ascites will have SBP at the time of hospitalization. There is no typical presentation of SBP, and signs such as abdominal pain, fever, or leukocytosis are frequently absent. The diagnosis is established by the finding of >250/mL polymorphonuclear cells in the ascites or the growth of organisms in a culture of ascites fluid. SBP should be differentiated from secondary bacterial peritonitis as a consequence of bowel perforation or nonperforating abdominal abscess (Algorithm 47.1).

SBP should be treated with prompt parenteral antibiotics. Second- and third-generation cephalosporins (cefotaxime 1 g IV q8hr or ceftriaxone 1 g q24hr) have proven effective in the management of SBP. Renal dysfunction occurs in as many as one-third of patients with SBP despite adequate antibiotic treatment. Discontinuation of diuretics and the administration of IV albumin (25%) given at a dose of 1.5 g/kg body weight on day 1 and 1 g/kg on day 3 was shown in a randomized, controlled studies to reduce the rates of renal dysfunction. This intervention should be strongly

ALGORITHM 47.1   Assessment of Cirrhotic Ascites

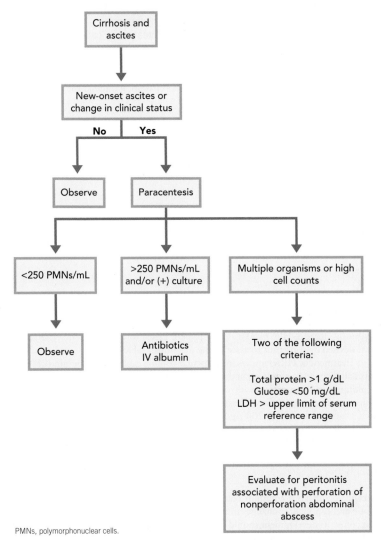

PMNs, polymorphonuclear cells.

considered in all patients with SBP and particularly those with jaundice and renal insufficiency.

Antibiotic prophylaxis (norfloxacin 400 mg PO daily) has been advocated in patients with a previous episode of SBP and in those with ascitic fluid protein <1.5 g/dL and at least one of the following criteria: serum creatinine >1.2 mg/dL, serum urea nitrogen >25 mg/dL, Na <130 mEq/L, or bilirubin >3 mg/dL.

| TABLE 47.1 | Diagnostic Criteria for the Hepatorenal Syndrome |

Major criteria
    Advanced, chronic hepatic failure and portal hypertension
    Serum creatinine >1.5 mg/dL or 24-hr urine creatinine clearance
      <40 mL/min
    Absence of shock, massive gastrointestinal or renal fluid losses, exposure to
      nephrotoxic agents, hypovolemia, or ongoing sepsis
    No sustained improvement in renal function following diuretic withdrawal and
      volume expansion with 1.5 L of isotonic saline
    Proteinuria <500 mg/dL
    No evidence of obstructive uropathy or parenchymal renal disease

Minor criteria
    Urine volume <500 mL/day
    Urine sodium <10 mEq/L
    Urine osmolality >plasma osmolality
    Urine RBCs <50 per HPF
    Serum sodium <130 mEq/L

HPF, high-power field; RBC, red blood cell.

THE HEPATORENAL SYNDROME

The hepatorenal syndrome (HRS) is a clinical diagnosis based on the development of progressive renal failure in cirrhosis. The syndrome can be subdivided into a rapidly progressive (type 1 HRS) and a slower (type 2 HRS) form. Diagnostic criteria have been devised by consensus to assist in the diagnosis (Table 47.1).

    Treatment of HRS requires intravascular volume expansion. Albumin (25%) is a particularly potent volume expander and support for its role is provided by the success of albumin in conjunction with vasoactive agents in improving HRS compared to vasoactive agents and saline. The coadministration of albumin with vasoactive agents such as octreotide (100 to 200 μg SC q8hr) and midodrine (7.5 to 12.5 mg q8hr) or terlipressin (a vasoconstrictor not currently approved in the US) has been studied for the treatment of HRS in clinical trials of varying quality.

ENCEPHALOPATHY

Encephalopathy is a common complication of cirrhosis. Early symptoms are often subtle and can include changes in mood and insomnia that can progress to agitation and coma. Its development should prompt a search from precipitants that commonly include infection, gastrointestinal hemorrhage, or medication exposures. The mediators of hepatic encephalopathy are unknown and serum ammonia is, at best, a casual marker of hepatic encephalopathy.

    Treatment options include cathartics (lactulose 30 mL PO q2–8hr or lactulose retention enemas) or enterically active antibiotics (neomycin 500 mg PO q6hr or rifaximin 550 mg bid). In a randomized, double-blind placebo controlled study in which 90% of patients were receiving lactulose; the addition of rifaximin significantly reduced the risk of recurrent episodes of hepatic encephalopathy.

TABLE 47.2	Guidelines for the Management of Variceal Hemorrhage

Resuscitate hypovolemic shock
Assessment of airway and intubation if airway protection necessary
Octreotide 50 μg IV bolus followed by 50 μg/hr IV infusion
Blood and urine culture; diagnostic paracentesis
Prophylactic parenteral antibiotics
Upper endoscopy
TIPS, BRTO, or Blakemore tube for variceal bleeding refractory to endoscopic
  management

BRTO, balloon-occluded retrograde transvenous obliteration; TIPS, transjugular intrahepatic portosystemic shunt.

VARICEAL HEMORRHAGE

Variceal hemorrhage has an annual incidence rate of 20% in patients with cirrhosis, and each episode carries a 20% to 40% mortality rate. There is no typical presentation of variceal bleeding and it should be suspected in those with known chronic liver disease and gastrointestinal hemorrhage. The initial steps in the management of acute variceal bleeding involve treatment of shock and protection of the airway (Table 47.2). Volume resuscitation in the form of packed red blood cells should be privileged to other blood products. Octreotide (50 μg IV bolus followed by 50 μg/hr IV infusion) should be started. Diagnostic paracentesis should be performed and prophylactic parenteral antibiotics should be given; the latter intervention is associated with decreased risk of rebleeding.

Upper endoscopy should be performed promptly, as both band ligation and sclerotherapy can result in effective hemostasis for esophageal varices. TIPS is an option for esophageal variceal bleeding that is refractory to endoscopy or for bleeding gastric varices. Early TIPS placement (within 24 to 48 hours following hospitalization for variceal hemorrhage) in patients with Child's class B and C cirrhosis has also been advocated as a strategy that prolongs survival.

Balloon-occluded retrograde transvenous obliteration (BRTO) is another potential therapy that may be particularly helpful in the management of bleeding gastric or ectopic varices. Balloon tamponade devices (Blakemore tube) can also be inserted temporary in cases where TIPS or endoscopy is either delayed or unsuccessful. Nonselective β-blockers (e.g., propranolol, nadolol, or carvedilol) are effective at reducing the risk of initial and recurrent variceal bleeding; however, they should be introduced only after acute bleeding is controlled and the patient is hemodynamically stable.

TRANSJUGULAR INTRAHEPATIC PORTOSYSTEMIC SHUNT

TIPS is a channel created between the hepatic vein and the intrahepatic portion of the portal vein. It is placed to reduce portal pressure in patients with complications related to portal hypertension, most commonly variceal hemorrhage or refractory ascites. Contraindications to TIPS placement can include pulmonary hypertension, right-sided heart failure, severe encephalopathy, polycystic liver disease, or tumor within the path of the TIPS.

SUGGESTED READINGS

Bass NM, Mullen KD, Sanyal A, et al. Rifaximin treatment in hepatic encephalopathy. *N Engl J Med*. 2010;362(12):1071–1081.

> *A multicenter, randomized, placebo-controlled study revealed that rifaximin at a dose of 550 mg twice daily significantly reduced the risk of an episode of hepatic encephalopathy in study subjects with cirrhosis of which 90% were on concomitant lactulose.*

Garcia-Pagan JC, Caca K, Bureau C, et al. Early use of TIPS in patients with cirrhosis and variceal bleeding. *N Engl J Med*. 2010;362(25):2370–2379.

> *A provocative multicenter study that showed that patient with advanced liver disease (Child's class B and C) undergoing TIPS early after variceal bleeding had improved survival. The rate of survival at 6 weeks was 97% in the TIPS group compared with 67% in the group that received medical therapy only.*

Garcia-Tsao G, Bosch J. Management of varices and variceal hemorrhage in cirrhosis. *N Engl J Med*. 2010;362(9):823–832.

Gines P, Angeli P, Lenz K, et al. EASL clinical practice guidelines on the management of ascites, spontaneous bacterial peritonitis, and hepatorenal syndrome in cirrhosis. *J Hepatol*. 2010;53(3):397–417.

> *Practice guidelines from the European Association for the Study of the Liver.*

Runyon BA. Management of adult patients with ascites due to cirrhosis: an update. *Hepatology*. 2009;49(6):2087–2107.

> *Updates practice guidelines for the management of cirrhotic ascites from the American Association for the Study of Liver Diseases.*

Salerno F, Guevara M, Bernardi M, et al. Refractory ascites: pathogenesis, definition and therapy of a severe complication in patients with cirrhosis. *Liver Int*. 2010;30(7):937–947.

48 Upper Gastrointestinal Bleeding

Chandra Prakash Gyawali

Acute upper gastrointestinal bleeding (UGIB) is a common medical emergency that frequently results in emergency department evaluations and intensive care unit admissions. The annual incidence of acute UGIB is estimated to range between 80 and 90 cases per 100,000 population, carrying a mortality rate of 6% to 12%. In recent years, the incidence has declined in younger populations, possibly because of lower *Helicobacter pylori* incidence and widespread use of proton pump inhibitors (PPIs). Concurrently, incidence has risen in older populations from increased use of nonsteroidal anti-inflammatory drugs (NSAIDs). Common causes of acute UGIB are listed in Table 48.1.

One of the first assessments in any patient with acute gastrointestinal bleeding is determining the severity of the bleeding episode (Algorithm 48.1). Bleeding is considered massive with loss of one-fifth to one-fourth of the circulating volume if a previously normotensive or hypertensive patient develops resting hypotension. In the absence of resting hypotension, evidence of postural or orthostatic hypotension (drop of systolic blood pressure of 15 mm Hg or increase in heart rate of 20 beats per minute) indicates loss of 10% to 20% of the circulating volume. Bleeding is considered minor

TABLE 48.1	Etiology of Upper Gastrointestinal Bleeding

Peptic ulcer disease (accounts for ~50%)
    Gastric ulcers
    Duodenal ulcers
    Gastric erosions and gastritis

Esophageal and/or gastric varices (accounts for 10%–20%)
Stress ulcers
Mallory–Weiss tear
Esophagitis and esophageal ulcers
Vascular abnormalities (angiodysplasia, Dieulafoy lesion, telangiectasia)
Portal hypertensive gastropathy
Neoplasms, benign and malignant
Hemobilia (bleeding into bile ducts)
Hemosuccus (bleeding into pancreatic ducts)
Aortoenteric fistula

ALGORITHM 48.1 | **Initial Management of Acute Gastrointestinal (GI) Bleeding**

Resuscitation
- Establish two large-bore IVs or central line
- Obtain blood for blood typing, CBC, CMP, INR, PTT
- Infuse isotonic saline, Ringer's lactate, or 5% hetastarch
- Blood transfusion: O negative if extremely urgent
- Oxygen by nasal canula

Factors propagating bleeding
- Discontinue anticoagulants (warfarin, heparin), thrombolytic agents
- Discontinue antiplatelet agents if possible (aspirin, clopidogrel)
- Discontinue antithrombotic agents[a] if possible
- Correct prolonged PT/INR with FFP infusions and/or vitamin K injection
- Correct prolonged PTT with protamine infusion if necessary

Level of bleeding[b]
- Hematemesis, coffee ground emesis indicate upper GI bleeding
- Melena usually indicates upper GI bleeding but can originate more distally
- Maroon stool, red blood in the stool typically indicate lower GI bleeding
- Any bleeding in the presence of hemodynamic compromise can be upper GI in origin

Etiology of bleeding[b]
- Presence of cirrhosis may indicate variceal bleeding
- Hypotension or shock preceding bleeding may indicate ischemic colitis
- Recent polypectomy may indicate postpolypectomy bleeding
- Prior aortic graft surgery may indicate aortoenteric fistula
- Prior radiation therapy may indicate radiation enteritis or proctopathy
- Prior emesis may indicate Mallory–Weiss tear

CBC, complete blood cell count; CMP, complete metabolic panel; INR, international normalized ratio; PTT, partial thromboplastin time; PT, prothrombin time; FFP, fresh-frozen plasma; GI, gastrointestinal. [a]Antithrombotic agents can also propagate bleeding and include glycoprotein IIb/IIIa receptor antagonists (abciximab [ReoPro], eptifibatide [Integrilin], tirofiban [Aggrastat]), and direct thrombin inhibitors (argatroban, bivalirudin). [b]These will dictate the nature of further investigation.

if neither of these conditions is met, indicating loss of <10% of circulating volume. In all instances, two large-bore intravenous (IV) lines or a central line is urgently placed and normal saline or Ringer's lactate solution is administered intravenously. Rapid repletion of circulating volume is crucial when massive blood loss ensues, and transfusion of packed red blood cells needs to be arranged. Therefore, blood is drawn for blood cell count, metabolic profile, coagulation parameters, blood typing, and cross-matching. When type-specific blood is not immediately available, O-negative blood may need to be transfused, using rapid infusing devices if necessary. Oxygen is administered by nasal cannula to improve oxygen-carrying capacity of blood, and vital signs and urine output are constantly monitored.

Factors propagating bleeding can be rapidly assessed during this initial evaluation. Patients receiving heparin infusion, thrombolytic therapy, or newer antithrombotic agents (Algorithm 48.1) need to be assessed to determine if it is safe to temporarily discontinue these medications. Oral anticoagulants are held, and the anticoagulation reversed with vitamin K and/or fresh-frozen plasma, if possible.

Once the patient is stabilized hemodynamically, further evaluation can resume (Algorithm 48.1). A history of hematemesis or coffee-ground emesis establishes the diagnosis of UGIB. Melena (passage of dark, tarry, sticky, foul-smelling stool) typically indicates a proximal gut source for blood loss, but melena can develop from bleeding sites as far distal as the proximal or even middle colon. Nevertheless, the presence of melena points to upper endoscopy as the starting point of investigation of the bleeding episode. An upper gastrointestinal source of bleeding may be identified in as many as 10% to 11% of patients presenting with hematochezia and altered hemodynamic parameters. Therefore, in the presence of significant hemodynamic compromise, upper gastrointestinal tract evaluation is indicated even if the bleeding presentation resembles lower gastrointestinal bleeding.

Aspiration of bloody gastric contents through a nasogastric tube establishes the diagnosis of UGIB and can help triage the need for emergent endoscopy. The aspiration of brighter shades of red blood may indicate ongoing bleeding, wherein urgent endoscopy with endoscopic therapy may lower morbidity. On the other hand, dark blood or coffee grounds that clear quickly on nasogastric tube lavage may indicate that active bleeding has ceased, and elective endoscopy within 24 hours may be adequate (Table 48.2). Early indicators for the need for intensive care unit admission include massive bleeding, hemodynamic compromise, variceal bleeding, bleeding onset while hospitalized for an unrelated illness, and the presence of factors that predict a poor outcome (Table 48.3). Hemoccult testing of clear nasogastric aspirates has very little value in the assessment of acute UGIB. If the nasogastric aspirate is clear, or clears quickly with a tap water lavage, the nasogastric tube can be removed; with bloody aspirates that do not clear, the nasogastric tube may provide an assessment of the acuity and ongoing nature of bleeding.

Acute UGIB consists of two broad categories: acute variceal UGIB and acute nonvariceal UGIB (Algorithm 48.2). These categories require differing investigative and therapeutic approaches and may be associated with varied short- and long-term morbidity and mortality. For instance, variceal UGIB is associated with a higher rate of rebleeding (30% to 40% vs. 15% to 20% for nonvariceal bleeding) and a significantly higher mortality (20% to 30% vs. 6% to 9%, respectively). Acute nonvariceal UGIB that develops in patients hospitalized for an unrelated illness is associated with worse morbidity and mortality (estimated at 35%) compared with patients admitted through emergency departments for acute bleeding.

TABLE 48.2	Triage of Patients with Acute Upper Gastrointestinal Bleeding

Admission to intensive care unit
  Hypotension at presentation
  Moderate-to-severe bleeding onset while admitted for an unrelated illness
  Ongoing hemodynamic instability despite resuscitation
  Absence of adequate hematocrit increase despite blood transfusion
  Low initial blood cell count (hematocrit <25% with cardiopulmonary disease
    or stroke, <20% otherwise)
  Bright or dark red NG tube aspirate, especially if it does not clear with lavage
  Prolonged coagulation parameters (prothrombin time >1.2 times the control
    value)
  Myocardial infarction, stroke, or other systemic complications of rapid blood
    loss
  Any unstable comorbid disease, including altered mental status
  Variceal bleeding
  Evidence of active oozing, spurting, or visible vessel on endoscopy

Admission to regular hospital floor
  Stable hemodynamic parameters after initial resuscitation
  Mild hematocrit drop <5% from baseline and/or baseline hematocrit >30%)
  Stable coagulation parameters
  Coffee grounds on NG tube aspirate that clears with lavage
  No systemic complications from blood loss
  No bleeding source found on upper endoscopy
  Nonvariceal bleeding source without active bleeding; bleeding lesion with a
    clean or pigmented base

Emergent or urgent upper endoscopy
  Suspected or known variceal bleeding
  Hemodynamic instability despite resuscitation
  Bright red or dark red NG aspirate, especially if it does not clear with lavage
  Absence of appropriate hematocrit increase despite blood transfusion

NG, nasogastric.

TABLE 48.3	Factors of Predicting Poor Outcome After Acute Upper Gastrointestinal Bleeding

Age >65 yr
Comorbid medical illnesses (liver disease, COPD, renal failure, coronary artery
  disease, malignancy)
Variceal bleeding
Systolic blood pressure <100 mm Hg at presentation
Large peptic ulcers >3 cm
Active bleeding (spurting blood vessel) at endoscopy
Multiple units of blood transfusion
Onset of acute bleeding when hospitalized for unrelated illness
Need for emergency surgery for bleeding control

COPD, chronic obstructive pulmonary disease.

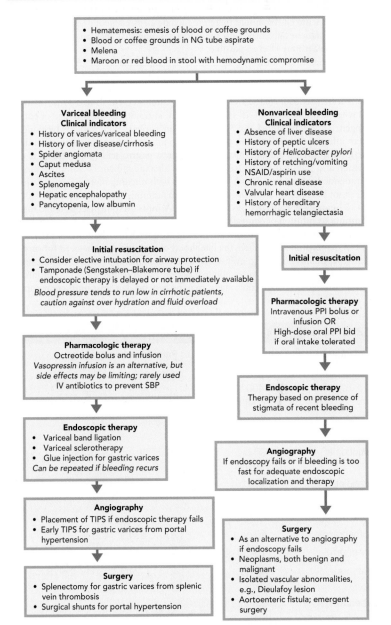

ALGORITHM 48.2   Management of Acute Upper Gastrointestinal (GI) Bleeding

- Hematemesis: emesis of blood or coffee grounds
- Blood or coffee grounds in NG tube aspirate
- Melena
- Maroon or red blood in stool with hemodynamic compromise

Variceal bleeding
Clinical indicators
- History of varices/variceal bleeding
- History of liver disease/cirrhosis
- Spider angiomata
- Caput medusa
- Ascites
- Splenomegaly
- Hepatic encephalopathy
- Pancytopenia, low albumin

Nonvariceal bleeding
Clinical indicators
- Absence of liver disease
- History of peptic ulcers
- History of *Helicobacter pylori*
- History of retching/vomiting
- NSAID/aspirin use
- Chronic renal disease
- Valvular heart disease
- History of hereditary hemorrhagic telangiectasia

Initial resuscitation
- Consider elective intubation for airway protection
- Tamponade (Sengstaken–Blakemore tube) if endoscopic therapy is delayed or not immediately available

Blood pressure tends to run low in cirrhotic patients, caution against over hydration and fluid overload

Initial resuscitation

Pharmacologic therapy
Octreotide bolus and infusion
Vasopressin infusion is an alternative, but side effects may be limiting; rarely used
IV antibiotics to prevent SBP

Pharmacologic therapy
Intravenous PPI bolus or infusion OR
High-dose oral PPI bid if oral intake tolerated

Endoscopic therapy
- Variceal band ligation
- Variceal sclerotherapy
- Glue injection for gastric varices
Can be repeated if bleeding recurs

Endoscopic therapy
Therapy based on presence of stigmata of recent bleeding

Angiography
- Placement of TIPS if endoscopic therapy fails
- Early TIPS for gastric varices from portal hypertension

Angiography
If endoscopy fails or if bleeding is too fast for adequate endoscopic localization and therapy

Surgery
- Splenectomy for gastric varices from splenic vein thrombosis
- Surgical shunts for portal hypertension

Surgery
- As an alternative to angiography if endoscopy fails
- Neoplasms, both benign and malignant
- Isolated vascular abnormalities, e.g., Dieulafoy lesion
- Aortoenteric fistula; emergent surgery

NG, nasogastric; IV, intravenous; SBP, spontaneous bacterial peritonitis; TIPS, transjugular intrahepatic portosystemic shunt; NSAIDs, nonsteroidal anti-inflammatory drugs; PPI, proton pump inhibitor.

Initial management of acute variceal UGIB includes IV infusion of octreotide, and IV PPI administration is considered routine in nonvariceal UGIB. Early clinical evaluation of acute UGIB should therefore include an assessment to determine which category the patient falls into, with the understanding that such an assessment may not always be accurate or even possible.

The initial mode of therapy for acute UGIB is pharmacologic (Algorithm 48.2). Octreotide, a somatostatin analogue, lowers splanchnic and portal venous pressure in the short term, with slowing or cessation of variceal UGIB. Early administration of octreotide is encouraged (25 to 50 μg bolus, followed by 50 to 100 μg/hr infusion) when acute variceal UGIB is suspected. IV antibiotics with coverage of enteric pathogens are administered for 7 to 10 days in patients with variceal bleeding to prevent infectious complications, particularly spontaneous bacterial peritonitis. In all other instances, PPIs are administered to suppress gastric acid (Table 48.4), as clot formation and stabilization are facilitated in an alkaline milieu. IV administration is recommended for the first 72 hours in patients with ongoing bleeding or in patients who cannot tolerate oral administration. IV bolus administration (omeprazole, 40 mg every 12 hours IV or equivalent) is favored, but IV infusion (omeprazole, 6 to 8 mg/hr by continuous infusion or equivalent) has been advocated by some for rapid ongoing bleeding. Double-dose PPI (omeprazole, 40 mg or equivalent) administered twice daily has been demonstrated to reduce the likelihood of rebleeding or the need for surgery in acute peptic ulcer bleeding, even when endoscopic therapy was not administered. Stable patients without active ongoing bleeding can tolerate oral PPI administration, and double-dose, two times daily, may be beneficial at least until endoscopy is

TABLE 48.4	Doses of Antisecretory Medication	
Medication	Oral therapy (mg)	Parenteral therapy (mg)
Cimetidine[a]	300 qid 400 bid 800 qhs	300 q6hr
Ranitidine[a]	150 bid 300 qhs	50 q8hr
Famotidine[a]	20 bid 40 qhs	20 q12hr
Nizatidine[a]	150 bid 300 qhs	
Omeprazole	20 qd	
Esomeprazole	40 qd	20–40 q24hr
Lansoprazole	15–30 qd	30 q12–24hr
Pantoprazole	40 qd	40 q12–24hr or 80 IV, then 8 mg/hr infusion
Rabeprazole	20 qd	

[a]Dosage adjustment required in renal insufficiency.
qid, four times daily; bid, two times daily; qhs, at bedtime; qd, daily.

performed; some centers administer this higher dose for 5 days. PPI therapy is also used in the prophylaxis of erosive upper gut disease in predisposed patients on aspirin or NSAIDs, especially when there are risk factors for peptic ulcer disease. Although the use of PPI with clopidogrel may result in decreased clopidogrel effect *in vitro,* recent large, randomized, placebo-controlled studies suggest that the interaction does not appear to translate into worse vascular outcomes.

A crucial adjunct to pharmacologic therapy is endoscopy (Algorithm 48.2), both for definitive diagnosis of the bleeding lesion and for administration of endoscopic therapy to lower the risks for rebleeding, other morbidity including surgery, and mortality. Timing of endoscopy depends on the degree of bleeding, whether bleeding is ongoing, and the patient's overall condition (Table 48.2). Urgent endoscopy is generally indicated in any patient with significant or ongoing bleeding. Hemodynamic parameters should be in the process of being normalized when endoscopy is performed. Conscious sedation can be administered when hemodynamic stability is achieved and the patient is no longer hypotensive. Rapid bleeding or the presence of blood or clots within the upper gastrointestinal tract may preclude complete examination. Administration of a prokinetic agent such as metoclopramide (5 to 10 mg IV) or erythromycin (250 mg IV) may induce gastric-emptying and allow a cleaner endoscopic field. Lavage using large-bore, double-lumen orogastric tubes can be performed to clear the stomach of blood and clots. Positioning the patient so that the intraluminal blood pool is away from the area of interest during endoscopy can be useful. In some instances, especially if large volumes of luminal blood or massive intraluminal clots are encountered, endoscopy may need to be repeated at a later time or angiography used for bleeding localization. Therapy administered during endoscopy can include variceal band ligation, sclerotherapy, or glue injection for variceal UGIB and epinephrine injection, thermal cautery, bi- or monopolar cautery, hemoclip deployment, and sclerosant injection for nonvariceal UGIB. Rebleeding rates are typically high in variceal bleeding, up to the order of 30% to 40%. Rebleeding rates approximate 15% to 20% in nonvariceal bleeding, stratified by the presence or absence of stigmata of recent hemorrhage in the case of peptic ulcer bleeding (Table 48.5).

Short- and long-term outcomes of therapy depend on the cause of the lesion. Rebleeding rates are typically high with variceal bleeding. Nonselective β-blocker therapy is initiated if the patient tolerates the approach. Repeat variceal band ligation or sclerotherapy can be considered when bleeding recurs. When access to definitive therapy is not immediately available, placement of a Sengstaken–Blakemore or similar tube can tamponade the varices and temporarily stabilize the patient (Table 48.6). Rebleeding refractory to endoscopic therapy is managed by the placement of a transjugular

TABLE 48.5	Outcome After Endoscopic Therapy of Peptic Ulcers	
Endoscopic finding	Risk for rebleeding (%) after treatment	Mortality (%) after treatment
Clean ulcer base	<5	2
Flat pigmented spot	10 (<1)	3 (<1)
Adherent clot	22 (5)	7 (<3)
Visible vessel	43 (15)	11 (<5)
Active bleeding	55 (20)	11 (<5)

Modified from Laine L, Petersen WL. Bleeding peptic ulcer. *N Engl J Med.* 1994;331:717–727.

TABLE 48.6 | Balloon Tamponade for Variceal Bleeding

Indications

    Temporary control of variceal bleeding (gastric, esophageal, or both)

    Access to endoscopic or radiologic therapy not immediately available to stabilize patient for transport

    Efficacy is thought to be better when combined with pharmacologic therapy (Algorithm 48.2)

Equipment

    Sengstaken–Blakemore tube (three lumen), Minnesota tube (four lumen), Linton–Nachlas tube (gastric balloon alone), or similar tube

    Nasogastric tube when three-lumen tube or gastric balloon alone is used

    Soft restraints

    Traction mechanism (typically a football helmet, weights, or orthopedic traction system)

    Manometer

    Tube clamps, surgical scissors

    Topical anesthetic, tube connectors, syringes

Technique

    Patient needs to be intubated and sedated, with soft restraints in place

    Test balloons, check intraluminal pressures at full inflation with a manometer

    Gastric lavage till clear through nasogastric tube, which is then removed

    Introduce lubricated tube through mouth

    When gastric juice or blood is aspirated through gastric lumen, check tube position radiographically

    With manometer attached to measuring port, fill gastric lumen with air in 100-mL increments to recommended volume for particular tube (typically 450–500 mL)

    If rapid pressure increase is noted on manometer, tube may have been inflated in esophagus; deflate immediately, advance tube, reinflate

    Clamp air inlet for gastric balloon, pull back, and then secure to traction device

    If esophageal balloon inflation is desired, inflate esophageal balloon to 30–45 mm Hg pressure as measured by manometer on measuring port

    Further traction can be applied if bright red blood continues to be aspirated through gastric port

    With three-lumen tubes, place nasogastric tube so the tip is 3–4 cm above esophageal balloon and then connect to intermittent suction

    Deflate balloons for 5 min every 5–6 hr to reduce risk of pressure necrosis

    Keep balloons inflated for up to 24 hr as needed

    Efficacy is around 80% when correctly placed

Complications

    Complications occur in 15%–30%; mortality rate is around 6%

    Major complications include asphyxia, airway occlusion, esophageal rupture, esophageal, and gastric pressure necrosis

    Aspiration pneumonia, epistaxis, and pharyngeal erosions are other complications

ALGORITHM 48.3   Management of Peptic Ulcers

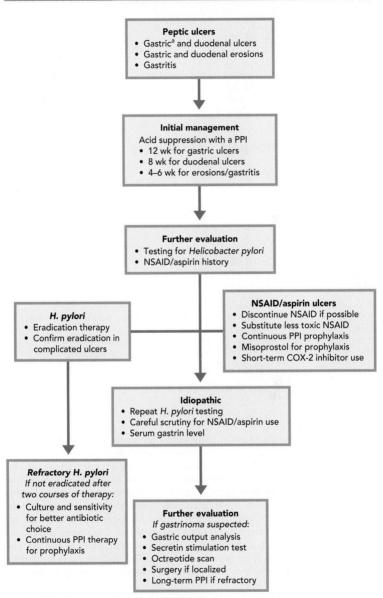

Peptic ulcers
- Gastric[a] and duodenal ulcers
- Gastric and duodenal erosions
- Gastritis

Initial management
Acid suppression with a PPI
- 12 wk for gastric ulcers
- 8 wk for duodenal ulcers
- 4–6 wk for erosions/gastritis

Further evaluation
- Testing for *Helicobacter pylori*
- NSAID/aspirin history

H. pylori
- Eradication therapy
- Confirm eradication in complicated ulcers

NSAID/aspirin ulcers
- Discontinue NSAID if possible
- Substitute less toxic NSAID
- Continuous PPI prophylaxis
- Misoprostol for prophylaxis
- Short-term COX-2 inhibitor use

Idiopathic
- Repeat *H. pylori* testing
- Careful scrutiny for NSAID/aspirin use
- Serum gastrin level

Refractory H. pylori
If not eradicated after two courses of therapy:
- Culture and sensitivity for better antibiotic choice
- Continuous PPI therapy for prophylaxis

Further evaluation
If gastrinoma suspected:
- Gastric output analysis
- Secretin stimulation test
- Octreotide scan
- Surgery if localized
- Long-term PPI if refractory

PPI, proton pump inhibitor; NSAID, nonsteroidal anti-inflammatory drug; COX-2, cyclooxygenase-2.
[a]Evaluation with endoscopy or barium contrast study is repeated at 3 months in all patients with gastric ulcers to confirm healing. If the ulcer is not completely healed, multiple biopsy samples are taken to exclude other nonpeptic causes, including malignancy.

TABLE 48.7	Regimens for *Helicobacter pylori* Eradication	
Medications	Dose	Comments[a]
Clarithromycin Amoxicillin PPI[b]	500 mg bid 1 g bid bid	First line
Pepto-Bismol Metronidazole Tetracycline PPI[b] or H2RA[c]	524 mg qid 250 mg qid 500 mg qid bid	First line in penicillin-allergic patients Salvage regimen if three-drug regimen fails
Clarithromycin Metronidazole PPI[b]	500 mg bid 500 mg bid bid	Alternate regimen, if four-drug therapy is not tolerated
Levofloxacin Amoxicillin PPI[b]	250 mg bid 1 g bid bid	Alternate salvage regimen
Rifabutin Amoxicillin PPI[b]	300 mg qd 1 g bid bid	Alternate salvage regimen

[a]Duration of therapy: 10–14 days. When using salvage regimens after initial treatment failure, choose drugs that have not been used before.
[b]Standard doses for PPI: omeprazole, 20 mg; lansoprazole, 30 mg; pantoprazole, 40 mg; rabeprazole 20 mg, all twice daily. Esomeprazole is used as a single 40 mg dose once daily.
[c]Standard doses for H2RA: ranitidine, 150 mg; famotidine, 20 mg; nizatidine, 150 mg; cimetidine, 400 mg, all twice daily.
bid, twice daily; PPI, proton pump inhibitor; qid, four times daily; H2RA, H$_2$-receptor antagonists.

intrahepatic portosystemic shunt. Gastric varices related to portal hypertension are managed with a transjugular intrahepatic portosystemic shunt earlier in the course, and those resulting from splenic vein thrombosis may require splenectomy for successful management. Rebleeding from peptic ulcers can be treated endoscopically, reserving angiographic measures (such as embolization) or surgery for repeated endoscopic failures. Eradication of *H. pylori* accelerates healing of peptic ulcers (Algorithm 48.3, Table 48.7). When NSAIDs or aspirin are the etiologic factors, discontinuation and substitution of a less toxic NSAID or a cyclooxygenase-2 inhibitor, continuous acid suppression with a PPI, or the addition of a mucosal protective agent such as misoprostol may reduce the risk for recurrence of bleeding. Bleeding from neoplastic lesions responds poorly to endoscopic or angiographic hemostasis, and surgery is frequently required. Isolated vascular lesions such as Dieulafoy lesion can be successfully treated endoscopically, angiographically, or surgically with low likelihood for recurrence. On the other hand, angiodysplasia or telangiectasia can redevelop after endoscopic ablation or may be present elsewhere in the luminal gut, and blood loss frequently recurs.

SUGGESTED READINGS

Barkun A, Bardou M, Marshall JK. Consensus recommendations for managing patients with nonvariceal upper gastrointestinal bleeding. *Ann Intern Med.* 2003;139:843–857.

Bhatt DL, Cryer BL, Contant CF, et al. Clopidogrel with or without omeprazole in coronary artery disease. *N Engl J Med.* 2010;363:1909–1917.

Cheung FKY, Lau JYW. Management of massive peptic ulcer bleeding. *Gastroenterol Clin N Am.* 2009;38:231–243.

Ferguson CB, Mitchell RM. Nonvariceal upper gastrointestinal bleeding: standard and new treatment. *Gastroenterol Clin North Am.* 2005;34:607–621.

Laine L, Peterson WL. Bleeding peptic ulcer. *N Engl J Med.* 1994;331:717–727.

Lanza FL, Chan FKL, Quigley EM, et al. Guidelines for prevention of NSAID-related ulcer complications. *Am J Gastroenterol.* 2009;104:728–738.

Leontiadis GI, McIntyre L, Sharma VK, et al. Proton pump inhibitor treatment for acute peptic ulcer bleeding. *Cochrane Database Syst Rev.* 2004;3:CD002094.

Zaman A, Chalasani N. Bleeding caused by portal hypertension. *Gastroenterol Clin North Am.* 2005;34:623–642.

49 Lower Gastrointestinal Bleeding

Chandra Prakash Gyawali

Acute lower gastrointestinal bleeding (LGIB) is traditionally defined as bleeding originating distal to the ligament of Treitz. Acute LGIB is about one-fifth as frequent as acute upper gastrointestinal bleeding (UGIB), with an annual incidence of hospitalization estimated at 44 per 100,000 population. Similar to trends with acute UGIB, the incidence is higher among older populations; overall, incidence of LGIB is increasing while that of UGIB is decreasing in the general population. In contrast to UGIB, acute LGIB is associated with less hemodynamic compromise, fewer transfusion requirements, and lower mortality (5%). Typically, acute LGIB is self-limiting, but bleeding can be intermittent and recurrent. Similar to acute UGIB, patients who develop acute LGIB while hospitalized for an unrelated illness have a worse outcome, with an estimated mortality rate of 23%. In recent years, advances in endoscopic and radiologic techniques in actively bleeding patients (such as hemoclip use and superselective embolization of the bleeding vessel) have reduced the need for emergent surgery, leading to lowered rebleeding and morbidity rates in acute LGIB.

Presentation can range from scant bright red blood around formed stool or on toilet tissue to massive uncontrolled bloody bowel movements with hemodynamic compromise and shock. The color of bloody stool has been demonstrated to be a good predictor of the location of the bleeding source in patients without hemodynamic collapse. Patients pointing to a bright red or a dark red color on a color card had the highest positive predictive value for acute LGIB in one study, higher than physician reports of the same color data. Colonic bleeding is clinically indistinguishable from small bowel bleeding, but because colonic sources (Table 49.1) are identified more frequently than small bowel sources and because the colon is much more accessible than the small bowel for investigative procedures, the work-up initially focuses on the colon. Bloody diarrhea is sometimes interpreted as acute LGIB by patients, and a few questions usually resolve the issue. If the presentation is bloody diarrhea rather than acute LGIB, stool culture, including culture for *Escherichia coli* O157:H7, and the stool *Clostridium difficile* toxin test are ordered. Parasitic infestations such as amebiasis may need to be considered and ameba serology ordered, when relevant. In immunosuppressed patients, cytomegalovirus colitis can present with bloody diarrhea. Bleeding presentations of inflammatory bowel disease (Crohn's disease, ulcerative colitis) are more often bloody diarrhea than acute LGIB. The upper gastrointestinal tract can also be the source of bright or dark red blood in the stool if bleeding is massive. The small bowel is investigated if an alternate source is not apparent or identified elsewhere in the luminal gut. Therefore, the spectrum of acute LGIB is broad.

TABLE 49.1	Causes of Acute Lower Gastrointestinal Bleeding

Colonic sources
  Diverticulosis
  Angiodysplasia
  Neoplasia includes large polyps and cancers
  Postpolypectomy bleeding
  Colitis includes inflammatory and infectious causes
  Ischemia
  Anorectal causes includes hemorrhoids and anal fissure
  Radiation proctopathy and colopathy
  Aortoenteric fistula (rare)
  Dieulafoy lesion (rare)
  Rectal varices (rare)

Small bowel sources
  Angiodysplasia
  Neoplasia includes cancers, stromal tumors, and lymphoma
  Enteritis includes inflammatory and infectious causes
  Radiation enteritis and enteropathy
  Meckel's diverticulum
  Aortoenteric fistula (rare)

Initial resuscitation and early management of acute gastrointestinal bleeding do not vary by location (see Algorithm 48.1, Chapter 48). In addition to the placement of two large-bore intravenous lines, infusions of normal saline, Ringer's lactate solution, or blood products may be appropriate depending on severity of bleeding and acuity of presentation. Anticoagulants, antiplatelet agents, and medications that affect the coagulation cascade are discontinued if possible. When clotting parameters are significantly abnormal, fresh-frozen plasma, vitamin K, and protamine are administered as indicated.

Certain clinical and laboratory features at presentation may identify patients at risk for higher short-term morbidity, including continued and recurrent bleeding, hemodynamic compromise, syncope, aspirin or anticoagulant use, more than two comorbid medical conditions, and continued bleeding 4 hours after initial presentation. Others have identified prolongation of prothrombin time >1.2 times the control value and altered mental status as additional predictors of poor outcome. These characteristics are useful in making triage decisions, especially in identifying patients who could benefit from admission to an intensive care unit and patients who need urgent investigative procedures (Table 49.2).

As many as 10% of hemodynamically unstable patients presenting with bright shades of blood in their stool may have a bleeding source within reach of an upper endoscope. It is important that these patients be evaluated with the initial intent to exclude an upper source, as upper endoscopy is infinitely easier to perform than colonoscopy in the setting of an acute bleed. A nasogastric tube can be placed and aspiration performed, looking for a bloody aspirate. However, a clear aspirate does not exclude bleeding just distal to the pylorus, and if suspicion is high, an upper endoscopic examination is indicated. Patients with acute bleeding in the setting of past aortic graft

TABLE 49.2 Triage of Patients with Acute Lower Gastrointestinal Bleeding

Admission to intensive care unit
  Hypotension (systolic blood pressure <115 mm Hg) at presentation
  Moderate-to-severe bleeding onset while admitted for an unrelated illness
  Ongoing hemodynamic instability despite resuscitation
  Absence of adequate hematocrit increase despite blood transfusion
  Low initial blood count (hematocrit <25% with cardiopulmonary disease or
    stroke, <20% otherwise)
  Prolonged coagulation parameters (prothrombin time ≥1.2 times the control
    value)
  Myocardial infarction, stroke, or other systemic complications of rapid blood
    loss
  Any unstable comorbid disease, including altered mental status
  Ongoing significant bleeding 4 hr after presentation
  Evidence of active oozing, spurting, or visible vessel on endoscopy
  Requirement of angiography for localization or control of bleeding

Admission to regular hospital floor
  Stable hemodynamic parameters after initial resuscitation
  Mild hematocrit drop <5% from baseline and/or baseline hematocrit >30%
  Stable coagulation parameters
  No systemic complications from blood loss
  Absence of ongoing bleeding 4 hr after presentation

Emergent *upper* endoscopy in patients with bloody stool
  Bright red or dark red blood in stool with hemodynamic compromise
  Bloody NG aspirate
  Suspicion of aortoenteric fistula (distal duodenum needs to be evaluated)

NG, nasogastric.

repair need an emergent upper endoscopy for evaluation of the distal duodenum, the commonest location for an aortoenteric fistula.

Further evaluation of the patient depends on several factors: the severity and acuity of bleeding, hemodynamic state of the patient, coagulation parameters, and investigative facilities available at the institution. In patients with minimal bleeding with historical features suggesting a distal source (red blood coating outside of formed stool, pain with defecation, tenesmus, passage of fresh clots), inspection of the perianal area, anal canal, rectum, and sometimes the distal colon may be a useful initial step. This can be achieved with anoscopy and/or flexible sigmoidoscopy. However, sigmoidoscopy rarely replaces full colonoscopy after a bowel preparation, as a concurrent more proximal bleeding source cannot be excluded with this approach alone.

Colonoscopy may provide a high rate of identification of the bleeding source if performed within the first 24 hours (45% to 95%), but the feasibility and quality of bowel preparation will impact whether colonoscopy can be successfully performed (Algorithm 49.1). Bowel preparation may not be possible unless the patient is hemodynamically stable and able to use the bathroom. Therapeutic maneuvers may not be safe unless coagulation parameters have been brought close to normal. If a bleeding lesion is identified during colonoscopy, therapeutic measures including epinephrine

ALGORITHM 49.1 Investigation of Acute Lower Gastrointestinal Bleeding

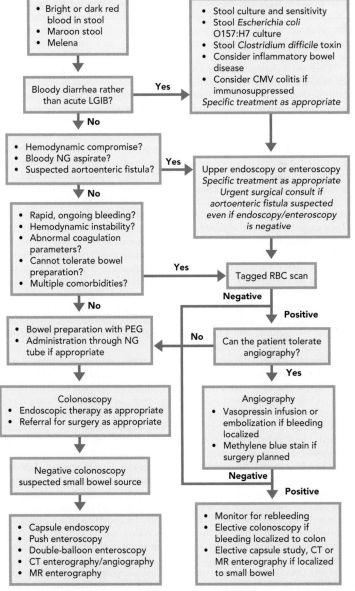

LGIB, lower gastrointestinal bleeding; CMV, cytomegalovirus; NG, nasogastric; RBC, red blood cell; PEG, polyethylene glycol; CT, computed tomography; MR, magnetic resonance.

injection, thermal therapy, and mechanical therapy with hemoclips can be successfully attempted. Sometimes, a definitive lesion cannot be identified, but bleeding can be localized to a segment of bowel. At other times, a potential bleeding lesion (such as diverticulosis or angiodysplasia) is visualized but without active bleeding or stigmata of recent hemorrhage. This provides only circumstantial evidence for localization of the bleeding source, unless a prior radiologic study localized bleeding to the same area of the colon as the potential bleeding lesion on colonoscopy. Early colonoscopy has been demonstrated to shorten the duration of hospitalization and reduce treatment costs.

When early colonoscopy cannot be performed because of rapid bleeding, hemodynamic instability, significantly impaired coagulation parameters, comorbid illnesses, or inability to tolerate a bowel preparation, a tagged red blood cell (RBC) scan helps triage actively bleeding patients to more invasive procedures such as mesenteric angiography and angiotherapy. In the research setting, bleeding rates as low as 0.1 to 0.5 mL/min are picked up by tagged RBC scans, but in the clinical setting, only 45% of tagged RBC scans demonstrate extravasation. Rapidly positive scans have the highest accuracy and predict the best likelihood of identification of the bleeding site at subsequent angiography. A positive tagged RBC scan may identify a population of acute LGIB patients with higher in-hospital morbidity and rebleeding. Delayed positive scans have a much lower sensitivity in accurately localizing the bleeding source, as intestinal peristalsis may impact the reading. A high rate of false localization (22% to 42%) makes a tagged RBC scan unreliable in localizing bleeding for subsequent surgery. The test continues to be used as a screening test prior to more invasive testing such as angiography, although some suggest that the test unnecessarily delays more definitive studies and reduces chances of early bleeding localization. If a rapidly bleeding site is identified on angiography, vasopressin can be infused after selective catheterization of the bleeding vessel. This may induce vasoconstriction and cessation of bleeding. Alternatively, selective embolization of the bleeding vessel can be attempted. Complications of angiography can be dye-related (renal failure), procedure-related (hematoma formation, retroperitoneal bleeding, intestinal ischemia), or as a result of vasopressin infusion (arrhythmias, myocardial infarction).

When blood is seen throughout the colon as well as within the terminal ileum, or if a potential colonic source is not evident despite a careful and adequate examination, the bleeding source could reside in the small bowel. Conventional contrast radiologic studies such as the small bowel follow-through series or enteroclysis have a very low yield for identification of a bleeding source in this setting. Capsule endoscopy has now become the test of choice in situations in which a small bowel source of bleeding is suspected. The drawbacks of capsule endoscopy include the fact that real-time reading is not possible, accurate localization of findings is almost impossible, and no therapeutics can be administered. Actively bleeding sources identified in the small bowel have required surgery in the past, either for surgical resection or for endoscopic therapy during intraoperative enteroscopy. More recently, newer endoscopic techniques such as double-balloon enteroscopy have been developed that allow reach of almost the entire small bowel for endoscopic therapy, but these may be associated with a higher degree of morbidity and complications than routine endoscopic procedures. These studies can be considered in refractory situations or in obscure gastrointestinal bleeding (Table 49.3).

Newer tests that have been studied include computed tomographic angiography, wherein arterial-phase images may demonstrate vascular abnormalities such as angiodysplasia or may even demonstrate extravasation of contrast into the bowel lumen

TABLE 49.3	Obscure Lower Gastrointestinal Bleeding[a]

Approach
  Consider repeating endoscopic procedures: push enteroscopy, colonoscopy, capsule endoscopy
  If bleeding is rapid and severe with hemodynamic compromise, repeat tagged RBC scan

Consider angiography
  During bleeding episode to localize bleeding by demonstration of contrast extravasation
  During nonbleeding interval to identify characteristic angiographic patterns of potential bleeding lesions such as angiodysplasia and neoplasia
  CT or MR angiography are options, but therapy (vasopressin infusion, embolization) is not possible
Consider CT or MR enterography to look for luminal or mural small bowel lesions

Consider double-balloon enteroscopy, a new technique that may allow visualization of the entire small bowel

Consider intraoperative enteroscopy:
  Healthy individuals with significant bleeding recurrences and a potential small bowel source
  Radiologic studies or advanced endoscopic studies demonstrating a potential small bowel source amenable to endoscopic therapy
  For localization of a likely small bowel source for surgical resection

Provocative measures (administration of heparin, thrombolytic agents, or vasodilators) are very rarely used and should not be recommended except in very refractory situations, in patients without comorbidities, under very close observation by experienced personnel

---

[a]Obscure LGIB consists of persistent or recurrent bleeding, with no bleeding source evident on conventional endoscopy.
RBC, red blood cell; CT, computed tomography; MR, magnetic resonance; LGIB, lower gastrointestinal bleeding.

in patients with rapidly bleeding sources. Although computed tomographic angiography may provide a less invasive option than conventional angiography, this option has not been systematically studied as a diagnostic option in acute LGIB. Computed tomography and magnetic resonance enterography may allow detailed evaluation of the small bowel wall and mucosa for potential bleeding lesions and inflammation. These newer and advanced radiologic options can be considered both in refractory situations and in obscure gastrointestinal bleeding (Table 49.3).

Diverticulosis and angiodysplasia account for >50% of colonic bleeding sources. Diverticular bleeding is arterial bleeding and therefore presents with clinically significant painless episodes of bright red blood in the stool. Bleeding spontaneously ceases in >80% of patients, but a quarter may develop recurrent bleeding. Multiple recurrences of diverticular bleeding are an indication for resection of the offending segment of colon. Bleeding from angiodysplasia can be slow and more persistent and may be associated with iron deficiency anemia. Endoscopic ablation of bleeding lesions may decrease the rate of bleeding, but patients typically require iron repletion and

TABLE 49.4 **Management of Vascular Lesions**[a]

Initial management

Endoscopic ablation when possible, using thermal cautery, argon plasma coagulation, or laser:
  Lesions accessible with conventional endoscopy
  Double-balloon enteroscopy in specialized cases
  Numerous lesions may not be amenable to endoscopic therapy

Iron repletion
  Oral iron therapy, ferrous sulfate 325 mg tid or equivalent
  Intravenous or parenteral iron repletion when oral iron is not tolerated or inadequate

Intermittent blood transfusions

Surgery: rare, only for isolated, discrete, limited vascular lesions such as hamartoma or Dieulafoy lesion

Refractory situations

Continue above measures

Consider adding medications with anecdotal and limited evidence in decreasing blood loss:
  ε-Aminocaproic acid
  Combination estrogen–progesterone hormone therapy
  Danazol
  Octreotide by subcutaneous injection

---

[a]Vascular lesions include angiodysplasia, telangiectasia, hamartoma, arteriovenous malformation, nevus, and Dieulafoy lesion.
tid, three times daily.

supplementation (Table 49.4). In refractory situations, medications with anecdotal or limited evidence can be considered, but these approaches can be associated with serious thrombotic complications. Hemorrhoids account for 5% to 10% of episodes of acute LGIB and are the most common cause of bright red blood in the stool or toilet tissue in the ambulatory patient. Other causes are less common and include neoplasia, colitis, Meckel's diverticulum, and radiation proctopathy. Angiodysplasias are the most common small bowel cause of acute LGIB. Other small bowel causes include tumors, including stromal tumors, lymphoma, and, rarely, adenocarcinoma, inflammatory disorders including Crohn's disease, and ulcers/erosions from nonsteroidal anti-inflammatory drug use.

One of the dilemmas in patients with acute LGIB is making a clinical determination as to whether the lesion identified on diagnostic testing is indeed the source for the patient's bleeding episode. This is particularly important as active bleeding or stigmata of recent bleeding are not always identified on potential bleeding lesions. At times, more than one potential bleeding lesion may be identified. Criteria have been suggested to assess the level of diagnostic certainty in interpreting diagnostic tests in acute LGIB, which may help determine the nature of definitive management or follow-up needed, especially when surgery is recommended on the basis of results of diagnostic tests (Table 49.5).

TABLE 49.5	Levels of Diagnostic Certainty in Interpreting Test for Acute Lower Gastrointestinal Bleeding

Definitive evidence of a bleeding source
  Active oozing or bleeding visualized at colonoscopy or angiography
  Stigmata of recent bleeding (adherent clot, nonbleeding visible vessel) identified on colonoscopy
  Positive tagged RBC scan associated with either of above

Circumstantial evidence of a bleeding source
  Single potential bleeding source on colonoscopy with fresh blood in the same segment
  Single potential bleeding source on colonoscopy or angiography in the same area as a positive tagged RBC scan
  Bright or dark red blood on objective stool testing, single potential source (without endoscopic stigmata) on colonoscopy, negative upper endoscopy, and capsule endoscopy
  Bright or dark red blood, maroon stool, or melena on objective stool testing, single potential source (without endoscopic stigmata) on capsule endoscopy, negative upper endoscopy, and colonoscopy

Equivocal evidence of a bleeding source
  "Hematochezia" unconfirmed by objective testing, potential sources (without endoscopic stigmata) on colonoscopy or capsule endoscopy

RBC, red blood cell.

SUGGESTED READINGS

Currie GM, Kiat H, Wheat JM. Scintigraphic evaluation of acute lower gastrointestinal hemorrhage: current status and future directions. *J Clin Gastroenterol.* 2011;45:92–99.

Davila RE, Rajan E, Adler DG, et al. ASGE guideline: the role of endoscopy in the patient with lower GI bleeding. *Gastrointest Endosc.* 2005;62:656–660.

Green BT, Rockey DC. Lower gastrointestinal bleeding—management. *Gastroenterol Clin North Am.* 2005;34:665–678.

Lanas A, Garcia-Rodriguez LA, Polo-Tomas M, et al. Time trends and impact of upper and lower gastrointestinal bleeding and perforation in clinical practice. *Am J Gastroenterol.* 2009;104:1633–1641.

Strate LL, Naumann CR. The role of colonoscopy and radiological procedures in the management of acute lower intestinal bleeding. *Clin Gastroenterol Hepatol.* 2010;8:333–343.

Zuckerman GR, Prakash C, Askin MP, et al. AGA technical review on the evaluation and management of occult and obscure gastrointestinal bleeding. *Gastroenterology.* 2000;118:201–221.

50 Acute Pancreatitis

Mrudula Kumar and Daniel K. Mullady

BACKGROUND

Acute pancreatitis is inflammation of the pancreas associated with varying degrees of autodigestion, edema, necrosis, and hemorrhage of pancreatic tissue. The principal symptom is abdominal pain, mainly in the epigastric region. Nausea and vomiting are common. In a patient with characteristic abdominal pain, the diagnosis is confirmed by elevated serum amylase and lipase levels (greater than three times normal) and/or evidence of pancreatic inflammation on cross-sectional imaging. There are many causes of acute pancreatitis, but gallstones and alcohol account for nearly 70% of cases (Table 50.1). The clinical course varies from mild, self-limited episodes to severe pancreatitis with associated multiorgan dysfunction, local complications such as infected peripancreatic fluid collections, or extrapancreatic complications such as venous thrombosis. Up to 20% of patients presenting with pancreatitis have a severe course. The overall mortality rate from the presence of severe pancreatitis with infectious complications is approximately 10% to 20% and can increase to more than 50% in the presence of persistent organ failure. Predicting severity is of highest importance, and all patients should be treated as severe until proven otherwise with aggressive intravenous fluid (IVF) resuscitation and pain control.

EVALUATION

The evaluation of a patient with suspected pancreatitis should begin with a careful history with attention to symptom onset, prior pancreatitis, alcohol use, gallstone disease, and review of medications. On physical examination, patients typically have epigastric tenderness but can have a diffusely tender abdomen. Bowel sounds may be absent indicative of ileus. Patients may also have systemic inflammatory response syndrome (SIRS) with fever, tachycardia, and tachypnea. Findings suggesting severe disease include diminished breath sounds, hypoxia, and altered mental status. Cullen's sign (periumbilical ecchymosis) and Grey Turner's sign (flank ecchymosis) are rare findings and indicate hemorrhagic pancreatitis.

Per the Atlanta Symposium, the diagnosis of acute pancreatitis requires two of the following: (1) abdominal pain, (2) amylase and/or lipase elevation greater than three times the upper limit of normal, and (3) pancreatic inflammation on cross-sectional imaging. Serum lipase levels are more sensitive in the diagnosis of acute pancreatitis and remain elevated for longer than serum amylase. Other initial laboratory values should include liver function tests, complete blood cell count, serum urea nitrogen

TABLE 50.1	Causes of Acute Pancreatitis	
Common	**Uncommon**	**Rare**
Gallstones	Pancreas divisum	Malignancy
Alcohol	Autoimmune pancreatitis	Hereditary
	Hypertriglyceridemia	Vascular (e.g., ischemia)
	Medications	Abdominal trauma
	Iatrogenic (post-ERCP)	Toxins (e.g., scorpion bite)
	Sphincter of Oddi dysfunction	Hypercalcemia
	Idiopathic	Infection (e.g., mumps, coxsackie viral infection)

ERCP, endoscopic retrograde cholangiopancreatography.

(BUN), and creatinine. Elevations in liver enzymes (particularly transaminases) with or without associated hyperbilirubinemia suggest the presence of bile duct stones or compression of the common bile duct by pancreatic edema.

An abdominal ultrasonography should be performed, especially in suspected gallstone pancreatitis, to assess for cholelithiasis or choledocholithiasis. Cross-sectional imaging is not mandatory as part of the initial evaluation but can be performed if there is concern for complications. Contrast-enhanced computed tomography (CECT) is the best modality for evaluating pancreatic inflammation, necrosis, and peripancreatic fluid collections. The most common findings on imaging in uncomplicated pancreatitis are enlargement of all or part of the pancreas with blurring of the margins and inflammatory changes. CECT done at the initial presentation may underestimate disease severity, as it can take up to 72 hours for necrosis to develop. Therefore, CECT should be delayed unless there is a concern for other complications or if the diagnosis is in doubt.

For recurrent acute pancreatitis (two or more episodes), a detailed work-up, including IgG4, triglyceride, and calcium levels, is warranted. A thorough review of patient's medication profile should be examined, as iatrogenic causes account for 2% of pancreatitis. An endoscopic ultrasonography can be performed to evaluate for pancreatic cancer in patients who do not have an identified etiology. Empiric cholecystectomy should be considered in patients with no identifiable cause for recurrent acute pancreatitis, even if liver function tests and gallbladder imaging are normal.

PREDICTION OF SEVERITY

Early prediction of severity in acute pancreatitis is vitally important in identifying patients at increased risk for morbidity and mortality. This can be challenging as there is no single, reliable way to predict severity. Current severity indices are based on clinical and radiographic parameters. An important clinical factor is persistent organ failure at >48 hours. Persistent pain, respiratory failure, and renal failure generally indicate severe disease.

Various grading and scoring systems have been developed to risk-stratify acute pancreatitis patients. Historically, the Ranson criteria and Glasgow scoring systems

TABLE 50.2	BISAP Score for Predicting Severity and Complications in Acute Pancreatitis

BUN >25
Impaired mental status
Systemic inflammatory response
Age >60
Pleural effusion
Calculate within 24 hr; increased risk for complications in patients with score of ≥3

BUN, serum urea nitrogen.

have been used, but these are cumbersome and can take 48 hours to complete. More recently, the Acute Physiology and Chronic Health Examination II (APACHE II) has been used to predict severity in acute pancreatitis, but it is not pancreas specific. Patients with an APACHE II score >8 usually have severe disease. A new prognostic scoring system, the bedside index for severity in acute pancreatitis (BISAP), has been proposed as a simple method for early identification of patients at risk for in-hospital mortality and is as accurate as other scoring systems (Table 50.2). One point is assigned for each of the following signs within 24 hours of presentation: BUN level >25 mg/dL, impaired mental status, SIRS, age >60, and pleural effusion on imaging studies. A BISAP score ≥3 is associated with an increased risk of complications. Other single factors on admission that are associated with a severe course include hemoconcentration (hematocrit >44%), obesity, C-reactive protein (CRP) >150 mg/dL, albumin <2.5 mg/dL, calcium <8.5 mg/dL, and early hyperglycemia (Table 50.3).

The CT severity index is a scoring system based on an unenhanced CT grading system (A–E) and percent necrosis (Table 50.4). Pancreatic necrosis appears as a sharply demarcated region that does not enhance after intravenous (IV) contrast. A score of >6 indicates severe disease and a poorer prognosis. There are a variety of local complications that can be diagnosed on cross-sectional imaging in severe acute pancreatitis (Table 50.2). Early findings include pancreatic necrosis and acute fluid collections that are almost always sterile. Other complications that can occur at various stages include peripancreatic artery pseudoaneurysm (e.g., gastroduodenal, hepatic, and splenic arteries) and venous thrombosis (e.g., portal, superior mesenteric, and

TABLE 50.3	Other Single Factors on Admission Associated with Severe Acute Pancreatitis

Hematocrit >44%
Obesity
C-reactive protein >150 mg/dL
Albumin <2.5 mg/dL
Calcium <8.5 mg/dL
Early hyperglycemia

TABLE 50.4	CT Grading of Acute Pancreatitis: CT Severity Index[a]	
Grade[b]	Findings	Score
A	Normal pancreas: normal size, sharply defined, smooth contour, homogeneous enhancement, retroperitoneal peripancreatic fat without enhancement	0
B	Focal or diffuse enlargement of the pancreas; contour may show irregularity, enhancement may be inhomogeneous but there is no peripancreatic inflammation	1
C	Peripancreatic inflammation with intrinsic pancreatic abnormalities	2
D	Intrapancreatic or extrapancreatic fluid collections	3
E	Two or more large collections of gas in the pancreas or retroperitoneum	4

Necrosis score based on contrast-enhanced CT

Necrosis (%)	Score
0	0
<33	2
33–50	4
≥50	6

[a]CT severity index equals unenhanced CT score plus necrosis score: maximum, 10; ≥6, severe disease.
[b]Grading based on findings on unenhanced CT.
CT, computed tomography.

splenic veins). Pancreatic necrosis can be sterile (Fig. 50.1A) or infected (Fig. 50.1B). Infected necrosis is a delayed complication, occurring at least 2 to 3 weeks after the onset of symptoms. Persistent fevers and leukocytosis without another source and the presence of gas in the necrotic area are clinical indicators of infected necrosis. The diagnosis can be confirmed with needle aspiration of the necrotic area, but the decision to proceed with invasive treatment is based on the patient's overall stability.

MANAGEMENT

Because early prediction of disease severity can be difficult, interventions can be delayed. In general, all patients should be treated as severe until proven otherwise. This section addresses the treatment strategies in severe acute pancreatitis including IVF, pain control, nutritional support, the role of endoscopic retrograde cholangiopancreatography (ERCP), use of antibiotics, and management of peripancreatic fluid collections (Table 50.5).

Hypovolemia is the principal etiology of pancreatic hypoperfusion and inflammation in acute pancreatitis. Thus, rapid restoration of intravascular volume must be the first therapeutic strategy. Recommendations regarding rate vary and should be individualized. In patients with signs of severe volume depletion, maximal fluid resuscitation of 500 to 1000 mL/hr should be initiated and can be decreased once

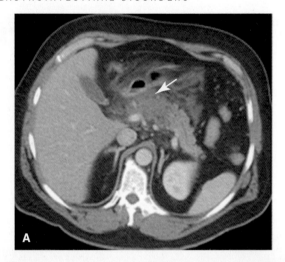

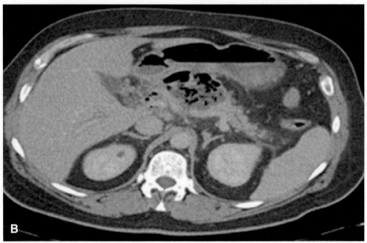

Figure 50.1. A: Necrotizing pancreatitis. Area of decreased attenuation in the pancreatic head and neck (*arrow*) represents necrosis in a patient with severe ethanol-induced pancreatitis. The body and tail are viable. **B:** Imaging in the same patient several weeks after presentation with gas within the fluid collection indicating infected necrosis.

evidence for hypoperfusion subsides. At the very least, a patient presenting with acute pancreatitis should be started on at least 250 to 300 mL/hr to maintain urine output of at least 0.5 mL/kg/hr. Although routine use of invasive intravascular monitoring is not recommended, it may be useful in severe disease. It is not mandatory to decrease the IVF rate in the presence of pulmonary edema, as this may be secondary to acute respiratory distress syndrome and not cardiogenic shock. Bowel rest should be maintained until pain and nausea have resolved. IV opiate pain medication should be

TABLE 50.5	Management of Severe Acute Pancreatitis in the Intensive Care Unit

- Supportive care: aggressive IVF, pain control
- Early ERCP (<48–72 hr) in patients with suspected concurrent cholangitis or biliary obstruction
- Early enteral nutrition via nasojejunal tube
- No role for antibiotics in infection prophylaxis
- Reserve drainage[a] for
  - Acute fluid collections with abdominal compartment syndrome
  - Suspected infected necrosis in an unstable patient (usually occurs 2–3 wk into illness)

---

[a]Current evidence supports "step-up" approach to peripancreatic fluid collections and infected necrosis (endoscopic or percutaneous drainage initially followed by surgery if necessary).
IVF, intravenous fluid; ERCP, endoscopic retrograde cholangiopancreatography.

administered for pain control, and it may be necessary to administer pain medications via a patient-controlled anesthesia pump.

In cases of gallstone pancreatitis, antibiotics should be initiated and biliary decompression via ERCP should be performed early (within the first 72 hours) if ascending cholangitis is suspected. In some cases in which patients are too unstable for sedation or in which ERCP is unavailable, a percutaneous transhepatic cholangiogram with catheter placement can be performed. Early ERCP does little to affect the course of pancreatitis but impacts the course of cholangitis. If a patient with acute pancreatitis has abnormal liver enzymes and an intact gallbladder, cholecystectomy should be performed during the same hospital stay or within 30 days of discharge.

The ideal approach to nutritional support is through early enteral feeding via a nasojejunal tube. Enteral nutrition preserves the intestinal mucosa and has the added benefit of potentially reducing incidence of bacterial translocation from the gut. Outcome studies have shown that enteral nutrition is associated with reduced central catheter infections, reduced sepsis, less need for surgical intervention, decreased length of hospital stay, and lower cost than total parenteral nutrition. The incidence of multiorgan failure and mortality is no different between parenteral and enteral nutrition.

Antibiotic prophylaxis is controversial. In general, antibiotics should not be used routinely in severe acute pancreatitis. Antibiotics are recommended if there is a concern for concurrent cholangitis. Early in the course of disease, patients with severe acute pancreatitis can be febrile and have leukocytosis from inflammation associated with pancreatitis, and antibiotics are not warranted for these signs alone. Antibiotics should not be given for pancreatic necrosis, as infected necrosis is a late complication that takes several weeks to develop. Overall, antibiotics may decrease infectious complications but have not been shown to decrease mortality.

The management of peripancreatic fluid collections is also controversial. Acute fluid collections (enzyme-rich pancreatic fluid and tissue debris in and around the pancreas) occur in up to 40% of patients with severe acute pancreatitis. They represent a serous or exudative reaction to pancreatic injury and inflammation. There is little role for draining acute fluid collections unless abdominal compartment syndrome is suspected. The majority of acute fluid collections resolve spontaneously. Those that persist gradually encapsulate over 4 to 6 weeks and include a spectrum of collections ranging from pseudocysts, which are mostly fluid, to walled off pancreatic necrosis, which is mostly debris. Drainage should be performed in those patients who become symptomatic (e.g., pain and gastric outlet obstruction) or who do not respond to antibiotics for infected collections.

Treatment of infected necrosis is based on the patient's clinical course. Unstable patients with infected necrosis or abdominal compartment syndrome usually require drainage of infected necrosis. Traditionally, this has been with exploratory laparotomy, debridement, and drain placement with associated high morbidity and mortality. Recently, there has been a move toward delayed intervention and minimally invasive approaches including direct endoscopic pancreatic necrosectomy and percutaneous drainage that are less morbid and likely as effective as surgery.

SUGGESTED READINGS

Al-Omran M, AlBalawi ZH, Tash Kandi MF, Al-Ansary LA. Enteral versus parenteral nutrition for acute pancreatitis. *Cochrane Database Syst Rev.* 2010;**20**(1):CD002837

Banks PA, Freeman ML. Practice guidelines in acute pancreatitis. *Am J Gastroenterol.* 2006;101:2379–2400.

Greer SE, Burchard KW. Acute pancreatitis and critical illness: a pancreatic tale of hypoperfusion and inflammation. *Chest.* 2009;136:1413–1419.

Pandol SJ, Saluja AK, Imrie CW, et al. Acute pancreatitis: bench to bedside. *Gastroenterology.* 2007;132:1127–1151.

Papachristou GI, Muddana V, Yadav D, et al. Comparison of BISAP, Ranson's, APACHE-II, and CTSI scores in predicting organ failure, complications, and mortality in acute pancreatitis. *Am J Gastroenterol.* 2010;**105**(2):435–441.

Pezzilli R, Zerbi A, DiCarlo V, et al. Practical guidelines for acute pancreatitis. *Pancreatology.* 2010;10:523–535.

van Santvoort HC, Besselink MG, Bakker OJ, et al. A step-up approach or open necrosectomy for necrotizing pancreatitis. *N Engl J Med.* 2010;362:1491–1502.

51

Status Epilepticus
Rajat Dhar

DEfiNITION

Status epilepticus (SE) is formally defined as any seizure lasting more than 30 minutes or repetitive seizures for this period without return to baseline level of consciousness in between. As most seizures stop without treatment within 2 to 3 minutes, any seizure lasting more than 5 minutes is unlikely to stop spontaneously and requires treatment. There is also greater risk of neuronal injury as seizures persist beyond 30 minutes so aggressive prompt intervention (especially for convulsive seizures) is paramount. SE is classified by seizure type (generalized vs. partial, either simple or complex) and manifestations (tonic-clonic vs. focal motor vs. nonconvulsive). It occurs in more than 100,000 persons each year in the United States. Mortality is between 5% and 30% for SE, varying with type and duration, but outcome is largely determined by etiology (Table 51.1). Causes can be divided into acute processes, either in the central nervous system or systemically, or chronic disorders such as preexisting epilepsy or an old stroke or brain tumor. It is imperative to evaluate and manage the underlying etiology as well as control seizures.

INITIAL MANAGEMENT OF STATUS EPILEPTICUS

The first priorities are stabilization of the airway, breathing, and circulation. Not all patients with incipient SE require intubation, but all require close attention to patency of the airway. The head should be positioned to avoid obstruction and an artificial airway may be placed. Placing an oral airway may be challenging in a patient with teeth clenched, but a nasal airway can usually be inserted. Oxygen can be applied via nasal cannula or face mask. Many patients with SE will maintain oxygen saturation with these basic measures and continue to ventilate. It is common for patients with seizures to develop an acute lactic acidosis that resolves as SE is controlled. Hypertension is more common than hypotension in the early stages of SE whereas hemodynamic support and invasive monitoring is often required later as treatment intensifies.

Benzodiazepines are usually the first-line agents to stop persistent seizures (Algorithm 51.1). Lorazepam can be given in 2 to 4 mg aliquots repeated every 2 to 3 minutes to a maximum of 0.1 mg/kg IV. If IV access is not immediately available, then rectal diazepam gel (0.2 mg/kg in adults, usually 10 to 20 mg) can be used. Midazolam can also be squirted into the mouth (5 to 10 mg, with rapid buccal absorption). Such agents will be effective in 50% or more of SE cases treated early. The duration of anticonvulsant action of these agents is relatively short (longest for

TABLE 51.1	Causes of Status Epilepticus
Causes	Evaluation
Acute symptomatic CNS lesion Encephalitis/meningitis Cerebrovascular (ischemic stroke, ICH, SAH, CVST) Traumatic brain injury Global hypoxic-ischemic brain injury (post cardiac arrest) drowning/asphyxiation Hypertensive encephalopathy/PRES	Brain imaging (head CT, MRI); lumbar puncture
Chronic CNS lesion Existing stroke Brain tumor (primary or metastatic, paraneoplastic)	Brain imaging (head CT, MRI)
Toxic/metabolic derangement Drug intoxication or overdose (TCA, amphetamine) Drug withdrawal (alcohol, benzodiazepines) Iatrogenic: medications (beta-lactams, theophylline, others) Hypoglycemia $\pm$ hyperglycemia Electrolytes (hyponatremia, hypocalcemia) Febrile seizures (in young children)	Drug screen and drug history, EKG; glucose level; electrolytes
Epilepsy Noncompliance with AEDs Recent change in dose or AED Psychogenic seizures ("pseudo-status")	Medication history; serum AED levels

CNS, central nervous system; CT, computed tomography; MRI, magnetic resonance imaging; AED, antiepileptic drugs; ICH, intracerebral hemorrhage; SAH, subarachnoid hemorrhage; CVST, cerebral venous sinus thrombosis; TCA, tricyclic antidepressant; PRES, posterior reversible encephalopathy syndrome; EKG, electrocardiogram.

lorazepam), so a longer-acting antiepileptic drugs (AED) should be given concurrently or immediately after benzodiazepines in cases of SE. *Phenytoin* is the most commonly used AED, as it is available IV with rapid onset of action. A dose of 18 to 20 mg/kg should be given at a maximum rate of 50 mg/min. Rapid infusions of phenytoin can cause bradycardia, arrhythmias, hypotension, and even cardiac arrest. It can also cause *purple glove* syndrome and infusion site reactions. Therefore, acute IV administration may be preferred using *fosphenytoin* (a prodrug that is dose in "phenytoin equivalents" or PE and can be given at a rate of 150 mg PE per minute through a peripheral IV without infusion problems) if central access is not available. If seizures are still not controlled after initial phenytoin load then an additional 5 to 10 mg/kg can be given. A phenytoin level should be drawn 1 hour after loading is complete and further IV or enteral doses given as necessary to maintain total blood levels of 15 to 25 μg/mL.

ALGORITHM 51.1   Initial Management of Status Epilepticus

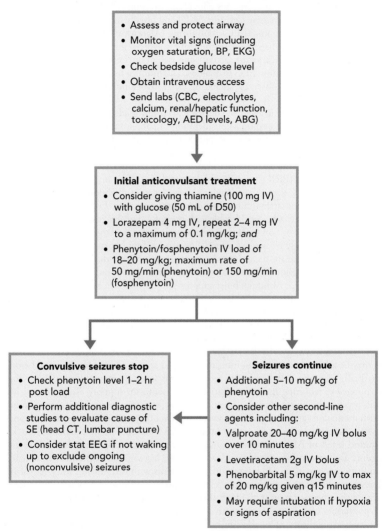

- Assess and protect airway
- Monitor vital signs (including oxygen saturation, BP, EKG)
- Check bedside glucose level
- Obtain intravenous access
- Send labs (CBC, electrolytes, calcium, renal/hepatic function, toxicology, AED levels, ABG)

Initial anticonvulsant treatment
- Consider giving thiamine (100 mg IV) with glucose (50 mL of D50)
- Lorazepam 4 mg IV, repeat 2–4 mg IV to a maximum of 0.1 mg/kg; *and*
- Phenytoin/fosphenytoin IV load of 18–20 mg/kg; maximum rate of 50 mg/min (phenytoin) or 150 mg/min (fosphenytoin)

Convulsive seizures stop
- Check phenytoin level 1–2 hr post load
- Perform additional diagnostic studies to evaluate cause of SE (head CT, lumbar puncture)
- Consider stat EEG if not waking up to exclude ongoing (nonconvulsive) seizures

Seizures continue
- Additional 5–10 mg/kg of phenytoin
- Consider other second-line agents including:
- Valproate 20–40 mg/kg IV bolus over 10 minutes
- Levetiracetam 2g IV bolus
- Phenobarbital 5 mg/kg IV to max of 20 mg/kg given q15 minutes
- May require intubation if hypoxia or signs of aspiration

BP, blood pressure; EKG, electrocardiogram; CBC, complete blood cell count; AED, antiepileptic drugs; ABG, arterial blood gas; CT, computed tomography; EEG, electroencephalogram.

REFRACTORY STATUS EPILEPTICUS

A proportion of patients presenting with SE (20% to 30%) will fail to respond to both benzodiazepines and phenytoin (or another second-line agent, such as IV valproate or phenobarbital). By this time, seizures have usually persisted for 60 minutes, if not longer. This subgroup is designated to have *refractory status epilepticus* (RSE) that carries a significantly higher mortality and worse functional outcome. Most will require continuous infusions of anesthetic anticonvulsants to control RSE. These patients need to be admitted to the intensive care unit (ICU) and usually require ventilatory support and electroencephalographic (EEG) monitoring (Algorithm 51.2). SE that begins as convulsive (e.g., generalized tonic-clonic) often evolves into a state of dissociation between ongoing electrical seizure activity and lack of obvious motor expression; such nonconvulsive RSE requires EEG to diagnose and monitor its treatment. Subtle motor manifestations may be observed, including facial myoclonus, tonic eye deviation, or nystagmus.

Choice of anesthetic agent to control RSE is not guided by strong comparative evidence. It should be based on a consideration of patient factors including hemodynamic stability, seizure severity and duration, and goal of treatment (i.e., seizure cessation vs. burst suppression), as well as local (physician and institutional) experience. The major choices are compared in Table 51.2. There is a definite risk of "propofol-related infusion syndrome (PRIS)" with the high cumulative doses of propofol required in RSE; this manifests as metabolic acidosis, hyperkalemia, rhabdomyolysis, renal failure, bradycardia, and arrhythmias (including cardiac arrest). Even in the absence of PRIS, hypotension can be considerable with propofol. For this reason, midazolam is a reasonable first-line option for RSE if seizure cessation is the target on EEG. Propofol or pentobarbital may be used as second-line agents if midazolam either fails to control seizures or there are breakthroughs or recurrent seizures during maintenance or weaning of the infusion. These two agents are better able to induce a burst suppression pattern on EEG. Although burst suppression has not been associated with better outcome (than seizure control alone) in RSE, it may be reasonable to target this goal in more resistant/recurrent cases. Volatile anesthetics have been used in limited series and require specialized equipment and monitoring. Their major advantages are short half-life and ability to rapidly induce burst suppression.

Once the EEG goal has been achieved (seizure cessation and/or burst suppression), it may be advisable to maintain infusion rates and seizure control for 24 hours before gradually weaning. Many patients requiring this level of intervention will develop hypotension requiring fluid resuscitation and vasopressor support. Respiratory drive will be severely inhibited or abolished and all patients require mechanical ventilation with meticulous attention paid to prevention of ventilator-associated pneumonia and other nosocomial infections, a major source of ICU mortality in these patients. If background levels of AEDs are not maintained then seizures will recur when anesthetic agents are weaned off. Phenytoin, levetiracetam, lacosamide, valproate, topiramate, and/or other agents should be continued in patients with RSE during and after use of anesthetic infusions. Free phenytoin levels should be monitored frequently, if possible, with a therapeutic target in the high therapeutic range (1.5 to 2.5 μg/mL). Induced hypothermia offers another alternative in resistant cases (e.g., failure of midazolam) and may avoid the use of long-lasting barbiturates or the risks of propofol. This has only been shown effective in a small series where temperature was lowered to between 31°C and 35°C (titrated to EEG response). The major advantage is rapid offset of metabolic suppression once temperature is normalized (in comparison to pentobarbital, which persists for days after infusion is stopped). *Ketamine,* an glutamine-autognone-receptor antagonist, has also shown anecdotal promise in controlling RSE and has the advantages of working independent of gamma-aminobutyric acid (GABA) receptors, which are downregulated after prolonged seizures, and also not worsening hemodynamic instability.

ALGORITHM 51.2 Treatment of Refractory Status Epilepticus

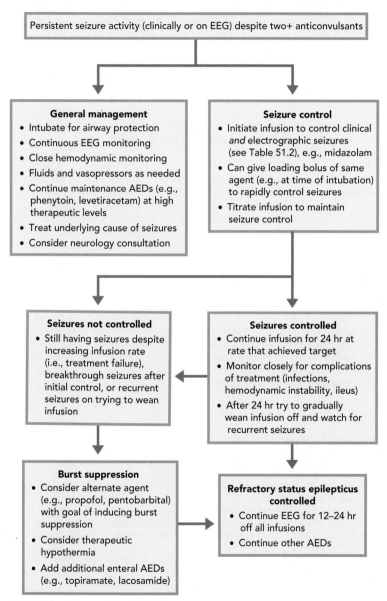

Persistent seizure activity (clinically or on EEG) despite two+ anticonvulsants

General management
- Intubate for airway protection
- Continuous EEG monitoring
- Close hemodynamic monitoring
- Fluids and vasopressors as needed
- Continue maintenance AEDs (e.g., phenytoin, levetiracetam) at high therapeutic levels
- Treat underlying cause of seizures
- Consider neurology consultation

Seizure control
- Initiate infusion to control clinical *and* electrographic seizures (see Table 51.2), e.g., midazolam
- Can give loading bolus of same agent (e.g., at time of intubation) to rapidly control seizures
- Titrate infusion to maintain seizure control

Seizures not controlled
- Still having seizures despite increasing infusion rate (i.e., treatment failure), breakthrough seizures after initial control, or recurrent seizures on trying to wean infusion

Seizures controlled
- Continue infusion for 24 hr at rate that achieved target
- Monitor closely for complications of treatment (infections, hemodynamic instability, ileus)
- After 24 hr try to gradually wean infusion off and watch for recurrent seizures

Burst suppression
- Consider alternate agent (e.g., propofol, pentobarbital) with goal of inducing burst suppression
- Consider therapeutic hypothermia
- Add additional enteral AEDs (e.g., topiramate, lacosamide)

Refractory status epilepticus controlled
- Continue EEG for 12–24 hr off all infusions
- Continue other AEDs

EEG, electroencephalogram; AED, antiepileptic drugs.

TABLE 51.2	Anesthetic Infusions for Refractory Status Epilepticus			
	Midazolam	Propofol	Pentobarbital	Volatile anesthetics
Mechanism	Benzodiazepine (GABA)	Unclear (GABA modulation)	Barbiturate (GABA)	Polysynaptic GABA
Loading dose[a]	0.2 mg/kg	1–2 mg/kg	5 mg/kg	N/A
Starting infusion	0.05 mg/kg/hr	1–2 mg/kg/hr (15–30 μg/kg/min)	1 mg/kg/hr	N/A
Infusion range	0.05–0.8 mg/kg/hr	1–15 mg/kg/hr (15–250 μg/kg/min)	0.5–10 mg/kg/hr	0.8%–2.0%
Half-life	1–2 hr[b]	<1 hr[b]	15–40 hr	<1 hr
Adverse effects	Hypotension, tachyphylaxis	Hypotension, "infusion syndrome," lipemia	Hypotension, bradycardia, poikilothermia, pulmonary infections	Hypotension, ileus

GABA, gamma-aminobutyric acid.
[a]May repeat loading dose boluses till seizures controlled.
[b]May accumulate with prolonged infusions.

SE in comatose survivors of cardiac arrest (i.e., *postanoxic* SE) is usually an ominous sign of diffuse cerebral damage. Especially when accompanied by myoclonic jerking, the presence of SE is one of the most consistent predictors of death/nonrecovery after cardiac arrest. Myoclonus may be transiently controlled by agents such as valproate, clonazepam, or levetiracetam, but SE is usually refractory and aggressive measures should be withheld pending discussion of prognosis with the family.

SUGGESTED READINGS

Abou Khaled KJ, Hirsch LJ. Advances in the management of seizures and status epilepticus in critically ill patients. *Crit Care Clin.* 2007;22:637–659.

Bassin S, Smith TL, Beck TP. Clinical review: status epilepticus. *Crit Care.* 2002;6:137–142. Available from http://ccforum.com/content/6/2/137

Chen JW, Wasterlain CG. Status epilepticus: pathophysiology and management in adults. *Lancet Neurol.* 2006;5:246–256.

Claassen J, Hirsch LJ, Emerson RG, et al. Treatment of refractory status epilepticus with pentobarbital, propofol, or midazolam: a systematic review. *Epilepsia.* 2002;43:146–153.

Corry JJ, Dhar R, Murphy T, et al. Hypothermia for refractory status epilepticus. *Neurocrit Care.* 2008;9:189–197.

Lowenstein D. The management of refractory status epilepticus. An update. *Epilpesia.* 2006;47(Suppl. 1):35–40.

52

Acute Ischemic Stroke
Michael A. Rubin

Stroke is the third leading cause of death in the United States and a leading cause of disability. Approximately 85% of all strokes are ischemic. Although most strokes can be managed in a hospital ward, many cases of acute ischemic stroke warrant intensive care. Patients who have undergone thrombolysis are usually admitted to an intensive care unit (ICU) or step down unit for monitoring for hemorrhagic complications and blood pressure management. Large coritcol strokes or strokes affecting the brainstem require close neurologic monitoring in a critical care setting due to the potential need for osmotic therapy or surgical decompression. Furthermore, bilateral cortical or brainstem insult can lead to decreased alertness or loss of bulbar muscle control requiring intubation and ventilation.

PRESENTATION

Stroke is a sudden loss of adequate perfusion to a segment of the brain causing irreversible damage. Its presentation varies considerably and may be as subtle as minor sensory loss or as impressive as the complete loss of motor function (except for eye movements) as seen in the locked-in syndrome. Thalamic and brainstem infarctions may cause a nonspecific alteration of mental status that may be difficult to distinguish from metabolic or infectious encephalopathy. Clinical diagnosis is usually possible if the onset history and pattern of deficits match a typical stroke syndrome. Suspicion of stroke should always lead to a head computed tomography or magnetic resonance imaging (MRI) to evaluate for an intracranial hemorrhage or other structural lesion such as neoplasia or abscess. Other pathologies that may mimic stroke include postictal "Todd's paralysis," complicated migraine, and psychosomatic disorders.

MANAGEMENT

General critical care management is similar to other ICU patients: maintain homeostasis of acid–base physiology, oxygenation, euvolemia, euglycemia, and so on. Variations include inhibiting fever (which has been shown to worsen outcome in stroke) and avoiding the practice of permissive hypercapnia (due to potential elevation of intracranial pressure). Aspirin (or another antiplatelet agent) should be given to ischemic stroke patients within 48 hours. The aspiring/dypiradmal combination is considered by some to be a superior agent, but combining clopidogrel and aspirin has shown to be deleterious and therefore should not be given unless there is another indication for the combination such as a coronary stent. The Academy of Neurology no longer recommends heparin for acute ischemic stroke, although there are rare occasions that it may be considered. Anticoagulation for atrial fibrillation is indicated, but does not have to be started in the setting of an acute stroke. Enoxaprin has been shown to be superior in preventing deep venous thrombosis (but not necessarily the occurrence of pulmonary embolus) and should be given within 24 hours of stroke. Seizure prophylaxis is not indicated in ischemic stroke and some agents, in fact, have been shown to worsen outcome. However, suspicion of seizure should be evaluated and treated if appropriate. For ischemic strokes <3 hours old, intravenous thrombolysis with tissue plasminogen activator (tPA) is the intervention of choice in selected patients. In addition, a recent study (from the European cooperative acute stroke study (ECASS) group) has shown benefit of thrombolysis up to 4.5 hours with additionally criteria (Table 52.1).

Stroke often causes reactive hypertension, that is, a physiologic self-induction of hypertension to perfuse the ischemic penumbra. High blood pressure should be tolerated up to 220/120 mm Hg unless there is evidence of ongoing end-organ damage (acute myocardial infarction, dissecting aneurysms, heart failure, renal failure) or if tPA was given. For the first 24 hours after thrombolysis, systolic blood pressure is kept under 180 and diastolic BP under 105 mm Hg to avoid hemorrhagic complications. Labetalol, nicardipine, or hydralazine can be used; nitrates are avoided because of their potential for venous dilatation and subsequent intracranial pressure elevation. Some centers extend the rational of hypertension preserving penumbra to the point that they *induce* hypertension. Although this approach is debated, most stroke physicians would at least consider pressure induction if a clear decrease in blood pressure is associated with worsening neurologic symptoms.

Determining the cause of stroke is necessary to guide therapy for secondary prevention. Telemetry, echocardiography, brain MRI, carotid Doppler study, and various forms of angiography may be used. Proper use and interpretation of these diagnostic tests should be done by or with the consultation of a stroke physician, given the increasing complexity of stroke management. General methods of the past, such as universal anticoagulation and carotid endarterectomy, have changed to more complex algorithms and will likely evolve even further.

CEREBRAL EDEMA

A large acute ischemic stroke typically causes cytotoxic edema. Edema, especially in young patients without age-related cerebral atrophy, may have dire consequences requiring close monitoring and aggressive interventions. Some strokes may cause compression of the cerebral ventricular system and lead to obstructive hydrocephalus requiring the placement of a ventriculostomy. Edema will create pressure differentials between the cerebral compartments created by dural folds leading to herniation syndromes. Cerebellar infarction is notorious for compressing the fourth ventricle and brainstem and causing catastrophic herniation. The peak effect typically occurs within 3 to 5 days, but in severe cases, rapid deterioration can occur within the first 2 days with the mortality rate close to 80%. Risk factors for deterioration within the first day include patients of younger age, those with larger infarcts, or those treated with thrombolysis. Simple measures such as keeping the head elevated at 30 or more degrees, avoiding hypotonic solutions (which lead to hyponatremia and worsening cerebral edema) and careful monitoring may be sufficient. In more advanced cases, osmotic therapy, external ventricular drainage, or decompressive posterior craniectomy may be necessary.

TABLE 52.1	Indications and Contraindications for Thrombolysis

Indications

Acute onset of focal neurologic symptoms in a defined vascular territory, consistent with ischemic stroke

Clearly defined onset of stroke less than 3 hr prior to planned start of treatment (if patient awakens with symptoms, onset is defined at "last seen normal")

Age 18 or older

No evidence of intracranial hemorrhage, nonvascular lesions (e.g., brain tumor, abscess) or signs of advanced cerebral infarction such as sulcal edema, hemispheric swelling, or large areas of low attenuation consistent with acute stroke on CT.

Contraindications

Onset of stroke greater than 3 hr prior to planned start of treatment

Rapidly improving symptoms or mild symptoms (relative)

If MCA stroke, an obtunded or comatose state may be a relative contraindication

Seizure at onset of stroke symptoms or within 3 hours prior to tPA administration

Clinical presentation suggestive of subarachnoid hemorrhage regardless of CT result

Hypertension, SBP > 185 mm Hg or DBP > 110 mm Hg.

Minor ischemic stroke within 1 month or major ischemic stroke or head trauma within the last 3 months

History of intracerebral or subarachnoid hemorrhage if recurrence risk is substantial

Untreated cerebral aneurysm, arteriovenous malformation, or brain tumor

Gastrointestinal or genitourinary hemorrhage within the last 21 days

Arterial puncture at a noncompressible site within the last 7 days or lumbar puncture within the last 3 days

Major surgery or major trauma within the last 14 days

Clinical presentation suggestive of acute myocardial infarction or post-MI pericarditis

Patient taking oral anticoagulants and INR >1.7

Patient receiving heparin within the last 48 hr and having an elevated aPTT

Patient receiving low-molecular-weight heparin within the last 24 hr

Pregnant, or anticipated pregnant, female

Known hemorrhagic diathesis or unsupported coagulation factor deficiency

Received tPA less than 7 days previously

Glucose <50 or >400 mg/dL

Platelet count <100,000/mm^3

INR >1.7 or elevated aPTT

Positive pregnancy test

Additional contraindications for 4.5-hr window

Combination of previous stroke *and* diabetes

Need for intravenous drip to obtain SBP <185 or DBP <110

tPA, tissue plasminogen activator; CT, computed tomography; MCA, middle cerebral artery; SBP, systolic blood pressure; DBP, diastolic blood pressure; BP, blood pressure; MI, myocardial infarction; INR, international normalized ratio; aPTT, activated partial thromboplastin time.

ALGORITHM 52.1 Management of Malignant Cerebral Edema due to Stroke

Stage 1: Initial intensive care and monitoring
- Monitoring of vitals and mental status at least every 2 hr
- Keep the head of bed at 30 degrees elevation
- Avoid jugular compression by keeping head midline
- Maintain normothermia and euglycemia
- Avoid hypotonic solutions
- Permissive hypertension, treat only SBP > 220 or DBP > 120
- Intubation for airway protection (GCS <9 or bulbar weakness).

Stage 2: Osmotic therapy for intracranial hypertension
- Avoid hypercarbia (ascertain adequate minute ventilation, treat fever)
- Give intravenous boluses of mannitol (see chapter 60)
- Consider hypertonic saline if mannitol is unsuccessful or contraindicated.

Stage 3: Surgery for cerebral edema; consult neurosurgeon for possible decompressive hemicraniectomy
- Allow surgical evaluation *before* offering to family
- Continue osmotic therapy and medical management

Stage 4: Experimental techniques (induced hypothermia)

SBP, systolic blood pressure; DBP, diastolic blood pressure; GCS, Glasgow Coma Scale.

Interventions for cerebral edema range from medical methods to surgical treatments. As with all significant interventions, the intensivist must establish early a clear understanding of the patient's and family's wishes regarding the degree of interventions desired. See chapter 60 on osmotic therapy for further details. Algorithm 52.1 demonstrates a stepwise approach to manage these patients, beginning with intubation for airway protection, osmotic therapy, considering for decompressive craniectomy, and lastly, with experimental techniques such as induced hypothermia.

Several trials have been completed to evaluate the utility of decompressive hemicraniectomy in large cortical strokes. Each showed a mortality benefit, but individually did not show significance in morbidity. All three studies were intentionally stopped early so that the data could be pooled into one analysis. Those aged 60 years and less had a significant improvement in both mortality and return to a functional state with minimal assistance. Some argue that this treatment should be reserved for patients with nondominant hemisphere infarctions, as they will have preserved language function. Others will not consider the procedure in those older than 60 years, but we would argue that the age chosen for the study was somewhat arbitrary and those close to the age in otherwise good health should be considered for intervention. If the intervention is being considered, early consultation with a neurosurgeon is advised, as the benefit is likely limited to early edema.

SUGGESTED READINGS

Adams HP Jr, del Zoppo G, Alberts MJ, et al. Guidelines for the early management adults with ischemic stroke: a guidline from the American Heart Associaton/American Stroke Association Stroke Council. *Stroke.* 2007;38:1655–1711.
An evidence-based review and most up-to-date guidelines for the management of patients with acute ischemic stroke.

Andrews PJ. Critical care management of acute ischemic stroke. *Curr Opin Crit Care.* 2004;10: 110–115.
A retrospective and prospective review on the management of acute stroke in the critical care setting.

del Zoppo GJ, Saver JL, Jauch EC, et al. Expansion of the time window for treatment of acute ischemic stroke with intravenous tissue plasminogen activator: a science advisory from the American Heart Association/American Stroke Association. *Stroke.* 2009;40;2945–2948.
Update on new time window for tPA.

Gupta R, Connolly ES, Mayer S, et al. Hemicraniectomy for massive middle cerebral artery territory infarction: a systematic review. *Stroke.* 2004;35:539–543.
An excellent review of factors to account for when deciding whether to proceed with decompressive hemicraniectomy for hemispheric malignant infarction.

53 Aneurysmal Subarachnoid Hemorrhage

Rajat Dhar

Subarachnoid hemorrhage (SAH) comprises bleeding into the subarachnoid space (containing cerebrospinal fluid [CSF]) surrounding the brain and the spinal cord. The most common etiology of SAH is aneurysmal rupture, although other etiologies may be responsible (Table 53.1), and 10% to 20% are cryptogenic; a large proportion of these have a *perimesencephalic* pattern of bleeding (localized around the brainstem without extension into the lateral Sylvian fissures and no frank intraventricular or parenchymal hemorrhage). This form of SAH is felt to be benign and likely venous in origin. Although SAH comprises 10% or less of all acute cerebrovascular events, it affects a younger population and carries with it significant mortality (20% to 30% within 30 days) and persistent neurologic morbidity (due to the initial bleed and effects of delayed ischemia, discussed later). Risk factors for aneurysmal rupture include hypertension, cigarette smoking, heavy alcohol use, polycystic kidney disease, and a history of aneurysms/SAH in first-degree relatives. Patients with SAH should ideally be managed in centers with expertise in both neurocritical care and endovascular/surgical management of intracranial aneurysms (Algorithm 53.1).

DIAGNOSIS AND INITIAL MANAGEMENT

Patients with SAH usually present with sudden severe headache that reaches maximum intensity within seconds (i.e., "thunderclap headache"). This may be associated with syncope or persistent alteration in the level of consciousness. Meningismus develops over a few hours. The diagnosis is confirmed by noncontrast computed tomography (CT) of the head that has greater than 95% sensitivity if performed within 24 hours of symptom onset. Those presenting in a delayed fashion (headache onset >24 hours) or with negative CT findings despite clinical suspicion should undergo lumbar puncture to evaluate for red blood cells and *xanthochromia* (the yellow discoloration of centrifuged CSF seen with blood breakdown). It is critical to fully evaluate any patient with a sudden or new headache for SAH, as delayed diagnosis places them at risk for aneurysmal rebleeding, with a mortality approaching 50%. Those with confirmed SAH but negative initial angiogram should undergo repeat angiography (or CT angiography) in 1 to 3 weeks to exclude a missed aneurysm.

Acute hydrocephalus, from obstruction to CSF flow, is seen in half of the patients and may require urgent ventriculostomy if mental status is impaired. Once the patient

ALGORITHM 53.1 Initial Evaluation and Management of Patients with Subarachnoid Hemorrhage

Patient has subarachnoid hemorrhage
- Presents with sudden onset of the worst headache of his or her life ± LOC
- Noncontrast head CT shows blood (hyperdensity) in the basal cisterns, Sylvian fissure, and sulci of the brain; blood may also be present in the ventricles
- Lumbar puncture shows xanthochromia in a patient with negative head CT

- Admission to intensive care unit, preferably specialized neuro-ICU
- Bed rest, airway protection, maintain MAP < 110 mm Hg to prevent rebleeding, monitor vitals, frequent neurologic examinations, EKG, chest radiography
- Institute anticonvulsant prophylaxis, laxatives, pain, and anxiety control
- Order **cerebral angiography**
- Place EVD if signs of hydrocephalus (drowsiness, large ventricles on head CT)

Aneurysm or other vascular malformation found → **No**
- Consider digital subtraction angiography if initially used CTA or MRA
- Consider other cause (trauma, PMSAH)
- Repeat angiography in 1–3 wk

Yes

Treat aneurysm/vascular malformation to prevent rebleeding
- Consult neurosurgery and neurointerventionalist to determine optimal treatment plan (clipping vs coiling of aneurysms, embolization and resection of AVM)
- Immediate treatment of aneurysms is strongly recommended
- Evacuation of hematoma if focal deficits complicated by herniation or increased ICP

Aneurysm "protected" (clipped or coiled successfully)

Initial preventative measures for vasospasm
- Maintain euvolemia
- Permissive hypertension (hold antihypertensives)
- Nimodipine 60 mg orally or enterally every 4 hr

Monitor closely for common complications
- Frequent neurologic examination
- Monitoring of ICP if appropriate
- Frequent monitoring of vitals, heart rhythm, electrolytes
- Place Foley catheter to monitor input and output closely
- See Algorithm 53.2

LOC, loss of consciousness; CT, computed tomography; ICU, intensive care unit; MAP, mean arterial pressure; EKG, electrocardiography; EVD, external ventricular drain; CTA, CT angiography; MRA, magnetic resonance angiography; PMSAH, perimesencephalic SAH; AVM, arteriovenous malformation; ICP, intracranial pressure.

TABLE 53.1	Cause of Subarachnoid Hemorrhage
Etiology	Clues/Comments
Intracranial aneurysm	Most common cause of spontaneous SAH, usually presents with "thunderclap headache," diffuse hemorrhage on imaging
Arteriovenous malformation	Often associated with intraparenchymal bleeding
Trauma	Blood usually more focal, located around cerebral convexity
Perimesencephalic	Angiogram negative, blood confined to cisterns around brainstem
Arterial dissection	Only if dissection extends intracranially
Coagulopathy	May be focal (with minor trauma) or diffuse, angiogram negative
Venous thrombosis	Often associated with edema and parenchymal hemorrhage
Pituitary apoplexy	Sudden headache with visual complaints and ophthalmoplegia
Reversible cerebral vasoconstriction syndrome	Focal SAH, often at convexity
	Angiogram reveals diffuse segmental vasoconstriction
	Associated with certain medications, postpartum, drug abuse

SAH, subarachnoid hemorrhage.

has been diagnosed and stabilized, cerebral angiography (conventional or, in some centers, CT angiography) should be performed to evaluate for an aneurysm or other vascular lesion. Measures to prevent contrast-induced nephropathy should be instituted in those at risk. The severity of SAH is graded using either the Hunt and Hess or World Federation of Neurosurgical Societies' scales (Table 53.2). Survival is inversely proportional to grade, with grade V patients who do not improve with initial stabilization (sometimes with ventriculostomy to drain CSF if hydrocephalus is present) invariably do poorly. The amount of blood on admission CT scan is also graded using the Fisher or modified Fisher scales (Table 53.3); higher-grade patients are at greater risk for vasospasm.

The risk of *rebleeding* is as high as 20% in the first 24 to 48 hours after SAH. Along with ventricular arrhythmias, this is the most common cause of early death after SAH. Early treatment of the ruptured aneurysm is critical to prevent rebleeding and may be accomplished by surgical clipping (with craniotomy) or endovascular approach with coiling. The patient's age, clinical condition, and anatomy of the aneurysm will inform the preferred treatment, in discussion between the neurosurgeon and endovascular specialist (e.g., interventional neuroradiologist). Prior to definitive aneurysmal treatment, blood pressure should be aggressively controlled to prevent further bleeding; mean arterial pressure (MAP) should be kept below 110 mm Hg. Short-acting antihypertensives (e.g., labetalol, nicardipine) and analgesics are preferred. Blood pressure can be liberalized after successful aneurysm treatment; higher blood pressure postoperatively also promotes cerebral perfusion.

TABLE 53.2	Clinical Grading Scales
Grade	Criteria

Hunt and Hess grading system
1	Asymptomatic or mild headache
2	Moderate to severe headache, nuchal rigidity, or cranial nerve palsy
3	Confusion, lethargy, and/or mild focal neurologic deficit
4	Stupor and/or hemiparesis
5	Comatose, posturing

World Federation of Neurosurgical Societies' Scale
I	GCS 15, no motor deficit
II	GCS 13–14, no motor deficit
III	GCS 13–14 or motor deficit
IV	GCS 7–12
V	GCS 3–6

GCS, Glasgow coma scale.

Aneurysmal rupture often triggers a cascade involving release of catecholamines and cytokines. This sympathetic hyperactivity may induce cardiopulmonary dysfunction. Electrocardiographic changes are common and elevated troponin (with levels usually <5 to 10 μg/L) is seen in 20% to 30%. Ten percent of patients (especially those with severe SAH and elevated cardiac enzyme levels) will have *stunned myocardium* with wall motion abnormalities or globally depressed systolic and/or diastolic function on acute echocardiography. Coronary angiography (if performed but usually not required) is invariably unrevealing (i.e., no obstructive lesion). This form of "stress-induced cardiomyopathy" is reversible and often resolves within 1 to 2 weeks. All patients require close cardiac monitoring and some may even require inotropes to support cardiac function. Pulmonary edema with hypoxemia is seen in 10% to 20% and may be cardiogenic as well as neurogenic.

TABLE 53.3	CT Grading Scales for Risk of Vasospasm			
Amount of SAH in basal cisterns		IVH	Fisher grade	Modified Fisher grade
Diffuse or localized, thick		Present	3	4
Diffuse or localized, thick		Absent	3	3
Diffuse or localized only thin SAH		Present	4	2
Only thin SAH		Absent	2	1
No SAH		Present	4	2
No SAH		Absent	1	0

SAH is considered thick if it completely fills at least one cistern or fissure. IVH is considered present if there is blood in both lateral ventricles.
SAH, subarachnoid hemorrhage; IVH, intraventricular hemorrhage.

COMPLICATIONS OF SUBARACHNOID HEMORRHAGE

A number of concerns still exist for the patient with SAH after the ruptured aneurysm has been secured. *Seizures* most often occur early after SAH (either at ictus or prior to hospitalization ~5% to 10%). However, there is an approximately 5% additional risk of seizures in-hospital and, despite lack of evidence for their benefit, many experts recommend anticonvulsant prophylaxis for patients after SAH. This can either be given for just the immediate perioperative period (3-day total course) or be continued till hospital discharge. Levetiracetam at a dose of 1000 mg twice daily is a commonly used regimen. It may be worth evaluating those remaining (or becoming) poorly responsive after SAH with electroencephalographic monitoring to exclude subclinical seizures.

Hyponatremia is a common complication of SAH, occurring in 30% of patients, most often 4 to 10 days after admission. It may be due to syndrome of inappropriate antidiuretic hormone secretion (SIADH, euvolemic) and/or cerebral salt wasting (CSW, hypovolemic). Distinguishing between the two is important (but often challenging), as therapeutic strategies are different: avoid excess water intake with SIADH and replace volume with isotonic or hypertonic saline solutions in CSW. Total fluid restriction should never be utilized in hyponatremia after SAH, as it has been shown to elevate the risk of cerebral infarction. As SIADH and CSW often overlap, it is advisable to assess volume status, and unless hypovolemia can be confidently excluded, then saline replacement (either with normal or hypertonic saline infusions) is the safer approach (which can be accompanied by oral fluid restriction of 1 to 1.5 L/day). All patients with SAH should have daily measurements of serum sodium as well as close monitoring of fluid "ins and outs." They should not receive hypotonic fluids and diuretics should be restricted, as hypovolemia also promotes cerebral ischemia. Central *fever* is also commonly seen and may be part of a systemic inflammatory response ("SIRS"), making true infection difficult to diagnose in these patients.

CEREBRAL VASOSPASM AND DELAYED CEREBRAL ISCHEMIA

Cerebral infarction as a result of delayed ischemia is the major source of secondary disability after SAH. Arterial narrowing (i.e., vasospasm) is seen on angiography in a majority of SAH patients between 4 and 21 days after bleeding (peaking around days 7 to 10) and is more likely in those with greater thickness of SAH (estimated by the modified Fisher scale; Table 53.3). Some patients with vasospasm will remain asymptomatic, but others will develop neurologic deficits found to be related to reductions in cerebral blood flow (CBF) below ischemic thresholds. This reduction in CBF and oxygen delivery may be worsened by hypovolemia, hypotension, and anemia. For this reason, patients with SAH are kept euvolemic by adjustment of intravenous fluids and normotensive (avoiding blood pressure–lowering medications). The optimal hemoglobin level and the role of transfusion are less clear. All patients should receive nimodipine, a calcium channel antagonist that has demonstrated efficacy in improving neurologic outcome (at a dose of 60 mg every 4 hours enterally, continued for 21 days). The dose may be halved and given q2h if excessive drops in blood pressure after each dose necessitate. Some centers employ transcranial Doppler to screen for developing vasospasm, as an increase in velocities in the basal cerebral vessels suggests a decrease in their caliber. Prophylactic hypervolemia or hypertensive therapy is not effective in either improving cerebral perfusion or preventing deficits from vasospasm.

ALGORITHM 53.2 | **Management of Complications After Subarachnoid Hemorrhage**

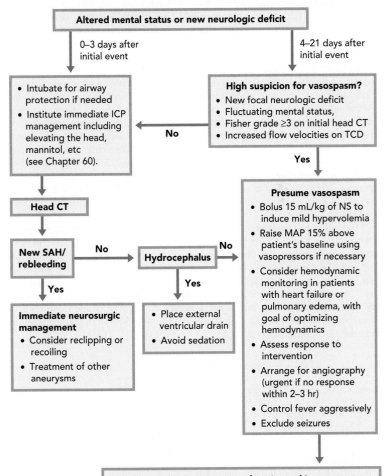

ICP, intracranial pressure; CT, computed tomography; TCD, transcranial Doppler; SAH, subarachnoid hemorrhage; NS, normal saline; MAP, mean arterial pressure.

Any alteration in neurologic status (development of new neurologic deficits or alteration in mentation) after SAH requires prompt evaluation for ischemia (Algorithm 53.2). If apparent confounders have been excluded (usually with head CT to rule out hydrocephalus, new bleeding, or cerebral edema), then hemodynamic augmentation to raise blood pressure should be initiated. Metabolic derangements including hyponatremia (see earlier), fever, hypoxemia or hypercapnia, and seizures can also cause neurologic worsening mimicking symptomatic vasospasm. "Triple H" therapy (hypervolemia, hypertension, and hemodilution) is instituted, with a fluid bolus and vasopressors titrated to raise MAP 10% to 15% above the patient's baseline. Hemodilution is now generally avoided unless polycythemia is present. In cases of cardiac failure, inotropic support may be helpful in reversing neurologic deficits. Noninvasive cardiac monitoring may be helpful in optimizing hemodynamics (cardiac index, stroke volume, and pulse pressure variability). Patients with suspected delayed cerebral ischemia should undergo angiography to evaluate for vasospasm (which may further confirm the clinical suspicion). Angiography also allows endovascular therapies to be administered, including intra-arterial injections of vasodilators (e.g., verapamil, nimodipine, nicardipine, milrinone) and balloon angioplasty of accessible (proximal) segments. While vasodilators usually offer only transient relief of arterial narrowing, angioplasty durably reverses vasospasm (and sometimes deficits), usually without requiring retreatment.

Hemodynamic augmentation should be titrated to clinical effect (i.e., reversal of new/worsening deficits) rather than a specific blood pressure target. High doses of vasopressors may be required for induced hypertension. Close observation for complications from this therapy (e.g., pulmonary edema, arrhythmias, cardiac injury, worsening cerebral edema, or hemorrhagic transformation of an established infarct) is mandatory. Once clinical response is achieved, this goal MAP should be maintained for at least 48 to 72 hours before cautious and gradual weaning of MAP and vasopressors is attempted. Improvement on a repeat angiogram may be helpful in guiding when to wean therapy in more complex cases.

SUGGESTED READINGS

Bederson JB, Connoly ES, Batjer HH, et al. Guidelines for the management of aneurysmal subarachnoid hemorrhage. *Stroke.* 2009;40:994–1025.

Diringer MN. Management of aneurysmal subarachnoid hemorrhage. *Crit Care Med.* 2009;37: 432–440.

Keyrouz SG, Diringer MN. Clinical review: prevention and therapy of vasospasm in subarachnoid hemorrhage. *Crit Care.* 2007;11:220. Available from http://ccforum.com/content/11/4/220

Suarez J, Tarr RW, Selman WR. Aneurysmal subarachnoid hemorrhage. *N Engl J Med.* 2006;354: 387–396.

54 Intracerebral Hemorrhage

Ahmed Hassan

Intracerebral hemorrhage (ICH), accounting for 10% to 15% of all strokes, is caused by rupture of a blood vessel into the brain parenchyma. It usually presents with headache, altered level of consciousness, and focal neurologic symptoms. There are several etiologies of ICH: hypertension, trauma, cerebral amyloid angiopathy, vascular malformations, bleeding disorders, anticoagulants, sympathomimetic substances (amphetamines and cocaine), tumors, and cerebral vein thrombosis. Hypertensive hemorrhage, the most common etiology of ICH, is most frequently located at branch points of perforating arteries in the deep gray matter (basal ganglia/thalamus), pons, or cerebellum. ICH due to trauma usually presents as a parenchymal contusion. Cerebral amyloid angiopathy typically causes lobar hemorrhage in nonhypertensive elderly patients and has an increased risk of recurrence. Anticoagulation raises the risk and severity of ICH and rebleeding in any of these settings.

ICH may cause damage to the brain by several mechanisms. Hematoma interrupts the neuronal pathways, and blood and its breakdown products can be highly toxic and can contribute to seizures, electrolyte derangements, fever, and autonomic changes. A recently ruptured vessel is also prone to rebleed. Finally, elevated intracranial pressure (ICP) due to the hematoma and subsequent edema may damage other areas of the brain and result in herniation. All of these possible mechanisms of injury make ICH the subtype of stroke with the highest morbidity and mortality (35% to 50% at 30 days).

Patients with ICH are at high risk for early deterioration and should initially be cared for in an intensive care setting (Table 54.1). Enlarging hematoma manifests with headache, vomiting, and a decreased level of consciousness as ICP rises, although none of these findings are specific; thus, rapid neuroimaging with noncontrast computed tomography (CT) is recommended to distinguish ICH from ischemic stroke. If there is clinical or radiographic suspicion of underlying structural lesions (e.g., vascular malformations, tumor, or cerebral vein thrombosis), CT angiography and venography, contrast-enhanced CT, contrast-enhanced magnetic resonance imaging, magnetic resonance angiography, and venography may be useful.

PREVENTION OF HEMATOMA EXPANSION AND REBLEEDING

Even in the absence of coagulopathy, ICH is prone to expand and/or recur, usually in the first 12 to 24 hours. All anticoagulants and antiplatelet agents should be stopped.

TABLE 54.1	Issues to Address During Management of Intracerebral Hemorrhage

- Hematoma expansion/rebleed
- Cerebral perfusion/blood pressure
- Cerebral edema
- Seizures
- Indications for surgical intervention

Normal coagulation should be restored with vitamin K and fresh-frozen plasma (Table 54.2). Patients with a severe coagulation factor deficiency or severe thrombocytopenia should receive appropriate factor replacement or platelets. Recombinant factor VIIa or prothrombin complex concentrate may be considered to reverse anticoagulation in those at risk of volume overload or lung injury, but they have not been shown to improve outcomes compared with fresh-frozen plasma and may carry a greater risk of thromboembolic events.

MAINTAINING CEREBRAL PERFUSION: BLOOD PRESSURE MANAGEMENT

High blood pressure (BP) was thought to contribute to rebleeding; however, there is no convincing evidence that lowering BP improves outcome. A higher BP may be necessary to provide adequate blood flow to the brain while ICP is elevated, particularly in chronically hypertensive patients with impaired autoregulation; aggressive BP management may cause hypoperfusion. Even in normotensive patients, ICH may lead to transient hypertension resolving spontaneously over a few days. A modest (~15%) reduction in BP does not seem to worsen neurologic outcome. However, ongoing damage to other organs (heart or kidneys) is a compelling indication to treat elevated BP. If mean arterial pressure is above 130 to 140 mm Hg or end-organ damage is present, short-acting agents are used to gently lower BP. Nitrates are avoided because of the risk of cerebral vasodilatation with worsening edema. Addressing pain may also help to control elevated BP (Algorithm 54.1).

TABLE 54.2	Stabilizing Coagulation Status After Intracerebral Hemorrhage

- Discontinue all antiplatelet and anticoagulant medications
- Reverse anticoagulation or correct coagulopathy:
  - Vitamin K 10 mg IV or enterally daily for 3 days
  - Fresh-frozen plasma 15–20 mL/kg
  - Platelet and coagulation factor replacement as needed for thrombocytopenia and coagulation factor deficiency, respectively
- Consider prothrombin complex concentrate or recombinant factor VIIa for coagulopathic patients needing an urgent surgical procedure or those at risk for volume overload
- Follow coagulation panel frequently, keep corrected for 24–48 hr

IV, intravenous.

ALGORITHM 54.1 Blood Pressure Management After Intracerebral Hemorrhage

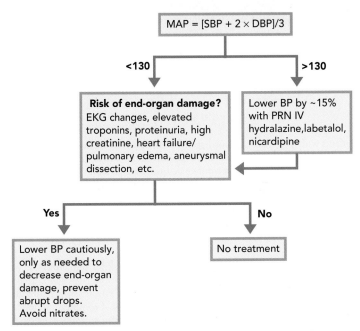

MAP, mean arterial pressure; SBP, systolic blood pressure; DBP, diastolic blood pressure; EKG, electrocardiogram; PRN, as needed; IV, intravenous; BP, blood pressure.

TREATMENT OF CEREBRAL EDEMA

Cerebral edema in ICH can occur as a result of the direct effects of hematoma volume and edema, as well as hydrocephalus due to intraventricular hemorrhage (IVH) or ventricular compression. In patients with a decreased level of consciousness (Glasgow Comma Scale score ≤8), clinical evidence of cerebral herniation, or those with significant IVH or hydrocephalus, ICP monitoring with a ventricular or parenchymal catheter should be considered. (See ICP treatment Algorithm 60.1 in Chapter 60.)

SEIZURES

The primary neuronal damage and blood products increase seizure risk after ICH. Seizures occur in 5% to 15% of these patients, usually in the first few days of hospitalization. Prophylactic anticonvulsant therapy is not indicated in ICH, but in patients with depressed mental status out of proportion to the degree of brain injury, continuous electroencephalography should be considered. Patients with clinical seizures and patients with mental status changes and electrographic seizures should be treated with anticonvulsant therapy.

TABLE 54.3	Indications for Neurosurgical Intervention After Intracerebral Hemorrhage

- Posterior fossa or temporal lobe hemorrhage >3 cm
- ICH causing hydrocephalus or brainstem compression
- Hydrocephalus or IVH requiring EVD
- Complicated cases requiring ICP monitoring

ICH, intracerebral hemorrhage; EVD, external ventricular drain; IVH, intraventricular hemorrhage; ICP, intracranial pressure.

NEUROSURGICAL INTERVENTION

In patients with a cerebellar hemorrhage who are deteriorating neurologically or who have brainstem compression and/or hydrocephalus from ventricular obstruction, surgical removal of the hemorrhage is recommended as soon as possible (Table 54.3). In most other cases of ICH, the utility of surgical evacuation remains controversial. For patients with supratentorial lobar hemorrhage >30 mL and within 1 cm of the surface, evacuation by standard craniotomy may be considered, although strong evidence is lacking.

GENERAL CARE

Patients with ICH, like all critically ill patients, are at risk for numerous complications including myocardial infarctions, heart failure with pulmonary edema, deep vein thrombosis (DVT), aspiration pneumonia, urinary tract infections, pressure ulcers, and orthopedic complications (contractures etc.). Sequential compression devices in addition to elastic stockings should be used from admission, and subcutaneous low-molecular-weight heparin or unfractionated heparin for DVT prophylaxis can be started after 48 hours if there is no evidence of hematoma expansion. Spontaneous lobar ICH in particular carries a relatively high risk of recurrence, thus avoidance of long-term anticoagulation for nonvalvular atrial fibrillation in these patients is recommended. In the presence of a clear indication for anticoagulation (e.g., mechanical heart valve) or antiplatelet therapy (e.g., coronary artery stents), it is reasonable to restart anticoagulation in nonlobar ICH in 2 to 4 weeks and antiplatelet therapy in all ICH 1 to 2 weeks after documentation of cessation of bleeding.

SUGGESTED READING

American Heart Association Stroke Council and Council on Cardiovascular Nursing. Guidelines for the management of spontaneous intracerebral hemorrhage: a guideline for healthcare professionals from the American Heart Association/American Stroke Association. *Stroke.* 2010;41;2108–2129.

55 Coma

Michael A. Rubin

Coma is a state of persistent unresponsiveness. It can occur because of a primary neurologic disorder or as a complication of a systemic pathology. Either way, there must be a disruption of the normal function of either the reticular activating system in the brainstem or both cerebral hemispheres. The underlying cause of coma may be immediately apparent on the basis of the initial history and examination; however, in other situations, it may take days to discern the cause of the severe encephalopathy. Although coma is an extremely serious situation, an extensive evaluation may result in finding the cause and providing the treatment of coma recovery.

EVALUATION AND MANAGEMENT OF COMA

Although the depressed mental states along the spectrum that leads to coma have been described by terms such as *stupor, lethargy,* and *obtundation,* the terms are used differently by various sources and are usually not specific enough. When following a patient's response to therapy, a more detailed description is valuable and has higher interrater reliability. The amount of stimulation required to elicit a response and what the response is should be identified. The Glasgow Coma Scale is widely used as a standard method to describe neurologic function in a quick and concise manner (Table 55.1), and it carries prognostic value for patients with traumatic brain injury.

Initial Evaluation and Stabilization

Concurrent with the investigation of the cause of coma, appropriate resuscitative measures should be provided. Intubation is usually necessary for airway protection; fluids and/or vasopressors are instituted for hypotension; warming blankets may be required for hypothermia. Laboratory tests including a rapid blood glucose test, arterial blood gases, electrolyte panel, chemistries, blood counts, cultures, toxin screens, and thyroid and liver function tests should be ordered. In addition, brain imaging is important to evaluate for a surgical cause of coma. Other tests such as lumbar puncture and electroencephalography may be useful depending on the presentation. The initial examination during stabilization should guide the priorities of the work up. For example, pupillary abnormalities suggest an underlying intracranial structural lesion with elevated intracranial pressure requiring expedient head computed tomography and neurosurgery consultation. The presence of fever, nuchal rigidity, or skin rash should prompt lumbar puncture and antimicrobial therapy.

Many emergency departments employ a "coma cocktail," including intravenous administration of thiamine, glucose, and naloxone. Thiamine protects against the potentially fatal Wernicke encephalopathy and should be given to all patients with

TABLE 55.1	Glasgow Coma Scale

Best eye opening	
Spontaneous	4
With voice only	3
With pain only	2
None at all	1
Best verbal response	
Coherent speech	5
Confused intelligible speech	4
Inappropriate words	3
Incomprehensible sounds	2
No verbal output	1
Best motor response	
Follows commands	6
Localizes pain stimuli[a]	5
Withdraws to pain stimuli	4
Decorticate posturing	3
Decerebrate posturing	2
No movements at all	1

[a]Localizing pain stimuli refers to gaze deviation, head turning, or hand movements toward the stimulus.

unexplained coma or suspicion of long-term alcohol abuse and/or malnutrition. Glucose is withheld until hypoglycemia is confirmed and thiamine has been given. Naloxone is useful as a therapeutic agent in the reversal of opioid toxicity, whereas flumazenil is equally effective in a benzodiazepine overdose. Caution should be exercised as rapid reversal in long-term users could precipitate seizure.

General and Neurologic Examination

After the initial assessment and stabilization of the patient, a more thorough evaluation may proceed. History of present and recent illness should be discussed with the caregivers or relatives. Much can be learned from clinical records from outside facilities as to the time course involved in the progression of the disease and any precipitating events. The cause may be apparent from the history; in some cases, the general physical examination may reveal signs of underlying diseases (such as rashes, liver failure stigmata, murmurs, etc).

The neurologic examination is focused on evaluating the function of the structures previously mentioned (brain stem and bilateral hemispheres) whose dysfunction is responsible for coma. This includes level of alertness and awareness, cranial nerve reflexes, motor function, and respiratory pattern. Consciousness is assessed by recording response to increasing intensities of stimuli. One begins with the name softly, then loudly, then with a gentle shake. If these fail to arouse the patient, a painful stimulus (supraorbital pressure, sternal rub, or temporomandibular pressure) should be applied. Also note if the stimulation must be repeatedly applied to maintain alertness or if the patient stays awake once aroused. If family is present, be sure to inform them the purpose of your examination, especially if painful stimuli are being applied.

ALGORITHM 55.1 — Oculovestibular Testing (Cold Calorics)

Inspect both ears and ascertain:
- Tympanic membranes are intact
- The EAC not obstructed
- Nob lood, CSF, or brain tissue in the EAC

- Lift the head of the patient to 30 degrees
- An assistant holds the eyelids of the patient open

- Insert a soft catheter into the EAC
- Instill 30–50 mL of ice-cold water over a minute
- Observe for eye movements or nystagmus for 2–3 min after the instillation.

Eye movements present
- If intact, the eyes deviate toward cold water
- Wait for the eyes to return to midline ≈3 min
- Repeat on the other side

Eye movements absent
- Wait for 3 min
- Repeat on the other side

EAC, external auditory canal; CSF, cerebrospinal fluid

During the brainstem examination, most of the cranial nerves are assessed. The pupillary changes to light should be recorded in millimeters for each eye, both directly and consensually. The pattern of pupillary response can be very useful in localization of the level of the cerebral insult. Spontaneous eye movements such as nystagmus and wandering movements should be noted. If a patient is unable to follow commands and the cervical spine is stable, extra ocular movements are assessed by performing the oculocephalic maneuver. Rapidly rotate the head in all directions and observe for contralateral deviation of the eyes. In addition, cold caloric testing (the oculovestibular reflex) can be done (Algorithm 55.1), but it does tend to be extremely noxious in those with some level of awareness. For the corneal reflex, drip sterile saline or gently apply a cotton swab. One can test the facial nerve by observing the grimace to a painful stimulus such as temporomandibular pressure. The ninth and tenth nerves responsible for gag and cough can be assessed during oral and endotracheal suctioning.

The motor system examination includes observation and description of spontaneous movements, and movements to command and noxious stimuli (deep nail bed pressure or a sharp proximal pinch) such as localization or withdraw should be noted. A posturing movement may occur spontaneously or with stimulation. Decorticate (flexor) posturing, elbow and wrist flexion with lower extremity extension, is typically less ominous than decerebrate (extensor) posturing, in which all extremities extend simultaneously. Although spinal reflexes may be affected by cortical influences, they should not be confused with withdrawal or purposeful movements. The so-called triple flexion response refers to flexion at the hip, knee, and ankle in response to pain applied to the foot and is generated by the spinal column. Distinguishing withdrawal from a triple flexion can be challenging, but stimulating the leg with a pinch in addition to the feet may help. In addition, triple flexion tends to be stereotypical; regardless of the amount of stimulation applied, the response is the same, which is different from that of a cortically initiated withdraw. Myoclonic jerks, often a sign of anoxic encephalopathy, suggest a poor outcome. Amplitude, tone, and rhythm of abnormal movements may help distinguish seizure from myoclonus, posturing, and shivering, although often electroencephalography is warranted.

Various respiratory patterns depending on the cerebral structural damage and/or underlying metabolic abnormality may be exhibited. Cortical impairment can lead to Cheyne–Stokes breathing in which there are periods of hypoventilation followed by corrective hyperventilation. Damage to the midbrain can lead to hyperventilation. Apneustic breathing is seen in pontine injuries, in which sharp inspiration is followed by an expiratory pause. Medulla damage can cause ataxic breathing with an irregular breathing pattern. Pain, pulmonary, and acid–base balance must first be evaluated in the case of hyperventilation, but it is common in primary central neurologic pathology associated with coma.

Diagnostic Studies in Coma

A nonfocal neurologic examination should prompt investigation of toxic/metabolic, infectious, or hypoxic/ischemic causes of coma, whereas any focality warrants urgent brain imaging and/or cerebrospinal fluid studies. It is imperative to consider the laboratory profile in the context of the history. For example, someone who was seen to clench their chest before abruptly losing consciousness who happens to have mild uremia should still be evaluated for cardiac ischemia and pulmonary embolism. If the results of laboratory tests do not aid in determining the cause, electroencephalography should be considered. A list of common causes is presented in Table 55.2.

Ongoing Management of Patients in Coma

In addition to treating the underlying cause, several management principles should be initiated to maximize the chance of recovery. Mechanical ventilation with monitoring of arterial blood gases ensures adequate oxygenation and ventilation. Hypotension should be avoided; vasopressors are used as needed. Daily electrolyte replacement and normovolemia are important. Full nutrition, preferably by enteral feedings, should be instituted as soon as possible. Other essential steps in routine critical care include gastric ulcer prevention, thromboembolism prevention, skin care, and oral care.

Conditions That May Be Mistaken for Coma

There are a few conditions in which a patient may seem unarousable and unresponsive but has an intact consciousness. Injury to certain parts of the pons may cause "locked-in syndrome" in which patients cannot move any muscles, except for those controlling vertical gaze and blinking; however, they retain full consciousness. Severe Guillain–Barré syndrome or parkinsonism may cause a similar scenario where motor examination is limited or absent but higher cortical function is retained. In addition to historical clues, careful neurologic examination of the brainstem reflexes can help avoid mistaking these conditions for coma. Occasionally, patients may present with psychogenic unresponsiveness, but they display purposeful resistance to eye-opening

TABLE 55.2	Causes of Coma

Drugs and toxins
  Opiates, alcohol, sedatives, amphetamines, barbiturates, tranquilizers, bromides, salicylates, acetaminophen, lithium, anticholinergics, lead, methanol, ethylene glycol, carbon monoxide, arsenic

Metabolic and systemic
  Anoxia or hypoxia, hypercapnia, hypotension, hypoglycemia, hyperglycemia, diabetic ketoacidosis, hypernatremia, hyponatremia, hypercalcemia, hypocalcemia, hypermagnesemia, hypothermia, hyperthermia, Wernicke encephalopathy, hepatic failure, uremia, Addisonian crisis, myxedema

Infectious/inflammatory
  Bacterial, viral, or fungal meningitis/meningoencephalitis, acute disseminated encephalomyelitis, syphilis, sepsis, malaria, Waterhouse–Friderichsen syndrome, typhoid fever

Structural brain lesions
  Subarachnoid hemorrhage, intraparenchymal hemorrhage, ischemic infarctions, global cerebral hypoperfusion, cerebral venous sinus thrombosis, traumatic brain injury, hydrocephalus, basilar occlusion, central pontine myelinolysis, large hemispheric masses, pituitary apoplexy, cerebral abscess or multifocal infection, chemotherapy-induced leukoencephalopathy

Other
  Nonconvulsive status epilepticus, locked-in syndrome, catatonia, hypertensive encephalopathy, heat stroke, psychogenic coma

and actively attempt to suppress subconsciously mediated eye movements. While it is a rare example, extreme catatonia can mimic coma.

ASSESSING PROGNOSIS IN COMA

Prognosis is highly dependent on the underlying cause. Metabolic and toxic disturbances can often be reversed leading to a good prognosis despite a minimal Glasgow Coma Scale score. Comorbidities, age, the extent of the underlying disease, and depth and duration of coma may also contribute. Anoxic brain injury following cardiac arrest, prolonged hypotension, or respiratory failure results in coma with a varying outcome. A panel of the American Academy of Neurology has issued guidelines on determining outcome following cerebral anoxia (Algorithm 55.2); these guidelines do not apply to coma resulting from other reasons. The most useful findings predictive of a poor outcome include extensor posturing or no motor response, fixed and dilated pupils, and myoclonic movements. Neurospecific enolase and abnormal somatosensory evoked potentials are also useful in determining a poor prognosis, but if present do not predict the amount of recovery.

Prognosis in Patients with Prolonged Coma

Regardless of the cause of comma, patients in a prolonged comma are less likely to recover. Often coma evolves into a "persistent vegetative state" in which a patient

ALGORITHM 55.2 Assessing Prognosis Following Anoxic Brain Injury

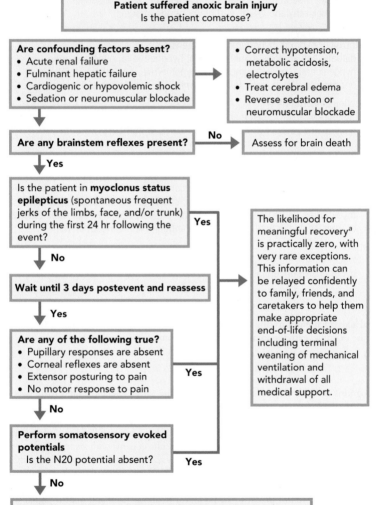

Patient suffered anoxic brain injury
Is the patient comatose?

Are confounding factors absent?
- Acute renal failure
- Fulminant hepatic failure
- Cardiogenic or hypovolemic shock
- Sedation or neuromuscular blockade

→

- Correct hypotension, metabolic acidosis, electrolytes
- Treat cerebral edema
- Reverse sedation or neuromuscular blockade

Are any brainstem reflexes present? — **No** → Assess for brain death

↓ **Yes**

Is the patient in **myoclonus status epilepticus** (spontaneous frequent jerks of the limbs, face, and/or trunk) during the first 24 hr following the event? — **Yes** →

↓ **No**

Wait until 3 days postevent and reassess →

↓ **Yes**

Are any of the following true?
- Pupillary responses are absent
- Corneal reflexes are absent
- Extensor posturing to pain
- No motor response to pain

— **Yes** →

↓ **No**

Perform somatosensory evoked potentials
Is the N20 potential absent? — **Yes** →

↓ **No**

The likelihood for meaningful recovery[a] is practically zero, with very rare exceptions. This information can be relayed confidently to family, friends, and caretakers to help them make appropriate end-of-life decisions including terminal weaning of mechanical ventilation and withdrawal of all medical support.

Based on neurologic criteria alone, the prognosis cannot be determined. If patient remains in comatose or a vegetative state for another 3 mo, then meaningful recovery[a] is very unlikely.

[a]Meaningful recovery is defined here as the absence of severe disability requiring constant nursing support, a vegetative state, or death. Many patients, families, and caretakers may consider less severe forms of disability to be outside a desirable state of meaning recovery.

Adapted with permission from Wijdicks EF, Hijdra A, Young GB, et al. Quality Standards Subcommittee of the American Academy of Neurology. Practice parameter: prediction of outcome in comatose survivors after cardiopulmonary resuscitation (an evidence-based review): report of the Quality Standards Subcommittee of the American Academy of Neurology. *Neurology.* 2006;67:203–210.

may show normal sleep–awake cycles but lacks overt signs of conscious, awareness, or responsiveness. If such state lasts for 12 months after brain trauma or 3 months in other cases, the chance for meaningful recovery is minimal. Recent consensus has created other levels of persistent inhibited function such as the minimally conscious state. Brain function is widely distributed and likewise injury can cause a spectrum of residual function. Brain death is a different clinical entity and should not be confused with a type of coma.

SUGGESTED READINGS

Wijdicks EF. Neurologic complications in critically ill patients. *Anesth Analg.* 1996;83:411–419.

Wijdicks EF, Hijdra A, Young GB, et al. Quality Standards Subcommittee of the American Academy of Neurology. Practice parameter: prediction of outcome in comatose survivors after cardiopulmonary resuscitation (an evidence-based review): report of the Quality Standards Subcommittee of the American Academy of Neurology. *Neurology.* 2006;67: 203–210.

56 Declaration of Brain Death

Rajat Dhar

THE CONCEPT OF BRAIN DEATH

Death may be legally determined by either cardiorespiratory or cerebral criteria, the latter (i.e., brain death) emerging as an important concept with the advent of intensive care unit care and artificial ventilation in the 1950s and being first formally delineated in the 1960s. *Brain death* is defined as the irreversible cessation of all brain functions, including the brainstem. The specific laws and policies governing determination of death by neurologic criteria vary among countries, states, and different medical institutions, albeit based on this overarching concept. The person is declared dead at the time that final determination of brain death has been made. Although it does not require consent of the family or surrogate decision makers, it is always preferable to explain the process explicitly at all stages of testing. Physicians should be sensitive to both religious and ethnic perspectives of the family, as well as allowing them time to process an often sudden catastrophic loss. The diagnosis of (brain) death is an absolute prerequisite for organ and tissue donation, and the role of the intensivist extends to stabilizing the potentially brain-dead patient to both allow safe testing while avoiding further organ injury should the person become an organ donor. Donation should not be discussed with the family prior to determination of death to avoid the appearance of a conflict of interest. The United States and other countries require physicians to contact local organ procurement agencies as soon as a patient is deemed to be a potential organ donor (i.e., any patient with severe brain injury who has lost significant brainstem function), even before the final confirmation of brain death.

DIAGNOSING BRAIN DEATH

In essence, brain death comprises irreversible coma (of known etiology), accompanied by loss of all brainstem reflexes, and absent respiratory drive. It may result from a variety of severe brain injuries, most commonly cerebral trauma, hemorrhage (subarachnoid, subdural, or intracerebral), and hypoxic-ischemic injury after cardiac arrest. Cerebral edema with raised intracranial pressure resulting from large brain tumors, meningitis or encephalitis, hydrocephalus, or fulminant liver failure may also progress to brain death. The particular etiology for coma should be known in each patient (from history or with adjunctive brain imaging), and brain death should never be diagnosed without a clear cause capable of inducing the observed degree of cerebral dysfunction. Any confounders must be carefully excluded, chief among these are hypothermia and drug intoxication. Overdose of a variety of medications (including barbiturates, tricyclic antidepressants, baclofen, and lidocaine) can mimic a brain-dead state with absent brainstem reflexes. The metabolic milieu must also be normalized as much as possible to avoid confounding from systemic disturbances including hypoglycemia, hypotension, severe electrolyte imbalances, or acid–base disorders that could result in cerebral dysfunction. Any sedation or neuromuscular blockade must have been allowed to wear off before testing (the latter can be tested by train-of-four stimulation). Patients in a locked-in state from lesions in the ventral pons may appear unresponsive, are unable to move to stimulation, and lack some brainstem function, but on closer testing are able to respond (with vertical eye movements or blinking) and have reactive electroencephalography (EEG) (a somewhat similar picture may be seen with high cervical spine injuries). Severe Guillain–Barré syndrome may induce a complete de-afferented state where the patient cannot move, respond, and can even lose brainstem and respiratory functions. Careful history, examination, and sometimes ancillary testing will exclude such confounding cases.

Once confounders have been excluded, homeostasis normalized (temperature, electrolytes, acid-base), and shock resuscitated, then the process of brain death testing can begin (Algorithm 56.1). Remember to document the temperature and blood pressure at the time of each examination. First an unresponsive comatose state without motor response should be verified. Central painful stimulation (e.g., supraorbital ridge, temporomandibular joint (TMJ) should elicit neither eye opening nor purposeful or reflexive movements (i.e., posturing of the upper extremities). There should be no spontaneous movements in the cranial nerve territory and no signs of seizure activity. All brainstem reflexes must then be tested on both sides to verify complete cessation of all brainstem function. This includes absence of midbrain function by lack of pupillary constriction to bright light; pupils should be mid-position or dilated. Pontine function is assessed with corneal reflex and cold water caloric testing of vestibular-ocular reactivity. Medullary failure is documented with lack of cough reflex to deep suctioning. To confirm stable absence of brain function, this whole sequence of testing should be repeated between 1 and 24 hours after the first examination. Short intervals are appropriate in catastrophic conditions in which devastating injury is clearly seen on imaging and condition has been unchanged before testing (new recommendations suggest one examination may be adequate in such a case). A longer duration is recommended in children and in patients with postcardiac arrest in whom imaging is usually normal and the early examination can fluctuate. Testing should also be deferred till after rewarming from induced hypothermia if utilized in such patients. At some institutions, only certain ("qualified") personnel can perform either all or parts of the brain death testing. In complicated cases, regardless, it is advisable to have assistance from a neurologist or neurosurgeon in the determination of death by neurologic criteria.

Clinical confirmation of complete cerebral death requires absence of spontaneous respiratory efforts despite adequate stimuli of hypercapnia and academia. The *apnea test* is required to complete determination of death by neurologic criteria, and time of death is set when the patient fails to breath and a blood gas demonstrates adequate academia (usually pH <7.28 to 7.30) and hypercapnia ($PaCO_2$ above 60 mm Hg and/or rise by 20 mm Hg from baseline). Two things should be done before performing the apnea test. Preoxygenation for at least 10 minutes on 100% FiO_2 will minimize the risk of desaturation during testing. A baseline blood gas should be reviewed and ventilator settings adjusted to obtain a $PaCO_2$ in the normal range (ideally 40–45 mm Hg) with a pH as close to normal as possible. Proper apnea testing may be impossible in significant CO_2 retainers or those who are markedly acidotic from

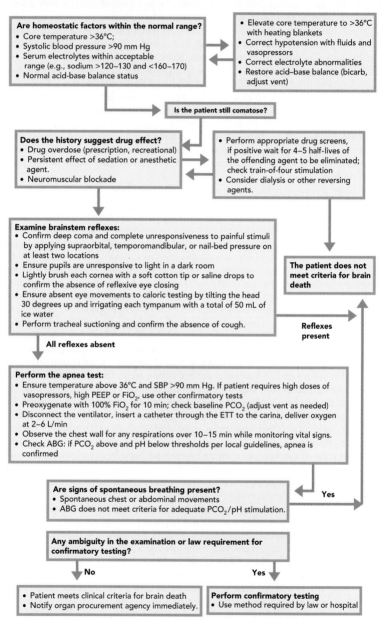

ALGORITHM 56.1 Approach to Determination of Death by Neurologic Criteria

Are homeostatic factors within the normal range?
- Core temperature >36°C;
- Systolic blood pressure >90 mm Hg
- Serum electrolytes within acceptable range (e.g., sodium >120–130 and <160–170)
- Normal acid–base balance status

→

- Elevate core temperature to >36°C with heating blankets
- Correct hypotension with fluids and vasopressors
- Correct electrolyte abnormalities
- Restore acid–base balance (bicarb, adjust vent)

Is the patient still comatose?

Does the history suggest drug effect?
- Drug overdose (prescription, recreational)
- Persistent effect of sedation or anesthetic agent.
- Neuromuscular blockade

→

- Perform appropriate drug screens, if positive wait for 4–5 half-lives of the offending agent to be eliminated; check train-of-four stimulation
- Consider dialysis or other reversing agents.

Examine brainstem reflexes:
- Confirm deep coma and complete unresponsiveness to painful stimuli by applying supraorbital, temporomandibular, or nail-bed pressure on at least two locations
- Ensure pupils are unresponsive to light in a dark room
- Lightly brush each cornea with a soft cotton tip or saline drops to confirm the absence of reflexive eye closing
- Ensure absent eye movements to caloric testing by tilting the head 30 degrees up and irrigating each tympanum with a total of 50 mL of ice water
- Perform tracheal suctioning and confirm the absence of cough.

The patient does not meet criteria for brain death

Reflexes present

All reflexes absent

Perform the apnea test:
- Ensure temperature above 36°C and SBP >90 mm Hg. If patient requires high doses of vasopressors, high PEEP or FiO_2, use other confirmatory tests
- Preoxygenate with 100% FiO_2 for 10 min; check baseline PCO_2 (adjust vent as needed)
- Disconnect the ventilator, insert a catheter through the ETT to the carina, deliver oxygen at 2–6 L/min
- Observe the chest wall for any respirations over 10–15 min while monitoring vital signs.
- Check ABG: if PCO_2 above and pH below thresholds per local guidelines, apnea is confirmed

Are signs of spontaneous breathing present?
- Spontaneous chest or abdominal movements
- ABG does not meet criteria for adequate PCO_2/pH stimulation.

Yes

Any ambiguity in the examination or law requirement for confirmatory testing?

No   Yes

- Patient meets clinical criteria for brain death
- Notify organ procurement agency immediately.

Perform confirmatory testing
- Use method required by law or hospital

PCO_2, partial pressure of arterial carbon dioxide; ETT, endotracheal tube; PEEP, positive end-expiratory pressure; SBP, systolic blood pressure.

metabolic derangements; ancillary testing (see later) should then be performed in lieu. Occasionally, ventilator self-cycling may falsely suggest the persistence of patient respiratory effort; changing from flow-triggered to pressure-triggered breaths (or a higher threshold) usually abolishes this artifact.

For apnea testing, the patient is disconnected from the ventilator and a suction catheter (with thumb-hole taped closed) attached to oxygen at a flow rate of 2 to 3 L/min is placed through the endotracheal tube down to the level of the carina. The chest should be exposed and the patient observed for visible respiratory efforts over a 10- to 15-minute duration (to allow adequate CO_2 retention to occur). A blood gas must be obtained before placing the patient back on the ventilator. Many patients will become hemodynamically unstable as acidemia develops, so be prepared to titrate up any vasopressors. If desaturation occurs, then increase the flow of oxygen to 6 L/min; should the patient not tolerate further testing (due to refractory hypotension or desaturation), then they should be placed back on the ventilator (although an arterial blood gas [ABG] can be obtained at that time, and if it meets criteria for hypercapnia and acidemia and no respiratory efforts were seen, the apnea test is still positive). Patients who are hemodynamically unstable and require high doses of vasopressors at baseline or those with hypoxemic respiratory failure (requiring high FiO_2 and/or positive end-expiratory pressure) may not tolerate apnea testing, and rather than risk instability and even cardiac arrest during the procedure, such patients may benefit from substituting a confirmatory test for apnea testing.

Certain reflexive and spontaneous movements may be seen in a significant proportion of those declared dead by cerebral criteria. These are likely generated by spinal motor generators and do not invalidate an otherwise complete and clear diagnosis of brain death. Common movements include triple flexion of the lower limb (at the ankle, knee, and hip), either spontaneously or in response to stimulation. Deep tendon and abdominal reflexes are often preserved. Fine jerking of the finger or toe may be observed in some cases, and rarely more complex movements are seen. The *Lazarus sign,* with abdominal flexion, adduction, and flexion of the arms, can be extremely startling to both family and health care personnel present; it may also raise questions about the correctness of the diagnosis of death. It is commonly triggered by neck flexion but has also been seen with hypoxic stimulation of cervical neurons during apnea testing or with hypotension. When brain perfusion scans are performed on patients with such movements, they invariably have confirmed lack of cerebral function. Reassuring those present is the most important part of managing these phenomena.

CONFIRMATORY TESTING

If the aforementioned sequence of clinical tests (including negative apnea test) confirms the absence of all brain function, then death can be pronounced without any ancillary tests (at least in adults and children older than 1 year). In cases in which testing cannot be completed, due to patient instability (for apnea testing) or impediment to full brainstem testing (e.g., eye swollen shut or missing), or in rare cases in which family dissent or historical ambiguity necessitates it, ancillary tests can be performed to confirm the state of total brain failure (Table 56.1). Such testing can never supersede clinical examination; for example, if someone manifests respiratory effort during apnea testing, it is inappropriate to then perform a confirmatory test to negate that finding.

The most common method of confirming brain death is by demonstrating a lack of effective intracranial perfusion. This can be achieved by nuclear scintigraphy or

TABLE 56.1	Confirmatory Tests Used to Declare Brain Death		
Method	Finding	Pros	Cons
Electroencephalography	Isoelectric Lack of reactivity to stimuli	Safe Bedside	Prone to artifacts Only test cortical function Affected by sedation and hypothermia
Cerebral angiography	No filling of intracranial arteries (high-pressure injection)	Reliable Not affected by sedation or temperature	Requires transportation Contrast injection
Nuclear scintigraphy	Absence of uptake ("empty light bulb")	Safe Bedside	None, preferred test (reliable, high specificity)
Transcranial Doppler ultrasonography	Absence of diastolic or reverberating flow with high pulsatility index—two studies, bilateral anterior + posterior	Safe Bedside	Requires bone windows and skilled technician Absence of signal does not equate with brain death

cerebral angiography. CT angiography and transcranial Doppler are being tested as simpler alternatives to conventional angiography. Although these are not confounded by sedation or metabolic disturbances, they do require stable blood pressure. Alternatively, isoelectric and nonreactive EEG is often used as an ancillary test but may be confounded by artifacts and sedation, so it is not suitable in all situations.

CARE OF THE POTENTIAL BRAIN-DEAD ORGAN DONOR

A few important metabolic and hemodynamic derangements are commonly seen as a result of herniation with brain death. Sympathetic failure can trigger a state of neurogenic shock with hypotension (although a transient state of hypertension and tachycardia may occur as the patient progresses to brain death, with abrupt catecholamine release). Vasopressors may be required to maintain systemic perfusion. Neurogenic pulmonary edema can occur, usually with rapid herniation, whereas cardiac injury from catecholamine excess can complicate pulmonary congestion. Diabetes insipidus occurs frequently and loss of excess free water can precipitate hypovolemia and exacerbate hypotension. If large volumes (>300 mL/hr) of dilute urine output are seen (in the absence of recent mannitol doses), especially with a rising serum sodium level, vasopressin agonists should be given to stop water loss. Desmopressin can be administered as a bolus of 1 to 4 μg IV or SQ with a half-life of approximately 12 hours. Alternately, vasopressin 2 to 5 units can be given IV or SQ and a vasopressin infusion is started, both to maintain blood pressure (infusion of $\leq$0.04 U/min) and prevent polyuria.

SUGGESTED READINGS

Report of the Quality Standards Subcommittee of the American Academy of Neurology. Practice parameters: determining brain death in adults. Available from http://www.aan.com/professionals/practice/pdfs/pdf_1995_thru_1998/1995.45.1012.pdf with an update at: http://www.aan.com/practice/guideline/uploads/433.pdf and http://www.aan.com/practice/guideline/index.cfm?fuseaction=home.view&guideline=431

Wijdicks EF. The diagnosis of brain death. *N Engl J Med.* 2001;344:1215–1221.

Wood KE, Becker BN, McCartney JG, et al. Care of the potential organ donor. *N Engl J Med.* 2004;351:2730–2739.

57 Delirium and Sedation
Michael A. Rubin

Delirium is the most common neurologic problem among all critically ill patients, affecting 60% to 80% of the population. Delirium is associated with worse intensive care unit (ICU) mortality, higher length of stay, and a risk of permanent cognitive disability. Some data even show worse mortality in the long term. Cognition is the most metabolically demanding process in the human organism and is easily disturbed by systemic or neurologic pathology, medications, or the routine of ICU care. Often, sedation induces a state of delirium that lingers longer than expected or desired.

Delirium is defined as an *acute* change in global cognitive function affecting attention, arousal, orientation, or perception. The course is usually fluctuating and symptoms often worsen at night ("sundowning") even in those without any preexisting dementia. Knowing a patient's baseline cognitive ability is essential as delirium must be distinguished from dementia (a chronic problem of impaired cognition) and neurologic emergencies (herniation) producing an acutely decreased level of alertness (Algorithm 57.1). There are two types of delirium: hypoactive and hyperactive. Patients with hyperactive delirium, previously called ICU psychosis, may be loud, agitated, and/or combative, eliciting a high degree of attention from staff. They often require medical and physical restraint and may not perceive the medical staff as trying to care for their well-being. Although hypoactive delirium is more common, particularly among the elderly, it tends to be overlooked. These patients may be quiet or sleepy yet profoundly confused and disoriented. Monitoring for both types should be routine in all ICUs; the etiology of both types is often the same. Although they may be more difficult on the medical staff, patients with hyperactive delirium have a better prognosis.

A useful conceptual model of delirium regards it as the product of two factors: *susceptibility* and *insult*. Susceptibility refers to underlying risk factors, such as age, history of dementia, sensory impairments, etc. (Table 57.1). Each individual has a certain cognitive reserve and is able to sustain a certain amount of disturbance before becoming delirious. Insults, such as infections, organ dysfunction, and metabolic derangements, are new factors in acutely worsening brain function. The sum of susceptibility and insults needs to cross a threshold to cause delirium. Of note, even after insult removal, a susceptible brain will take longer to return to its cognitive baseline than a brain of a healthier person. Elderly patients with dementia may take weeks to recover from even a minor infection. This is an important consideration when deciding dosage of psychoactive medications and expectations for recovery of cognitive function.

ALGORITHM 57.1   Diagnosis and Management of Altered Mental Status

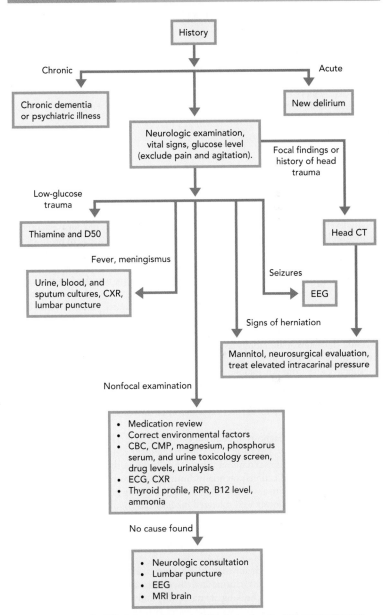

CT, computed tomography; EEG, electroencephalography; CXR, chest radiography; CBC, complete blood cell count; CMP, complete metabolic panel; electrocardiography; RPR, rapid plasma regain; MRI, magnetic resonance imaging.

TABLE 57.1	Risk Factors for Delirium

Age
Baseline dementia or cognitive impairment
Psychiatric comorbidity
History of alcohol or drug abuse
Low albumin/malnutrition
Psychosocial stress (e.g., death of spouse)
Hearing or visual impairment
Sleep deprivation
History of multiple medical problems

WORK-UP

The work-up of altered mental status in the ICU begins with knowledge of their baseline cognitive function, including known dementia and level of functional independence. Dementia is highly underdiagnosed; often people's living arrangement and activity level can be useful data. The time line of the delirium is of course essential to distinguish the cause from a primary neurologic insult to the sequelae of medications, abnormal sleep patterns, and metabolic disturbance. It is essential to see delirium as both an indication of an evolving pathology and a problem in itself that needs to be treated; giving a sedative without consideration of etiology may lead to masking a developing crisis.

The general and neurologic examinations guide the search for insults that cause delirium. Some causes may be obvious when you walk in the patient's room: fever, hypoxemia, or hypotension is easily assessed on any continuous ICU monitor. Hypoglycemia can likewise be rapidly assessed. The goal of the neurologic assessment is similar to that of coma in that discovery of focal signs helps differentiate a structural neurologic cause from a metabolic or infectious cause. Any asymmetry should raise concern for a focal lesion and may constitute an emergency. Subtle signs of seizure (eye or head deviation, rhythmic movements of the face or extremities) are sought. See Chapter 55 on coma for further explanation of the relevant neurologic examination.

The differential diagnosis of delirium is broad (Table 57.2). A careful examination, medication review, and basic laboratory studies will address most causes. Medications are among the most common causes of delirium in the ICU (Table 57.3). In addition to current medications potentially causing cognitive dysfunction, recently discontinued medicines with a withdrawal potential, new drug interactions, or change in the metabolism of previously well-tolerated medications should be addressed. Always be willing to reconsider a change in a patient's physiology; do not assume that a patient's cognition is drifting down just because of his or her presence in the ICU. Liver and renal dysfunction may alter medication levels; elderly patients may become delirious even with "therapeutic" levels.

Basic studies include chemistries, blood counts, electrolytes, urine and blood toxicology, ammonia, drug levels, urine analysis, electrocardiography, and chest radiography. Thyroid testing and checking of vitamin B_{12} and rapid plasma reagin levels are done to establish the reversible causes of dementia. Any suspicion for infection such as fever, meningismus, or leukocytosis should be pursued with blood cultures and lumbar

TABLE 57.2	Causes of Delirium
Vascular	Stroke, hemorrhage, reversible posterior leukoencephalopathy, vasospasm, migraine
Toxins	Medications, alcohol, illicit drugs, occupational exposures, withdrawal
Seizures	Aura, ictal state, nonconvulsive status epilepticus, postictal state
Other organs	Hepatic, uremia, cardiac disease, lung disease
Electrolytes	Hypoglycemia, hyponatremia, hypocalcemia, hypomagnesemia
Neoplastic	Primary tumor, metastases, carcinomatous meningitis, paraneoplastic syndromes
Infection	Urinary tract infection, pneumonia, meningitis/encephalitis, sepsis
Trauma	Direct trauma, edema, diffuse axonal injury, postconcussive syndrome
Autoimmune	Neuropsychiatric lupus, Hashimoto encephalopathy, CNS vasculitis, limbic encephalitis
Endocrine	Hypo/hyperthyroidism, hypopituitary state, hyper/hypoparathyroidism
Nutritional	Vitamin B_{12} deficiency, Wernicke encephalopathy (thiamine deficiency), Machiafava–Bignami disease

CNS, central nervous system.

TABLE 57.3	Medications that Can Cause Delirium
During use	**Withdrawal**
Anticholinergic agents	Appetite suppressants
Sedatives	Cough/cold remedies
Antiemetics	Alcohol (even without delirium tremens)
Antipsychotics	Selective serotonin reuptake inhibitors
Antispasmodics	Nicotine
Tricyclic antidepressants	Baclofen
Muscle relaxants	
Digoxin	
Cimetidine	
Anticonvulsants	
Corticosteroids	
Lithium	
Benzodiazepines	
Barbiturates	
Opioids	

TABLE 57.4	Nonmedication Causes of Delirium
Cause	Treatment
Disorientation	Frequent reorientation
Sleep cycle change	Provide stimulating activity, keep out of bed during day, no interruptions at night
Sensory deficits	Put on glasses, hearing aids
Poor communication	Communication devices
Catheters, restraints	Remove catheters, tubes, and restraints as early as possible
Dehydration	Assess for dehydration and hydrate
Malnutrition	Feed with parenteral nutrition if needed
Pain	Assess for and treat pain
Immobility	Remove restraints early, range-of-motion exercises, keep out of bed
Urinary retention	Place a bladder catheter or start scheduled catheterizations
Constipation	Disimpact if needed, start bowel routine
Fever	Antipyretics, scheduled if necessary
Infection	Search for and treat underlying infection
Hypoxemia, hypercarbia	Check arterial blood gases, ventilate or oxygenate as needed

puncture. Other causes of delirium (Table 57.4) should also be sought and corrected, if possible.

If the cause of delirium is not found, neurologic consultation should be obtained. Serious conditions can exhibit subtle findings or even nonfocal examination. For instance, strokes in the nondominant hemisphere can cause delirium in the absence of hemiparesis, or fluent aphasia may be mistaken for delirium. Nonconvulsive status epilepticus may have no symptoms except delirium (see Chapter 51). Lumbar puncture, electroencephalography, brain imaging, and more specific laboratory studies are usually needed at this point.

TREATMENT OF DELIRIUM

A methodical and thorough approach will help identify the cause of delirium in most cases and should guide the treatment. However, a useful technique to combat the contribution of delirium that is due simply to the routine of being in the ICU include family members bringing in familiar objects (glasses, hearing aids, clocks, calendars, photographs of friends, and family) and regular reorientation of the patient. Placing patients in rooms with natural light helps restore normal sleep–wake cycles, and if possible, limit stimulation at night. Next, approach the differential systematically. After a neurosurgical or neurologic cause has been evaluated and the remaining possibilities are metabolic and pharmacologic, eliminate any potential inciting medications. Likewise, address the metabolic dysfunction if possible.

If delirium persists despite treating possible causes or if treating of causes is not feasible, consider treating symptoms pharmacologically. This should not be the first choice, redirection is always the first option followed by soft restraints. If more extensive physical restraints leave the patient agitated and uncomfortable, then escalate to pharmacologic treatment. The goal should not be to make the patients unconscious but to treat them to the point that they are not a danger to themselves. Although hypoactive delirium should be monitored and evaluated, we would not recommend trying to improve level of consciousness in the acute setting with activating medications. Although no randomized controlled trials have been done to prove efficacy of any one agent for delirium, clinical experience has shown relative efficacy and superiority of antipsychotic medications. Although atypical antipsychotics are becoming more popular, haloperidol is still the most commonly used medication. It is given at 1 to 10 mg intravenously or intramuscularly repeated every 30 minutes until effect and then continuing at 25% of the effective dose every 6 hours. A scheduled regimen is more effective than as-needed dosing; elderly or small patients receive a smaller dose. Newer antipsychotics include quetiapine, risperidone, and olanzapine, all of which are given orally or enterally, and ziprasidone, which is also available in an intramuscular form.

Patients treated with antipsychotics need to be carefully monitored for fever or rigidity (indicating neuroleptic malignant syndrome), extrapyramidal symptoms (tremors, stereotypic movements, dystonia), and QT interval prolongation, which can lead to fatal arrhythmias. All patients should have a baseline and daily electrocardiogram. Benzodiazepines may be effective but are not the first-line sedative, as they tend to have lingering affects and disturb sleep architecture, which can worsen delirium. The exception is delirium caused by withdrawal from long-term use of alcohol, benzodiazepines, or barbiturates. An unfortunately common habit in the ICU is to overmedicate patients with sedatives and analgesics while undertreating delirium. A more prudent approach is to evaluate for delirium, pain, and anxiety separately and treat each specifically.

SEDATION IN THE INTENSIVE CARE UNIT

In critical care medicine, sicker patients are becoming more dependent on invasive devices, frequently necessitating pharmacologic sedation for patient comfort. Titrating to a predefined goal and avoiding oversedation is imperative. The risk of delirium after sedation is proportional to the amount of medications used. The modified Ramsey sedation scale (Table 57.5) is a commonly used tool in the ICU setting; another scale focusing more on agitation is the Richmond Agitation Sedation Scale Sedationag (Table 57.6). Having a sedation goal with frequent titration of medicines as part of institutional protocols eases communication between medical personnel and helps to avoid inappropriate over sedation.

TABLE 57.5	Modified Ramsey Sedation Scale
1	Patient anxious and agitated or restless or both
2	Patient cooperative, oriented, and tranquil
3	Patient responds to commands only
4	Asleep, brisk response to a light glabellar tap or loud auditory stimulus
5	A sluggish response to a light glabellar tap or loud auditory stimulus
6	No response to a light glabellar tap or loud auditory stimulus

TABLE 57.6	Richmond Agitation Sedation Scale
+4	Combative, violent, danger to staff
+3	Pulls or removes tube(s) or catheters; aggressive
+2	Frequent nonpurposeful movement, fights ventilator
+1	Anxious, apprehensive but not aggressive
0	Alert and calm
−1	Awakens to voice (eye opening/contact) >10 sec
−2	Light sedation, briefly awakens to voice (eye opening/contact) <10 sec
−3	Moderate sedation, movement or eye opening. No eye contact
−4	Deep sedation, no response to voice, but movement or eye opening to physical stimulation
−5	Unarousable, no response to voice or physical stimulation

Usual sedation protocols combine benzodiazepines and opioids. Continuous infusions may be beneficial in avoiding oversedation and withdrawal, but they may not be available in all situations. Propofol, with a very short half-life, is advantageous in situations in which frequent neurologic examinations are needed. However, because of the lipid components of propofol formulation and subsequent infection risk, propofol should only be used for the short term. The central alpha-2 agonist dexmedetomidine (Precedex®) allows for patients to be aroused for examinations but otherwise keeps them comfortably sedated. Sedation protocols differ and should be targeted to the specific patient population (neurologic, medical, or surgical ICU), in addition to having a built-in sedation target with parameters for modification for each individual patient. Our approach to neurologic patients requires that the minimum amount of sedation be used always, as the serial neurologic examination is the most important indicator of changes in cerebral physiology. However, a patient may be so ill from sepsis, acute respiratory distress syndrome, or recent surgery that any activity could worsen their condition, at which point a deeper level of sedation is needed. Although this will increase the likelihood of a longer time of awakening, the first priority is keeping the patient alive. Any paralyzed patient must also be kept on continuous sedation.

Sedation should be weaned as soon as possible. Daily weaning trials have been shown to decrease ventilation time; they also allow for better neurologic examinations. Ideally, to avoid withdrawal, patients should be switched to scheduled dosing of longer-acting drugs before discontinuing continuous sedation and should be slowly tapered thereafter.

SUGGESTED READINGS

Jacobi J, Frasier GL, Coursin DB, et al. Clinical practice guidelines for the sustained use of sedatives and analgesics in the critically ill adult. *Crit Care Med.* 2002;30:119–141.
   Updated (original version published in 1995) practice guidelines for sedation of adult patients in the intensive care setting with comprehensive review of literature.
Lacasse H, Perreault MM, Williamson DR. Systematic review of antipsychotics for the treatment of hospital-associated delirium in medically or surgically ill patients. *Ann Pharmacother.* 2006;40:1966–1973.
   Comprehensive review of data on available antipsychotics for the treatment of delirium.

58 Acute Spinal Cord Disorders

Michael A. Rubin

Acute spinal cord injury (SCI) results from numerous traumatic causes such as motor vehicle collisions, recreational activities, sports injuries, and work-related falls. In addition, many nontraumatic causes of myelopathy have been described (Table 58.1). SCI may lead to devastating life-long disability with major health, emotional, and financial impact, especially if one considers that injuries most commonly occur in the 20–30s when people have young families and are in their most financially productive years. Despite extensive public education campaigns, licensing requirements, and weapon control laws, SCI continues to increase in its prevalence.

Certain types of myelopathy can be reversed if addressed in a timely fashion; therefore, prompt recognition of clinical symptoms is imperative. The usual clinical presentation involves a triad of motor impairment (may be asymmetric), sensory loss, and sphincter dysfunction (urine retention, incontinence of stool and/or urine) with preservation of cerebral function (unless there is concomitant traumatic brain injury). Pain at the corresponding level of the spine is not always present. A group of syndromes has been well described that help localize the level of the injury (Table 58.2). Algorithm 58.1 presents a detailed initial approach to this serious medical emergency. In addition to surgical care and medical interventions for improving neurologic outcome, intensive care unit (ICU) management may be necessary for the systemic complications of SCI.

TRAUMATIC SPINAL CORD INJURY

Cervical cord injury is the most common type of traumatic SCI. Traumatic brain injury is found in up to a half of these patients; just as many may have injuries to other organs. Almost 50% of victims of cord trauma will present in spinal shock with flaccid areflexic paralysis and lack of sensation in all modalities, but it usually resolves within 48 hours. Spine stability is assessed with multiple-view radiography, computed tomography, and often magnetic resonance imaging (to evaluate for ligamentous injury) to direct surgical interventions or the use of a cervical collar for stabilization. Surgery may have to be done urgently or may be delayed if there is concern for cord edema. The surgical plan and the stability of the spine are important for critical care management, as limitations of movement while in bed and the ability to extend the neck are important to airway management. Immobilization, performed to limit secondary cord damage due to improper positioning of the unstable spine, carries its own risks, including increased intracranial hypertension, airway compromise, diminished chest wall mobility, pressure sores, and pain.

TABLE 58.1	Causes of Spinal Cord Injury

- Traumatic and degenerative (compression fractures, disc herniation)
- Vascular (infarcts, epidural hematoma, arteriovenous malformations)
- Infections (abscesses, myelitis, empyema, tuberculosis)
- Inflammatory/demyelinating (transverse myelitis, acute disseminating encephalomyelitis, multiple sclerosis)
- Neoplastic (tumors and metastases, postradiation)
- Other (vitamin B_{12} deficiency, syringomyelia, amyotrophic lateral sclerosis, spinal canal stenosis, spondylosis)—usually more chronic course

Neuroprotection

For those patients who present within 3 hours of traumatic injury, methylprednisolone infusion at 30 mg/kg followed by 5.4 mg/kg/hr for 24 hours may improve neurologic function. The infusion may be continued for 48 hours if the injury is 3 to 8 hours old; however, there is an increased risk of gastrointestinal bleeding and infection associated with prolonged infusion. Review of the studies supporting the use of methylprednisolone has led many to question the methodology; therefore, this protocol is considered a therapeutic option and no longer the standard of care. Other interventions have been studied such as GM-1 ganglioside and thyrotropin-releasing hormone.

Cardiovascular Management

Many patients with cervical or upper thoracic cord injury may develop neurogenic shock because of the interruption of the spinal sympathetic chain. Decreased sympathetic innervation to the heart and blood vessels results in cardiovascular depression with bradycardia, hypotension, and low systemic vascular resistance. Hemodynamic monitoring is advised, and treatment with fluids and vasopressors to preserve organ perfusion is essential. Vasopressors with chronotropic/inotropic features (norepinephrine, dopamine) are preferred to augment cardiac function as well as to increase vascular tone. The optimal blood pressure goal is unclear; experimental data show that hypotension further worsens SCI due to hypoperfusion. We recommend targeting mean arterial

TABLE 58.2	Spinal Cord Syndromes

- Complete transection—loss of bilateral motor and sensory function below level
- Hemisection—Brown–Sequard syndrome—loss of ipsilateral motor and proprioception/vibration; contralteral loss of pain and temperature
- Central cord—impairment of hands and arms more than legs
- Anterior cord—loss of all modalities except proprioception/vibration
- Posterior cord—preservation of motor and pain/temperature, loss of proprioception/vibration
- Cauda equina—extremely painful, asymmetric, lower motor neuron findings, late urinary retention
- Conus medularus—less painful, symmetric, mixed upper and lower motor neuron findings, early urinary retention

ALGORITHM 58.1 **Initial Approach to a Patient with Suspected Spinal Cord Injury/Acute Myelopathy**

Suspect SCI or myelopathy:
- New onset of weakness (both legs or all four extremities)
- Sensory deficits
- Intact cerebral function
- Sphincter dysfunction (check rectal tone and catheterize the bladder).

↓

Initial stabilization:
- Immobilize patient with cervical or thoracic cord lesions
- Address airway, breathing, and circulation

↓

Obtain proper imaging:
- CT of spine if suspect bone abnormalities (fractures)
- MRI of spine if soft tissue or cord itself may be involved (hematoma, abscess, neoplasms)

Trauma:
- Neurosurgery consult
- Consider MP load 30 mg/kg followed by 5.4 mg/kg/hr for 23 hr

Epidural hematoma:
- Neurosurgery consult
- Immediately reverse anticoagulation with FFP and vitamin K

Epidural abscess:
- Neurosurgery consult
- Vancomycin and ceftriaxone
- Look for source (blood cultures, CT)

Tumor or metastases:
- Neurosurgery consult
- Dexamethasone 10 mg IV, followed by 4 mg IV q6h
- Look for primary source

Demyelinating lesions:
- Neurology consult
- MP 1 g IV daily for 5 days

Spinal cord infarct:
- Neurology consult
- Consider anticoagulation (if known embolic source)
- Keep mean arterial pressure > 70–80 mm Hg

SCI,spinal cord injury; CT, computed tomography; MRI, magnetic resonance imaging; MP, methylprednisolone; FFP, fresh-frozen plasma; IV, intravenous.

pressure of 70 to 80 mm Hg. Atropine should be kept at bedside; transcutaneous pacing may be needed in rare cases of symptomatic refractory bradycardia.

Airway and Breathing

Endotracheal intubation is recommended for those cord trauma victims who have associated traumatic brain injury with Glasgow Coma Scale score of <8 or signs of elevated intracranial pressure. Any airway compromise due to focal edema, fractures, and/or hemorrhages of the neck may also require intubation. Only physicians with advanced airway skills should attempt intubation with an unstable spine; fiber-optic intubation is often required, as the cervical spine often cannot be extended. Measures should be taken to avoid hypotension during intubation, and succinylcholine is contraindicated in SCI of >24 hours. Neurosurgeons should be at bedside to help with immobilization of the spine if a cervical collar must be removed.

Close respiratory monitoring in a critical care setting is necessary, as SCI victims encounter multiple pulmonary complications (neurogenic pulmonary edema, pneumonia, atelectasis, pleural effusions, pulmonary embolism) and are prone to respiratory failure even days after the initial injury. Patients with extensive operative courses and/or prone positioning may have massive fluid shifts in the first few postoperative days and can develop rapid pulmonary edema as fluid is mobilized. In a patient with limited neck mobility, this situation is potentially dangerous. With lesions above C3 level, diaphragmatic function is lost, often resulting in apnea and respiratory arrest; most patients need mechanical ventilation. With lesions between C3 and C5, diaphragmatic function is partially preserved; however, intercoastal muscles may be compromised, leading to diminished lung volumes, poor cough, and hypoventilation.

Thromboembolism Prevention

The majority of patients with SCI eventually develop deep venous thromboses (DVTs), with the highest risk in the first 3 months after the injury; however, there is no current indication for asymptomatic inferior vena cava (IVC) filter placement. Weekly surveillance Doppler studies are optional. Pneumatic compression devices and elastic stockings should be applied as soon as possible; adding pharmacologic means of prevention (low-molecular-weight heparin or adjusted dose unfractionated heparin) may be delayed until surgical plans are finalized and there is no risk of bleeding. Therapeutic anticoagulation should be withheld for 3 to 7 days after surgery, which may require the placement of an IVC filter in the case of DVT or pulmonary embolism.

Gastrointestinal Management

Acute gastroparesis may require gastric suctioning and administration of prokinetic agents to avoid aspiration. Ileus and constipation commonly complicate the course in patients with SCI; bowel regimen (e.g., scheduled laxatives, suppositories every other day) should be instituted early to prevent fecal impaction. H_2-antagonists or proton pump inhibitors are given for stress ulcers and gastrointestinal bleeding prophylaxis.

Skin

As quadriparesis and paraparesis obviously limit motion, this patient population is prone to pressure ulcers. Frequent alteration of position to allow pressure relief and meticulous care of wounds is necessary. Low-air-loss suspension beds and automatically rotating beds may diminish the incidence of decubitus ulcers and facilitate healing of existing ulcers.

Other Issues

Spasticity and contractures become a major problem for these patients within weeks after the injury. Early physical and occupational therapy should be initiated; baclofen, diazepam, and dantrolene are useful agents for spasticity. Pulmonary, urinary tract, and cutaneous infections are common. Universal precautions for ventilator-associated pneumonia should be instituted. Urinary retention is seen commonly and may require self-catheterization or in-dwelling catheters. Pain and depression are seen in most patients and should be addressed promptly. A pain management specialist is often helpful, and psychological support systems are essential.

NONTRAUMATIC MYELOPATHY

Most patients with nontraumatic SCI do not require an ICU admission, unless the upper cord is involved. It is important to identify those at risk for respiratory failure or hemodynamic instability and treat them with the same supportive care as earlier. Furthermore, the nontraumatic causes of myelopathy may have other interventions such as resection of abscess, endovascular therapy for vascular malformations, and steroids or intravenous immunoglobulin for inflammatory disorders.

SUGGESTED READINGS

Early acute management in adults with spinal cord injury: a clinical practice guideline for health-care professionals. *J Spinal Cord Med.* 2008;31:403–479.
> *Guidelines from the Consortium for Spinal Cord Medicine*

Stevens RD, Bhardwaj A, Kirsch JR, et al. Critical care and perioperative management in traumatic spinal cord injury. *J Neurosurg Anesthesiol.* 2003;15:215–229.
> *An excellent evidence-based review on multifaceted approach to patients with traumatic spinal cord injury.*

59 Neuromuscular Disorders in the Critically Ill

Rajat Dhar

The neuromuscular system encompasses the connections between the motor neurons in the spinal anterior horn and the effector muscles that allow us to move and breathe. Disorders of this system usually lead to generalized weakness and may be best divided into those with onset prior to hospital admission and those developing in patients admitted to the hospital/intensive care unit (ICU) for another illness. They are also classified on the basis of neurologic localization (Table 59.1). Occasionally a disorder with onset prior to admission may not be recognized till a patient is admitted for another problem (e.g., aspiration pneumonia) or develop as a secondary feature of a multisystem disorder (e.g., vasculitis, porphyria).

NEUROMUSCULAR RESPIRATORY FAILURE

Respiratory muscles may be affected in almost any of the acute neuromuscular disorders, but most commonly in Guillain–Barré syndrome (GBS), myasthenia gravis (MG), and amyotrophic lateral sclerosis (ALS). In fact, some patients with ALS present with isolated or predominant respiratory involvement without much extremity weakness, which can make the diagnosis challenging. Weakness of the respiratory system (diaphragm as well as intercostal muscles of the chest wall) leads to impaired ventilation as well reduced cough and clearance of secretions. Accessory muscles, including the sternocleidomastoid and scalenes, may compensate in part, but hypercapnic respiratory failure will result from progressive weakness. Hypoxemia may develop due to atelectasis and airway plugging from retained secretions. However, it is critical not to rely on arterial blood gas (ABG) evidence of hypercapnia or hypoxemia (or oxygen desaturation) as markers of imminent neuromuscular respiratory failure (NMRF), as these will occur late in the course as severe decompensation is imminent. There are a number of clinical markers that occur much earlier, and should be closely tracked in patients with acute quadriparesis with suggestion of respiratory involvement (Table 59.2). Observing the patients breathe (especially when lying flat), speak, lift their head, and cough can provide important information.

Ancillary testing involves bedside spirometry to measure negative inspiratory force (NIF) and forced vital capacity (FVC). NIF is the maximal inspiratory pressure generated after forceful exhalation, as measured with a mouthpiece attached to a pressure gauge; it is normally -50 to -70 cm H_2O. Values below -30 suggest significant

TABLE 59.1	Causes of Neuromuscular Respiratory Failure by Localization	
Localization of disorder	Onset prior to ICU admission	ICU-acquired weakness
Muscle	Inflammatory myopathies Acid maltase deficiency Mitochondrial myopathies Myotonic dystrophy Periodic paralysis	Critical illness myopathy Acute necrotizing myopathy Rhabdomyolysis (incl. drugs) Electrolytes ($\downarrow PO_4$, $\downarrow K$)
Neuromuscular junction	Myasthenia gravis Lambert–Eaton syndrome Botulism, Tick paralysis Organophosphate toxicity	Prolonged neuromuscular blockade Hypermagnesemia
Peripheral nerve/ root	Guillain–Barré syndrome Multifocal motor neuropathy Porphyria, Vasculitis, CMT Heavy metals and toxins HIV, Diphtheria, Lyme disease Paraproteinemia, Paraneoplastic	Critical illness polyneuropathy Phrenic nerve injury
Anterior horn cell	Amyotrophic lateral sclerosis Poliomyelitis (West Nile virus)	
Central (Spinal cord/brain)	Acute myelopathy (ischemic, compressive, inflammatory) Brainstem infarction	Spinal cord ischemia (e.g., postoperative), epidural abscess Central pontine myelinolysis

ICU, intensive care unit; CMT, Charcot–Marie Tooth (inherited neuropathy); HIV, human immunodeficiency virus.

weakness. FVC measures the amount of air exhaled and normally exceeds 3 to 4 L. Values less than 30 mL/kg require close monitoring. A consistent downward trend or values less than 20 mL/kg may signal impending respiratory failure and warrant evaluation for preemptive intubation and ventilation. Spirometry can be performed at regular intervals (one to four times per day) in patients with progressive weakness, but not too frequently as to induce fatigue. Facial weakness may prevent the patient forming a tight seal around the mouthpiece, making results artifactually low; a facemask pressed tightly against the lips may overcome this limitation. The trend and overall clinical evaluation should guide decision making and not any isolated FVC or NIF values.

Intubation of patients with NMRF should be performed prior to acute decompensation and ideally before hypercapnia, significant atelectasis, or aspiration develop. Neuromuscular blocking agents (NMBs) should be avoided if possible; succinylcholine can precipitate lethal hyperkalemia in patients with denervation and nondepolarizing NMBs can cause prolonged paralysis in MG. A trial of noninvasive ventilation

TABLE 59.2	Signs of Impending Neuromuscular Respiratory Failure
Sign	**Red flag**
Clinical	
Progressive weakness	Quadriplegia, inability to lift head off bed
Bulbar involvement	Dysphagia, weak voice, bifacial weakness
Weak cough	Trouble expelling secretions, "wet" voice
Respiratory complaints	
Dyspnea	Complains of respiratory fatigue
Tachypnea	Unable to speak in full sentences, count to 20
Orthopnea	Nocturnal desaturations, prefers to sit up
Accessory muscle use	Using neck & abdominal muscles
Abdominal paradox	Inward motion of abdomen with inspiration
Signs of distress	
Tachycardia	Restless
Diaphoresis	Staccato speech
Monitoring	
Vital capacity (VC) testing (bedside)	VC < 15–20 mL/kg, falling, drop by 30% Desaturation (late sign)
Arterial oxygen saturation	Hypercapnia = hypoventilation (late sign)
Arterial blood gas: $PaCO_2$	Atelectasis, Pneumonia
Chest radiographs	

(i.e., bilevel positive airway pressure [BiPAP]) may be considered in select patients with NMRF as long as mental status and airway reflexes are preserved. Some patients with neuromuscular failure may not have diaphragmatic weakness requiring ventilatory support but enough bulbar weakness to necessitate intubation for airway protection. Such patients, of course, will not benefit from BiPAP and will also not require much ventilator support once intubated. The use of BiPAP in GBS may be unsuccessful partially for this reason (i.e., failure of airway protection) and also because these patients usually progress rapidly beyond the support that non-invasive positive pressure ventilation (NIPPV) is able to easily provide. Overventilation (to fully normalize PCO_2) should be avoided in those with chronic retention, otherwise alkalemia will develop, impairing subsequent weaning. Decisions about tracheostomy should be deferred in GBS and MG patients till after immunomodulatory treatment (with plasmapharesis or intravenous immunoglobulin [IVIG]) is completed, as rapid improvement can be seen. Decisions on tracheostomy and weaning can also be facilitated by daily measurements of FVC and NIF on the ventilator (FVC > 7–10 mL/kg and NIF < –20 cm H_2O). It is advisable to wait for 24 hours of spontaneous breathing (with an ABG to exclude CO_2 retention) in patients recovering from NMRF prior to extubation as delayed fatigue can occur.

GUILLAIN–BARRÉ SYNDROME

GBS is an acute inflammatory demyelinating polyneuropathy that is the most common cause of flaccid paralysis worldwide. It is a monophasic autoimmune process often triggered by an upper respiratory or gastrointestinal infection. Clinical hallmarks include symmetric proximal and distal muscle weakness in the legs and arms associated with areflexia and frequent bulbar, facial, and respiratory muscle involvement. *Dysautonomia* is seen in more than half of the patients with GBS and may manifest as wide fluctuations in blood pressure, tachycardia and/or bradycardia (sometimes leading to cardiac arrest), and gastrointestinal symptoms including ileus. Cautious should be exercised in treating blood pressure due to potential lability and atropine may be kept at the bedside as suctioning may induce bradycardia. Sensory complaints and back pain are common in GBS, although patients with acute para- or quadriparesis and sensory dysfunction (especially a "sensory level") should be evaluated for spinal cord compression or other causes of myelopathy. The diagnosis of GBS is supported by finding elevated protein levels in cerebrospinal fluid (CSF) without pleocytosis. Nerve conduction studies (NCS) and electromyography (EMG) may be obtained to assist with diagnosis and prognosis, but may be relatively normal if performed early in the course. The incidence of NMRF requiring intubation is 30% and almost half of these patients require tracheostomy for prolonged ventilation. Treatment is with IVIG (total dose 2 g/kg over 2 to 5 days) or plasmapharesis, and although it may be delayed, recovery is the rule. ICU stay is most prolonged in those with complete quadriplegia and axonal changes (e.g., reduced motor amplitudes) on EMG/NCS.

MYASTHENIA GRAVIS

MG is an autoimmune disease where antibodies are directed against the acetylcholine receptor (Ach-R) at the neuromuscular junction. This impairment of neuromuscular synaptic transmission leads to fatigable weakness with predominant ocular (ptosis, restriction of ocular movements with diplopia) and bulbar involvement. NMRF occurs with diaphragmatic involvement and is the hallmark of *myasthenic crisis,* which occurs in 20% of patients with MG. There is often an identifiable precipitant such as intercurrent infection, surgery (including thymectomy), or medications (commonly antibiotics, see Table 59.3). Worsening of MG is seen in a subset of patients shortly after initiating corticosteroid therapy (especially at doses more than 20 mg/day) and may precipitate crisis. The diagnosis of MG is primarily clinical, confirmed either by presence of Ach-R antibodies in the serum or the finding of "decrement" (of motor amplitudes) on repetitive nerve stimulation. Treatment of MG consists of cholinesterase inhibitors (pyridostigmine) and immunosuppression (including corticosteroids). Crises are usually treated with IVIG or plasmapharesis (as in GBS). Recovery is usually more rapid

TABLE 59.3	Medications that can Aggravate Weakness in Myasthenia Gravis
Antibiotics	Aminoglycosides, ciprofloxacin, clindamycin, erythromycin, azithromycin, tetracyclines, polymyxin B, colistin
Antiarrhythmics	Quinidine, procainamide, lidocaine, β-blockers, calcium channel blockers
Hormones	Corticosteroids
Neuromuscular blockers	Succinylcholine, vecuronium, pancuronium, etc.
Other	Lithium, phenytoin, quinine, statins

ALGORITHM 59.1 Managing Neuromuscular Respiratory Failure

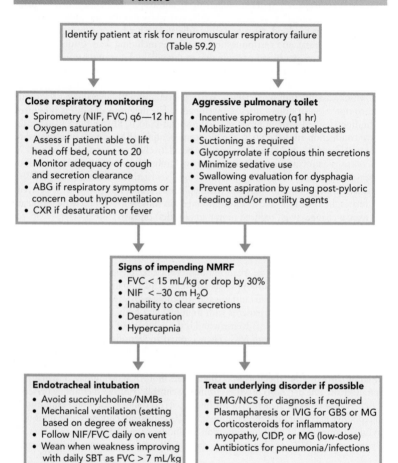

Identify patient at risk for neuromuscular respiratory failure
(Table 59.2)

Close respiratory monitoring
- Spirometry (NIF, FVC) q6—12 hr
- Oxygen saturation
- Assess if patient able to lift head off bed, count to 20
- Monitor adequacy of cough and secretion clearance
- ABG if respiratory symptoms or concern about hypoventilation
- CXR if desaturation or fever

Aggressive pulmonary toilet
- Incentive spirometry (q1 hr)
- Mobilization to prevent atelectasis
- Suctioning as required
- Glycopyrrolate if copious thin secretions
- Minimize sedative use
- Swallowing evaluation for dysphagia
- Prevent aspiration by using post-pyloric feeding and/or motility agents

Signs of impending NMRF
- FVC < 15 mL/kg or drop by 30%
- NIF < −30 cm H_2O
- Inability to clear secretions
- Desaturation
- Hypercapnia

Endotracheal intubation
- Avoid succinylcholine/NMBs
- Mechanical ventilation (setting based on degree of weakness)
- Follow NIF/FVC daily on vent
- Wean when weakness improving with daily SBT as FVC > 7 mL/kg
- Delay tracheostomy 1–2 weeks

Treat underlying disorder if possible
- EMG/NCS for diagnosis if required
- Plasmapharesis or IVIG for GBS or MG
- Corticosteroids for inflammatory myopathy, CIDP, or MG (low-dose)
- Antibiotics for pneumonia/infections

NIF, negative inspiratory force; FVC, forced vital capacity; ABG, arterial blood gas; CXR, chest x-ray; NMB, neuromuscular blocking drug; SBT, spontaneous breathing trial; EMG/NCS, electromyography and nerve conduction studies; IVIG, intravenous immunoglobulin; GBS, Guillain–Barré syndrome; MG, myasthenia gravis; CIDP, chronic inflammatory demyelinating polyneuropathy

than in GBS and most patients do not require prolonged ventilation or tracheostomy (Algorithm 59.1).

In patients on high doses of pyridostigmine, there may be concern that increasing weakness is a sign of cholinergic toxicity and not worsening MG. Cholinergic crisis will usually be associated with excessive salivation, muscle cramping, diarrhea, and fasciculations, peaking shortly after drug dosing. This is a rare toxidrome in MG but can be excluded by discontinuing the medication and reevaluating. Pyridostigmine can exacerbate pulmonary secretions and is usually held during periods of respiratory failure. Imaging of the chest may be obtained when a new patient with MG is stabilized to evaluate for thymoma. However, thymectomy should be delayed till after crisis has resolved to avoid exacerbation postoperatively.

ICU-ACQUIRED WEAKNESS

Patients who are critically ill often develop neuromuscular weakness that not only prolongs duration of mechanical ventilation, but may also contribute to residual disability in survivors. There has been considerable confusion and overlap in terminology and classification of such disorders. Dysfunction at both the level of the peripheral nerve and muscle occurs commonly (even in the same patient) and can be hard to distinguish clinically or even with EMG/NCS. The term "ICU-acquired weakness" may be preferable to label the clinical syndrome in the absence of electrodiagnostic or pathologic testing. The diagnosis is often suspected in the setting of failure to wean after recovery from critical illness (most often sepsis and acute respiratory distress syndrome). Weakness can be assessed by testing muscle groups in the upper and lower extremities when a patient awakens from sedation and encephalopathy; it may be suspected even in uncooperative patients when painful stimulation elicits a grimace but limited limb movement.

Critical illness polyneuropathy (CIP) reflects noninflammatory axonal nerve damage as a result of sepsis; it may be best viewed as another end-organ failure resulting from cytokine-mediated systemic inflammatory response with nerve edema and tissue hypoxia. It may be exacerbated by hyperglycemia, and attempts at intensive glucose control have yielded reductions in CIP. Myopathy has been related to corticosteroid and NMB exposure and was first described in a patient with status asthmaticus. Creatine kinase (CK) levels may be elevated early in the course but are often normal by the time weakness is recognized. The pathologic hallmark is selective loss of the thick (myosin) muscle filaments. It is difficult to clinically distinguish CIP from myopathy, as sensory loss (absent in myopathy) is hard to test in ICU patients and the pattern of weakness (both proximal and distal muscles) is similar in both. NCS will show reduced motor amplitudes in both states. Evaluation of motor units with EMG may help (as neuropathic and myopathic changes in unit morphology are different) but weak encephalopathic ICU patients rarely cooperate adequately to allow recruitment of motor units. Muscle biopsy will show the hallmark of "myosin loss myopathy" but is not mandatory in cases of ICU-acquired weakness. Once a clinical diagnosis has been made, supportive care (and avoiding additional precipitants) is required for both subtypes. Biopsy (muscle ± nerve) may be useful if the patient does not improve or there is suspicion of an underlying systemic disorder (e.g., inflammatory myopathy with elevated CK, nerve vasculitis). Restricting use of neuromuscular blockers (or monitoring level of paralysis, if used), daily sedative holidays, and early mobilization of ICU patients may minimize the risk of these disorders, as may intensive insulin therapy.

SUGGESTED READINGS

Chalela JA. Pearls and pitfalls in the intensive care management of Guillain-Barré syndrome. *Semin Neurol.* 2001;21:399–405.

Dhar R, Stitt L, Hahn AF. The morbidity and outcome of patients with Guillain-Barré syndrome admitted to the intensive care unit. *J Neurol Sci.* 2008;264:121–128.

Gorson K. Approach to neuromuscular disorders in the intensive care unit. *Neurocrit Care.* 2005;3:195–212.

Lawn ND, Fletcher DD, Henderson RD, et al. Anticipating mechanical ventilation in Guillain-Barré syndrome. *Arch Neurol.* 2001;58:893–898.

Schweickert WD, Hall J. ICU-acquired weakness. *Chest.* 2007;131:1541–1549.

60 Traumatic Brain Injury and Elevated Intracranial Pressure

Ahmed Hassan

Severe head trauma is a leading cause of morbidity and mortality worldwide, especially among young adults. Almost 2 million people sustain a traumatic brain injury (TBI) in the United States each year; the most common causes are falls, motor vehicle accidents, and assault. Yet the reduction of mortality rates in severe TBI from 50% to 25% over the last 25 years emphasizes the impact of improvements in medical and surgical management, particularly in prevention of secondary brain injury, which occurs hours to days after the initial trauma.

The Glasgow Coma Scale (GCS) is widely used for classification and prognosis (Table 60.1). An assessment of eye opening/level of consciousness and motor and verbal responses is performed and recorded. According to this scale, head injuries are classified as mild (GCS, 14–15), moderate (GCS, 9–12), and severe (GCS, 3–8).

Initial management focuses on airway, breathing, and circulation. Those patients with GCS ≤ 8 usually require endotracheal intubation and mechanical ventilation. In cases of ongoing bleeding and hypotension, fluid resuscitation, hemotransfusion, and/or vasopressors to maintain adequate perfusion should be initiated. Because approximately 15% of patients with TBI have an associated spinal cord injury, an effort should be made to stabilize and immobilize the spine.

Once the initial steps have been performed, a noncontrasted head computed tomography (CT) and plain films of the spine to assess the magnitude and type of injury should be obtained. The range of head injuries extends from simple scalp lacerations and skull fractures to contusions, hemorrhagic insults (epidural, subdural, intraparenchymal, and subarachnoid hemorrhages), and diffuse axonal injury. Neurosurgical consultation should be sought emergently as certain types of TBI require immediate operative treatment.

Further management of head injury is based on prevention, recognition, and aggressive treatment of secondary insults to the brain, including hypoxia, hypotension, hypoperfusion, and elevated intracranial pressure (ICP).

MANAGEMENT OF PATIENTS WITH SEVERE TBI

Patients with severe TBI should be monitored in the intensive care unit for ICP and cerebral perfusion pressure (CPP) monitoring. ICP monitoring is indicated in all cases of severe TBI (GCS ≤ 8) with an abnormal CT scan (Table 60.2). ICP can be measured

TABLE 60.1	**Glasgow Coma Scale**
Best eye opening	
Spontaneous	4
With voice only	3
With pain only	2
None at all	1
Best verbal response	
Coherent speech	5
Confused intelligible speech	4
Inappropriate words	3
Incomprehensible sounds	2
No verbal output	1
Best motor response	
Follows commands	6
Localizes pain stimuli[a]	5
Withdraws to pain stimuli	4
Decorticate posturing	3
Decerebrate posturing	2
No movements at all	1

[a]Localizing pain stimuli refers to gaze deviation, head turning or hand movements towards the stimulus.

using either a ventricular catheter, which has the advantage of CSF drainage, or a parenchymal catheter. Routine ventricular catheter exchange or prophylactic antibiotic use for ventricular catheter placement is not recommended. CPP is the difference between mean arterial pressure (MAP) and ICP. MAP is accurately measured by direct cannulation of one of the arteries (e.g., radial, femoral).

ICP CONTROL

Elevated ICP (>20 mm Hg) after head injury is associated with unfavorable outcomes. In approximately half of those who die after severe TBI, increased ICP resulting in herniation is the primary cause of death. In all patients who have ICP monitors,

TABLE 60.2	**Indications for ICP and CPP Monitoring**

Patients with GCS ≤ 8 and an abnormal CT scan (i.e., hematoma, contusion, swelling, herniation, or compressed basal cisterns).
Patients with a normal CT scan and at least two of the following on admission:
  Age > 40
  Unilateral or bilateral motor posturing
  Systolic BP < 90 mm Hg

ICP, intracranial pressure; CPP, cerebral perfusion pressure; GCS, Glasgow Coma Scale; CT, computed tomography; BP, blood pressure.

ALGORITHM 60.1 Management of Elevated Intracranial Pressure

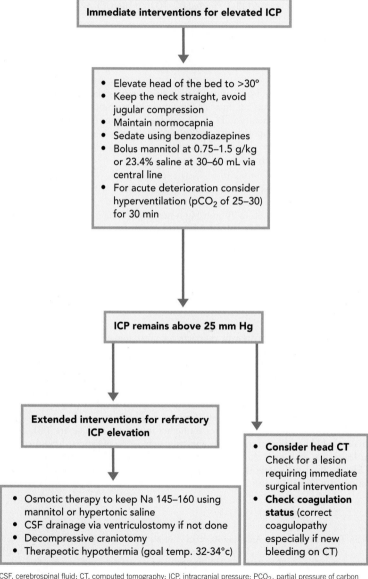

Immediate interventions for elevated ICP

- Elevate head of the bed to >30°
- Keep the neck straight, avoid jugular compression
- Maintain normocapnia
- Sedate using benzodiazepines
- Bolus mannitol at 0.75–1.5 g/kg or 23.4% saline at 30–60 mL via central line
- For acute deterioration consider hyperventilation (pCO$_2$ of 25–30) for 30 min

ICP remains above 25 mm Hg

Extended interventions for refractory ICP elevation

- Osmotic therapy to keep Na 145–160 using mannitol or hypertonic saline
- CSF drainage via ventriculostomy if not done
- Decompressive craniotomy
- Therapeotic hypothermia (goal temp. 32-34°c)

- **Consider head CT** Check for a lesion requiring immediate surgical intervention
- **Check coagulation status** (correct coagulopathy especially if new bleeding on CT)

CSF, cerebrospinal fluid; CT, computed tomography; ICP, intracranial pressure; PCO$_2$, partial pressure of carbon dioxide

TABLE 60.3	CPP Management

Keep MAP above 80 mm Hg until CPP can be measured.
Use normal saline boluses and vasopressors if needed.
Once ICP monitor is inserted, CPP goal 60–70 mm Hg (CPP = MAP − ICP).
Control ICP, see Algorithm 60.1
Use vasopressors to keep CPP within goals while correcting hypovolemia.

MAP, mean arterial pressure; CPP, cerebral perfusion pressure; ICP, intracranial pressure.

universal measures should be instituted, including elevating the head of bed to >30 degrees, keeping the chin midline, and maintaining normocarbia, normothermia, and euvolemia. For refractory ICPs (>20 mm Hg for >5 min), sedation, osmotherapy, hyperventilation, hypothermia, and surgical decompression should be considered (Algorithm 60.1). Hyperventilation is recommended only as a brief temporizing measure for symptoms of herniation.

CPP THRESHOLD

Maintenance of CPP at 60 to 70 mm Hg is necessary to maintain adequate cerebral blood flow; reduction below these level increases risk for ischemia. CPP may drop because of a decrease in MAP, an increase in ICP, or by a combination of these two mechanisms. Maintenance of CPP at 60 to 70 mm Hg is achieved by administering fluids to maintain euvolemia and in refractory cases, vasopressors to augment MAP (Table 60.3).

GENERAL CARE

Up to 25% of TBI patients will experience a posttraumatic seizure within 7 days of injury, thus seizure prevention with anticonvulsants is indicated for 7 days after TBI. Continuation of prophylaxis should not extend beyond 1 week as it does not affect the development of late posttraumatic seizures. Sequential compression devices in addition to elastic stockings should be used from admission, and subcutaneous low-molecular-weight heparin or unfractionated heparin for DVT prophylaxis can be started 48 hours after documentation of cessation of bleeding.

Because metabolic expenditures are higher in patients with severe TBI, caloric intake should be adjusted to provide approximately 140% of expected requirements. At least 15% of calories should be supplied as protein. Early feeding (within 48 to 72 hours of insult) is important, resulting in a trend toward fewer infectious complications and lower mortality.

SUGGESTED READING

Brain Trauma Foundation; American Association of Neurological Surgeons; Congress of Neurological Surgeons. Guidelines for the management of severe traumatic brain injury. *J Neurotrauma*. 2007;24(Suppl 1):S1–S106.

61 Neurologic Approach to Central Nervous System Infections

Michael A. Rubin

Central nervous system (CNS) infections can progress from initiation to life-threatening in a matter or hours; therefore, any suspicion should prompt rapid evaluation and treatment. The classic triad of headache, fever, and meningismus may only be seen in half of the patients with bacterial meningitis and only some will have a focal neurologic deficit and peripheral leukocytosis. Pachymeningitis (infection of the dural folds) may have a much more indolent course, consequently, an extended history of symptoms does not rule out meningitis. In immunocompromised patients, the index of suspicion is even higher, as any one of these symptoms may be the sole manifestation of infection. In addition to the devastation caused by the infection, abscess may form and seizures may occur. Provoked seizures often lead to status epilepticus, so a low threshold should be kept for electroencephalography (EEG) and appropriate treatment. Furthermore, neurosurgical procedures, indwelling hardware, and penetrating skull injuries complicate the treatment of meningitis.

Blood cultures and a coagulation profile should promptly be done and those who are immunocompromised or have depressed level of consciousness, papilledema, or focal neurologic deficit should have a head computed tomography prior to lumbar puncture (LP) due to the risk of herniation with a mass lesion (see Table 61.1). Correct coagulopathy prior to LP to prevent forming an epidural hematoma. Opening pressure should always be measured and the standard lab profile sent as shown in Table 61.2. Although antimicrobials may reduce the yield of cerebrospinal fluid (CSF) cultures, a reliable gram stain is still possible and treatment should not be delayed for LP, although blood cultures should be drawn prior to administration of antimicrobials. Treatment should be appropriate for age and other risk factors and should remain broad until the offending organism is identified (see Algorithm 61.1). If able to treat early, bacterial meningitis should be treated also with dexamethasone for the first 2 to 4 days, especially in the case of *streptococcus pneuomonia*. It is wise to save CSF in the lab for future studies since after the cell count, protein, and glucose are known, an index of suspicion may be raised for the likely class of organisms and extra agglutination or polymerase chain reaction (PCR) tests might be useful. Table 61.2 lists the various CSF patterns according to cause. For further review of risk factors, pathogens, antimicrobial treatment, and duration, see Chapter 34.

TABLE 61.1	Contraindications to Lumbar Puncture
Absolute	Relative
Space-occupying lesion in the posterior fossa Presence of midline shift Effacement of the cisterns or fourth ventricle Skin infection in the area of puncture Lumbar epidural abscess or empyema	International normalized ratio above 1.4 Platelet count below 50,000/μL

MENINGITIS

Leptomeningitis is the most common type of CNS infection, with mortality reaching 60%; delay in proper recognition and immediate treatment can lead to death.

Bacterial Meningitis

A preceding pneumonia, otitis media, or acute sinusitis is common; do not assume that the infection is a spontaneous event. An accurate history may elucidate the source and allow a more narrow differential diagnosis. The usual empiric regiment includes ceftriaxone (or meropenim) and vancomycin with possible addition of amplicillin. Common organisms in the adult population include *Streptococcus pneumoniae, Neisseria meningitidis,* and *Staphylococcus aureus.* In the elderly or immunocompromised *Listeria monocytogenes* should be considered and those with neurosurgical hardware or penetrating skull injuries should also be covered for aerobic gram-negative bacilli. Patients should be monitored closely for complications including septic shock, cerebral edema, hydrocephalus, venous sinus thrombosis, seizures, disseminated intravascular

TABLE 61.2	Cerebrospinal Fluid (CSF) Findings Suggestive of Infection		
CSF parameter	Bacterial meningitis	Viral meningitis	Fungal meningitis
Opening pressure (mm H_2O)	>180	Often normal	Variable
White cell count	1000–10,000	<300	50–200
Percent neutrophils	>80	<20	Usually <50
Protein	100–500	Often normal	Variably elevated
Glucose	<40	>40	Usually <40
Gram stain (% positive)	60–90	0	0
Culture (% positive)	70–85	50	25–50

Adapted from Zunt and Marra (1999), with permission.

ALGORITHM 61.1 Approach to Treatment of Suspected Infection of the Central Nervous System

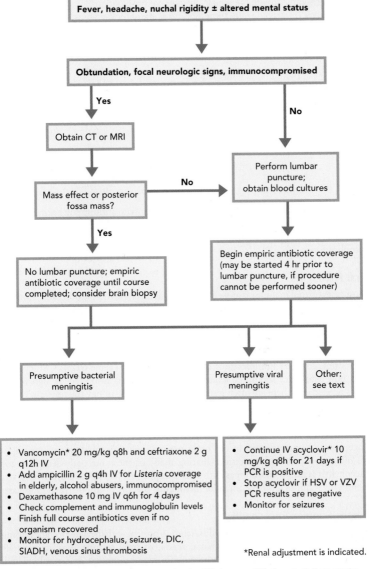

Fever, headache, nuchal rigidity ± altered mental status

↓

Obtundation, focal neurologic signs, immunocompromised

Yes ↓   **No** ↓

Obtain CT or MRI

↓

Mass effect or posterior fossa mass? —**No**→ Perform lumbar puncture; obtain blood cultures

Yes ↓

No lumbar puncture; empiric antibiotic coverage until course completed; consider brain biopsy

Begin empiric antibiotic coverage (may be started 4 hr prior to lumbar puncture, if procedure cannot be performed sooner)

↓

Presumptive bacterial meningitis   **Presumptive viral meningitis**   **Other: see text**

- Vancomycin* 20 mg/kg q8h and ceftriaxone 2 g q12h IV
- Add ampicillin 2 g q4h IV for *Listeria* coverage in elderly, alcohol abusers, immunocompromised
- Dexamethasone 10 mg IV q6h for 4 days
- Check complement and immunoglobulin levels
- Finish full course antibiotics even if no organism recovered
- Monitor for hydrocephalus, seizures, DIC, SIADH, venous sinus thrombosis

- Continue IV acyclovir* 10 mg/kg q8h for 21 days if PCR is positive
- Stop acyclovir if HSV or VZV PCR results are negative
- Monitor for seizures

*Renal adjustment is indicated.

CT, computed tomography; MRI, magnetic resonance imaging; IV, intravenous; DIC, disseminated intravascular coagulation; SIADH, syndrome of inappropriate antidiuretic hormone secretion; PCR, polymerase chain reaction; HSV, herpes simplex virus; VZV, varicella-zoster virus.

TABLE 61.3	Noninfectious Causes of Meningitis

Medications and toxins
    Nonsteroidal anti-inflammatory medications (ibuprofen, ketorolac)
    Chemotherapy agents (especially intrathecal preparations)
    Antibiotics (metronidazole, trimethoprim-sulfamethoxazole, isoniazid)
    Vaccinations
    Intravenous immunoglobulin G
    Intravenous contrast

Neoplastic (leptomeningeal metastases)

Autoimmune or inflammatory disorders
    Systemic lupus erythematosus
    Sjögren syndrome
    Primary central nervous system angiitis
    Behçet disease

coagulation, hearing loss, and syndrome of inappropriate antidiuretic hormone secretion. Often neurologic consultation on meningitis is valuable not just for information on treatment of the infection but also for identification of the associated neurologic complications.

Viral Meningitis

Most cases of viral meningitis are self-limiting and carry a favorable outcome. However, herpes simplex meningitis can have a high morbidity but may be treated with acyclovir.

Noninfectious Aseptic Meningitis

If all microbiology tests have negative results and there is no clinical improvement with antibiotics, consider noninfectious causes of meningitis (Table 61.3). CSF cytology with flow cytometry should be requested if malignancy is suspected. A high volume tap is needed and there are often restrictions on what time of day the tests can be run.

ENCEPHALITIS

Encephalitis is an infection of the brain parenchyma. Encephalitis and meningitis are often two ends of a spectrum, sharing many of the same pathogens. Bacterial encephalitis is not as common as with viral encephalitis. Just as the treatment of viral meningitis is limited, the treatment of meningitis, therapy is supportive in most cases.

Herpes Simplex Encephalitis

Herpes simplex virus (HSV) encephalitis tends to present with focal neurologic findings such as hemiparesis, dysphasia, aphasia, ataxia, or focal seizures that are generally of short (<1 week) duration. Xanthochromia may be present as a result of mild hemorrhage into the subarachnoid space; otherwise, CSF findings are similar to those of viral meningitis. Further studies may increase the index of suspicion for HSV such as temporal lobe findings on magnetic resonance imaging or epileptic activity as seen on EEG in those same regions. Prompt diagnosis and treatment of this infection is of paramount importance given its significant morbidity and mortality; acyclovir should be given intravenously for the entire duration of treatment. Because refractory seizures or status epilepticus are commonly seen, patients with altered mental status should undergo EEG.

Arthropod-Borne (Arboviral) Encephalitis

Encephalitides of the arthropod-borne type include St. Louis encephalitis, California encephalitis, Japanese B encephalitis, Eastern and Western equine encephalitis, and West Nile encephalitis. Treatment of these infections is generally supportive.

BRAIN ABSCESS

Brain abscess arises from one of following three sources: direct spread (such as from an infected sinus), hematogenous spread from another source, or penetrating trauma. Neurosurgical patients are at risk in the months or even years after a procedure and ventricular peritoneal shunt infection is not uncommon even if placed in a meticulously sterile manner. Most brain abscesses are bacterial and often polymicrobial, although fungal infections are also possible, especially in the immunocompromised patient. Common aerobes include *Streptococcus* species (including *viridans* in endocarditis patients), *Staphylococcus* species (especially after surgical procedures), *Pseudomonas* species, and *Enterobacter* species (otitis media). Anaerobic abscesses (*Bacteroides* and *Actinomyces* species) may arise from oral sources (dental carriers) and abdominal or pelvic infections. Neutropenic patients and transplant recipients have a particular predilection for *Aspergillus* abscesses. Toxoplasmosis is the most common intracranial infection in patients with acquired immune deficiency syndrome (AIDS).

The presentation of a brain abscess typically involves headache lateralizing to the side of the abscess, accompanied by focal neurologic signs and, occasionally, meningismus. Evidence of elevated intracranial pressure (papilledema, vomiting, or depressed level of consciousness) may also be present. Diagnosis of brain abscess relies primarily on neuroimaging with a contrast agent. The typical abscess appears as a ring-enhancing lesion with surrounding cerebral edema. Abscesses resulting from hematogenous spread (septic emboli due to endocarditis) may present as multiple lesions. Abscesses due to direct invasion from the facial sinuses or dental infections will typically affect the frontal lobes.

The workup for the source includes blood and urine cultures, echocardiography, and possibly further body imaging. Toxoplasma titers are checked in immunocompromised patients. When a possible abscess is localized, definitive characterization may require stereotactic aspiration followed by empiric antibiotic coverage until specific organisms and sensitivities have been determined.

Antimicrobial coverage for brain abscesses varies with the presumptive source of infection. Empiric treatment for a hematogenous source includes vancomycin and metronidazole. Abscess originating from a sinus, otogenic, or oral source requires metronidazole and either penicillin G or ceftriaxone. Neurosurgical patients with postoperative abscess require vancomycin and a third generation cephalosporin (ceftazidime or cefepime). Immunocompromised hosts (including neutropenic and recent posttransplant patients) require amphotericin B for additional fungal coverage. A total course of 6 to 8 weeks is standard in all cases.

FUNGAL INFECTIONS

Fungal CNS infections (meningoencephalitis, brain abscess, or granuloma) are usually encountered as opportunistic infections in the immunosuppressed hosts. Amphotericin B (1 mg/kg daily intravenously) is the first-line agent for most infections, and because of poor CNS penetration flucytosine (25 mg/kg every 6 hours orally) is added. Both medications require renal adjustment; patients should be closely monitored, as risk of side effects is high. After a 4- to 6-week course, a suppressive phase with a triazole is continued for at least 6 weeks. Infectious disease specialist consult is highly recommended.

INFECTIONS RELATED TO NEUROSURGERY

Infections following neurosurgery include meningitis, encephalitis, ventriculitis, abscess, and hardware infection. These typically occur within weeks of surgery, although vulnerability to infections remains for years. Ventriculoperitoneal shunt infections may present with symptoms of hydrocephalus (increasing headaches, vomiting, lethargy) and abdominal distention; otherwise, symptoms are similar to other types of CNS infections. Neurosurgical consultation is mandatory.

In addition to the usual workup, shunts are assessed with imaging to determine their functional status and tapped to identify the organism. Infected hardware must be removed if possible. The most common organisms causing postneurosurgical infection include *Staphylococcus* species and gram-negative organisms. It is unknown if additional benefit is provided by directly infusing antibiotics into an externalized shunt or temporizing ventriculostomy.

THE IMMUNOCOMPROMISED PATIENT

The immunocompromised population includes patients with AIDS, solid-organ or bone marrow transplantation recipients, and those receiving chemotherapy or immunosuppressants for autoimmune conditions. The most common infections include toxoplasmosis, cryptococcal meningitis or encephalitis, fungal abscess (*Aspergillus*), and progressive multifocal leukoencephalopathy (JC virus). Special CSF testing includes PCR testing for *Toxoplasma,* JC virus, Epstein–Barr virus, and cytomegalovirus, as well as *Cryptococcus* and *Histoplasma* antigen testing. The Venereal Disease Research Laboratory test should also be requested, given the higher incidence of neurosyphilis in AIDS patients. An infectious diseases consult is strongly recommended if CNS infection is suspected in an immunocompromised patient.

SUGGESTED READINGS

Pruitt AA. Infections of the nervous system. *Neurol Clin.* 1998;16:419–447.
   An excellent review of comprehensive approach to infections of the central nervous system with special attention to the immunocompromised patients.
Tunkel AR, Hartman BJ, Kaplan SL, et al. Practice guidelines for the management of bacterial meningitis. *Clin Infect Dis.* 2004;39:1267–1284.
   Current recommendations for the diagnosis and management of bacterial meningitis representing data published through May 2004.

Ziai WC, Lewin JJ 3rd. Advances in the management of central nervous system infections in the ICU. *Crit Care Clin.* 2006;22:661–694.

Most recent review of management of various acute central nervous system infections in the critical care setting.

Zunt JR, Marra CM. Cerebrospinal fluid testing for the diagnosis and central nervous system infection. *Neurol Clin.* 1999;17:675–689.

A detailed review of various methods of testing cerebrospinal fluid for suspected infection of the central nervous system.

62 Thrombocytopenia in the Intensive Care Unit

Warren Isakow

Thrombocytopenia is a very common occurrence in the intensive care unit (ICU), occurring in as many as 60% of patients. The normal platelet count ranges between 150,000 and 450,000/μL. In the ICU, it is important to recognize that the absolute platelet count is important, but trends in the platelet count, specifically a decline by more than one-half, may be evidence of a serious clinical problem such as heparin-induced thrombocytopenia (HIT), which requires urgent attention. A systematic approach to the diagnosis allows for the common causes to be detected early and enables rational use of platelet transfusions (Algorithm 62.1). Platelet survival in the circulation is approximately 7 to 10 days, and one-third of the platelets are sequestered in the spleen under normal circumstances.

Recognition of thrombocytopenia normally occurs after a complete blood count is drawn, but it is important to remember that mucocutaneous bleeding is a classic sign of thrombocytopenia. Bleeding from thrombocytopenia normally occurs only once the platelet count is <50,000/μL in postsurgical patients; spontaneous bleeding can occur with counts <5000/μL. The diagnostic approach starts with a thorough history and physical examination, followed by examination of the peripheral smear. A pathophysiologic approach to thrombocytopenia enables all common causes to be rapidly screened for and facilitates recognition of potential causes (Table 62.1). Careful attention should be paid to prescription and over-the-counter drugs (Table 62.2).

The common causes of thrombocytopenia in an ICU setting are as follows:

- Drug-induced (heparin, H_2-receptor blockers, GP2b3a inhibitors, antibiotics, alcohol)
- Sepsis
- Massive bleeding
- Thrombocytopenia with microangiopathic hemolytic anemia (thrombocytopenic thrombotic purpura [TTP], hemolytic uremic syndrome [HUS], disseminated intravascular coagulation [DIC]).

Clinical recognition of the cause is vital, as the therapies differ considerably depending on the etiology. For example, a patient with thrombocytopenia secondary to bleeding should be treated with platelets compared with a patient with TTP/HUS, in whom platelet transfusion is generally contraindicated. A few common conditions will be discussed, and readers are encouraged to refer to *Suggested Reading* for further details.

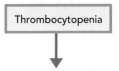

ALGORITHM 62.1   **Diagnostic Algorithm for Thrombocytopenia**

Thrombocytopenia

History and physical examination
- Drugs
- Current bleeding
- Neurologic symptoms and signs
- Recent viral illness
- Gastrointestinal bleeding
- Family history
- Travel history (malaria)
- EtOH use
- Splenomegaly
- Lymphadenopathy
- Petechiae
- Fundal hemorrhage

Peripheral smear
- Pseudothrombocytopenia (artifact)
- Schistocytes (TTP)
- Spherocytes (hemolysis)
- Left shift, bands (sepsis)
- Blasts (leukemia)
- Large platelets (peripheral destruction)
- Macrocytosis (liver disease, EtOH)

Review of complete blood count
- Concomitant cytopenias

Decreased platelet production

Increased platelet destruction

Increased platelet sequestration

EtOH, alcohol; TTP, thrombocytopenic thrombotic purpura.

TABLE 62.1	Pathophysiologic Classification of Thrombocytopenia	
Decreased production	Increased destruction	Increased sequestration
Aplastic anemia	Immunologic	Hypersplenism from any cause:
Hematologic malignancies	ITP	Cirrhosis
Lymphoma	Heparin-induced (HIT)	Portal hypertension
Leukemia	Drug-induced (see Table 62.2)	Congestive heart failure
Myelodysplasia	HIV	Hematologic malignancies
Metastatic malignancy	Autoimmune disease	Lipid storage disorders
Nutritional (vitamin B_{12} and folate)	Infectious	
Drugs (see Table 62.2)	Posttransfusion purpura	
Chemotherapy and radiation	Antiphospholipid antibody syndrome	
Alcohol	Nonimmunologic	
Viral infections	DIC	
HIV	HUS/TTP	
Mumps	HELLP syndrome	
Parvovirus	Preeclampsia/eclampsia	
Varicella	Malignant HTN	
Rubella	Sepsis	
Epstein–Barr	Cardiac valves (prosthetic endocarditis)	
Hepatitis C	Burns	
	Massive bleeding	

HIV, human immunodeficiency virus; ITP, immune thrombocytopenic purpura; HIT, heparin-induced thrombocytopenia; DIC, disseminated intravascular coagulation; HUS, hemolytic uremic syndrome; TTP, thrombotic thrombocytopenic purpura; HELLP, hemolysis, elevated liver enzyme levels and a low platelet count; HTN, hypertension.

IMMUNE THROMBOCYTOPENIC PURPURA

Immune thrombocytopenic purpura (ITP) is a condition caused by autoantibodies directed against the platelets surface glycoproteins. Binding of the antibodies results in accelerated platelet removal by the spleen. *Evans syndrome* refers to ITP together with autoimmune hemolytic anemia. The diagnosis of ITP is made by exclusion; checking for antiplatelet antibodies has no role in the diagnosis. Treatment consists of corticosteroids, intravenous immunoglobulin, anti-RhD antibodies, rituximab, danazol, cyclophosphamide, azathioprine, or splenectomy.

HEPARIN-INDUCED THROMBOCYTOPENIA

Type 1 Heparin-Induced Thrombocytopenia

Platelet counts often decline modestly in the first few days after starting therapy with a heparin product. This is a spontaneously resolving reversible decline with a platelet nadir above $100,000/\mu L$. This condition is not normally associated with complications.

TABLE 62.2	Common Drugs Associated with Thrombocytopenia	
Decreased production	Immune-mediated destruction	Unknown mechanism
Chemotherapeutic agents	Abciximab (all GP2b3a inhibitors)	Fluconazole
Busulfan	Amphotericin B	Ganciclovir
Cyclophosphamide	Aspirin	Nitrofurantoin
Cytosine arabinoside	Carbamazepine	Rifampin
Daunorubicin	Chloroquine	Valganciclovir
Methotrexate	Cimetidine	
6-Mercaptopurine	Clopidogrel	
Vinca alkaloids	Digoxin	
Estrogens	Eptifibatide	
Ethanol	Heparin	
Linezolid	Meropenem	
Thiazide diuretics	Phenytoin	
	Piperacillin	
	Quinine	
	Ranitidine	
	Trimethoprim/sulfamethoxazole	
	Valproic acid	
	Vancomycin	

Type 2 Heparin-Induced Thrombocytopenia

This is a much more serious disorder that occurs when patients develop antibodies against the heparin-platelet factor-4 complex. It can be induced by exposure to unfractionated or low-molecular-weight heparins. Important clues to the diagnosis include a >50% decline in the platelet count 5 to 10 days after being exposed to heparin for the first time. A more rapid decline in platelet counts can occur with prior heparin exposures. The platelet count is often well below $100,000/\mu L$ without clinical evidence of bleeding. In addition, patients may develop erythema or necrosis at heparin injection sites and systemic symptoms such as fever, wheezing, and tachycardia from heparin boluses. The major clinical problem with continued heparin exposure is not bleeding but devastating thrombotic complications in up to 50% of patients. These thromboses can be venous or arterial and can result in life-threatening complications such as limb ischemia, deep venous thrombosis, pulmonary embolism, myocardial infarction, cerebral sinus thrombosis, stroke, as well as mesenteric and renal infarction. When this diagnosis is suspected, all sources of heparin products should be immediately stopped, a serologic test (enzyme-linked immunosorbent assay [ELISA]) for heparin-dependent antibodies should be requested and the patient should be started on a direct thrombin inhibitor. The current ELISA for heparin-platelet factor-4 antibodies is highly sensitive but has low specificity. A more specific functional assay that measures platelet degranulation and serotonin release in response to heparin-platelet factor-4 complexes is also available at some centers to help confirm the diagnosis; however, therapy with a direct thrombin inhibitor should not be delayed if there is significant clinical concern for HIT. Currently available direct thrombin inhibitors include lepirudin (renally metabolized), argatroban (hepatically metabolized), and bivalirudin

(Food and Drug Administration approved for use in patients with HIT or suspected HIT undergoing percutaneous coronary interventions). Appropriate dosing of the thrombin inhibitors is critical to avoid bleeding complications and should be discussed with an ICU pharmacist. Platelets should not be given to patients with HIT unless there is life-threatening bleeding. Once the platelet count has demonstrated recovery to >100,000/μL, warfarin therapy should be initiated and the direct thrombin inhibitor should be continued until therapeutic anticoagulation with warfarin has been achieved.

SEPSIS-INDUCED THROMBOCYTOPENIA

Sepsis-induced thrombocytopenia is usually multifactorial and caused by marrow suppression, increased platelet destruction, drugs used to treat the septic patient, and associated DIC. Treatment is supportive and possible offending drugs should be stopped. Specific infections tend to cause thrombocytopenia, and physicians should be aware of the common culprits, according to their geographic location. In Missouri, ehrlichiosis needs to be considered and travelers should be screened for malaria. DIC is recognized by the combination of microvascular thrombosis and bleeding, thrombocytopenia, coagulopathy, and low fibrinogen levels. Treatment of this complication is supportive with therapy directed at the underlying cause and occasional use of platelets, fresh-frozen plasma, and cryoprecipitate for the actively bleeding patient.

THROMBOTIC THROMBOCYTOPENIC PURPURA

The diagnostic pentad of TTP is as follows:

- Microangiopathic hemolytic anemia
- Thrombocytopenia
- Renal failure
- Fever
- Altered mental status

However, all five criteria are met in <40% of patients. The major differential diagnosis is DIC. Both TTP and DIC are associated with thrombocytopenia, microangiopathic hemolytic anemia, and schistocytes. In DIC, there is often an associated coagulopathy with prolonged prothrombin time, activated partial thromboplastin time, and thrombin time, which should all be normal in TTP. In addition, fibrinogen levels in DIC are low and FDP levels are high, which should not be seen in TTP. The degree of thrombocytopenia is often more severe in TTP than in DIC, and the associated elevation in lactate dehydrogenase levels is also more profound.

Management of patients with TTP is challenging. Importantly, platelet transfusions in these patients are contraindicated in the absence of life-threatening bleeding, as they can precipitate vaso-occlusive crises of vital organs, such as the brain and myocardium. This disorder is caused by an acquired deficiency of ADAMTS13, which normally cleaves von Willebrand factor multimers. Absence of ADAMTS13 activity results in large circulating multimers of von Willebrand factor, which cause platelets to adhere to the endothelium with resultant thrombosis, thrombocytopenia, and shearing of red cells as they pass the thrombi, which causes a microangiopathic hemolytic anemia. The syndrome is most commonly precipitated by infections (*Escherichia coli* O157:H7 enteritis, human immunodeficiency virus) or drugs (ticlopidine, cyclosporin, tacrolimus, clopidogrel). Treatment consists of plasma exchange or fresh-frozen plasma/intravenous immunoglobulin if plasma exchange is not immediately available. The assay for ADAMTS13 plays no role in diagnosis in the acute setting.

PLATELET TRANSFUSIONS

The indications for transfusing platelets depend on the cause of the thrombocytopenia and the presence of bleeding. As previously noted, transfusions should be avoided in TTP and HIT unless the patient is experiencing life-threatening bleeding. For other causes, platelets should be transfused prophylactically when the platelet count is <10,000/μL to prevent spontaneous intracranial bleeding. For major surgery, the counts should be >100,000/μL; for minor procedures, the counts should be >50,000/μL.

SUGGESTED READINGS

Akca S, Haji-Michael P, de Mendonca A, et al. Time course of platelet counts in critically ill patients. *Crit Care Med.* 2002;30:753–756.
    This prospective, observational multicenter cohort study identified late thrombocytopenia (day 14) as being predictive of death and related changes in platelet count over time to patient outcome.

Arepally GM, Ortel TL. Clinical practice. Heparin-induced thrombocytopenia. *N Engl J Med.* 2006;355:809–817.
    An excellent recent review of the incidence, diagnostic algorithm, and therapies available.

Cines DB, Bussel JB. How I treat idiopathic thrombocytopenic purpura. *Blood.* 2005;106:2244–2251.
    A thorough review of the topic for clinicians.

George JN. Clinical practice. Thrombotic thrombocytopenic purpura. *N Engl J Med.* 2006;354:1927–1935.
    An excellent review of the topic for clinicians.

Lo GK, Juhl D, Warkentin TE, et al. Evaluation of pretest clinical score (4T's) for the diagnosis of heparin-induced thrombocytopenia in two clinical settings. *J Thromb Haemost.* 2006;4:759–765.
    A prospective study evaluating the diagnostic utility of a clinical scoring system for HIT based on using the 4 T's: Severity of the thrombocytopenia, timing of the thrombocytopenia, presence of thrombosis, and evaluating other causes of thrombocytopenia.

Rice TW, Wheeler AP. Coagulopathy in critically ill patients: Part 1: Platelet Disorders. *Chest.* 2009;136:1622–1630.
    An excellent clinically focused 2 part review of the common coagulopathies and platelet disorders encountered in the ICU.

Sekhon SS, Vivek R. Thrombocytopenia in adults: a practical approach to evaluation and management. *South Med J.* 2006;99:491–498.
    A concise review for clinicians with relevant suggestions for daily clinical practice.

Strauss R, Wehler M, Mehler K, et al. Thrombocytopenia in patients in the medical intensive care unit: bleeding prevalence, transfusion requirements, and outcome. *Crit Care Med.* 2002;30:1765–1771.
    Prospective observational study in a university hospital, found that 44% of patients developed ICU acquired thrombocytopenia. These patients had higher mortality, more bleeding, and greater transfusion requirements.

Vanderschueren S, De Weerdt A, Malbrain M, et al. Thrombocytopenia and prognosis in intensive care. *Crit Care Med.* 2000;28:1871–1876.

Prospective observational cohort study which identified thrombocytopenia as a readily available risk marker for mortality, independent of severity of disease indices.

Vincent JL, Yagushi A, Pradier O. Platelet function in sepsis. *Crit Care Med.* 2002;30:S313–S317.

A review of the multifactorial etiology of thrombocytopenia in septic patients and the role of platelets in modulating sepsis.

63

Acute Management of the Bleeding Patient/Coagulopathy

Yen-Michael S. Hsu and Brenda J. Grossman

Bleeding in the intensive care unit (ICU) is common and associated with several known etiologies. Initial evaluation of the patient by history and physical examination will usually lead to a cause of bleeding. A patient bleeding from a single site will most likely have a structural defect (e.g., site of trauma, gastrointestinal bleed), whereas a patient bleeding from multiple mucosal surfaces or from puncture sites most likely has a derangement in the coagulation or fibrinolytic systems of hemostasis. No history of bleeding suggests an acquired reason for bleeding, whereas a lifelong history of bleeding suggests a genetic or congenital etiology. Determining the cause of bleeding in the patient is paramount to rapid management and control of the bleeding.

Hemostasis is a tightly regulated process that involves complex interactions between circulating cellular proteins, blood cells, and vascular endothelial cells. This process can be divided into two phases: primary and secondary hemostasis. *Primary hemostasis* refers to a process that requires interactions between intact platelets, endothelial cells, and von Willebrand factor (vWF), which leads to the formation of a platelet plug. Abnormal primary hemostasis typically results in bleeding from mucosal surfaces (e.g., epistaxis, gastrointestinal bleeding, vaginal bleeding, or hematuria) and skin (petechia or prolonged bleeding at venipuncture sites). *Secondary hemostasis* refers to the formation of the fibrin clot and is achieved through the activation of coagulation proteins. Any significant deficiency in coagulation proteins or interference with their activations, and hence the formation of the fibrin clot, will lead to excessive bleeding. Abnormal secondary hemostasis may be clinically manifested by spontaneous bleeding from deep tissue sites (e.g., intraperitoneal bleeding, hemarthroses, and intramuscular hematomas). This chapter focuses on the identification and the management of bleeding that are primarily due to abnormalities in secondary hemostasis. Thrombocytopenia-related bleeding would be addressed in a separate chapter. Structural bleeding, such as gastrointestinal bleeding, is addressed in Chapters 48 and 49.

COAGULATION

Coagulation and subsequent fibrin formation have been historically represented as occurring by two distinct pathways (Fig. 63.1). The extrinsic or tissue factor (TF) pathway is classically triggered by tissue injury and release of TF into circulation, which then activates factor VII. The intrinsic pathway or contact activation pathway

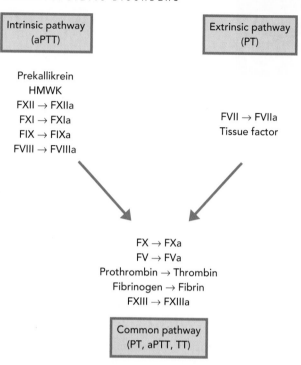

Figure 63.1. Classical Model of Hemostasis. The classical coagulation cascade is depicted as two distinct pathways converging on a common pathway. Although the pathways are not distinct *in vivo*, the distinct pathways can be measured *in vitro*. Disorders of the intrinsic pathway are measured by the activated partial thromboplastin time (aPTT), and disorders of the extrinsic pathway are measured by the prothrombin time (PT). HMWK, high-molecular-weight kininogen; FV/VII/VIII/IX/X/XI/XII, factors V/VI/VIII/IX/X/XII.

classically occurs in response to blood contact with an artificial or a negatively charged surface. Each pathway is depicted as the sequential activation of coagulation factors in the presence of calcium and phospholipids and converges onto a common pathway to form thrombin. Thrombin, in turn, cleaves fibrinogen to form fibrin and thus a clot is formed. These pathways do not act independently *in vivo*, but this concept is useful in for laboratory diagnosis and treatment of coagulpathies; defects in the extrinsic pathway are measured by the prothrombin time (PT) and defects in the intrinsic pathway by the activated partial thromboplastin time (aPTT).

More recently, a cell-based model of thrombin generation has been proposed to show the *in vivo* interaction between the classical pathways. This model proposes that the TF pathway initiates activation whereas the contact activation pathway amplifies the activation.

Screening Test for Coagulation

Initial testing to determine the cause of bleeding should include a PT, aPTT, and platelet count. If these fail to elucidate the cause of bleeding, further testing for platelet

TABLE 63.1	Rapid Interpretations of Abnormal Prothrombin Time and/or Activated Partial Thromboplastin Time in a Bleeding Patient	
PT result	aPTT result	Possible interpretation and associating conditions/coagulopathy
Normal	Normal	Platelet dysfunction, thrombocytopenia, factor XIII deficiency, α2-antiplasmin deficiency, plasminiogen activator inhibitor-1 deficiency
Prolonged	Normal	Liver diseases (early), factor VII deficiency/defect
Normal	Prolonged	Hemophilia A/B/C, Lupus anticoagulant[a]
Prolonged	Prolonged	Liver disease (end stage), vitamin K deficiency, warfarin therapy, disseminated intravascular coagulopathy, isolated fibrinogen, factor II, V, or X deficiency/defect

[a]Although Lupus anticoagulant is the most common cause for an isolated prolonged aPTT, it is not associated with bleeding.

function and deficiencies in the fibrinolytic pathway may be necessary. Table 63.1 lists the interpretation of the most common patterns of coagulation screening test.

Further Test to Assess Acute Bleeding

Thrombin Time (TT): It measures the conversion of fibrinogen to fibrin. Prolonged results occur when

- heparin or a direct thrombin inhibitor is in the test system;
- fibrinogen is decreased or abnormal;
- therapeutic fibrinolysis or fibrinogen degradation products (FDP) are present; and
- liver disease is severe.

Mixing Studies: These studies are conducted to determine the cause of a prolonged aPTT or PT.

These tests are performed to distinguish between factor deficiencies and inhibitors of coagulation. A 50:50 mix of patient's plasma and pooled normal plasma is tested immediately and after 1 hour incubation at 37°C. Figure 63.2 depicts the interpretation of mixing studies.

Platelet Function Test (e.g., PFA-100): In the presence of a normal platelet count and a hemoglobin level of at least 10 g/dL, PFA-100 is useful in detecting platelet dysfunction. Further laboratory testing such as platelet aggregation tests may be needed to characterize the platelet defect but will not alter the initial therapy.

COMMON ACQUIRED DISORDERS OF COAGULATION IN CRITICAL CARE SETTING

Vitamin K Deficiency and Warfarin Therapy

Causes
- Inadequate oral vitamin K intake
- Antibiotics

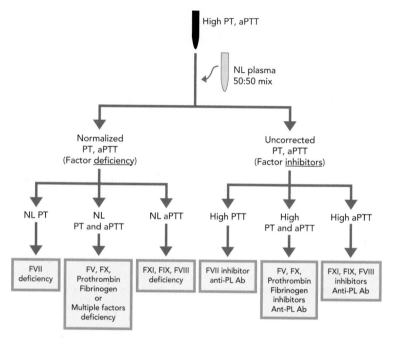

Figure 63.2. Mixing Analysis of Elevated Prothrombin Time (PT) and Activated Partial Thromboplastin Time (aPTT) in a Bleeding Patient. Patient's plasma is mixed with normal pooled plasma at 1:1 ratio, followed by subsequent retesting of PT and aPTT. Normalization of PT or aPTT suggests a factor deficiency. However, if mixing study does not correct the prolongation, this favors the presence of factor-specific or nonspecific inhibitors. NL, normal; FV/VI/VIII/IX/X/XI, factors V/VI/VIII/IX/X; anti-PL Ab, anti-phospholipid antibody.

- Generalized fat malabsorption
- Warfarin therapy

Pathophysiology

Vitamin K is a cofactor for γ-glutamyl carboxylation, which is required for the function of factors II, VII, IX, and X, protein C, and protein S. Therefore, patients with vitamin K deficiency often present with prolonged PT and elevated international normalized ratio (INR). Major sources of vitamin K are green and leafy vegetable, oil, and colonic flora. With daily requirement of 100 to 200 μg of vitamin K, a healthy adult has 1 week of vitamin K reserve with a restrictive diet.

Diagnosis

Measuring vitamin K–independent coagulation factors (i.e., factor V) is useful to distinguish vitamin K deficiency from liver disease. Vitamin K levels are not routinely measured. Ultimately, the diagnosis is made by a shortening of the PT in response to treatment with vitamin K. Failure to correct the PT after vitamin K administration suggest an alternative cause of bleeding.

Management

Vitamin K therapy may be given through intravenous (IV), subcutaneous (SC), or enteral routes. In a critically ill bleeding patient, the enteral route should generally be avoided because of high likelihood of gut dysfunction, whereas the SC route should be avoided in patients with perfusion defects or edema. There is a risk of anaphylaxis with IV administration of vitamin K; therefore, this route should be restricted in those situations where the SC or enteral routes are not feasible and the risk of anaphylaxis is considered justified. Unfortunately, in the critically ill patient, this is the most reliable route. A dose of 1 to 2 mg should be given either daily until the PT has corrected or for 3 days. Patients with milder forms of vitamin K deficiency may be treated with oral vitamin K of 5 to 20 mg, depending on the severity of deficiency. The effect of vitamin K supplement should be observed within 24 hours. In the setting of life-threatening bleeding (e.g., intracranial bleeding), fresh-frozen plasma (FFP) should be given at the initial dose of 10 to 15 mL/kg with concurrent slow administration of 10 mg of IV vitamin K.

Liver Disease

Causes

- Shock liver due to hypoperfusion
- Acute hepatitis
- Chronic liver disease
- Acute liver injury

Pathophysiology

Liver is the major organ that produces coagulation factors (except vWF and factor VIII) and fibrinolytic proteins. It is also important in clearing activated factors and inhibitors of coagulation. Insults to the liver are associated with bleeding abnormalities caused by factor deficiencies and accumulation of activated factors and inhibitors of coagulation, which may interfere with platelet function. In addition, hypersplenism is often associated with liver cirrhosis and portal hypertension and may cause thrombocytopenia.

Diagnosis

PT, aPTT, and INR are often elevated. In the absence of additional coagulation factor inhibitors, the abnormal clotting time may be corrected *in vitro* by the 50:50 mixing study. Measuring factor V and factor VII levels may help differentiate liver disease from vitamin K deficiency. Both factors are deficient in liver disease, whereas only factor VII is deficient in vitamin K deficiency.

Management

FFP, cryoprecipitate (rich source of fibrinogen), and platelets should be used in the setting of active bleeding. In general, a platelet count of $100,000/\mu L$, a fibrinogen level of >100 mg/dL, and PT <1.5 times normal control should be adequate to achieve hemostasis. The initial dose of FFP should be 10 to 15 mL/kg ($\sim$4 to 6 units). For thrombocytopenic patient, one unit of single donor platelets (or four units of random platelet concentrates) should be given with a posttransfusion platelet count dictating further dosing. Cryoprecipitate is usually given in pools of 10 units, which generally contain 2000 mg of fibrinogen in 150 mL. In rare cases, where bleeding is not controlled after adequate resuscitation with blood products, recombinant factor VIIa (RFVIIa) might be considered. RFVIIa has been associated with clinically significant thrombosis and should be used with caution. There is no well-defined study for the

TABLE 63.2	Underlying Conditions Commonly Associated with Disseminated Intravascular Coagulation
Sepsis	Abruptio placentae
Trauma	Uterine atony
CNS injury	Fat emboli
Heat stroke	Tumor lysis syndrome
Burns	Acute hemolytic transfusion reaction
Venomous snakebites	

CNS, central nervous system.

dosing in off-label use of RFVIIa; however, 20 to 90 μg/kg should provide adequate hemostatic control. In the absence of active bleeding, prophylactic FFP, cryoprecipitate, or platelet transfusion has not been shown to reduce bleeding risk or improve outcome.

Disseminated Intravascular Coagulation

Cause

There are many causes of disseminated intravascular coagulation (DIC) (Table 63.2). Most conditions associated with DIC can be categorized into conditions in which there is tissue damage, neoplasia, infection, or obstetric emergencies.

Pathophysiology

DIC is a consumptive coagulopathy with rapid and enhanced systemic activation of normal coagulation. Through consumption of coagulation and fibrinolytic factors and their inhibitors, an imbalance in this tightly regulated process occurs. Excessive fibrin clots are formed in small and mid-size blood vessels causing thrombotic occlusions and ultimately end-organ damage. Coagulation factors are quickly exhausted without adequate physiologic compensation and bleeding occurs.

Diagnosis

DIC is characterized by a prolonged PT/aPTT/TT, thrombocytopenia, and microangiopathic hemolytic anemia. The level of fibrinogen may be normal due to pathologic compensation in the early disease stage; however, significant hypofibrinogenemia is found in severe DIC. D-dimer and other FDP are useful to distinguish DIC from other coagulopathies with thrombocytopenia and by prolonged coagulation screening test.

Management

Primary goal of management is to treat the underlying disease causing DIC. Sometimes this is all that takes to stop the process. However, in most cases, this is not easily or rapidly accomplished and the patient will need further support. Resuscitation to maintain adequate perfusion is necessary, as acidosis will only exacerbate the coagulopathy. The role of FFP, cryoprecipitate, and platelets is unclear. In a bleeding patient, platelet transfusions (usually as a single-donor platelet or 4 to 6 platelet concentrates) are generally given to keep the platelet count above 50,000/μL and cryoprecipitate (usually in pools of 10 units) to keep the fibrinogen above 60 mg/dL. The role of antithrombin III concentrates and heparin is controversial in most cases of DIC. Heparin has been useful in cases of subacute DIC associated with acute promyelocytic leukemia, abdominal aortic aneurysm, and purpura fulminans.

Uremic Bleeding

Causes

Bleeding in patients with uremia is multifactorial, including intrinsic platelet dysfunction and abnormal platelet–vessel wall interactions. In addition, anemia contributes to increase bleeding because platelets flow more centrally in the vessel, making it less likely that they would interact with the injured vessel wall.

Pathophysiology

Accumulation of toxin (e.g., guanidinosuccinic acid) in plasma inhibits normal platelet activation and aggregation. Increase levels of nitric oxide and prostacyclan are found in patients with uremia as compared to nonuremic individuals and these negatively impact platelet adhesion to endothelium and platelet–platelet interactions. Defects in platelet function have been attributed to the environment in which the platelets exist, as incubation of platelets from a uremic patient into normal plasma corrects the dysfunction whereas placement of platelets from nonuremic individual into uremic plasma causes the defect to occur.

Diagnosis

Patients with uremia usually present with mucosal bleeding, such as gingival bleeding, epistaxis, and hematuria. Less commonly, central nervous system and severe gastrointestinal bleeding may occur. In addition to laboratory changes associated with decrease renal function, patients may present with a decrease in hemoglobin and mild thrombocytopenia. The most common laboratory abnormality, although not routinely performed, is decreased platelet aggregation in response exogenous agents. PT and aPTT are usually normal.

Management

Hemodialysis or peritoneal dialyses are the most effective methods to improve platelet function in patients with uremia. Red blood cell transfusions to correct anemia have been shown to decrease bleeding in the acute situation. Desmopressin (DDAVP) at a dose of 0.3 μg/kg IV or SC every 24 hours (or 10 units of cryoprecipitate when DDAVP has been ineffective or contraindicated) may temporarily control the bleeding. Platelet transfusions will not be effective in the setting of uremia. Once uremia is corrected, the patient's endogenous platelets should be functional.

MORE COMMON CONGENITAL DISORDERS OF COAGULATION

Hemophilia A and B

Cause

Hemophilia is a genetic deficiency in factor VIII or IX. Most individuals inherit the gene causing the deficiency, but up to 30% of deficiencies are caused by a spontaneous mutation. *Hemophilia A,* the most common type, is an X-linked genetic disorder that affects 1 in 5000 male births and up to 80% of all hemophilia individuals. The severity of hemophilia is categorized into mild, moderate, and severe forms correlating with the level of factor VIII deficiency (6%–30%, 2%–5%, and <1%, respectively). *Hemophilia B* is also an X-linked genetic disorder and has an incidence of 1 in 25,000 male birth worldwide, which contributes to 20% to 25% of the hemophilia cases. Hemophilia B is a deficiency of the factor IX protein. In contrast to factor VIII, which has a half-life of 8 to 12 hours, factor IX has longer half-life (24 to 25 hours) and wider tissue distribution.

Pathophysiology

In general, factor VIII and factor IX levels of ≥30% are needed for normal coagulation. With decreasing amounts of these factors, *in vivo* hemostasis is impaired. Primary hemostasis or platelet function is normal.

Diagnosis

Individuals with hemophilia will have an isolated prolongation in the aPTT. Those with severe hemophilia present with a lifelong history of spontaneous bleeding, which may include hemarthroses. Up to 30% of patients will present without a family history of bleeding. Individuals with moderate hemophilia will usually have an excessive bleeding history if trauma or surgery has occurred. Individuals with mild hemophilia might present with a prolongation in the aPTT without a history of excessive bleeding. The final diagnosis is made with the finding of decreased factor VIII or IX levels in patient's plasma.

Management

Treatment depends on the severity of the hemophilia and severity of bleeding.

Hemophilia A: DDAVP may be used to increase factor VIII levels by three- to fivefold in patients with mild and moderate forms of hemophilia A and should be tried in cases of mild bleeding. The typical dose, given intravenously or subcutaneously, is 0.3 μg/kg. The expected rise in factor VIII should occur within 5 to 8 hours. Patients with severe hemophilia and any bleeding will require factor concentrates for factor replacement. Factor VIII concentrates are either viral-inactivated plasma-derived or recombinant products. Both are effective and an individual choice is usually made on the basis of availability. Factor VIII concentrate is dosed by the patient's weight. A unit of factor VIII should increase the plasma level of factor VIII by 2% per kg of body weight. The goal of replacement therapy in patients with minor bleeding is a factor VIII level of 25% to 30%; with moderate to severe bleeding, it is 50%; and with surgical or life-threatening bleeding, it is 75% to 100%. Factor VIII concentrate has a half-life of 8 hours and levels should be monitored during treatment. Dosing is usually repeated every 8 to 12 hours, depending on the measured plasma levels of factor VIII. Treatment should be continued until the bleeding is stabilized. In the surgical patient, factor replacement is typically continued for 10 to 12 days after the procedure.

Some patients with hemophilia A will develop inhibitors to factor VIII, which will prevent the concentrates from working. In these patients, RFVIIa at a dose of 90 to 120 μg/kg every 2 hours may be given until hemostasis is achieved. These patients may consume an enormous amount of concentrates and should be managed by a hematologist experienced in the management of patients with inhibitors.

Hemophilia B: Plasma-derived and recombinant factor IX products are available for replacement therapy. Each unit of factor IX concentrate should raise the plasma factor IX level by 1% per kg of body weight. Factor IX half-life is 24 hours and therefore dosing should occur at 18- to 24-hour intervals. The subsequent doses are usually half the initial dose, but monitoring of plasma levels will help to adjust the dose as necessary. The goal of plasma levels of factor IX is similar to those noted earlier for factor VIII. Patients with inhibitors to factor IX should be treated with RFVIIa as noted earlier for patients with inhibitors to factor VIII.

von Willebrand Disease

Causes

von Willebrand disease (vWD) is a genetic disease caused by a deficiency or qualitative defect in vWF. It is inherited in an autosomal-dominate manner; therefore, men and women are equally affected.

Pathophysiology

vWF is a carrier molecule for factor VIII and normal levels are needed to maintain adequate levels of factor VIII in circulation. In addition, vWF is necessary for platelet adhesion to vessel wall at sites of injury and thus essential for normal platelet function. There are several types of vWD ranging from mild to severe quantitative disorder and several types with qualitative defects.

Diagnosis

Patients with vWD present with mucocutaneus bleeding (e.g., bleeding from gums, menorrhagia in women) and easy bruising. vWF antigen, Ristocetin cofactor activity and factor VIII levels are measured to determine the type of vWD. Types I (mild) and III (severe) are quantitative defects of vWF, whereas type II (several different defects) is a qualitative defect. von Willebrand multimer studies may be necessary to determine the type of vWD.

Management

DDAVP, which promotes the release of vWF, has been shown to be beneficial in raising the vWF in type 1 and certain type 2 vWD patients. It should not be used in individuals diagnosed with type IIb vWD or type III. If individuals are refractory to DDAVP or are severely deficient in vWF (type III vWD), Humate-P® or Wilate® should be given. The initial dose in severe bleeding or surgery is 40 to 60 Ristocetin cofactor units/kg, followed by 20 to 40 Ristocetin cofactor units/kg every 12 to 24 hours to keep vWF levels at 50 to 100 IU/dL for 7 to 14 days. For milder bleeding and surgery, an initial dose of 30 to 60 Ristocetin cofactor units/kg should be given, followed by 20 to 40 Ristocetin cofactor units/kg every 12 to 48 hours to keep the vWF above 30 IU/dL for 3 to 5 days. Antifibrinolytic agents, (e.g., aminocaproic acid, tranezamic acid) may be helpful adjuvant treatments to achieve hemostasis in patients bleeding from mucosal surfaces.

SUGGESTED READINGS

Hoffman M. A cell-based model of coagulation and the role of factor VIIa. *Blood Rev.* 2003;17:51–55.
A succinct review highlighting the importance of the cellular control of hemostasis in vivo.
Levi M, Hugo TC. Disseminated intravascular coagulation. *N Engl J Med.* 1999;341:586–592.
Review of diagnosis and management of DIC.
Levi M, Levy JH, Andersen HF, et al. Safety of recombinant activated factor VII in randomized clinical trials. *N Engl J Med.* 2010;363:1791–1800.
Analysis of thrombotic events in 35 randomized trials of off label use of recombinant VIIa.
MacLaren R, Wilson SJ, Campbell A, et al. Evaluation and survey of intravenous vitamin K1 for treatment of coagulopathy in critically ill patients. *Pharmacotherapy.* 2001;21:175–182.
Observational study and survey of vitamin K usage in ICU patients.
Mannucci PM. Treatment of von Willebrand's disease. *N Engl J Med.* 2004;351:683–694.
Review of laboratory diagnosis and treated of VWD.

Mannucci PM, Tuddenham EG. The hemophilias—from royal genes to gene therapy. *N Engl J Med.* 2001;344:1773–1779.

    Review of history, biology and treatment of hemophilias, including discussion plasma-derived and recombinant products.

Marks PW. Coagulation disorders in the ICU. *Clin Chest Med.* 2009;30:123–129.

    Review of mechanisms, laboratory abnormalities and management of coagulation disorder in ICU patients.

Noris M, Remuzzi G. Uremic bleeding: closing the circle after 30 years of controversies. *Blood.* 1999;94:2569–2574.

    Review of mechanism of bleeding in uremia.

Stravitz RT. Critical management decisions in patients with acute liver failure. *Chest.* 2008;134:1092–1102.

    Review of etiology, treatment and management of complications of acute liver failure.

64 Transfusion Practices

James C. Mosley, III and Morey A. Blinder

Anemia is a common problem in the intensive care unit (ICU) setting. In the critically ill patient, oxygen delivery and oxygen consumption may be impaired by factors such as decreased cardiac output, decreased red cell mass, decreased circulating blood volume from red blood cell (RBC) loss, and altered acid–base status. Causes of anemia in this setting are varied and include overt blood loss from bleeding or hemolysis, a functional decrease in usable iron, and decreased erythropoietin production.

Anemia is traditionally treated with infusions of RBCs to increase oxygen-carrying capacity and tissue delivery of oxygen. Various studies have estimated that more than 40% of all ICU patients receive blood transfusions and that more than 66% of these transfusions were not for replacement.

There is great variability in transfusion parameters and guidelines from center-to-center, and yet the optimal management of anemia in the ICU setting is not well defined. One approach compares a "transfusion-trigger" for a hemoglobin level <10 g/dL, a more "restrictive" pattern of transfusions for a hemoglobin value of <7 g/dL only. Although results vary, most studies have noted no increased mortality from the "restrictive" transfusion threshold of 7 g/dL, suggesting that hemoglobin levels of 7 to 9 g/dL are well tolerated in the critically ill patient. Furthermore, a trend toward increasing morbidity and mortality in groups with the more aggressive transfusion threshold for hemoglobin levels <10 g/dL has been noted. However, under circumstances of acute coronary syndromes, a clear trend toward increased survival has been demonstrated with transfusions for hemoglobin levels <10 g/dL. Nevertheless, transfusion practices must take into account systemic organ dysfunction that may affect oxygen delivery, anticipated blood losses, and overall patient morbidity, resulting in patient and situation-specific use of RBCs. It is currently recommended that, except in the circumstance of an acute coronary syndrome, patients be transfused for hemoglobin values of <7 g/dL, with a goal of maintaining hemoglobin levels of 7 to 9 g/dL.

DOSING AND ADMINISTRATION

Each unit of packed RBCs is approximately 300 mL and is generally given during 2 to 3 hours. One unit of packed RBCs is expected to increase hemoglobin by approximately 1 g/dL and raise the hematocrit by approximately 3% in a healthy individual without ongoing blood loss or destruction. Prior to transfusions, the patients' blood should be tested for ABO status, but type O-negative RBCs can be given in emergency situations.

TABLE 64.1	Blood Products	
Product	Indications	Comments
Packed red blood cells	• Increase oxygen-carrying capacity in patients with anemia • Can be used to increase blood volume in acute loss	• Transfusions to keep Hgb 7–9 g/dL in ICU setting • Data support higher levels in ACS
Platelets	• Thrombocytopenia with high risk of bleeding • *Not* indicated in presence of increased destruction without bleeding	• Prophylactic transfusion only if platelet count <10,000/μL. • Thresholds for procedures vary by institution
Fresh-frozen plasma	• Bleeding in setting of factor deficiency or coagulopathy • Warfarin reversal • Severe DIC	• Dosage ranges from 5–15 mL/kg, but generally start with 2 units and recheck PT/PTT
Cryoprecipitate	• Fibrinogen deficiency	• Contains fibrinogen as well as vWF, factors VIII, and fibronectin
Humate-P	• vWD types 2B, 2N, 3	• A specific vWF-containing factor VIII concentrate
Factors VIII and IX concentrates	• Hemophilia A and B treatment, respectively	• Virally inactivated • Recombinant technologies have eliminated infectious risks
Recombinant Factor VIIa	• Bleeding complications in acquired hemophilia A and B • Factor VII deficiency	• Recombinant • Used for surgery and acute bleeding in hemophilia

Hgb, hemoglobin; ICU, intensive care unit; ACS, acute coronary syndrome; DIC, disseminated intravascular coagulation; PT/PTT, prothrombin time/partial thromboplastin time; vWF, von Willebrand factor; vWD, von Willebrand disease.

TYPES OF RBC PRODUCTS

Table 64.1 presents some of the various blood products and their indications. Included in this section is further discussion of common products.

Whole Blood

Whole blood is currently used in autologous donation situations (prior to surgery, and so forth). Whole blood contains all normal constituents of human plasma, including RBCs, platelets, and plasma proteins.

Packed RBCs

Packed RBCs contain approximately 200 mL of RBCs resuspended in a preservative solution. Each bag has a hematocrit of approximately 55% to 60% and approximately 200 mg of iron.

Gamma-Irradiated

External-beam radiation is applied to the unit of blood to produce gamma-irradiated blood. This allows for destruction of donor T lymphocytes for prevention of graft-versus-host disease in stem cell transplant patients and severely immunocompromised patients.

Cytomegalovirus Antibody-Negative

Cytomegalovirus (CMV) antibody-negative blood is used in patients who are known to be CMV-negative and at high risk for complications if infected with CMV (e.g., transplant patients and pregnant patients). Leukocyte reduction is also a relatively effective method for reducing risk of CMV infection. Leukocyte reduction is performed most often at the time of product collection.

Washed RBCs

The donor cells are processed with normal saline to remove as much of the donor serum as possible. This is most commonly used in patients who are immunoglobulin A (IgA)-deficient and at a high risk for anaphylaxis during transfusions, as well as in paroxysmal nocturnal hemoglobinuria patients to deplete complement.

RISK OF TRANSFUSIONS

Transfusion of blood products carries risks. These risks can be divided on the basis of whether the complication is short term (related to each unit that is transfused) or long term (proportional to the total number of units that a patient receives over his or her lifetime).

Short-Term Transfusion Risks

Acute Hemolytic Reactions

The most serious and immediately life-threatening complication of transfusions is an acute hemolytic reaction. This is due to antibodies, usually immunoglobulin M, in the recipient's serum against major antigens present on the donor RBCs, and occurs with an estimated frequency of 1 in 250,000 to 1 in 1,000,000. This is initially manifested acutely as fever, dyspnea, tachycardia, back pain, hypotension, chills, and chest pain, within the first several minutes of the transfusion. If an acute hemolytic reaction is suspected, *the infusion should be stopped immediately*, and the blood bank notified. Algorithm 64.1 outlines management strategies for acute hemolytic reactions.

Delayed Hemolytic Reactions

Delayed hemolytic reactions usually occur more than 24 to 48 hours, and up to 7 to 10 days, after a transfusion. Delayed reactions result from antibodies in the recipient's serum that are directed toward minor antigens on the donor's RBCs, which are produced by an anamnestic response. This usually manifests as an asymptomatic but sudden decrease in hemoglobin concentration, with laboratory evidence of hemolysis, including a positive direct Coombs test and increased indirect bilirubin concentration.

ALGORITHM 64.1 Management of Acute Hemolytic Reaction

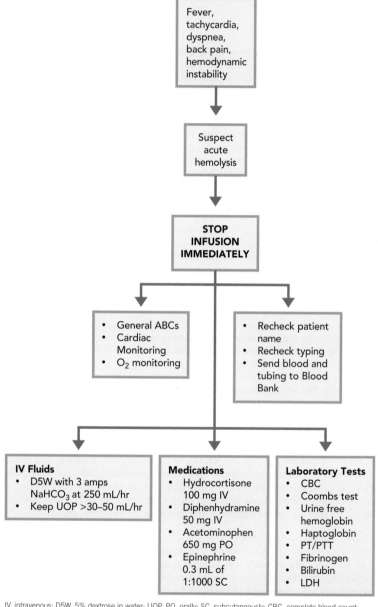

IV, intravenous; D5W, 5% dextrose in water; UOP, PO, orally; SC, subcutaneously; CBC, complete blood count; PT/PTT, prothrombin time/partial thromboplastin time; LDH, lactate dehydrogenase.

Nonhemolytic Febrile Reactions

Nonhemolytic febrile reactions occur in approximately 1% of transfusions and are the result of antibodies in the recipient's serum against white blood cells in the donor's product. This manifests acutely as an increase in body temperature and is more common in patients who have been previously alloimmunized by numerous transfusions. This reaction is treated with antipyretic medications.

Allergic Reactions

Allergic reactions occur because of transfused allergens in the donor's product, with symptoms such as urticaria and bronchospasm; they occur in approximately 1 in 100 transfusions. This condition is treated with antihistamine medications. However, a potentially severe form may be encountered in IgA-deficient individuals who can have anaphylactic reactions to serum from non–IgA-deficient donors. This is best prevented with washed RBCs, but can be treated with high-dose corticosteroids, airway protection, and antihistamines.

Transfusion-Related Acute Lung Injury

Transfusion-related acute lung injury (TRALI) occurs by a poorly understood mechanism, but an immune antibody-mediated process has been established in a majority of cases. A nonimmune mechanism has been postulated as well. Data from animal models and recent clinical studies suggest that both processes occur and that TRALI may be the end result of diffuse neutrophil activation and capillary leak by these mechanisms. TRALI presents with diffuse capillary damage in the pulmonary vasculature with rapid-onset dyspnea, hypoxia, fever, and bilateral pulmonary infiltrates resembling acute respiratory distress syndrome, in the absence of volume overload or heart failure. Treatment is supportive as most cases are self-limiting, but patients may require mechanical ventilation.

Bacterial Infection

Blood units can be contaminated with bacterial agents, including cold-growing organisms such as *Yersinia enterocolitica*, as well as various gram-negative organisms. Incidence of bacterial infection has dramatically decreased since the introduction of disposable plastic blood bags.

Long-Term Transfusion Risks

Viral Infections

Infectious complications of blood transfusions are located in Table 64.2. All blood products are currently screened for hepatitis B, hepatitis C, human immunodeficiency virus 1 and 2, and human T-lymphotropic virus I and II. Other infectious risks include viruses that are not screened for, such as CMV and parvovirus B19, and the prion transmitted Creutzfeldt–Jacob disease.

Iron Overload

Although not typically an issue in the ICU setting, secondary iron overload syndromes occur in proportion to the number of blood products a patient receives. Patients at highest risk include those with multiple transfusions over long periods of time (e.g., sickle-cell disease, thalassemias, myelodysplastic syndromes). Each milliliter of packed RBCs contains approximately 1 mg of iron. Patients who are repeatedly transfused in the absence of blood loss are at risk of overwhelming the body's ability to use iron with resultant deposition into tissues such as the myocardium, bone marrow, and liver.

TABLE 64.2	Transfusion-Associated Infections		
Virus	Risk factor (per million)	Estimated frequency (per unit)	No. of deaths (per million units)
Hepatitis A	1	1/1,000,000	0
Hepatitis B	7–32	1/30,000–1/250,000	0–0.14
Hepatitis C	4–36	1/30,000–1/150,000	0.5–17
HIV	0.4–5	1/200,000–1/2,000,000	0.5–5
HTLV I and II	0.5–4	1/250,000–1/2,000,000	0
Parvovirus B19	100	1/10,000	0

HIV, human immunodeficiency virus; HTLV, human T-lymphotropic virus.
Adapted from Goodnough et al. (1999), with permission.

SUGGESTED READINGS

Drews RE. Critical issues in hematology: anemia, thrombocytopenia, coagulopathy, and blood product transfusions in critically ill patients. *Clin Chest Med.* 2003;24:607–622.
A systematic review of diagnosis, evaluation, and treatment of blood and bleeding disorders commonly encountered in the critical care setting.

Goodnough LT, Brecher ME, Kanter MH, et al. Transfusion medicine: first of two parts. Blood transfusion. *N Engl J Med.* 1999;6:438–441.
A review article on principles of basic transfusion medicine, including complications and indications for transfusion.

Herbert PC, Wells G, Blajchman MA, et al. A Multicenter, randomized, controlled clinical trial of transfusion requirement in critical care. *N Engl J Med.* 1999;6:409–417.
A randomized trial of 838 ICU patients to receive transfusions for hemoglobin levels of less than 10 g/dL, or 7 g/dL. Overall 30-day mortality was similar in the two groups, but there was significantly less in-hospital mortality in patients transfused for hemoglobin levels less than 7 g/dL (22.2% vs. 28.1%, p 0.05), demonstrating that a "restrictive" transfusion strategy is well tolerated and potentially superior to liberal transfusion strategies.

McLellan SA, McClelland DB, Walsh TS. Anaemia and red blood cell transfusion in the critically ill patient. *Blood Rev.* 2003;17:195–208.
A review of anemia and transfusion strategies in critically ill patients.

Pajoumand M, Erstad BL, Camamo JM. Use of Epoetin Alfa in critically ill patients. *Ann Pharmacother.* 2004;38:641–648.
A review of the use of Epoetin Alfa for reduction of red blood cell transfusions in critically ill patients with anemia.

Triulzi DJ. Transfusion-related acute lung injury: an update. *Hematology Am Soc Hematol Educ Program.* 2006;497–501.
Review of current research and proposed mechanisms of TRALI.

Uy GL. Transfusion medicine. In: Lin TL, ed. *Hematology and Oncology Subspecialty Consult.* Baltimore: Lippincott, Williams & Wilkins; 2004:73–79.
Book chapter focusing on basic transfusion medicine and practical information about blood products and proper use.

Vincent JL, Baron JF, Reinhart K, et al. Anemia and blood transfusion in critically ill patients. *JAMA.* 2002;12:1499–1507.
A prospective observational study of patients in European ICUs evaluating the prevalence of anemia and transfusion use in this setting.

Hypercoagulable States

James C. Mosley, III

Hypercoagulable states are a heterogeneous group of inherited or acquired disorders that predispose individuals to the inappropriate formation of a clot in the venous or arterial circulation. The inappropriate formations of thrombi occur in the presence of Virchow's triad of hypercoagulability, stasis, and endothelial damage. Embolization of these clots can occur, resulting in pulmonary embolism (PE) in the case of venous embolic disease, or emboli to vital organs in the setting of arterial thrombosis.

Various manifestations of hypercoagulability are demonstrated in the intensive care unit (ICU) setting. Patients are at an increased risk of venous thromboembolic disease because of their prolonged immobilization, the numerous procedures that they are exposed to, and their underlying disease states. Patients in the ICU setting may have only transient risk factors for thromboembolic disease, or may also have underlying conditions that increase their risk. Listed in Table 65.1 are common causes of hypercoagulability.

DEEP VENOUS THROMBOSIS AND PULMONARY EMBOLISM

Deep venous thrombosis (DVT) and PE are very common in the ICU and are likely under-diagnosed. Some observational studies have demonstrated a 20% to 40% incidence of DVT in the ICU setting.

Diagnosis of DVT and PE in the ICU can be difficult (Algorithms 65.1 and 65.2). Various studies have demonstrated that 10% to 100% of DVTs diagnosed by ultrasound in this setting were not found on physical examination. Furthermore, patients in the ICU setting have a number of factors confounding the diagnosis, including their numerous comorbid conditions, inability to communicate symptoms, numerous procedures and medications, and inability to undergo various diagnostic tests. Table 65.2 lists the diagnostic modalities for DVT and PE.

Treatment of DVT and PE should commence when clinically suspected. As previously mentioned, diagnosis can be difficult in the ICU setting, but delay in treatment can lead to increased morbidity and mortality. Clinically suspected DVT or PE should be treated with weight-based unfractionated heparin or with low-molecular-weight heparin. Dosing guidelines for unfractionated heparin and alternatives are listed in Tables 65.3 and 65.4.

DVT prophylaxis decreases the incidence of PE and venous thromboembolism in the ICU patient. In general, all patients in the ICU should receive DVT prophylaxis if no contraindication exists.

TABLE 65.1	Causes of Hypercoagulability	
Acquired causes	**Inherited causes**
Trauma/surgery	Factor V Leiden mutation
Malignancy	Prothrombin G20210A mutation
Immobilization	Protein C deficiency
Nephrotic syndrome	Protein S deficiency
Obesity	Antithrombin deficiency
Pregnancy	Increased factor VIII activity
Oral contraceptive use	
Congestive heart failure	
Myeloproliferative disorders	
Antiphospholipid antibodies	
Lupus anticoagulant	
Anticardiolipin antibodies	

ARTERIAL THROMBOEMBOLISM

Acute arterial thrombosis can be secondary to embolization of material (e.g., from the atria in atrial fibrillation or from a proximal source secondary to a damaged artery), or an *in situ* formation of clot. Symptoms are generally related to the territory served by the artery that has thrombosed, and generally is noted as a painful, pale, and cool extremity, or an acute neurologic deficit in the case of a stroke. However, in the ICU setting, these symptoms may be masked by the patient's other comorbidities.

TABLE 65.2	Diagnostic Tests for Deep Venous Thrombosis (DVT) and Pulmonary Embolism (PE) in the Intensive Care Unit Setting	
Test	**Indication for testing**	**Key points**
Venous duplex ultrasound	Suspected DVT in extremities	• Good sensitivity and specificity for proximal DVT
Spiral computed tomography	Suspected PE	• Good sensitivity for large PEs • Contrast bolus predisposes to nephrotoxicity
Ventilation-perfusion scanning	Suspected PE	• Good sensitivity for PEs • Difficult to interpret in setting of recent pneumonia or other infiltrative process
Computed tomography angiography/ venography	Suspected DVT or PE	• Not widely available • Large bolus of contrast used

Adapted from Cook et al. (2005), with permission.

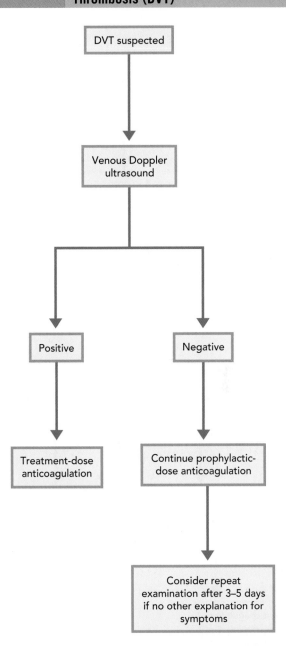

ALGORITHM 65.1   Algorithm for Diagnosis of Deep Venous Thrombosis (DVT)

ALGORITHM 65.2 **Algorithm for Diagnosis of Pulmonary Embolism (PE)**

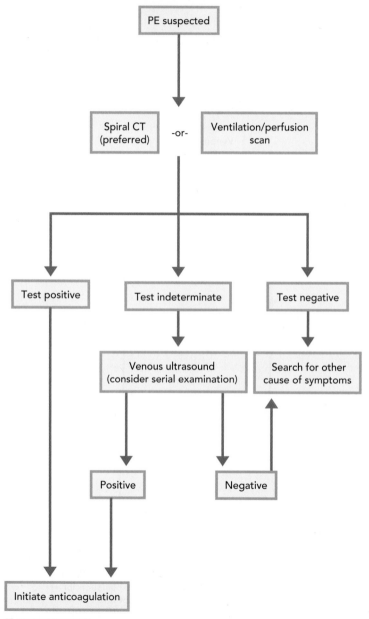

CT, computed tomography.

TABLE 65.3	Weight-Based Unfractionated Heparin Dosing

Initial Dose
Bolus 60–80 U/kg
Infusion 14–18 U/kg/hr

Adjustment: aPTT[a]

<40	2.000 units IV bolus and increase infusion rate by 2 U/kg/hr
40–44	Increase infusion rate by 1 U/kg/hr
45–70	No change
71–80	Decrease infusion by 1 U/kg/hr
81–90	Hold infusion for 30 min, decrease infusion rate by 2 U/kg/hr
>90	Hold infusion for 1 hr, decrease infusion rate by 3 U/kg/hr

IV, intravenous.
[a]aPTT should be drawn 6 hr after any adjustment to dose.

TABLE 65.4	Alternative Anticoagulants

Drug	Mechanism of action	Use	Prophylaxis dosing	Therapeutic dosing
Enoxaparin	Inactivation of factor Xa	Prophylaxis and treatment of DVT/PE	40 mg SC q24h	1 mg/kg SC q12h or 1.5 mg/kg SC q24h
Dalteparin	Inactivation of factor Xa	Prophylaxis and treatment of DVT/PE	5000 units SC q24h	100 U/kg SC q12h or 200 U/kg SC q24h
Fondaparinux	Inactivation of factor Xa	Prophylaxis and treatment of DVT/PE, HIT	2.5 mg SC q24h	7.5 mg SC q24h or 10 mg SC q24h if >100 kg
Lepirudin	Direct thrombin inhibitor	HIT	0.1 mg/kg/hr IV	0.4 mg/kg IV bolus, then 0.15 mg/kg/hr IV
Argatroban	Direct thrombin inhibitor	Treatment of thrombosis in HIT	2 μg/kg/min IV	

DVT, deep venous thrombosis; PE, pulmonary embolism; SC, subcutaneously; HIT, heparin-induced thrombocytopenia; IV, intravenous.

Clues from the physical examination can yield evidence as to the source of the thrombosis. Multiple sites of ischemia are typical of an embolic phenomenon (but can also be seen in the setting of vasculitis), whereas isolated ischemia is more typical of *in situ* thrombosis. Further evaluation of suspected arterial thrombosis can be performed with compression ultrasound, although computed tomography angiography is often more helpful.

Treatment of suspected arterial thrombosis should be instituted immediately, as delay in treatment can result irreversible damage due to ischemic tissue. Anticoagulation should be initiated as outlined in Tables 65.3 and 65.4, and surgical consultation should be sought for possible operative management.

HYPERCOAGULABILITY EVALUATION

Patients in the ICU have many transient risk factors for the development of thromboembolic disease. Because of this, most instances of thromboembolism do not warrant workup for an underlying hypercoagulable state. The optimal time for laboratory evaluation of hypercoagulable states is unclear, but is often undertaken approximately 6 weeks to 6 months after the event. Laboratory evaluation in the immediate days to weeks following a thrombosis can yield false results because of the increase in acute-phase reactants associated with acute clot formation, which can result in false-positive tests for hypercoagulable states. However, in the setting of recurrent thrombosis, cerebral vein or visceral vein thrombosis, and nonembolic arterial thrombosis, further evaluation is warranted. Minimal workup should include evaluation for lupus anticoagulant, anticardiolipin antibody, and fasting plasma homocysteine level. In cases marked by recurrent thrombosis or cerebral or visceral vein thrombosis, further workup should include a prothrombin G20210A mutation analysis as well as a factor V Leiden mutation analysis. Hematology consultation should be obtained for further evaluation and long-term treatment planning.

CONDITIONS ASSOCIATED WITH DECREASED PLATELETS AND HYPERCOAGULABILITY

There are occasional conditions that present with thrombocytopenia as well as hypercoagulability. Heparin-induced thrombocytopenia is a serious condition manifested by the formation of antibodies to platelets in response to heparin administration. This condition can cause thrombosis in the setting of severe thrombocytopenia, and is discussed in detail in Chapter 62.

Thrombotic thrombocytopenia purpura is another condition associated with hypercoagulability and thrombocytopenia. This serious condition is the result of a deficiency of or inhibitor to the von Willebrand factor cleaving protease, ADAMTS 13. It is manifested by thrombocytopenia, microangiopathic changes on peripheral blood smear (schistocytes), fever, mental status changes, and varying degrees of renal insufficiency. Treatment is emergent and requires immediate hematology consultation and plasma exchange. This condition is discussed further in the Chapter 61.

Disseminated intravascular coagulation can also present with thrombocytopenia and coagulopathy in the setting of hypercoagulability. Underlying conditions such as sepsis, ischemia, acidosis, and multiorgan failure can induce a consumptive coagulopathy, resulting in the formation of diffuse thrombi as well as diffuse hemorrhage.

SUGGESTED READINGS

Cook D, Douketis J, Crowther MA, et al. The diagnosis of deep venous thrombosis and pulmonary embolism in medical-surgical intensive care unit patients. *J Crit Care.* 2005; 25:314–319.
Review of current data investigating diagnostic modalities for DVT and PE with focus on patients in the critical care setting.

Geerts WH. Prevention of venous thromboembolism in high-risk patients. In: *American Society of Hematology Education Program Book.* Washington, D.C.: American Society of Hematology; 2006:462–466.
Review of prophylactic modalities for DVT in patients in various clinical circumstances.

Levine JS, Branch DW, Rauch J. The antiphospholipid syndrome. *N Engl J Med.* 2002;10: 752–763.
A review of the pathogenesis, diagnosis, and treatment strategies of the Antiphospholipid Antibody Syndrome.

Nachman RL, Silverstein R. Hypercoagulable states. *Ann Intern Med.* 1993;8:819–827.
A review of the major pathophysiologic mechanisms underlying inherited and secondary hypercoagulable states and review of the frequency, natural history, diagnosis, and management of the disorders.

Peles S, Pillot, G. Thrombotic disease. In: Pillot G, Chantler M, Magiera H, et al, eds. *Hematology and Oncology Subspecialty Consult.* Baltimore: Lippincott, Williams & Wilkins, 2004:25–32.
Edited book chapter describing hypercoagulable disease states, with focus on diagnosis and treatment strategies.

Rosenberg RD, Aird W. Vascular-Bed specific hemostasis and hypercoagulable states. *N Engl J Med.* 1999;20:1555–1564.
A review of the pathophysiologic mechanisms underlying coagulation disorders on a cellular level, describing the interaction of coagulation factors with vascular-bed–specific cellular signaling pathways.

Tabatabai, A. Disorders of hemostasis. In: Ahya SN, Flood K, Parajothi S, eds. *Washington Manual of Medical Therapeutics.* 30th ed. Baltimore: Lippincott, Williams & Wilkins, 2001:394–412.
Edited book chapter describing differential diagnosis, diagnostic strategies, and treatment modalities for hypercoagulable states, as well as bleeding disorders.

66 Maternal–Fetal Critical Care

Jeanine F. Carbone and Molly V. Houser

Although, most pregnant patients are young and healthy and less than 1% will require admission to the intensive care unit, the overall acuity of this patient population remains high. Most admissions will be secondary to obstetric complications such as hypertensive disorders from eclampsia/severe preeclampsia and hemorrhage. However, there are many other conditions for which a critical care practitioner should be prepared. To fully understand how to take care of this vulnerable patient population, it is important to understand the basic physiologic adaptations that occur in the mother in response to the demands of pregnancy (Table 66.1).

OXYGENATION AND RESPIRATORY SUPPORT DURING PREGNANCY

Normal physiologic changes of pregnancy increase oxygen delivery to the placenta and the fetus. Fetal oxygenation is dependent on maternal oxygen status. It is important to note that pregnancy is a chronically compensated state of respiratory alkalosis with a maternal pH of 7.40 to 7.47. Respiratory alkalosis is secondary to the increase in minute ventilation, which leads to a decrease in $PaCO_2$. This is compensated for by increased renal excretion of bicarbonate (normal value in pregnancy: 18 to 22 mEq/L).

Pregnancy itself increases oxygen consumption by 15% to 20%. Bearing in mind the physiologic changes in ventilation during pregnancy and the fetal oxygen dissociation curve, tighter parameters for oxygenation are required to maintain maternal and fetal well-being. The same respiratory support devices used in nonpregnant patients may be used in pregnant patients. Respiratory support should be aggressive, and the goal should be to maintain maternal SpO_2 ≥95% to 96% as to sustain adequate oxygen perfusion to the fetus. When determining necessity of intubation, airway edema related to pregnancy and decreased maternal reserve should be considered.

RESPIRATORY FAILURE

Diagnosis of respiratory distress may be difficult in the gravid patient, because about half of all pregnant women will have complaints of shortness of breath, fatigue, and decreased exercise tolerance. A careful evaluation of these symptoms is imperative to discern between normal pregnancy complaints and respiratory compromise. The most

TABLE 66.1	Physiologic Changes of Pregnancy
Cardiovascular	
Blood pressure	Decreased (reaches a nadir in the second trimester)
Heart rate	Increased (17%)
Cardiac output	Increased (40%)
Stroke volume	Increased (25%)
Systemic vascular resistance	Decreased (20%)
Hematologic	
Blood volume	Increased (40%–50%)
Coagulation factors	Increase in fibrinogen, vWF, clotting factors II, VII, VIII, IX, and X, and protein C resistance. Decrease in protein S
Red blood cell mass	Increased
White blood cell count	Increased
Hemoglobin	Decreased (12.5 g/dL at term)
Platelets	Decreased (secondary to hemodilution)
Renal	
Glomerular filtration rate	Increased (50%)
Renal plasma flow	Increased (50%–75%)
BUN and creatinine	Decreased
Urinary protein excretion	Increased
Pulmonary	
Tidal volume	Increased (40%)
Respiratory rate	Little to no change
Minute ventilation	Increased (40%)
Vital capacity	Unchanged
FEV_1	Unchanged
Residual volume	Decreased (20%)—secondary to elevated diaphragm
FRC	Decreased (20%)—secondary to elevated diaphragm
Inspiratory capacity	Increased (5%–10%)—secondary to decreased FRC

vWF, von Willebrand factor; BUN, blood urea nitrogen; FEV_1, forced expiratory volume in the first second of expiration; FRC, functional residual capacity.

common causes of respiratory failure in pregnancy are pulmonary embolus, pulmonary edema (secondary to preeclampsia, cardiomyopathy, or tocolytic induced), infection, and asthma. Clinical recognition and treatment of a pregnant patient in respiratory failure are extremely important, as maternal oxygen status affects fetal oxygen status. A change in fetal heart rate pattern may be one of the first signs of maternal respiratory failure. A general rule of thumb is to stabilize the maternal condition before considering delivery. If indicated, initiating mechanical ventilation in the mother will likely improve fetal condition (Algorithms 66.1 and 66.2).

ALGORITHM 66.1 **Differential Diagnosis for Respiratory Distress**

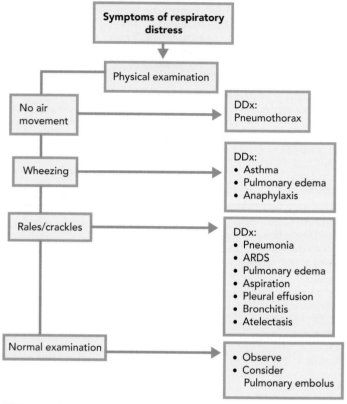

ARDS, acute respiratory distress syndrome; DDx, differential diagnosis.

AMNIOTIC FLUID EMBOLISM

Amniotic fluid embolism (AFE) is a rare but devastating obstetric disorder. Although uncommon with an incidence of about 1 in 20,000 deliveries, the maternal mortality rate can be as high as 60%. The pathophysiology of AFE is poorly understood. It appears to be due to an abnormal maternal immune response to fetal antigens, which is why AFE is sometimes referred to as an anaphylactoid syndrome of pregnancy. There are no known identifiable risk factors in pregnant women that predispose them to AFE. Classically, a pregnant women in labor, post–cesarean delivery, postdilation and evacuation, or 30 minutes postpartum will present with a sudden onset of acute hypoxia, acute hypotension ± cardiac arrest, followed by fetal hypoxia (if patient is antepartum), and consumptive coagulopathy. Unfortunately, for women who suffer from an AFE in its classic form, maternal death is the most common outcome (Algorithm 66.3).

ALGORITHM 66.2 Asthma

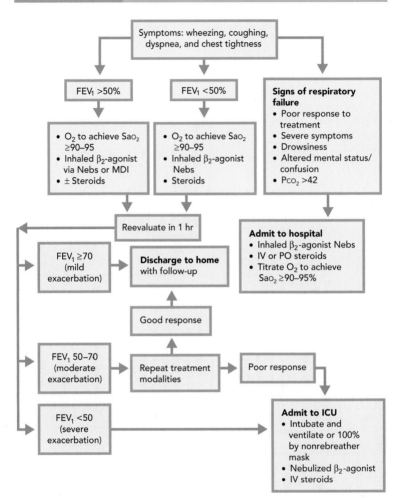

FEV₁, forced expiratory volume in the first second of expiration; Nebs, nebulizers; MDI, metered dose inhaler; Sao₂, oxygen saturation; ICU, intensive care unit.

VENOUS AIR EMBOLISM

Venous air embolism (VAE) is the entrapment of air from an open operative field into venous vasculature, producing systemic effects. It can occur at any time during delivery but most commonly seen with cesarean deliveries with an incidence ranging from 10% to 97%. VAE has been reported to be responsible for about 1% of all maternal deaths. There have also been case reports of VAE arising with oral genital sex during pregnancy and the use of home inflatable perineal stretching devices.

ALGORITHM 66.3   Amniotic Fluid Embolus

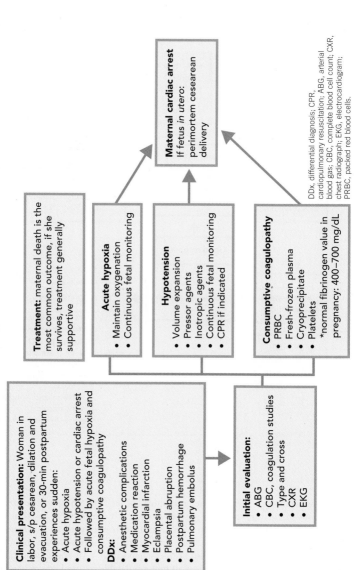

Clinical presentation: Woman in labor, s/p cesarean, dilation and evacuation, or 30-min postpartum experiences sudden:
- Acute hypoxia
- Acute hypotension or cardiac arrest
- Followed by acute fetal hypoxia and consumptive coagulopathy

DDx:
- Anesthetic complications
- Medication reaction
- Myocardial infarction
- Eclampsia
- Placental abruption
- Postpartum hemorrhage
- Pulmonary embolus

Initial evaluation:
- ABG
- CBC, coagulation studies
- Type and cross
- CXR
- EKG

Treatment: maternal death is the most common outcome, if she survives, treatment generally supportive

Acute hypoxia
- Maintain oxygenation
- Continuous fetal monitoring

Hypotension
- Volume expansion
- Pressor agents
- Inotropic agents
- Continuous fetal monitoring
- CPR if indicated

Consumptive coagulopathy
- PRBC
- Fresh-frozen plasma
- Cryoprecipitate
- Platelets
- *normal fibrinogen value in pregnancy: 400–700 mg/dL

Maternal cardiac arrest
If fetus *in utero*: perimortem cesearean delivery

DDx, differential diagnosis; CPR, cardiopulmonary resuscitation; ABG, arterial blood gas; CBC, complete blood cell count; CXR, chest radiograph; EKG, electrocardiogram; PRBC, packed red blood cells.

ALGORITHM 66.4 Venous Air Embolism (VAE)

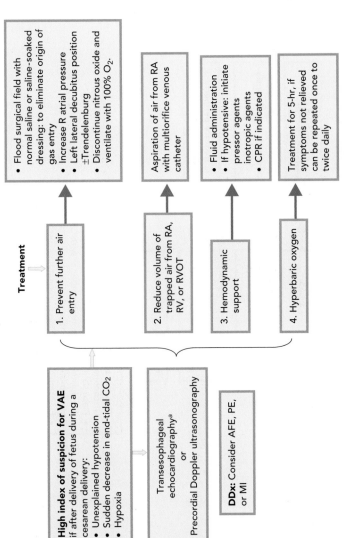

High index of suspicion for VAE
if after delivery of fetus during a
cesarean delivery:
- Unexplained hypotension
- Sudden decrease in end-tidal CO_2
- Hypoxia

Transesophageal
echocardiography[a]
or
Precordial Doppler ultrasonography

DDx: Consider AFE, PE,
or MI

Treatment

1. Prevent further air entry
- Flood surgical field with normal saline or saline-soaked dressing: to eliminate origin of gas entry
- Increase R atrial pressure
- Left lateral decubitus position ±Trendelenburg
- Discontinue nitrous oxide and ventilate with 100% O_2.

2. Reduce volume of trapped air from RA, RV, or RVOT
- Aspiration of air from RA with multiorifice venous catheter

3. Hemodynamic support
- Fluid administration
- If hypotensive: initiate pressor agents inotropic agents
- CPR if indicated

4. Hyperbaric oxygen
- Treatment for 5-hr, if symptoms not relieved can be repeated once to twice daily

[a]Most sensitive device for diagnosing VAE. RA, right atrium; RV, right ventricle; RVOT, right ventricular outflow tract; AFE, amniotic fluid embolism; PE, pulmonary embolism; MI, myocardial infarction; CPR, cardiopulmonary resuscitation.

ALGORITHM 66.5 **Differential Diagnosis for Pulmonary Edema in Pregnancy**

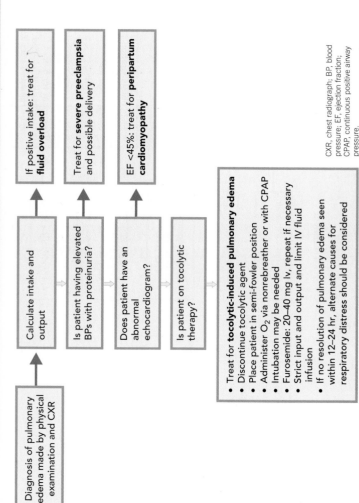

Diagnosis of pulmonary edema made by physical examination and CXR

↓

Calculate intake and output → If positive intake: treat for **fluid overload**

Is patient having elevated BPs with proteinuria? → Treat for **severe preeclampsia** and possible delivery

Does patient have an abnormal echocardiogram? → EF <45%: treat for **peripartum cardiomyopathy**

Is patient on tocolytic therapy?

Treat for tocolytic-induced pulmonary edema
- Discontinue tocolytic agent
- Place patient in semi-fowler position
- Administer O₂ via nonrebreather or with CPAP
- Intubation may be needed
- Furosemide: 20–40 mg Iv, repeat if necessary
- Strict input and output and limit IV fluid infusion
- If no resolution of pulmonary edema seen within 12–24 hr, alternate causes for respiratory distress should be considered

CXR, chest radiograph; BP, blood pressure; EF, ejection fraction; CPAP, continuous positive airway pressure.

ALGORITHM 66.6   Acute Renal Failure in Pregnancy

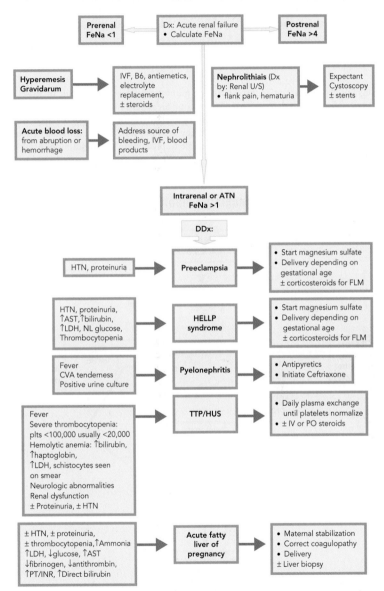

IVF, intravascular fluid; U/S, ultrasonography; ATN, acute tubular necrosis; FeNa, fractional excretion of Na$^+$; HELLP, hemolysis elevated liver enzymes and low platelets; TTP/HUS, thrombotic thrombocytopenic purpura/hemolytic uremic syndrome; CVA, costovertebral angle; Plts, platelets; HTN, hypertension; LDH, lactose dehydrogenase; AST, aspartate aminotransferase; PT/INR, prothrombin time/international normalized ratio; FLM, fetal lung maturity; NL, normal.

Symptoms of VAE are complaints of chest tightness, shortness of breath, hypotension, arrhythmias, and hypoxemia. Other conditions in pregnancy have similar clinical manifestations, so the differential diagnosis must include AFE, pulmonary embolism, pneumothorax, bronchospasm, pulmonary edema, and myocardial infarction (Algorithm 66.4).

PULMONARY EDEMA IN PREGNANCY

Pregnant women are at increased risk of pulmonary edema due to an increase in plasma volume and a decrease in colloid oncotic pressure. The most common causes of pulmonary edema in pregnancy are secondary to tocolytic use, cardiogenic causes, fluid overload, and preeclampsia. Tocolytic therapy accounts for 25% of pulmonary edema in pregnant patients, and it is most amenable to prevention by careful monitoring of tocolytic use in mothers having preterm labor. This complication can be seen during

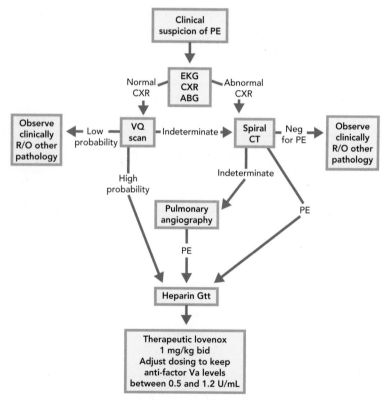

ALGORITHM 66.7 Pulmonary Embolism (PE)

EKG, electrocardiogram; CXR, chest radiograph; ABG, arterial blood gas; CT, computed tomography; R/O, rule out; VQ, ventilation-perfusion.

tocolytic use or after discontinuation. Patients with pulmonary edema often present with complaints of dyspnea, tachycardia oxygen desaturation, and tachypnea. On physical examination, bilateral crackles should always be present and sometimes an S3 gallop may be ascultated. It is important to note that an S3 gallop can also be a normal manifestation in pregnancy, especially in the third trimester, secondary to increased blood volume. Chest radiographs will usually demonstrate bilateral diffuse interstitial

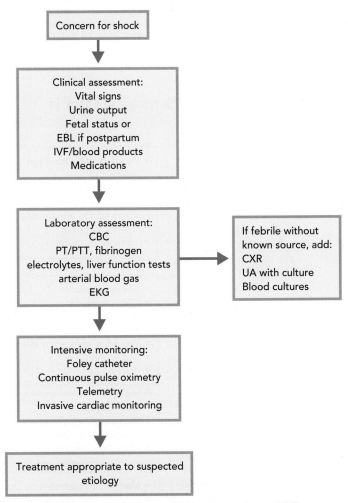

ALGORITHM 66.8 **Management of Shock in Pregnancy**

Concern for shock

↓

Clinical assessment:
Vital signs
Urine output
Fetal status or
EBL if postpartum
IVF/blood products
Medications

↓

Laboratory assessment:
CBC
PT/PTT, fibrinogen
electrolytes, liver function tests
arterial blood gas
EKG

→

If febrile without
known source, add:
CXR
UA with culture
Blood cultures

↓

Intensive monitoring:
Foley catheter
Continuous pulse oximetry
Telemetry
Invasive cardiac monitoring

↓

Treatment appropriate to suspected
etiology

EBL, estimated blood loss; IVF, intravascular fluid; CBC, complete blood cell count; PT/PTT, prothrombin time/partial thromboplastin time; EKG, electrocardiogram; CXR, chest radiograph; UA, urinalysis.

opacities with a reticular pattern, and echocardiogram will be normal (Algorithms 66.5, 66.6, and 66.7).

SHOCK IN PREGNANCY

The most common causes of shock in pregnancy are from hemorrhage and sepsis. The pathophysiology of shock in pregnancy falls into the same categories as that in nonpregnant patients, and treatment of each type of shock is essentially unchanged. Choice of antibiotics in septic shock should take fetal safety into consideration when alternative treatments are available. Regardless of the etiology of shock, therapy involves identifying and eliminating the originating cause, providing adequate fluid replacement, and improving cardiac function and circulation. Aggressive resuscitation of the mother usually adequately resuscitates the fetus (Algorithms 66.8 and 66.9).

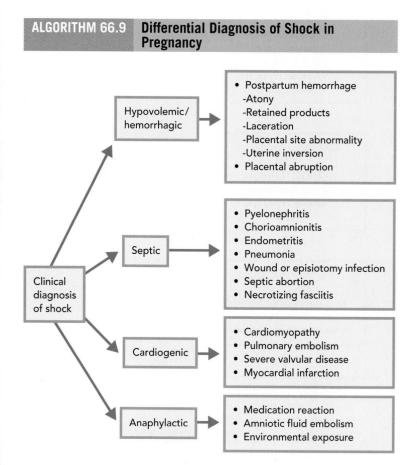

ALGORITHM 66.9 Differential Diagnosis of Shock in Pregnancy

SUGGESTED READINGS

Bandi VD, Munnur U, Matthay MA. Acute lung injury and acute respiratory distress syndrome in pregnancy. *Crit Care Clin.* 2004;20(4):577–607.

Clark SL. Amniotic fluid embolism. *Clin Obstet Gynecol.* 2010;53(2):322–328.

Cunningham FG, Leveno KJ, Bloom SL, et al. Maternal physiology. In: Cunningham FG, et al., eds. *Williams obstetrics.* New York, NY: McGraw-Hill, 2005:121–150.

Dildy GA, Belfort MA. eds. Critical care obstetrics. 4th ed. Malden, MA: Blackwell Science, 2004.

Foley MR, Strong TH, Garite TJ. Obstetric intensive care manual. In: Foley MR, Strong TH, Garite TJ, eds. New York, NY: McGraw-Hill, 2004:390.

Kim CS, Liu J, Kwon JY, et al. Venous air embolism during surgery, especially cesarean delivery. *J Korean Med Sci.* 2008;23(5):753–761.

Lombaard HP, Soma-Pillay P, Farrell el-M. Managing acute collapse in pregnant women. *Best Pract Res Clin Obstet Gynaecol.* 2009;23(3):339–355.

Martin JN Jr, Stedman CM. Imitators of preeclampsia and HELLP syndrome. *Obstet Gynecol Clin North Am.* 1991;18(2):181–198.

Martin SR, Foley MR. Intensive care monitoring of the critically ill pregnant patient. In: Creasy RK, et al., eds. Creasy and Resnik's maternal-fetal medicine principles and practice. Philadelphia, PA: Saunders Elsevier, 2009:1167–1194.

Sciscione AC, Ivester T, Largoza M, et al. Acute pulmonary edema in pregnancy. *Obstet Gynecol.* 2003;101(3):511–515.

Shaikh N, Ummunisa F. Acute management of vascular air embolism. *J Emerg Trauma Shock.* 2009;2(3):180–185.

Sheffield JS. Sepsis and septic shock in pregnancy. *Crit Care Clin.* 2004;20:651–660; viii.

Sibai BM. Imitators of severe preeclampsia. *Obstet Gynecol.* 2007;109(4):956–966.

Zeeman GG. Obstetric critical care: a blueprint for improved outcomes. *Crit Care Med.* 2006;34(9 Suppl):S208–S214.

Zeeman GG, Wendel GD Jr, Cunningham FG. A blueprint for obstetric critical care. *Am J Obstet Gynecol.* 2003;188(2):532–536.

67 Preeclampsia and Eclampsia

Molly J. Stout and Laura A. Parks

Preeclampsia is a disorder of pregnancy, characterized by hypertension and proteinuria that typically occurs after 20 weeks of gestation. It can also occur in the early postpartum period. Preeclampsia complicates approximately 12% to 22% of all pregnancies and is directly responsible for 17% of maternal deaths in the United States. Risk factors for preeclampsia include a history of preeclampsia in a prior pregnancy, primigravida, women younger than 20 years or older than 35 years, multifetal gestations, obesity, underlying chronic hypertension or chronic renal insufficiency, and connective tissue disorders.

The exact pathophysiologic mechanism for preeclampsia is unknown but likely has to do with dysregulation of placental factors such as regulators of angiogenesis, growth factors, cytokines, and regulators of vascular tone ultimately leading to poor perfusion to many organs including the central nervous system (CNS), kidneys, as well as the fetoplacental unit. It is notable that the underlying physiology of preeclampsia has to do with placental trophoblastic tissue and can occur in the absence of a fetus, as seen in women with a hydatidiform mole mole.

DIAGNOSIS

Preeclampsia can manifest with wide-ranging severity of disease, from asymptomatic hypertension and proteinuria to life-threatening neurologic, renal, or coagulopathic abnormalities. Hypertension is defined at blood pressure ≥ 140 systolic or ≥ 90 diastolic in a woman with previously normal blood pressure. Proteinuria is defined at urinary excretion of 300 mg of protein in a 24-hour urine collection. Severe preeclampsia is diagnosed if any of the following are present:

1. Blood pressure of ≥ 160 systolic or ≥ 110 diastolic on two occasions 6 hours apart
2. Proteinuria of ≥ 5 g in a 24-hour urine specimen (or 3+ on random urine dip on two occasions at least 4 hours apart)
3. Oliguria (>500 mL in 24 hours)
4. Neurologic or visual disturbances (including headache)
5. Pulmonary edema
6. Epigastric or right upper quadrant pain
7. Elevation in transaminases
8. Thrombocytopenia
9. Fetal growth restriction
10. Eclampsia—new-onset grand-mal seizures in a woman with preeclampsia

TABLE 67.1	End-Stage Complications in Patients with Preeclampsia/Eclampsia
System	Complications
CNS	Seizures, cerebrovascular hemorrhage, temporary cortical blindness
Cardiopulmonary	Critical hypertension, heart failure, cardiopulmonary arrest, pulmonary edema
Renal	Acute renal failure
Hepatic	Subcapsular hematoma, hepatic rupture with hemorrhage
Hematologic	Disseminated intravascular coagulation, hemolysis
Fetal	Fetal demise, placental abruption, intrauterine growth restriction, preterm delivery

CNS, central nervous system.

Mild preeclampsia can progress to severe preeclampsia quickly depending on the severity of disease, and women with mild preeclampsia must be monitored for development of criteria of severe preeclampsia. Severe, life-threatening complications are listed in Table 67.1.

The syndrome of hemolysis, elevated liver enzymes, and low platelets (hemolysis, elevated liver enzymes [HELLP] syndrome) is a life-threatening variant of severe preeclampsia. Women with HELLP syndrome may present with vague epigastric discomfort or mild nausea and vomiting. Notably, HELLP can be found in patients with minimal or absent hypertension and proteinuria. The laboratory findings in HELLP syndrome overlap with other life-threatening complications of pregnancy such as acute fatty liver of pregnancy and thrombotic thrombocytopenic purpura, which should be considered in the differential diagnosis. The main differential diagnosis of preeclampsia/eclampsia/HELLP syndrome is presented in Table 67.2, and several helpful laboratory tests are presented in Table 67.3. HELLP syndrome is associated with an increased risk for both maternal and fetal adverse outcomes including placental abruption, renal failure, recurrent preeclampsia, preterm delivery, and maternal or fetal death.

Eclampsia is defined as preeclampsia with generalized tonic-clonic seizures and/or coma. Approximately 50% of all cases of eclampsia are diagnosed during the antepartum period, 20% present with an intrapartum event, and the remaining 30% are diagnosed during the postpartum period. Although most postpartum seizures occur in the first 48 hours, cases have been reported as late as 3 weeks after delivery. Notably, nearly 15% of women with eclampsia initially present without hypertension and another 15% may lack proteinuria. Furthermore, the severity of hypertension and the amount of proteinuria in a preeclamptic patient are poor predictors of progression to eclampsia.

Women with underlying chronic hypertension or proteinuria present a diagnostic challenge. Worsening hypertension relative to measurements early in pregnancy or hypertension that becomes refractory to antihypertensive medications can be used as diagnostic clues. In addition, worsening proteinuria from previous urine dipsticks or a baseline 24-hour urine protein obtained early in pregnancy can also be used. Certainly, any development of end-organ damage or HELLP syndrome suggests superimposed severe preeclampsia.

TABLE 67.2	Key Differential Diagnosis of Severe Preeclampsia/ Eclampsia/HELLP

1. CNS
   a. Seizure disorder
   b. Hypertensive encephalopathy
   c. Cerebrovascular
      i. Intraventricular-intracerebral hemorrhage
      ii. Arterial embolism or thrombosis
      iii. Hypoxic ischemic encephalopathy
      iv. Angioma, atrioventricular malformation, or aneurysm
   d. Reversible posterior leukoencephalopathy syndrome
   e. Tumors
   f. Cerebral vasculitis
2. Thrombotic thrombocytopenic purpura
3. Acute fatty liver of pregnancy
4. Metabolic disease
   a. Hypoglycemia
   b. Hyponatremia

HELLP, syndrome of hemolysis, elevated liver enzymes, and low platelets.
Modified with permission from differential diagnosis figure. Sibai BM. Diagnosis, prevention, and management of eclampsia. *Obstet Gynecol.* 2005;105:402–410.

PATHOPHYSIOLOGY BY ORGAN SYSTEM

Vascular

Hemoconcentration and hypertension are the main vascular changes in preeclampsia. Women with preeclampsia may not develop the normal hypervolemia of pregnancy. Vascular reactivity mediated by alterations in prostaglandins, prostacyclin, nitric oxide, and endothelins cause intense vasospasm and intravascular contraction. Alterations in plasma oncotic pressure can cause third spacing of fluid manifested as edema. Careful attention to fluid status is required, as aggressive resuscitation with crystalloids or colloids can often cause pulmonary edema.

Hematologic

Hematocrit may be increased secondary to hemoconcentration. In the context of HELLP syndrome, hematocrit may be low due to hemolysis. Thrombocytopenia also characterizes HELLP syndrome.

Hepatic

Elevation of transaminases is often seen in severe preeclampsia. Hepatic hemorrhage with hepatic capsule irritation may cause right upper quadrant pain. Hepatic rupture is rare but is associated with catastrophic outcome.

Central Nervous System

Eclampsia and intracranial hemorrhage are associated with increased maternal mortality. Temporary blindness, headache, blurred vision, scotomata, and hyperreflexia are also CNS signs and symptoms of severe preeclampsia.

TABLE 67.3 Imitators of Preeclampsia/HELLP: Laboratory Findings

Laboratory finding	Normal pregnancy	Preeclampsia/HELLP	TTP	AFLP
Hematocrit	↓ 4%–7%	↑ with hemoconcentration ↓ with hemolysis	↓	↔
Platelet count	Slight ↓, but remains >150,000 μL	↓	↓	↔ to slight ↓
Fibrinogen	↑ (nl >300 mg/dL)	↔ or may ↓ with thrombocytopenia, DIC	↔	↓
PT and PTT	↔	↔ except in DIC	↔	↑
Serum creatinine	↓	↑	↑	↑
Serum uric acid	↓ 33%	↑	↑	↑
Urine protein	↑ but remains <300 mg/day Protein/creatinine ratio <0.19[a]	↑ >300 mg/day Protein/creatinine ratio >0.19[a]	↔ to ↑ ↔ to ↑	↔
Hepatic transaminases	↔	↑	↑	↑
WBC	Slight ↑	↔	↔	↑
LDH	↔	↑	↑	↑
Glucose	↔	↔	↔	↓
Ammonia	↔	↔	↔	↑
Bilirubin	↔	↑	↑	↑ (>5 mg/dL)

[a]Shown to correlate strongly with 24-hour urine protein quantity.

Modified with permission from Sibai BM. Imitators of severe preeclampsia/eclampsia. *Clin Perinatol.* 2004;31:835–852.

HELLP, syndrome of hemolysis, elevated liver enzymes, and low platelets; TTP, thrombotic thrombocytopenic purpura; AFLP, acute fatty liver of pregnancy; DIC, disseminated intravascular coagulation; PT, prothrombin time; PTT, partial thromboplastin time; WBC, white blood cell; LDH, lactate dehydrogenase; nl, normal.

Renal

Normal pregnancy physiology involves an increased glomerular filtration rate and renal blood flow resulting in decreased creatinine. Vasospasm in preeclampsia causes a reversal of this normal physiologic change, and oliguria and increased creatinine may occur.

Fetal

Intrauterine growth restriction, oligohydramnios, and placental infarctions may be seen as manifestations of preeclampsia.

TREATMENT

The definitive treatment of severe preeclampsia, eclampsia, and HELLP syndrome is delivery. The decision to proceed with delivery must balance maternal and fetal risks. Close attention should be initially paid to the medical stability of the mother, with consideration of specific target organs (Algorithm 67.1). Magnesium sulfate is the preferred antiseizure drug in the setting of preeclampsia/eclampsia. It is provided as an initial intravenous load of 4 to 6 g over 20 minutes, followed by continuous infusion of 2 g/hr. During seizures, the patient's airway should be protected and adequate oxygenation ensured. If seizures recur while the patient is receiving magnesium, a repeat (4 g) bolus of magnesium may be given. Other alternatives include intravenous administration of amobarbital or benzodiazepines (lorazepam or diazepam). Because magnesium undergoes renal clearance, serum levels should be assessed in any woman with evidence of impaired renal function and the dose adjusted as needed to sustain a blood level between 4 and 7 mEq/L (4.8 to 8.4 mg/dL, 2 to 4 mmol/L). Meticulous attention to pulmonary status and deep tendon reflexes on clinical examinations should be used in women on magnesium sulfate infusions to prevent magnesium intoxication, which in the most severe form can cause cadiorespiratory collapse. Phenytoin may be used in women with impaired renal function or compromised cardiopulmonary function. Seizure prophylaxis should continue for 24 hours after delivery and extended if the patient does not demonstrate evidence of improvement.

Once maternal stabilization is accomplished, the well-being of the fetus should be assessed using heart rate monitoring and ultrasonography, as emergency cesarean delivery is often necessary when the fetal status worsens. The priority of maternal stabilization is particularly important during periods of maternal seizures, which may be associated with impaired fetal oxygenation and nonreassuring fetal status. However, fetal status often improves with stabilization of maternal status.

The predominant cause of fetal morbidity and mortality is prematurity. Mild forms of preeclampsia may be expectantly managed to minimize the risk of prematurity and allow administration of corticosteroids for fetal lung maturity. However, severe preeclampsia involving eclampsia, persistent hypertension despite medical therapy, persistent CNS symptoms, pulmonary edema, HELLP syndrome, coagulopathy, oliguria, and acute renal failure require expedited delivery. When severe preeclampsia presents in the postpartum period, magnesium sulfate may still be used to prevent eclamptic seizures. Similarly, if preeclampsia is diagnosed in association with molar pregnancy, uterine evacuation and curettage are needed to remove retained placental fragments.

Unlike other hypertensive disorders, the course of preeclampsia/eclampsia is not influenced by antihypertensive therapy. Treatment with these medications is designed to prevent stroke and congestive heart failure. Furthermore, the preeclamptic patient

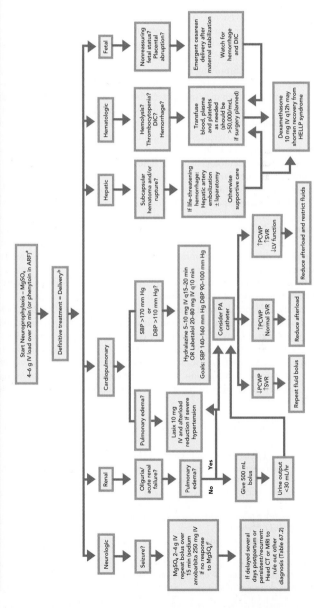

[a]The loading dose of magnesium is followed by MgSO₄ 2 g/hr with adjustment for therapeutic magnesium levels (4–7 mEq/L, 4.8–8.4 mg/dL).
[b]See exception in the text for a very preterm fetus (<32 wk) in a stable preeclamptic patient.
[c]Consider lorazepam or diazepam IV with careful attention to respiratory depression.

ARF, acute renal failure; SBP, systolic blood pressure; DBP, diastolic blood pressure; DIC, disseminated intravascular coagulation; IV, intravenous; CT, computed tomography; MRI, magnetic resonance imaging; PA, pulmonary artery; PCWP, pulmonary capillary wedge pressure; SVR, systemic vascular resistance; LV, left ventricle; HELLP, hemolysis, elevated liver enzymes, and low platelets.

is often edematous secondary to extravasation of fluid into the interstitial tissues in the setting of capillary leakiness and reduced oncotic pressure. This results in reduced intravascular volume despite the increase in total whole-body water that characterizes the disease. Therefore, vasodilatation should be performed carefully, as it may contribute to diminished organ perfusion, which may also impact uteroplacental perfusion and jeopardize the undelivered fetus. The use of furosemide should be reserved for the treatment of pulmonary edema. Antihypertensive drugs, including hydralazine, calcium channel blockers, or labetalol, are generally administered for the treatment of diastolic blood pressure levels of ≥ 110 mm Hg or systolic blood pressure levels >170 mm Hg. There is no clear evidence that one of these antihypertensive agents is superior to the others for improving maternal and/or fetal outcomes. Although not routinely indicated, head imaging using computed tomography or magnetic resonance imaging of preeclamptic women may reveal reversible posterior leukoencephalopathy. Conditions that may prompt providers to obtain CNS imaging studies in order to rule out cerebrovascular hemorrhage or other diseases include lateralizing signs, prolonged unconsciousness, papilledema, seizures while on magnesium sulfate, delayed presentation >48 hours after delivery, or an uncertain diagnosis of eclampsia with suspicion of alternative etiologies for neurologic abnormalities.

Most women with preeclampsia/eclampsia are expected to have a full recovery after delivery and removal of trophoblastic tissue. It is rare for patients to develop chronic renal failure or permanent neurologic deficits following preeclampsia. The recovery phase is heralded by the onset of increased diuresis, which can be expected within 24 hours after delivery but, in rare cases, can be delayed up to 1 week postpartum. Because of the high incidence of preeclampsia in pregnancy, the severe sequelae of the disease are among the most common indications for admission of a pregnant or postpartum patient to an intensive care unit. With thorough, prompt, and coordinated care by perinatal and critical care specialists, most patients will recover from preeclampsia/eclampsia without residual disease.

Unfortunately, evidence does not suggest the use of aspirin or other supplements for the prevention of preeclampsia. In addition, no screening test has been found to be reliable and cost-effective. Thus, the appropriate clinical and diagnostic judgment at the time of presentation is required. Women with multiple pregnancies complicated by preeclampsia, or early-onset disease, may suggest future health risks including a predisposition for chronic hypertension and metabolic syndrome. Age-appropriate screening tests should be used with the recognition of possible increased risk for disease later in life.

SUGGESTED READINGS

American College of Obstetricians and Gynecologists. *Diagnosis and Management of Preeclampsia and Eclampsia.* Washington, DC: American College of Obstetricians and Gynecologists, January 2002. Practice Bulletin 33.

Baxter JK, Weinstein L. HELLP syndrome: the state of the art. *Obstet Gynecol Surv.* 2004;59: 838–845.
  Review of the history, pathophysiology, clinical presentation, differential diagnosis, and management of HELLP syndrome.

Dekker G, Sibai B. Primary, secondary, and tertiary prevention of preeclampsia. *Lancet.* 2001;357:209–215.
  Review of risk factors for preeclampsia, methods of early detection, and the failure of primary and secondary prevention of the disease, highlighting the need for proper antenatal care and timed delivery in tertiary prevention.

Duley L, Henderson-Smart DJ, Meher S. Drugs for treatment of very high blood pressure during pregnancy. *Cochrane Database Syst Rev.* 2006;3:CD001449.

> *A review of 24 trials of medications used in the treatment of severe hypertension in pregnancy, demonstrating that hydralazine, labetalol, and calcium channel blockers are acceptable options.*

Isler CM, Barrilleaux PS, Rinehart BK, et al. Postpartum seizure prophylaxis: using maternal clinical parameters to guide therapy. *Obstet Gynecol.* 2003;101:66–69.

> *Prospective clinical study demonstrating that clinical criteria could be used successfully to shorten the duration of postpartum magnesium sulfate administration for seizure prophylaxis in preeclamptic patients.*

Lucas MJ, Leveno KJ, Cunningham FG. A comparison of magnesium sulfate with phenytoin for the prevention of eclampsia. *N Engl J Med.* 1995;333:201–205.

> *A randomized clinical trial demonstrating the superiority of magnesium to phenytoin in the prevention of eclampsia.*

Mabie WC. Management of acute severe hypertension and encephalopathy. *Clin Obstet Gynecol.* 1999;42:519–531.

> *Review of the pathophysiology and management of preeclampsia, briefly discussing the similarities and differences between eclampsia and hypertensive encephalopathy.*

Sibai BM. Imitators of severe preeclampsia/eclampsia. *Clin Perinatol.* 2004;31:835–852.

> *Review of disorders which should be included in the differential diagnosis of severe preeclampsia, focusing on acute fatty liver of pregnancy and thrombotic microangiopathies.*

Sibai BM. Diagnosis, prevention, and management of eclampsia. *Obstet Gynecol.* 2005;105:402–410.

> *Comprehensive review of eclampsia—timing of onset, cerebral pathology associated with the disease, differential diagnosis, maternal and perinatal outcomes, prevention, and management.*

Sibai BM, Mercer BM, Schiff E, et al. Aggressive versus expectant management of severe preeclampsia at 28 to 32 weeks gestation: a randomized controlled trial. *Am J Obstet Gynecol.* 1994;171:818–822.

> *A randomized trial demonstrating maternal and fetal safety with expectant management of severe preeclampsia less than 32 weeks, resulting in decreased neonatal morbidity.*

Walker JJ. Preeclampsia. *Lancet.* 2000;356:1260–1265.

> *Review of the pathophysiology, diagnosis, management, morbidity and mortality associated with preeclampsia.*

Zeeman GG. Obstetric critical care: a blueprint for improved outcomes. *Crit Care Med.* 2006;34:S208–S214.

> *Review of critical care issues in the obstetric patient and treatment options for preeclampsia and massive obstetric hemorrhage.*

68 Trauma Care for the Intensive Care Unit

Kevin W. McConnell and Douglas J.E. Schuerer

Care of the traumatically injured patient is a complex issue, given the multiple potential systems that are injured. This chapter reviews the initial evaluation and treatment of the trauma patient, then focuses on injuries that are most likely to cause early intensive care unit (ICU) death in this population. In addition, we review the management of the most likely problems that will result in an ICU admission. Any critical care of the trauma patient must be in conjunction with the various specialists that are needed for this population, including general surgery, neurosurgery, orthopaedic surgery, facial surgery, hand surgery, and rehabilitation medicine. This team approach is essential to ensure positive outcomes in the acutely injured patient. Another important factor in trauma care is that the trauma patient is often younger than the normal ICU population, and despite often initially becoming extremely ill, all have a high potential for recovery. Because of the brevity of this guide, it cannot be a thorough review of all traumatic injuries, but instead focuses on the most life-threatening ones that are related to eventual ICU care.

TRAUMA EVALUATION

The basic tenets of the initial resuscitation and management of the injured patient are described in the advanced trauma life support course. The course was designed to teach all physicians the basics of trauma care to better standardize and improve early interventions. Most trauma patients are initially evaluated in an emergency department, but transfers and other reasons may place a nonevaluated trauma patient directly in the ICU.

Primary Survey

The primary survey is commonly remembered as the ABCDEs of trauma. It is performed rapidly but completely and systematically to avoid missing injuries.

Airway

Assess for:

1. Obstruction, including foreign bodies, facial fractures, or bleeding. Begin measures to remove obstruction and establish airway.
2. Patency, which may be compromised because of head injury, intoxication, or swelling.

Note: Patients who are verbal without hoarseness or stridor usually have a patent airway, but this does not rule out future airway compromise. Maneuvers to obtain a definitive airway should begin immediately on recognition of the problem and before other lifesaving interventions.

Potential problems:

1. Swelling leading to delayed airway collapse.
2. Inability to obtain airway in a paralyzed patient; surgical airway a must.
3. Unknown laryngeal or tracheal disruption.

Breathing and Ventilation
Assess for:

1. Adequate chest wall excursion not limited by mental status, rib fractures, or pain.
2. Loss of or diminished breath sounds on either side from pneumothorax, hemothorax, pulmonary contusion, or other lung pathology.
3. Evidence of bruising or laceration to the chest.
4. Deviated trachea from tension pneumothorax or neck hematoma.

Potential problems:

1. Airway compromise and ventilation failure may be difficult to discern from one another.
2. Massive pulmonary injuries may falsely seem to be airway-related because of severe dyspnea.
3. Airway placement may worsen some pulmonary issues because of positive pressure ventilation (worsening pneumothorax).

Circulation with Hemorrhage Control
Assess for:

1. Blood volume and cardiac output
   a. Mental status deteriorates with increasing amounts of blood loss and progression of hemorrhagic shock.
   b. Ashen gray skin and poor capillary refill both imply poor circulation.
   c. Pulses are a marker of perfusion in the younger patient without vascular disease. Full and regular pulses are positive. Fast, thready, or diminished pulses likely delineate poor global flow or decreased flow to the affected extremity. Irregular pulses may indicate blunt cardiac injury.
2. Bleeding
   a. External blood loss is recognized readily and is best stopped by direct pressure. Multiple layers of gauze make tamponade more difficult. Tourniquets should not be used except in unusual circumstances.
   b. Occult bleeding from internal hemorrhage should be expected if patient has signs of shock.
   c. Potential sources are:
      i. Abdomen: bruising, tenderness, or distension.
      ii. Chest: decreased breath sounds, evidence of rib fractures.
      iii. Pelvis: unstable pelvis, pelvic bony pain.
      iv. Legs: femur fracture may have up to two units of blood in thigh.

Potential problems:

1. Patients on beta-blockade may not get tachycardic as a response to bleeding or anemia.
2. Elderly patients have less reserve and may decompensate quickly.
3. Children have more reserve and will not show signs of shock until severely volume-depleted.
4. Multiple occult sources for blood loss may exist in any one patient.

Disability or Neurologic Status

Rapid neurologic examination:

1. Glasgow Coma Score total score (3–15)
   a. Eye opening (1–4)
   b. Motor response (1–6)
   c. Verbal response (1–5)
2. Pupillary size and reactivity
3. Lateralizing signs
4. Spinal injury level

Potential problems:

1. Intoxication masking or reproducing a closed head injury.
2. Lucid intervals can be seen before compromise from intracranial lesions.

Exposure/Environmental Control

1. All clothing and dressings need to be removed to inspect for injuries and examination.
2. After assessment, patient should be covered as quickly as possible and warmth maintained. Hypothermia worsens bleeding and outcomes in trauma.

Resuscitation: During and continuing after the primary survey, resuscitation should be performed while completing each portion of the survey.

1. Airway: a definitive airway should be established if there is loss of the airway for any reason. If there is doubt or worsening of swelling, the airway should always be obtained early when it is safest.
2. Breathing and ventilation
   a. Add high-flow oxygen to all patients.
   b. If airway obtained, ensure continued ventilation with hand-bagging or a ventilator.
   c. Pneumothoraces and hemothoraces need to be released to permit adequate ventilation.
3. Circulation:
   a. Two large-bore intravenous (IV) lines should be obtained. If no peripheral IV access, consider a large-bore (not triple-lumen) catheter into a major vein.
   b. Adult interosseous needles are now available as well.
   c. Consider area of injury before placing IV access.

Adjuncts to the primary survey: Certain interventions are important in the resuscitation of the trauma patient. These are normally performed during the primary survey or immediately afterward.

1. Electrocardiographic monitoring: usually continuous on a monitor. Formal electrocardiogram may be needed if arrhythmias or possible ST segment changes present.

2. Pulse oximetry: helpful in assessing perfusion status and blood oxygenation trends.
3. Urinary catheter: assesses for blood and follow urine output. Risk of problems by not assessing for signs of urethral injury first (bruising at perineum, blood at meatus, high-riding prostate.)
4. Gastric catheter: assesses stomach contents for blood and evacuates stomach to lessen the risk of aspiration. Consider risk of intracranial injuries with nasogastric tube in patients with facial injuries.
5. Continuous blood pressure monitoring: may need arterial line if critically unstable, but this should not delay definitive care.
6. Chest plain films if major blunt or penetrating trauma; pelvic films if blunt trauma or penetrating wound to abdomen. Other films are determined after the secondary survey.

Secondary survey: The secondary survey is a thorough examination and assessment of the entire patient after the primary survey is complete and resuscitation is started. The following list is not exhaustive, but shows an example of what each body area examination should include.

1. History
   a. AMPLE History
      i. A – allergies
      ii. M – medications
      iii. P – past illness/pregnancy
      iv. L – last meal
      v. E – events of the injury
   b. Should include accident details or type of gun or knife used
2. Head: lacerations, bruises, eye injuries, vision
3. Maxillofacial: facial stepoffs, facial nerve injuries, intraoral mandible fractures
4. Neck: spine tenderness, trachea midline, hematomas
5. Chest: bruises, tenderness, change in breath sounds, crepitus, uneven chest excursion
6. Abdomen: bruising, tenderness, distention, evisceration of bowel or omentum.
7. Perineum: vaginal tears, rectal tone, hematomas, blood at meatus, rectal bleeding, and pregnancy test in female patients.
8. Limbs: distal pulses and capillary refill, tenderness, crepitus with movement, deformity of the limb.
9. Neurologic: detailed neurologic examination, especially levels of injury if paralysis.

Tertiary survey: Often patients admitted to the ICU have not been able to be fully assessed in the emergency department because of intoxication, head injury, or hemodynamic instability. It is therefore crucial that the ICU staff helps to perform a continual reassessment similar to the secondary survey as the patient stabilizes and is able to respond to the examiner. The tertiary survey must be done systematically and can often find undiagnosed fractures or other injuries.

Major Immediate Life-Threatening Conditions

After initial resuscitation, several immediately life-threatening conditions may be present, but may not be diagnosed at the time of initial resuscitation. These may become clinically apparent once the patient has arrived in the ICU for continued care.

Tension Pneumothorax

Tension pneumothorax often presents in delayed fashion, especially if the patient is on positive pressure ventilation. Blunt or penetrating injury to the chest and line insertions during resuscitation are often the cause.

Diagnosis:
>   Hypotension
>   Distended neck veins
>   Decreased breath sounds on one side
>   Chest x-ray (only if stable)

Treatment:
>   Needle decompression if unstable
>   Chest tube with closed suction drainage after needle decompression

Cardiac Tamponade

Most often cardiac tamponade is seen after penetrating injury to the heart, but can also develop from blunt injury from direct cardiac injury or broken ribs or sternum.

Diagnosis:
>   Hypotension
>   Distended neck veins
>   Equalization of pressures, if pulmonary artery catheter present
>   Diminished heart sounds
>   Echocardiography, if stable

Treatment:
>   Pericardiocentesis—may be repeated
>   Surgery is the definitive treatment

Blunt Cardiac Injury

Blunt trauma can cause several types of cardiac injury, including cardiac contusion, coronary artery dissection or transaction, valve injury, chordae tendineae rupture, septal defects, and pericardial tamponade.

Diagnosis:
>   Arrhythmias
>   Unexplained hypotension despite adequate resuscitation
>   Echocardiography
>   Cardiac enzymes (creatine phosphokinase, troponin) have *no proven benefit* in the diagnosis or treatment of blunt cardiac injury.

Treatment:
>   Inotropic agents
>   Supportive care
>   Surgery
>   Cardiac catheterization if coronary dissection

Massive Hemothorax

A massive hemothorax is a large collection of blood in the chest that can lead to hemorrhagic shock as well as tension-like physiology in the chest. It can be due to major pulmonary vascular injury or blunt aortic rupture.

Diagnosis:
>   Hypotension
>   Decreased breath sounds

Chest x-ray
Computed tomography (CT) scan of the chest with IV contrast if hemodynamically stable.
Treatment:
Chest tube
Resuscitation
Surgery

OTHER INJURIES REQUIRING ICU CARE

Hemorrhagic Shock

Hemorrhagic shock can quickly arise in the traumatically injured patient. A patient may have one bleeding focus or many. Differentiating this from distributive or spinal shock is also necessary, but shock secondary to continued bleeding should always be considered and treated first.

Major causes:
Liver or spleen injuries
Massive hemothorax
Exsanguinating peripheral arterial injuries
Pelvic fractures
Long-bone fractures
Retroperitoneal hematomas
Diagnosis:
Known or suspected bleeding diathesis
Anemia
Tamponade and tension pneumothorax ruled out
Treatment:
Rapid transfusion of blood and products as needed
Control of bleeding through surgery, splinting, or embolization

Distributive (Spinal) Shock

This type of shock develops after spinal cord injury and is due to loss of sympathetic innervation to the heart and distal vessels. It must be a diagnosis of exclusion after hemorrhagic and cardiogenic causes are ruled out.

Diagnosis:
Known spinal cord injury
Hypotension unresponsive to appropriate fluid resuscitation
Treatment:
Vasopressors and inotropes as needed

Flail Chest

Flail chest is secondary to massive blunt injury to the chest causing fracture of at least three contiguous ribs in two or more places. It results in paradoxical movement of the chest wall during inspiration. Pulmonary contusions are often underlying the injury.

Diagnosis:
Chest x-ray
CT scan of the chest
Physical examination (paradoxical motion and extreme tenderness)

Treatment:
    Pain control – consider thoracic epidural
    Pulmonary toilet
    Intubation and ventilation if needed
    Surgical stabilization may be helpful if slow improvement

Pulmonary Contusion

Pulmonary contusion is common finding in the ICU trauma patient and ranges from mild to severe. Treatment is supportive. Pulmonary contusions usually worsen during 48 hours before improving, and that time lag is important when making future treatment decisions regarding the pulmonary system. Although the trauma patient often has massive needs for resuscitation, in patients with isolated pulmonary contusion, care should be taken to avoid fluid overload.

Diagnosis:
    Chest x-ray
    CT scan of the chest
Treatment:
    Pulmonary toilet
    Oxygen
    Positive pressure ventilation if severe
    Intubation if needed
    Protective lung ventilation similar to patients with acute respiratory distress syndrome
    Oscillatory ventilation
    Consider placing affected side down if significant pulmonary hemorrhage

Spleen and Liver Injuries, Pelvic Hematomas

These are included together given the similarity of approach in these patients. For this group, the diagnosis is often known prior to ICU admission. The worst of these injuries that rendered the patient hemodynamically unstable have likely already been stabilized with packing or resection in the operation theater. Further management includes:

1. Serial assessment of blood counts and bleeding parameters
2. Continued resuscitation with appropriate fluids or products
3. If further bleeding continues, the patient likely requires further intervention with interventional radiology or surgery.
4. Need for pelvic stabilization to reduce venous bleeding in pelvic fractures

Head Injury

Often patients with multiple injuries also have head injuries. Intracranial injury care is reviewed elsewhere, but treatment strategies for the multiple injured patient are often different than those for isolated head injuries. The care of these patients must involve all of the specialty teams in the medical decision-making.

Cervical Spine Injury

Trauma victims are often brought to the ICU with their C-collar still in place. The collar should stay in place until an appropriate algorithm to exclude cervical spine injury has been followed. However, leaving the collar in place for an unnecessarily

ALGORITHM 68.1 Cervical Spine Evaluation Guidelines for Trauma Patients

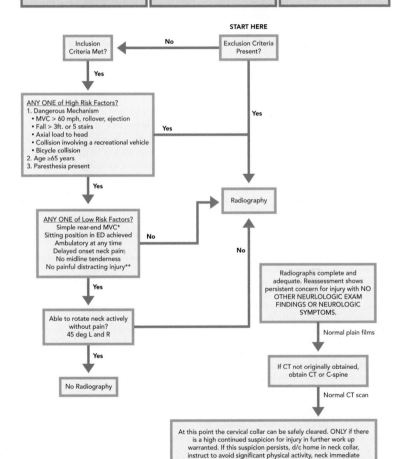

Inclusion to this decision making rule:
Adult with acute trauma to head or neck
GCS of 15, SBP>90, RR 10-24/min
Neck pain or no neck pain but ALL of the
following:
-visible injury above the clavicles
-non-ambulatory
-mechanism of injury present

Exclusion from this decision making rule:
GCS<15
unstable vital signs
age < 16 years
acute paralysis
known cervical vertebral disease
previous cervical spine surgery

• Simple rear end MVC excludes:
 -being pushed into oncoming
traffic
 -hit by bus or semi-trailer or larger
 -hit by a vehicle going >55mph

**Bony injury with pain scale rated
greater than 5/10

START HERE

Inclusion Criteria Met? ←—**No**—— Exclusion Criteria Present?

Yes

ANY ONE of High Risk Factors?
1. Dangerous Mechanism
 • MVC > 60 mph, rollover, ejection
 • Fall > 3ft. or 5 stairs
 • Axial load to head
 • Collision involving a recreational vehicle
 • Bicycle collision
2. Age ≥65 years
3. Paresthesia present

Yes →

Yes

ANY ONE of Low Risk Factors?
Simple rear-end MVC*
Sitting position in ED achieved
Ambulatory at any time
Delayed onset neck pain
No midline tenderness
No painful distracting injury**

No →

Radiography

No

Radiographs complete and
adequate. Reassessment shows
persistent concern for injury with NO
OTHER NEURLOGIC EXAM
FINDINGS OR NEUROLOGIC
SYMPTOMS.

Yes

Able to rotate neck actively
without pain?
45 deg L and R

Normal plain films

Yes

If CT not originally obtained,
obtain CT or C-spine

No Radiography

Normal CT scan

At this point the cervical collar can be safely cleared. ONLY if there
is a high continued suspicion for injury in further work up
warranted. If this suspicion persists, d/c home in neck collar,
instruct to avoid significant physical activity, neck immediate
medical attention if increased pain or neuro symptoms develop,
and refer for follow up in 1 week with Spine Service (Mower 2001)
NO FURTHER IMAGING NECESSARY UNLESS HIGH CLINICAL
SUSPICION WARRANTS IT.

prolonged period of time can lead to complications due to pressure wounds and difficulty with airway management. Algorithm 68.1 is the algorithm currently used in our institution. Recently updated evidence based guidelines are available at http://www.east.org/tpg/cspine2009.pdf.

LATER COMPLICATIONS

Although the traumatically injured ICU patient is apt to develop any of the common ICU complications, pulmonary emboli, and fat emboli are more common in this population. Careful thromboembolic prophylaxis must be initiated as soon as possible with careful screening for deep venous thrombosis throughout the hospital course. Fat emboli are associated with long-bone fractures, usually after repair, and can cause severe lung disease, but are treated as most respiratory distress patients with supportive care.

CONCLUSION

The traumatically injured patient often requires ICU care and monitoring. Recognizing the most common life-threatening concerns quickly is important in the care of these patients. The initial survey is important to systematically identify and treat those conditions as rapidly as possible. Continuous resuscitation is a key to the survival and ultimate recovery of these patients, as well as following and recognizing the endpoints of that resuscitation.

SUGGESTED READINGS

American College of Surgeons, Committee on Trauma. *Advanced Trauma Life Support for Doctors*, 8th ed. Chicago, IL: American College of Surgeons, 2008.

Dunham CM, Barraco RD, Clark DE, et al. Guideline for emergency tracheal intubation immediately after traumatic injury. *J Trauma*. 2003;54:391–416.

Pasquale M, Fabian T. Practice management guidelines of the screening of blunt cardiac injury. *J Trauma*. 1998;44:941–956.

Practice management guidelines for hemorrhage in pelvic fracture. Available at: http://www.east.org/tpg/pelvis.pdf. Accessed November 14, 2007.

Practice management guidelines for identification of cervical spine injuries following trauma. Available at: http://www.east.org/tpg/cspine2009.pdf. Accessed November 14, 2010.

Practice management guidelines for the nonoperative management of blunt injury to the liver and spleen. Available at: http://www.east.org/tpg/livspleen.pdf. Accessed November 14, 2007.

Practice management guidelines for Pulmonary Contusion—Flail Chest. Available at: http://www.east.org/tpg/pulmcontflailchest.pdf. Accessed November 14, 2010.

Schuerer DJ, Whinney RR, Freeman BD, et al. Evaluation of the applicability, efficacy, and safety of a thromboembolic event prophylaxis guideline designed for quality improvement of the traumatically injured patient. *J Trauma*. 2005;58:731–739.

Simon BJ, Cushman J, Barraco RD, et al. Pain management guidelines for blunt thoracic trauma. *J Trauma*. 2005;59:1256–1257.

Tishermam SA, Barie P, Bokhari F, et al. Clinical practice guideline: endpoints of resuscitation. *J Trauma*. 2004;57:898–912.

69

The Acute Abdomen

Jennifer L. Gnerlich, Robb R. Whinney, and
John P. Kirby

Acute abdominal pathology is a common event in the intensive care unit (ICU) setting, but the diagnosis is often delayed because of the absence of typical signs and
symptoms of peritonitis. Physical examination signs that define an acute abdomen,
such as global tenderness, rigidity, rebound, and guarding, are not always obvious in
the ICU setting when a patient has multiple ongoing medical issues. A retrospective
cohort study of medical ICU patients with abdominal pathology found surgical delay
was more likely to occur in patients with altered mental states, absence of peritoneal
signs, previous opioid analgesia, antibiotics, and mechanical ventilation. The delay in
diagnosis and management of an acute abdomen is associated with increased morality
rates. Therefore, learning to identify an acute abdomen in a critically ill patient with
masked physical symptoms is a life-saving skill.

PATIENT HISTORY

Obtaining a history from a patient in the ICU is frequently complicated by an altered
mental state, chemical sedation, or intubation. A careful review of the patient's medical
history, surgical history, allergies, and medications can provide a possible cause of the
abdominal pathology. If the patient is alert, the description of the pain, including quality and radiation, may help to focus the differential diagnosis. Most often, a patient is
not alert and important medical history must be obtained from family members. One
of the most important pieces of information influencing the differential diagnosis is
whether or not the patient has recently had an operation. The temporal relationship
of a change in abdominal examination from time of surgery can be suggestive of different pathologies. For example, a patient who recently underwent abdominal surgery
(<3 days) is at greater risk for bleeding and anastomotic leaks, whereas a patient who
is a week out of surgery is more likely to have an intra-abdominal abscess.

LABORATORY HISTORY

Laboratory tests are important adjuncts in the critical care setting, where most patients
cannot provide an accurate history or description of their current physical symptoms.
Following laboratory value trends can provide insight into an ongoing abdominal
process. An increasing trend in the white blood cell (WBC) count is usually a signal of infection or inflammation but is fairly nonspecific after a recent surgical procedure or in a patient receiving steroids. Conversely, an extreme WBC (35,000 to
40,000 cells/μL) can indicate a more severe infection, such as *Clostridium difficile*

colitis, and the workup should be done accordingly. A normal or decreasing WBC count can be misleading; thus, it is important to obtain a differential cell count and evaluate for a left shift. A decreasing WBC to leukopenic levels with a large left shift is concerning for overwhelming sepsis.

Abnormal liver function tests including fractionated bilirubin, alkaline phosphatase, and transaminase levels may localize the pathology to the gallbladder, biliary system, or liver, but are rarely diagnostic. Instead, they help guide further diagnostic strategies like appropriate imaging. Of note, in the critically ill patient, an acute increase in bilirubin may signify acalculous cholecystitis. Elevated amylase and lipase levels hone the diagnosis to pancreatitis, but be aware that an isolated amylase elevation may indicate a perforated viscus or ischemic bowel. Concomitant increase in both bilirubin and amylase suggests obstruction at the distal common bile duct or pancreatic duct. Although an elevated lactate level (>4 mmol/L) may signal the emergent condition of mesenteric ischemia with necrotic bowel it, less specifically, is the result of acidemia, hypoxia, hypovolemia, anemia, or renal failure or liver failure. Arterial blood gas should be obtained to determine if acidosis or hypoxemia is present and to quantify the base deficit. Abdominal compartment syndrome should be suspected when acidosis, hypoxemia, oliguria, and a distended abdomen are present. Bladder pressure can be transduced; a pressure >30 mm Hg may require emergent surgical decompression. Urine analysis is not specific, but microscopic hematuria or pyuria can suggest a urinary tract infection or a lower abdomen/pelvic infection.

PHYSICAL EXAMINATION

The physical examination is less reliable in a patient receiving analgesics, sedatives, or steroids and must focus more on changing physical examination signs rather than the traditional signs of peritonitis. In a patient whose clinical course is declining, it is important that the abdominal examination is performed serially and a digital rectal examination is completed.

Because abdominal pain may be difficult to elucidate in the critically ill patient, nonspecific signs such as tachycardia, hypotension, and fever raise concern for occult abdominal pathology. A sudden change in ventilatory settings, overbreathing the ventilator, or increasing airway pressures may signal a patient's attempt to compensate for a metabolic acidosis or indicate an elevation in intra-abdominal compartment pressure. An increase in nasogastric output, abdominal distention, absence of bowel movements, or abrupt intolerance of enteral feeds is concerning for a bowel obstruction, mesenteric ischemia, or an acute ileus due to an intra-abdominal infection. Because the nursing staff spends more extended periods of time with the patient, it is important to communicate with them about changes in the patient's condition, including the quantity and quality of bowel movements (*C. difficile* colitis or intestinal ischemia), drain output (abdominal sepsis, leak, or fistula), and wound drainage (intra-abdominal abscess or wound dehiscence). For a patient who has recently undergone an abdominal procedure, nonspecific signs would be concerning for some type of anastomotic leak (intestinal, biliary, pancreatic). For a patient who is about a week out of surgery, intra-abdominal sepsis, ischemia, or abscess should be considered.

An acute abdomen in the ICU setting may be of medical or surgical consequence, although there are some diagnoses that overlap (Table 69.1). To assist in differentiating abdominal pain in the critically ill patient in the ICU, the abdomen is best divided into six regions to help evaluate the source of the abdominal pathology (Table 69.2).

TABLE 69.1	Medical versus Surgical Causes of Acute Abdominal Pathology in the Intensive Care Unit
Medical	**Workup**
Acute renal failure (uremia)	↓UOP, UA (casts), ↑BUN and Cr, FeNa, renal ultrasound
Sickle cell crisis	↓Hematocrit, peripheral blood smear
Adrenal insufficiency/ addisonian crisis	BMP (↑ K^+, ↓ Na^+, ↓ glucose), plasma cortisol and ACTH, cosyntropin stimulation test
Spontaneous bacterial peritonitis	Ultrasound, paracentesis with Gram stain and culture
Diabetic ketoacidosis	Glucose, UA, BMP (Na^+ and K^+ levels), ABG (acidosis)
Gastroenteritis/enterocolitis	WBC,[a] stool ova/parasites
Esophagitis	EGD, barium swallow, pH monitoring
Hepatitis	LFTs, hepatitis panel (A, B, and C)
Peptic ulcer disease/ gastritis	EGD, barium swallow, pH monitoring, manometry
Nephrolithiasis/pyelonephritis	UA (pyuria, hematuria), renal ultrasound
Myocardial infarction	ECG, troponins
Pneumonia	Chest x-ray, sputum sample, WBC
Urinary tract infection	UA (bacteria, leukocyte esterase, nitrites)
Gynecologic disease	Pelvic examination, gonorrhea/chlamydia, ultrasound
Medical and surgical	**Workup**
Diverticulitis/IBD	WBC, CT scan,[b] flexible sigmoidoscopy/ colonoscopy
Clostridium difficile colitis	Stool toxin assay × 3, severely elevated WBC
Pancreatitis/pancreatic abscess	Amylase, lipase, ultrasound, CT scan to r/o necrosis
Intra-abdominal abscess	WBC, CT scan
Small/large bowel obstruction	WBC, lactate, plain film x-rays, CT scan
Choledocholithiasis	LFTs, RUQ ultrasound
Cholangitis	LFTs, WBC, RUQ ultrasound
Mallory-Weiss tear	EGD, hematocrit, coagulation studies
Surgical	**Workup**
Acute cholecystitis	WBC, LFTs, RUQ ultrasound
Acalculous cholecystitis	WBC, LFTs, RUQ ultrasound, HIDA scan
Perforated peptic or duodenal ulcer	Plain film x-rays (free air), upper GI series, CT scan
Acute appendicitis	WBC, CT scan with rectal contrast, ultrasound to r/o other pathology
Mesenteric ischemia and necrotic bowel	WBC, lactate, ABG (acidosis), CT scan
Colonic perforation	WBC, plain film x-rays (free air), CT scan

(continued)

TABLE 69.1	Medical versus Surgical Causes of Acute Abdominal Pathology in the Intensive Care Unit (*Continued*)
Surgical	**Workup**
Ruptured or leaking abdominal aortic aneurysm	Hematocrit, coagulation studies, CT angio (only need IV contrast)
Toxic megacolon	*C. difficile* stool toxin assay × 3, WBC, plain film x-rays, CT scan
Sigmoid or cecal volvulus	Plain film x-rays, CT scan
Boerhaave syndrome	Plain film x-rays, Gastrografin swallow
Wound dehiscence	WBC, wound culture, ultrasound, CT scan
Anastomotic leak (intestinal, biliary, pancreatic)	WBC, CT scan (if patient had a recent surgical procedure)
Abdominal compartment syndrome	↓UOP, WBC, lactate, ABG (acidosis), bladder pressures

[a]WBC should always be obtained with a differential cell count.
[b]CT scan should always be obtained with IV and oral contrast unless contraindication exists, i.e., abnormal renal function.
UOP, urine output; UA, urinalysis; BUN, blood urea nitrogen; Cr, creatine; BMP, blood metabolic profile; ACTH, corticotropin; ABG, arterial blood gas; WBC, white blood cell; EGD, esophagogastroduodenoscopy; ECG, electrocardiogram; CT, computed tomography; r/o, rule out; RUQ, right upper quadrant; HIDA, hepatobiliary iminodiacetic acid; GI, gastrointestinal; IV, intravenous.

The actual explanation of all possible acute abdominal emergencies and their diagnosis and treatment is beyond the scope of this chapter. An algorithm is provided to help guide management decisions for those patients in the ICU who may be experiencing intra-abdominal pathology (Algorithm 69.1).

RADIOGRAPHIC EXAMINATION

Imaging the abdomen helps to confirm or exclude intra-abdominal catastrophe. Initially, three plain film views of the abdomen (kidney/ureter/bladder, upright chest, and lateral decubitus) should be obtained. Air in the biliary tree or intestines, known as *pneumatosis*, suggests necrotic bowel and indicates the need for an emergent surgical consultation. Free air in the peritoneum or retroperitoneum suggests an intestinal or gastric perforation. However, in a patient who has recently undergone laparotomy, free air should be interpreted with caution as it may be the result of the procedure itself.

Abdominal ultrasound is noninvasive and is the imaging modality of choice for a patient with right upper quadrant symptoms or concerning liver function tests. Ultrasound can elucidate gallbladder pathology by demonstrating pericholecystic fluid, wall thickening, gallstones, ductal dilatation, or a distended gallbladder, indicating calculous or acalculous cholecystitis. If the concern for acalculous cholecystitis is high, then a hepatobiliary iminodiacetic acid (HIDA) scan will confirm the diagnosis. Abdominal ultrasound can also identify fluid in other areas, particularly around the pancreas or in

TABLE 69.2	Cause of Abdominal Pathology Based on Location	
I. Right upper quadrant	**II. Epigastrium**	**III. Left upper quadrant**
Acute cholecystitis	Pancreatitis	Splenic hemorrhage or abscess
Acalculous cholecystitis	Peptic ulcer disease/ gastritis	Peptic ulcer disease
Hepatitis	Perforated peptic or duodenal ulcer	Perforated peptic or duodenal ulcer
Choledocholithiasis	Mallory–Weiss tear	Pancreatitis
Cholangitis	Boerhaave syndrome	Pancreatic pseudocyst or abscess
Hepatic abscess	Esophagitis	Nephrolithiasis/ pyelonephritis
Pancreatitis	Gastroenteritis	Pneumonia (left lower lobe)
Peptic ulcer disease/ gastritis	Myocardial infarction	
Nephrolithiasis/ pyelonephritis	Pneumonia	
Appendicitis (women in pregnancy)		
Myocardial infarction		
Pneumonia		
IV. Right lower quadrant	**V. Periumbilical/ nonspecific**	**VI. Left lower quadrant**
Acute appendicitis	Small/large bowel obstruction	Sigmoid diverticulitis
Small/large bowel obstruction	Mesenteric artery ischemia or occlusion	Sigmoid volvulus
Cecal perforation	Ruptured or leaking abdominal aortic aneurysm	Colonic perforation
Cecal volvulus	Early appendicitis	Small/large bowel obstruction
Cecal diverticulitis	*Clostridium difficile* colitis or toxic megacolon	Enterocolitis
Enterocolitis	Wound dehiscence	Inflammatory bowel disease
Inflammatory bowel disease	Abdominal compartment syndrome	Nephrolithiasis
Nephrolithiasis	Intra-abdominal abscess	Urinary tract infection
Urinary tract infection	Anastomotic leak (intestinal, biliary, pancreatic)	Gynecologic disease
Gynecologic disease		

ALGORITHM 69.1 Diagnosis and Management of Acute Abdominal Pathology in the Intensive Care Unit

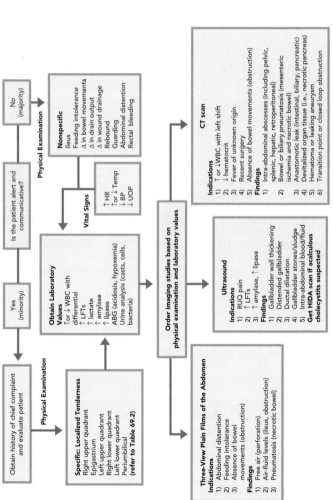

HR, heart rate; BP, blood pressure; UOP, urine output; WBC, white blood cell; LFT, liver function test; ABG, arterial blood gas; RUQ, right upper quadrant; HIDA, hepatobiliary iminodiacetic acid.

the pelvis. Although nonspecific, fluid in the pelvis can indicate an intra-abdominal pathology or be a consequence of aggressive resuscitative efforts.

Computed tomographic scanning (CT scan) with contrast is useful in identifying bowel thickening secondary to edema, dilated and fluid-filled intestines, fat stranding, and pneumatosis, all imaging signs concerning for necrotic bowel and requiring immediate surgical evaluation. CT scan can also demonstrate a transition point in a bowel obstruction for easier surgical management. In a recent surgical patient with sudden clinical deterioration and a drop in hematocrit, a CT scan can reveal an evolving hematoma or an acute bleed. Finally, CT scan is useful in identifying the location and size of intra-abdominal abscesses and in guiding management by either percutaneous drainage or laparotomy and washout.

SUGGESTED READINGS

Fink MP. Acute abdominal pain. In: Kruse JA, Fink MP, Carlson RW, eds. *Saunders Manual of Critical Care*. Philadelphia, PA: Elsevier Science, 2003:439–445.
  Short review of important physical exam findings, laboratory values, and imaging studies for the most common causes of an acute abdomen.
Gajic O, Urrutia LE, Sewani H, et al. Acute abdomen in the medical intensive care unit. *Crit Care Med*. 2002;30:1187–1190.
  Retrospective cohort study in a tertiary care center's medical intensive care unit that evaluated predictors of surgical delay for patients with an acute abdomen and the association between surgical delay and increased mortality in those patients.
Martin RF, Rossi RL. The acute abdomen: an overview and algorithms. *Surg Clin North Am*. 1997;77:1227–1243.
  Basic overview of managing a patient with an acute abdomen.
Martin RF, Flynn P. The acute abdomen in the critically ill patient. *Surg Clin North Am*. 1997;77:1455–1464.
  Overview of the diagnostic difficulties encountered in critically ill patient with an acute abdomen in the ICU and possible management strategies.
Sosa JL, Reines HD. Evaluating the acute abdomen. In: Civetta JM, Taylor RW, Kirby RR, eds. Critical care. 3rd ed. Philadelphia, PA: Lippincott, Williams & Wilkins, 1997:1099–1108.
  Textbook chapter reviewing the general approach to a patient with an acute abdomen in the ICU.

70 Management of the Organ Donor

Stephen R. Broderick and Varun Puri

The number of patients awaiting organ transplantation in the United States is significantly greater than the number of available organs, resulting in the death of many patients awaiting transplantation. A number of methods have been utilized in attempts to increase the donor pool. Recently, standardized and aggressive donor management protocols have been shown to increase the number of transplanted organs from potential donors. The use of organs from donation after cardiac death and extended criteria donors has also recently increased the number of available organs. The Health Care Financing Administration of the Department of Health and Human Services requires hospitals to contact the local organ-procurement organization when a patient is identified for whom death is imminent. In consultation with the intensive care unit (ICU) team, the organ-procurement organization establishes the criteria of donor suitability. Table 70.1 summarizes various criteria for establishing the suitability for organ donation.

After consent is obtained from the family, blood tests may be drawn to determine if a patient is a potential donor. However, invasive procedures to determine if a patient is suitable for organ donation should not be performed prior to the patient being declared brain dead. A summary of the process of obtaining consent for organ donation is summarized in Table 70.2. Of note, the establishment of brain death should be performed by two clinical examinations, apnea tests, and laboratory confirmation 24 to 48 hours apart by physicians trained in this area. (The specifics of the criteria for brain death are covered in Chapter 55.)

Once a patient has been found to be a suitable candidate for organ transplantation and has been declared brain dead, the goals of ICU care are to maintain end-organ function and viability.

Brain death is associated with widespread hemodynamic and metabolic dysregulation, which may have deleterious effects on organs intended for transplantation. Increasingly, the transplant community has been considering organ transplants using organs donated after cardiac death in the absence of brain death (Table 70.3). Several clinical problems apply both to the after-cardiac-death donors and to those with brain death, and these are discussed in the following sections and summarized in Algorithm 70.1.

NORMALIZE HEMODYNAMICS

Brain death may result in cardiac dysfunction and vasodilation, decreasing end-organ perfusion in the potential donor. The primary objectives of cardiovascular

TABLE 70.1	Criteria for Organ Donation

- Donor age
  Absolute contraindication → age >80
  Organ-specific contraindication → lungs, kidneys age >60
- Lack of significant past medical history
  No malignancy with high potential for recurrent or metastatic disease
  No significant system-specific disease (e.g., cardiac, pulmonary, liver)
  No primary brain tumors
  No significant infectious disease, including HIV, hepatitis, syphilis, toxoplasma.
    Routine serologic testing includes HIV, HTLV, hepatitis B, hepatitis C, CMV,
    syphilis, and toxoplasma
  No donor sepsis
  Cause of death not due to massive poisoning, with potential for transplanted
    organ nonfunction (acetaminophen, tricyclic antidepressants, carbon
    monoxide, cyanide, ethanol)

HIV, human immunodeficiency virus; HTLV, human T-cell leukemia virus; CMV, cytomegalovirus.

management of the potential donor are to maintain normovolemia, prevent hypotension, and optimize cardiac output.

Hypotension, defined as mean arterial blood pressure <60 mm Hg, is frequently encountered in brain-dead patients. Treatment should be initially directed at volume expansion to a central venous pressure of >12 mm Hg. Excessive volume losses due to hemorrhage is common in trauma victims. Crystalloid and colloid solutions, as well as blood products (packed red blood cells, fresh-frozen plasma) may be required to establish normovolemia. Persistent hypotension in the setting of adequate central venous pressure (CVP) should prompt placement of a pulmonary artery catheter (or other equivalent noninvasive monitor of cardiac function) to determine cardiac output and systemic vascular resistance.

Persistent hypotension may result from low systemic vascular resistance (<400 dynes/sec/cm) or a decrease in cardiac contractility. The use of vasoactive agents, namely dopamine, at a continuous infusion of 5 to 10 μg/kg/min or norepinephrine, 2 to 12 μg/min, may be necessary to maintain end-organ perfusion. Brain dead donors may exhibit depressed cardiac function for a number of reasons (following cardiac

TABLE 70.2	Obtaining Consent for Organ Donation

- Contact local OPO
- In conjunction with OPO, obtain verbal consent to perform non-invasive testing
  (blood sampling, ECG, radiology studies) to determine suitability for organ
  donation
- Establish the diagnosis of brain death (see Chapter 56)
- After brain death has been declared and in conjunction with OPO, obtain
  written family consent for donation
- In the absence of brain death, consider the option of "donation after cardiac
  death" or the so-called non-heartbeating donor

OPO, organ-procurement organization.

TABLE 70.3	Donation after Cardiac Death Donors: Maastricht Workshop Categories

- Dead on arrival
- Unsuccessful resuscitation
- Awaiting cardiac arrest/cessation of futile treatment
- Cardiac arrest in brain-dead donor

arrest, blunt cardiac trauma, or brainstem herniation). Brain death also directly leads to decreased ventricular function because of cardiac beta-receptor desensitization. The use of inotropic and chronotropic agents may be necessary to augment cardiac function to keep cardiac index >2 L/min/m^2. Agents of choice include continuous infusions of dopamine (as mentioned previously) or dobutamine (at 2 to 5 μg/kg/min).

There is now substantial evidence to support hormone replacement therapy in patients in whom hemodynamic stability is not achievable with volume, vasopressor, and inotropic therapy. While poorly understood, hormone therapy appears to counter the effects of a dysregulated hypothalamic–pituitary axis which results in a deficiency of thyroid hormone and cortisol. Hypotensive donors receiving >10 μg/kg/min of vasopressor should be treated with a combination of thyroid hormone (4.0 μg), methylprednisolone (15 mg/kg), vasopressin (1u), and insulin with continuous infusions administered until the time of procurement.

It is rare to encounter significant hypertension in brain-dead patients. If present, it is often related to brainstem herniation. Diastolic blood pressures >100 mm Hg should be treated to avoid arrhythmias. Sodium nitroprusside is the treatment of choice. Prolonged nitroprusside treatment should be avoided because of cyanide toxicity.

OPTIMIZE PULMONARY FUNCTION

Maintenance of pulmonary function using mechanical ventilation must be tailored to prevent atelectasis, pneumonia, pulmonary edema, and to maintain adequate gas exchange. Good oral hygiene can help prevent ventilator-associated pneumonias. Brain-dead patients often develop otherwise unexplained pulmonary edema, attributed to systemic inflammatory, and neurogenic responses. The use of positive end-expiratory pressure of 5 to 10 cm H_2O can offset this increased capillary permeability and maintain alveolar expansion. However, positive end-expiratory pressure levels >10 cm H_2O can result in impair venous return and negatively impact cardiac output. Hypervolemia should be avoided in patients who are potential lung donors. Judicious volume administration, often guided by central venous or pulmonary artery pressures, to achieve end-organ perfusion should be balanced against the accumulation of extravascular fluid in the lungs. Ventilator settings should be optimized to maintain arterial P_{CO_2} at 40 to 45 mm Hg and, whenever possible, at a fraction of inspired oxygen at ≤0.6 to minimize oxygen toxicity. Bronchodilator therapy may assist with airway clearance, prevention of atelectasis, and avoidance of pulmonary edema.

CORRECT ACID–BASE AND ELECTROLYTE DISTURBANCES

Brain-dead patients often develop polyuria, with urine outputs in excess of 500 mL/hr. This can be attributed to physiologic, osmotic, chemical (furosemide), and

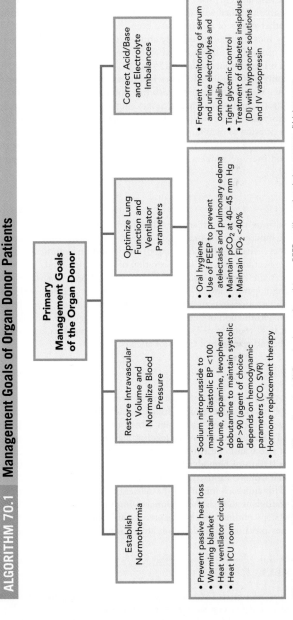

ALGORITHM 70.1   Management Goals of Organ Donor Patients

Primary Management Goals of the Organ Donor

Establish Normothermia
- Prevent passive heat loss
- Warming blanket
- Heat ventilator circuit
- Heat ICU room

Restore Intravascular Volume and Normalize Blood Pressure
- Sodium nitroprusside to maintain diastolic BP <100
- Volume, dopamine, levophend dobutamine to maintain systolic BP >90 (agent of choice depends on hemodynamic parameters (CO, SVR)
- Hormone replacement therapy

Optimize Lung Function and Ventilator Parameters
- Oral hygiene
- Use of PEEP to prevent atelectasis and pulmonary edema
- Maintain pCO$_2$ at 40–45 mm Hg
- Maintain FiO$_2$ <40%

Correct Acid/Base and Electrolyte Imbalances
- Frequent monitoring of serum and urine electrolytes and osmolality
- Tight glycemic control
- Treatment of diabetes insipidus (DI) with hypotonic solutions and IV vasopressin

ICU, intensive care unit; BP, blood pressure; CO, cardiac output; SVR, systemic vascular resistance; PEEP, positive end-expiratory pressure; IV, intravenous.

hypothermic diuresis, central diabetes insipidus (DI), or combinations of these. This diuresis can lead to profound hypernatremia, hypokalemia, and hyperosmolality. Frequent monitoring of serum and urine osmolality and electrolytes with correction to normal ranges is essential to prevent cardiac dysfunction. Tight control of blood sugars should also be instituted to prevent significant hyperglycemia-related osmotic diuresis. This is easily accomplished with a protocol-driven continuous insulin infusion.

When other causes of polyuria have been excluded, the diagnosis of DI can be established by measuring urine output, urine-specific gravity, urine and serum electrolytes, and osmolality. DI is established by three of the following criteria: urine output >500 mL/hr, serum sodium >155 mEq/L, urine-specific gravity <1.005, and serum osmolality >305 mOsm/L. When identified, DI should be treated by replacing 50% of the free water deficit rapidly with hypotonic saline or 5% dextrose in water. Frequent electrolyte and hemodynamic monitoring is essential to correct further imbalances. Refractory cases can be treated with intravenous vasopressin at an initial dose of 10 units with titration to maintain urine output of 150 to 300 mL/hr or 1-desamino-8-D-arginine vasopressin (DDAVP). Vasopressin decreases plasma hyperosmolality, increases blood pressure, reduces inotrope requirements, and helps to maintain cardiac output.

MAINTAIN NORMOTHERMIA

The hypothalamus controls thermoregulation in healthy individuals. The loss of hypothalamic function in the brain-dead patient, combined with deficient compensatory responses (shivering, vasoconstriction) often results in hypothermia in the organ donor. Passive heat loss and the administration of unwarmed fluids and blood products can exacerbate hypothermia. Hypothermia should be managed aggressively to avoid the coagulopathy, cardiac dysfunction, arrhythmia, and leftward shift of the oxyhemoglobin dissociation curve which may ensue. In addition, severe hypothermia prevents the determination of brain death. Measures to prevent hypothermia include warming the ICU room to >75°F, forced-air warming blankets, administration of warmed fluids, and warming of ventilator circuits.

SUMMARY

In summary, the management of a patient determined suitable for organ donation focuses on preservation of end-organ function and viability. Standardized aggressive donor management protocols have been shown to increase the rates of organ procurement and decrease donor lost to medical failures. After the necessary steps are performed to select and consent a patient for donation, maintenance of normothermia, normalization of hemodynamics, optimization of lung function, restoration of intravascular volume, and correction of acid–base and electrolyte disorders are paramount. This approach minimizes the deleterious effects of brain death on organs suitable for transplant and has the potential to improve long-term allograft function. Many of the steps outlined in this chapter are also suitable for preserving the viability of organs procured from donation after cardiac death in the absence of brain death.

SUGGESTED READINGS

Arbour R. Clinical management of the organ donor. *AACN Clin Issues.* 2005;16:551–580.
   An expanded and detailed guide to the topic of this chapter.

Dubose J, Salim A. Aggressive organ donor management protocol. *J Intensive Care Med.* 2008;23:367–375.

A review of protocol driven approaches to management of organ donors.

Kootstra G. Statement on non-heart-beating donor programs. *Transplant Proc.* 1995;27:2965.

Kutsogiannis DJ, Pagliarello G, Doig C, et al. Medical management to optimize donor organ potential: review of the literature. *Can J Anaesth.* 2006;53:820–830.

A lengthy review article discussing the evidence supporting management strategies for potential organ donors.

Pratschke J, Wilhelm MJ, Kusaka M, et al. Brain death and its influence on donor organ quality and outcome after transplantation. *Transplantation.* 1999;67:343–348.

A study that evaluates the influence of the duration of brain death on the eventual outcome of the transplantation procedure.

Whiting JF, Delmonico F, Morrissey P, et al. Clinical results of an organ procurement organization effort to increase utilization of donors after cardiac death. *Transplantation.* 2006;81:1368–1371.

A study that reviews the impact of increased use of DCD donors on the outcomes of transplantation.

Wood KE, Becker BN, McCartney JG, et al. Care of the potential organ donor. *N Engl J Med.* 2004;351:2730–2739.

A detailed review article on care of the potential organ donor.

71

Nutrition in the Intensive Care Unit

Beth E. Taylor and Robert Southard

The metabolic response to critical illness is characterized by changes in carbohydrate, fat, and amino acid metabolism. These metabolic changes cause an important shift from an anabolic state to a catabolic state characterized by severe macromolecular breakdown of essential proteins, fats, and carbohydrates. The malnutrition associated with critical illness can have a negative impact on multiple organ systems. This may lead to increased length of stay, increased susceptibility to infection, impairment in respiratory function, ventilator dependence, and overall increase in morbidity and mortality.

The goals of nutrition support in the intensive care unit (ICU) patient are to provide adequate calories and protein to keep up with ongoing losses, prevent or correct nutrient deficiencies, support wound healing, and promote immune function. It is essential when determining the nutritional needs of critically ill patients that one incorporates the severity of disease, organ system involvement, metabolic derangements, gastrointestinal function, and impact of different therapeutic procedures to gain an overall assessment of each individual's need.

In addition to the patient's present status, other components of the nutrition assessment should include preadmission dietary history (specifically, recent intake), recent antecedent weight loss, functional status, alcohol intake, and body mass index (BMI). The patient's BMI may be calculated using either pounds or kilograms (Table 71.1).

Several studies support the use of early feeding in the ICU patient with premorbid malnutrition based on admission, BMI (<18.5) or weight loss of >10% during the previous 6 months. Some evidence suggests, if enteral nutrition is to be used early, initiation of feeds within 48 hours of admission may lead to better wound healing and lower infection rates. Otherwise, initiation of nutrition support is indicated in the critically ill patient who is not expected to resume an oral diet in 7 to 10 days (Algorithm 71.1). It is important to understand the potential consequences of initiating feeds in patients who have been starved for a period of time. The addition of a large glucose load can cause a massive shift of intracellular electrolytes, specifically potassium, magnesium, and phosphorus. This shift places the patient at risk of the sequelae associated with low serum levels of these electrolytes. This phenomenon is known as *refeeding syndrome* and may lead to serious consequences, including death.

A nutrition-focused physical examination should consist of a review of oral health, skin turgor, and assessment for loss of muscle mass in the temporal, deltoid, and quadriceps muscle groups. Initial laboratory assessment should include a basic metabolic

TABLE 71.1	Body Mass Index Calculation

Weight (lbs) $\times$ 704/inches^2 or weight (kg)/m^2

70-kg 5'6" patient	70-kg 5'6" patient
$(70 \times 2.2) \times 704/(66)^2$	$5'6" = 66 \times 2.54 = 167.64$ cm
$154 \times 704/4356$	$167.64/100 = 1.67$ meters
$108416/4356$	$70/1.67^2$
24.88	$70/2.78$
	25.10

ALGORITHM 71.1	Timing of Nutrition Support (Assessment Should Begin within 48 Hours of Admission to the Intensive Care Unit)

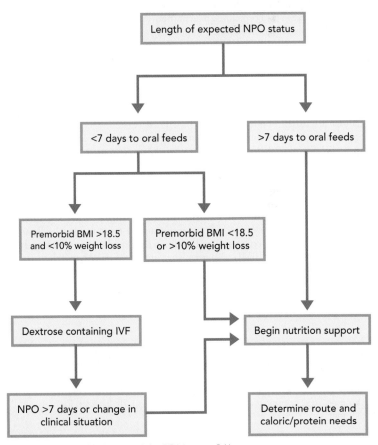

NPO, nothing by mouth; BMI, body mass index; IVF, intravenous fluids.

TABLE 71.2	Needs Estimated on Body Mass Index (BMI)
BMI	Energy (kcal/kg/day)
<15	35–40
15–19	30–35
20–25	20–25
26–29	15–17
29	15[a]

[a]Do not exceed 2000 calories per day for obese patients, allowing for mobilization of adipose stores for energy.

profile, magnesium, phosphate (for renal function and risk of refeeding syndrome), hepatic panel, and complete blood count.

Plasma albumin and prealbumin have a low sensitivity and specificity to changes in nutrition intake in the hospitalized patient. Both are affected by a plethora of factors. Levels are increased by corticosteroids, insulin, thyroid hormone, and dehydration. In contrast, levels are decreased by inflammatory mediators, severe liver and renal disease, malabsorption, and intravascular volume overload. In short, albumin and prealbumin levels in the critically ill patient reflect changes in protein synthesis, degradation, and distributive losses that are reflective of critical illness, not nutritional status.

Several equations exist to determine resting energy requirements in humans. The American Dietetics Association studied the reliability and validity of several predictive equations in a variety of hospitalized patients. These equations generate values within 10% of measured values in healthy subjects when compared with indirect calorimetry with a reliability of 70%. However, they are much less accurate in persons who are at extremes in weight or who are critically ill. Only two equations are designed for use in the critically ill patient, the 1992 Ireton-Jones equation and the 1998 Penn State equation; however, both are cumbersome to complete.

A more simple method for estimating caloric requirements in hospitalized patients has been developed using BMI (Table 71.2). The lower range in each category should be considered for initiation of nutrition support in insulin-resistant critically ill patients to decrease the risk of hyperglycemia and infection associated with overfeeding. In the critically ill obese patient (BMI ≥30) permissive underfeeding or hypocaloric feeding is recommended.

In general, protein needs are based on kilograms of ideal body weight, which can be determined using the Hamwi method (Table 71.3). The increased metabolic rate associated with critical illness along with several other potential factors including

TABLE 71.3	Hamwi Method to Determine Ideal Body Weight

Calculate ideal body weight[a]:
  Men: 106 pounds for first 5 feet plus 6 pounds for each inch above 5 feet
  Women: 100 pounds for the first 5 feet plus 5 pounds for each inch above 5 feet

[a]Conversion from pounds to kilograms: pounds ÷ 2.2.

TABLE 71.4	Recommended Daily Protein Intake[a]
Clinical condition	Protein needs (g/kg IBW/day[b]
Normal (nonstressed)	0.75
Critical illness/injury	1.00–1.50
Acute renal failure (undialyzed)	0.80–1.00
Acute renal failure (dialyzed)	1.20–1.40
Peritoneal dialysis	1.30–1.50
Burn/sepsis	1.50–2.00
CVVHD	1.70–2.50

[a]Clinical conditions are not additive; to calculate needs, use value that prescribes the highest protein needs.
[b]Lower protein requirements may be necessary in hepatic encephalopathy.
IBW, ideal body weight; CVVHD, continuous venovenous hemodialysis.

renal failure, extent of injury, presence of significant burns, and sepsis may significantly increase the requirements for protein (Table 71.4).

Once the decision to begin nutrition support has been made, the optimal delivery route needs to be determined and feeding initiated (Algorithm 71.2). At present, the general consensus is to feed enterally whenever possible.

Enteral nutrition may be beneficial in protecting gut mucosal integrity by maintaining villous height and supporting IgA producing immunocytes which comprise the gut-associated lymphoid tissue (GALT). Loss of integrity in the intestinal lumen may lead to the migration of bacteria to the portal and systemic circulation, thereby increasing the risk of systemic infection and potential for multi-organ dysfunction syndrome (MODS). If use of the enteral route is not feasible, total parenteral nutrition (TPN) should be considered as soon as possible in patients with evidence of protein–calorie malnutrition; or after 7 days in previously well-nourished patients. Each route has advantages and disadvantages and conditions in which it is contraindicated (Table 71.5).

Either gastric or small bowel feeding is acceptable in the ICU setting. In critically ill patients with gastric feeding intolerance (patient complaints of pain, vomiting, abdominal distention, or gastric residual >500 mL) placement of a small bowel feeding tube should be considered. Delivery of enteral feeding into the small bowel has been recommended as a strategy to reduce the risk of aspiration; however, randomized controlled studies of gastric versus small bowel feeding in ICU patients have been inconclusive. Unfortunately, patients who had significant risk factors for aspiration or who had gastric feeding intolerance were excluded from these studies. These patients may benefit from placement of a postpyloric feeding tube (Table 71.6). Although the short-term addition (24 to 72 hours) of prokinetic agents such as metoclopramide and erythromycin has been shown to temporarily improve gastric emptying and EN tolerance, longer use may lead to drug induced complications. Patients with severe acute pancreatitis fed via a small bowel feeding tube, as opposed to TPN, have been shown to have reduced infectious morbidity. Whether the tube feeding is provided pre- or postpyloric, other than increased gastric residual volume, the recommendations to troubleshoot complications are the same (Table 71.7).

The appropriate type of tube feeding formula to use in the critically ill patient continues to be debated. Based on the current evidence, whole-protein formulas are

ALGORITHM 71.2 Determination of Route and Initiation of Feeding

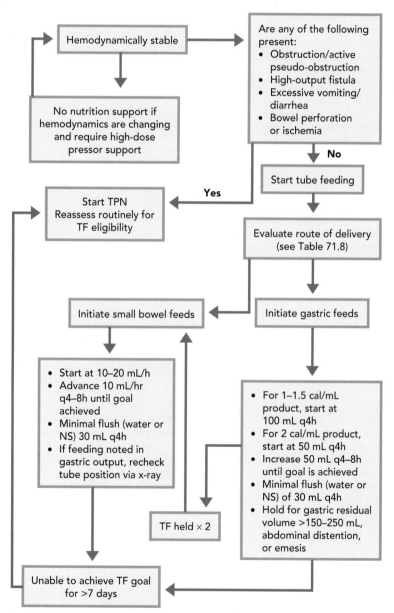

TPN, total parenteral feeding; TF, tube feeding; NS, normal saline.

TABLE 71.5	Advantages and Disadvantages of Enteral and Parenteral Nutrition	
Type of feeding	Advantages	Disadvantages
Enteral nutrition	Preserves gut mucosal integrity	Requires functional GI tract
	Less costly than TPN	More time to reach goal calories
	May blunt hypermetabolic response	Multiple contraindications (e.g., obstruction, fistula)
	Less infectious complications	
Parenteral nutrition	Does not require functioning GI tract	Intestinal atrophy
	Full support in <24 hr	Requires central IV access
		Increased rate of infectious complications

TPN, total parenteral nutrition; GI, gastrointestinal; IV, intravenous.

recommended unless symptoms of malabsorption are present, then a peptide-based product should be initiated. Studies using immune-modulating formulas (those enriched with glutamine, arginine, omega-3 fatty acids, antioxidants, or nucleotides) have been found to be positive in elective upper gastrointestinal surgical, head and neck cancer, burn, trauma, and ICU patients. No benefit of immune-modulating formulas has been established in patients with severe sepsis; in fact, caution should be used when providing products containing arginine to these patients. Advantage has been shown with the use of formulas containing antioxidants and omega-3 fatty acids for patients with pulmonary capillary leak syndromes (acute respiratory distress syndrome or acute lung injury). To receive optimal benefit from immune-modulating formulas,

TABLE 71.6	Gastric and Small Bowel Feeding Indications
Gastric feeding	Small bowel feeding
• Majority of ICU patients • Short gut (to maximize surface area fed) • Total laryngectomies (cannot aspirate)	• Delayed gastric emptying • Postoperative gastric ileus • Severe gastroesophageal reflux disease • Severe pancreatitis (unable to resume PO in 5–7 days) • Proximal gastrointestinal fistula • Intolerance to gastric feeds (despite prokinetic use); high gastric residual volumes, emesis • Supine positioning • Patients unable to protect their airway secondary to heavy sedation (Ramsey >5)

ICU, intensive care unit; PO, by mouth.

TABLE 71.7 Troubleshooting Tube Feeding Complications

Residuals: Gastric residual volume of 250 mL or more on more than one consecutive reading; or 500 mL on one reading.

- Clinically examine for signs of intolerance: abdominal distention, fullness, discomfort, or presence of emesis.
- Start a prokinetic agent: IV metoclopramide 10 mg q6h (if no renal failure present), for no >72 hr.
- Change to a more calorically dense product to decrease total volume infused.
- If a *Moss tube* is present, normal gastric output may reach 2 L/day because of drainage of proximal duodenum.
- Presence of a small amount of tube feeding from the gastric port is normal.
- Order a small bowel feeding tube.

Diarrhea: Quantify amount of stool. It is normal for a patient on tube feedings to have four to five soft formed stools per day.

- Review medications. Diarrhea may be secondary to an enteral medication. Try changing medication route to IV.
- Rule out the presence of *Clostridium difficile*.
- Try adding a soluble fiber to feeds (Benefiber 1 Tbsp TID) if patient fully resuscitated and without risk of bowel ischemia.
- Once infectious cause is ruled out, use an antidiarrheal agent (loperamide 2–4 mg q6h)
- KEEP FEEDING

Constipation: Difficulty passing or no bowel movement >3 days after feedings are at goal.

- Check for signs of dehydration, such as hypernatremia, prerenal azotemia, oliguria, low skin turgor, orthostatic hypotension
- Increase amount of free water.
- Rectal examination with disimpaction.
- Order KUB to rule out obstruction
- Once obstruction is ruled out, start bisacodyl suppository and/or enemas PRN.
- Start bowel regimen (docusate, 100 mg BID, and/or senna syrup, 5 mL BID).

IV, intravenous; TID, three times a day; KUB, kidney/ureter/bladder x-ray; PRN, as needed; BID, two times a day.

at least 50% to 60% of the patient's caloric goal should be provided. At present no recommendation can currently be made for use of probiotics via the enteral feeding route in the general ICU population because of lack of consistent outcome effect and heterogeneity of the bacterial strains studied. Insoluble fiber should be avoided in all critically ill patients and soluble fiber should only be used resuscitated, hemodynamically stable patients. Both forms should be avoided in any patient with severe dysmotility or at risk of bowel ischemia.

Critically ill patients presenting with injuries (traumatic brain injury) or conditions (severe dysphagia due to cerebral vascular accident) that will require >4 weeks of enteral support will benefit from early placement of long-term feeding access. For conditions requiring <4 weeks of therapy, placement of short-term feeding access via the nose or mouth should be instituted. Several options of both short- and long-term access and their associated risks are reviewed in Table 71.8.

TABLE 71.8	Short- and Long-Term Enteral Feeding Access

- *Salem sump nasogastric or orogastric:* a short-term feeding tube generally placed by the bedside nurse for decompression that may be used for feeding. The patient must have a functioning GI tract, adequate gastric-emptying, and low risk of aspiration. Nasally placed tubes carry the risk of sinusitis and nasal necrosis.
- *Nasoenteric feeding tube* for gastric or small bowel placement: a short-term, softer, more flexible tube with less risk of causing sinusitis or nasal necrosis, this tube may also be placed orally. Generally placed in patients for comfort. Small bowel tubes are placed in patients with poor gastric-emptying and have a high risk of reflux.
- *G-tube[a]* for surgical or percutaneous endoscopic gastrostomy: a long-term feeding tube for patients with a functioning GI tract and adequate gastric-emptying. G-tubes have a lower risk of aspiration when compared with above-the-diaphragm feeding access.
- *J-tube[a]* for surgical or percutaneous endoscopic jejunostomy: a long-term feeding tube indicated for patients with a functioning GI tract, poor gastric-emptying, and a high risk for reflux and aspiration.
- *G-J tube[a]:* a long-term feeding tube placed percutaneously or at time of laparotomy in patients for feeding into the distal duodenum with a gastric port for decompression.

[a]All tubes that transverse the two epithelial barriers of the skin and mucosa of the GI tract carry the risk of hemorrhage and infection at the incision site as well as peritonitis and risk of dislodgment. GI, gastrointestinal.

TABLE 71.9	Catheter Selection for Total Parenteral Nutrition (TPN)

- *Triple/quad lumen catheter:* used for in-hospital patients on TPN. The distal port is preferred for the infusion of TPN solution to maintain sterility and avoid contamination. Blood is drawn through the medial port and other infusions are performed through the proximal port(s).
- *PICC (peripheral inserted central catheter):* PICC lines are placed via the brachiocephalic vein. PICC lines have a long catheter (60 cm) with the tip positioned in the superior vena cava.
- *Tunneled catheter:* This is a silastic catheter (single-, double-, or triple-lumen) that is tunneled subcutaneously several centimeters from the insertion site before exiting the skin. If no infection is present, these catheters can stay in place indefinitely.
- *Hohn:* A percutaneously placed catheter used for patients requiring 6 months or less of TPN or IV medication. The distal port (red) is preferred for the infusion of TPN solution to maintain sterility and avoid contamination.
- *Implanted venous access device:* This is a subcutaneously implanted chamber attached to a silastic central venous catheter, either single- or double-lumen. Because the reservoir is implanted in the SQ, it must be accessed with a needle for drawing blood or administering TPN or other IV infusions. These catheters are generally reserved for patients receiving chemotherapy who require periodic infusions.

IV, intravenous.

TPN must be administered via a designated port of a central venous catheter to avoid potential complications associated with incompatibilities with intravenous medication administration. Parenteral nutrition via a peripheral intravenous line is not appropriate for the critically ill patient. Subclavian lines are preferred because of the ease in maintaining an occlusive dressing and the lower rate of infections. The least

TABLE 71.10	Electrolytes Administered Via the Total Parenteral Nutrition Solution	
Suggested electrolytes (per liter)	Conditions that may require alteration of amount provided	Electrolyte carriers
Sodium 60–150 mEq	• Renal function • Fluid status • GI losses • Traumatic brain injury	NaCl Na acetate $NaPO_4$
Potassium 40–120 mEq	• Renal function • GI losses • Metabolic acidosis • Refeeding	KCl K acetate KPO_4
Phosphate 10–30 mM	• Renal function • Refeeding • Bone disease • Hypercalcemia • Rapid healing[a] • Hepatic function	$NaPO_4$ KPO_4
Chloride 60–120 mEq	• Renal function • GI losses (gastric) • Acid-base status	NaCl KCl
Acetate 10–40 mEq	• Renal function • GI losses (small bowel) • Acid-base status • Hepatic function	NaAcetate KAcetate
Calcium 4.5–.2 mEq	• Hyperparathyroidism • Malignancy • Bone disease • Immobilization • Acute pancreatitis • Renal function	Ca Gluconate $CaCl_2$
Magnesium 8.1–24.3 mEq	• Renal function • Refeeding • Hypokalemia	Mg sulfate

[a]Rapid healing examples are burn, and young trauma patients who have rapid tissue generation. GI, gastrointestinal.

desirable is a femoral line that has been associated with a higher incidence of venous thrombosis. The choice of catheter type depends on the reason for TPN, expected duration of TPN, and the patient's overall status (Table 71.9).

When TPN is provided, the practitioner must be knowledgeable regarding the form in which electrolytes are provided, the normal amount recommended, and what conditions should precipitate an alteration in the amount provided (Table 71.10). One must be vigilant when prescribing the various electrolytes that are provided in TPN, as there are inherent risks associated with its administration. This is balanced with the need to avoid exceeding amounts, which may lead to precipitation within the TPN solution itself.

Clinicians often underestimate the importance of nutrition support in the ICU patient population. Early intervention by a nutrition support specialist as part of the multidisciplinary team is imperative to ensure that appropriate access is obtained and substrates provided. Understanding the massive catabolic state that exists with critical illness underscores the need for early and precise nutritional support. Early replacement of ongoing losses of micro- and macronutrients will aid in the patient's recovery once the critical illness has resolved and the anabolic building phase has commenced.

SUGGESTED READINGS

Dabrowski GP, Rombeau JL. Practical nutritional management in the trauma intensive care unit. *Surg Clin North Am.* 2000;80:921–932.
> *A practical overview of nutritional management of the trauma patient.*

Heyland DK, Dhaliwal R, Drover JW, et al. Canadian clinical practice guidelines for nutritional support in mechanically ventilated, critically ill adult patients. *J Parenter Enter Nutr.* 2003;27:355–373.
> *Canadian evidence-based practice guidelines for nutrition support in mechanically ventilated patients.*

Kreymann KG, Berger MM, Deutz NE, et al. ESPEN guidelines on enteral nutrition: intensive care. *Clin Nutr.* 2006;25:210–223.
> *Consensus guidelines based on review of the literature for enteral nutrition support in the critically ill with at least one organ failure.*

Kudsk KA. Effect of route and type of nutrition on intestine-derived inflammatory responses. *Am J Surg.* 2003;185:16–21.
> *This review article looked at the effects on the gastrointestinal from lack of feeding. Findings included an increase in proinflammatory markers and showed that the addition of glutamine reverses many of the defects seen in starvation in the critically ill.*

Marik PE, Zaloga G. Immunonutrition in high-risk surgical patients: a systematic review and analysis of the literature. *J Parenter Enter Nutr.* 2010;34:378–386.
> *In surgery patients, immunonutrition is associated with a reduction in risk of acquired infection and wound complications and a shorter LOS. However, there was not a mortality advantage.*

Martindale RG, McClave SA, Vanek VW, et al; American College of Critical Care Medicine; and the A.S.P.E.N. Board of Directors. Guidelines for the provision and assessment of nutrition support therapy in the adult critically ill patient: Society of Critical Care Medicine and American Society for Parenteral and Enteral Nutrition. *J Parenter Enter Nutr.* 2009;33:277. Executive Summary: *Crit Care Med.* 2009;37:1757.
> *Review of the literature and evidence based recommendations for nutritional support in the critically ill patient.*

Montejo JC, Minambres E, Bordege L, et al. Gastric residual volume during enteral nutrition in ICU patients: the REGANE study. *Intensive Care Med.* 2010;36:1386–1393.

Pontes-Arruda Alessandro, Aragao AM, Albuquerque JP, et al. Effects of enteral feeding with eicosapentaenoic acid, γ-linolenic acid, and antioxidants in mechanically ventilated patients with severe sepsis and septic shock. *Crit Care Med.* 2006;34:2325–2333.

> *This study showed that in patients with severe septic shock requiring mechanical ventilation who were tolerating enteral feeding, a diet rich in EPA, GLA, and antioxidants imparted improved ICU and hospital outcomes and was associated with decrease mortality.*

Singer P, Berger MM, Van den Berghe G, et al. ESPEN guidelines on parenteral nutrition: intensive care. *Clin Nutr.* 2009;28:387–400.

> *Consensus guidelines based on review of the literature for parenteral support in the critically ill patient, covering both parenteral macro- and micronutrients.*

72 Arterial Catheterization

Jeremy Kilburn

Arterial catheterization is the second most frequently performed invasive procedure in the intensive care unit after central venous catheterization. Indications for placing an arterial line include (a) frequent arterial blood gas measurements in patients with respiratory insufficiency, (b) direct arterial hemodynamic monitoring in patients on vasopressor or inotropic support, and less commonly, (c) for placement of an intra-aortic balloon pump or direct arterial administration of drugs (e.g., thrombolytics). Noninvasive arterial oxygen saturation is insufficient in unstable patients, and frequent direct measurement of the arterial pH, bicarbonate, and partial pressure of oxygen and carbon dioxide is often needed in patients on ventilator support or with suspected impending respiratory collapse. In unstable patients, noninvasive blood pressure monitors can be inaccurate, significantly underestimating blood pressure, necessitating the use of arterial lines for accurate hemodynamic monitoring.

Equipment required for catheterization includes (a) an intravascular catheter, (b) noncompliant tubing, (c) flush device with pressurized flush solution, (d) transducer, and (e) electronic monitoring equipment including a connecting cable and a monitor with an amplifier and display screen. Catheter sizes vary on the basis of arterial site (see following discussion) and, once inserted, are connected to the tubing. The tubing is connected to the transducer, which in turn is connected to the electronic monitor via a connecting cable. The noncompliant tubing transmits the pressure waveform from the artery to the transducer, which converts the pressure waveform to an electrical waveform. The electric waveform is amplified and displayed on the oscilloscope screen. The flush device allows continuous fluid infusion to prevent thrombus formation and is pressurized to prevent backup of high-pressure arterial blood into the tubing.

The most common site selected for arterial catheterization is the radial artery, followed by the femoral artery. Less common sites include the dorsalis pedis, brachial, and axillary arteries. Although both radial and femoral sites are acceptable and have a similar complication profile, the radial site is generally attempted first.

The radial and ulnar arteries are the distal branches of the brachial artery and are located on the lateral and medial sides of the wrists in anatomic position, respectively. They are connected to one another by the deep and superficial palmar arches in the hand. These arterial anastomoses are taken into consideration when a radial line is placed, as a potential complication of radial artery catheterization is thrombosis. If thrombosis occurs, collateral circulation from the ulnar artery through the palmar arches typically ensures adequate blood flow to the hand. Peripheral vascular disease that occludes the palmar arches could interrupt blood flow to the hand if radial artery thrombus occurs.

The modified Allen test is used in an attempt to identify patients who have compromised collateral palmar circulation. The test is performed by raising the patient's arm to 45 degrees, with the examiner compressing the radial and ulnar arteries with both hands. The patient is asked to repeatedly open and close the hand to drain the blood from it. When pallor develops, one artery is released and the time to palmar flushing is timed. Less than 7 seconds is considered positive, 8 to 14 seconds is equivocal, and 15 or more seconds is considered a negative test and evidence for a lack of adequate collateral circulation. The test is repeated with the other artery.

One study compared Allen test to Doppler ultrasound examination. The study found the test had a sensitivity of 87%, meaning that patients who had a positive Allen test also had ultrasound documentation of collateral flow 87% of the time. However, the negative predictive value was only 18%, meaning that only 18% of patients who had a negative Allen test had documented lack of collateral circulation by ultrasound. In addition, many patients in whom arterial lines are placed have decreased mental status and cannot participate in the test. Results may also be difficult to interpret for patients on vasopressor support. Thus, many centers have now abandoned the routine performance of the Allen test.

Two types of arterial catheters are commonly in use. The most basic is a catheter-over-needle apparatus. The other is also a catheter-over-needle, but with the addition of a guidewire. Peripheral sites, including the radial artery, are generally cannulated with a 20-gage Teflon catheter. Larger vessels such as the femoral artery are cannulated with an 18-gage Teflon catheter kit containing introducer needles and guide wire.

STEPS FOR RADIAL ARTERY CANNULATION

1. Position the supine patient's hand with 30 to 60 degrees of extension by propping the dorsal wrist surface on a rolled towel or other supporting structure with the ventral surface up.
2. Remove all objects from the wrist and cleanse the wrist's ventral surface with an antiseptic solution such as chlorhexidine or Betadine.
3. Drape the wrist in a sterile fashion and with sterile technique including sterile drapes, gloves, gown, and a mask (a reasonable rule is to gown and mask when placing objects in a patient that will remain in place and be a potential source of infection).
4. Palpate the radial artery on the patient's ventral wrist with the first two fingers of the nondominant hand 3 to 4 cm proximal to the crease at the base of the thenar eminence.
5. With the dominant hand, hold the catheter like a pencil between the first and second fingers.
6. While palpating gently with the nondominant hand, enter the skin at a 30- to 45-degree angle with the catheter tip just distal (relative to the patient) to the fingertips of the nondominant hand (see Figure 18.7 in Lin, 2001). Pressing too firmly on the radial artery can occlude flow and make cannulation difficult.
7. Advance the catheter toward the artery until a flash of blood enters the catheter tip.
8. If using a simple catheter-over-needle configuration, advance the tip of the needle slightly further into the artery to ensure that the tip of the catheter is in the arterial lumen (note: go to step 12 if using a device with a wire).
9. Drop the needle and catheter so that they lie flat on the skin (instead of at a 30- to 45-degree angle).

10. While holding the needle steady with the nondominant hand, advance the catheter gently forward into the artery lumen with a slight twisting motion.
11. Remove the needle; correct placement should result in pulsatile blood flow (if using a catheter without a wire go to step 15).
12. If using a catheter with a wire, when the flash of blood occurs, hold the catheter and needle steady and advance the wire into the arterial lumen, which should meet little resistance.
13. Now advance the catheter over the wire and into the arterial lumen.
14. Remove the needle and wire; correct placement should result in pulsatile blood flow.
15. Connect the catheter to the transducer tubing and flush device.
16. Secure the catheter securely to the skin, usually with suture or noninvasive device.
17. Cleanse the skin and catheter with antiseptic solution and cover with sterile dressing.

TIPS

If the initial attempt is unsuccessful, reposition the catheter and try again. A less steep angle may decrease your chance of traversing the artery. If further attempts are unsuccessful, try advancing the needle through the artery when the initial flash of blood is seen in the catheter tip. Next slowly withdraw the catheter until a flash of blood again occurs and attempt to advance a guidewire through the catheter and into the arterial lumen. Once the guidewire is in place, the catheter can be advanced over it. Deliberate palpation of the artery and focused technique will aid in a successful result. The artery often is transfixed initially with no blood flow. Thus, the catheter should always be withdrawn slowly as success is often achieved while withdrawing the catheter.

For *femoral artery cannulation,* a kit identical to the central venous catheterization kit is often used. The femoral artery lies in the femoral triangle bordered superiorly by the inguinal ligament, laterally by the sartorius muscle, and medially by the adductor longus muscle (see Fig. 73.4). From the lateral to medial positions in the triangle lie the femoral nerve, femoral artery, and femoral vein. The site should be cleaned and prepared in a sterile fashion. Similar to the radial artery, the femoral artery is palpated with the nondominant hand. Cannulation of the artery is performed in the same manner as venous cannulation (see Chapter 73), but when blood returns into the syringe and it is disconnected from the needle, pulsatile blood confirms arterial placement (although it may be nonpulsatile during cardiac arrest).

Complications of arterial line placement are listed in Table 72.1. The incidence of clinically significant complications is <5% at most centers. Thrombosis is the most common complication. The Thunder Project in 1993 by the American Association of Critical Care Nurses randomized 5193 patients with arterial lines to heparinized and nonheparinized flush solutions and followed catheter patency for up to 72 hours. The study found that arterial lines maintained with heparin had a greater probability of remaining patent than lines maintained without heparin. Multiple meta-analyses have confirmed lower thrombosis rates when lines are maintained with a continuous infusion of heparin, generally at a heparin concentration of 1 U/mL and a rate of 3 mL/hr. For patients with contraindications to heparin, a continuous infusion with sodium citrate or saline should be used.

Infection also occurs with arterial line placement, and its incidence can be minimized with careful sterile technique during catheter placement and routine catheter

TABLE 72.1	Complications of Arterial Cannulation

Thrombosis
Local or systemic infection
Hematoma
Pseudoaneurysm
Hemorrhage
Significant blood loss from frequent blood testing
Heparin-induced thrombocytopenia (for heparin-flushed lines)
Retroperitoneal hematoma (femoral lines)
Limb ischemia
Peripheral neuropathy
Insertion site pain

care. Catheter dressings should be changed approximately every 48 hours. Careful sterile technique should be used when drawing blood samples from the catheter. The incidence of catheter-related infections for arterial lines does not differ based on site (i.e., radial vs. femoral) if sterile technique is used. Also, catheters kept in place longer than 7 days have not demonstrated significantly higher rates of serious infections. In part due to higher pressure blood flow, arterial lines are less likely to become infected than central venous lines. For febrile patients, arterial lines do not necessarily need to be removed unless no other infectious source is identified. When catheters do become infected, the most common pathogen is *Staphylococcus epidermidis*. Catheters should be removed as soon as they are no longer needed.

SUGGESTED READINGS

American Association of Critical-Care Nurses. Evaluation of the effects of heparinized and non-heparinized flush solutions on the patency of arterial pressure monitoring lines: the AACN Thunder Project. *Am J Crit Care.* 1993;1:3–15.
  Randomized trial of 5139 patients with arterial lines assigned to heparinized and non-heparinized flush solutions and followed for up to 72 hours, showing lines maintained with heparin had a significantly greater probability of remaining patent over time than lines maintained with non-heparinized solutions.
Glavin RJ, Jones HM. Assessing collateral circulation in the hand: four methods compared. *Anesthesia.* 1989;44:594–595.
  Study comparing the Allen's test, ultrasound, pulse monitor, and pulse oximeter to detect collateral circulation in the hand, showing that none, when compared with ultrasound, reliably documented adequate ulnar collateral circulation.
Lin TL, Mohajer JM, Sakurai KA. eds. Accessing the Radial Artery. *The Washington Manual Internship Survival Guide.* 1st ed. Lippincott: William & Wilkins, 2001:165.
Thomas F, Burke JP, Parker J, et al. The risk of infection related to radial vs. femoral sites for arterial catheterization. *Crit Care Med.* 1983;10:807–812.
  Randomized study of 186 femoral or radial artery catheters, which found similarly low rates of infection between the two sites.

73 Central Venous Catheterization

Chad A. Witt

Central venous catheterization is commonly performed in the intensive care unit. Indications for central venous catheterization include administration of vasoactive medications, total parenteral nutrition, or other agents necessitating central venous access, central venous pressure monitoring, rapid large-volume fluid or blood product administration, and emergency venous access. Contraindications for central venous catheterization include known thrombosis of the target vessel and infection over the site of entry. There is no definitive cut-off for the performance of central venous catheterization in coagulopathic or thrombocytopenic patients, although the use of a micropuncture kit and/or correction with fresh-frozen plasma and/or platelet transfusion may be pertinent in this population prior to the procedure.

The most common complications of central venous catheterization include arterial puncture, pneumothorax, hydrothorax, hemothorax, air embolus, retroperitoneal hemorrhage, infections (central venous catheter-associated bacteremia, local site infection/cellulitis), and thromboembolic disease. Overall, the complication rate is related to the site of insertion, with the subclavian vein being less than the internal jugular vein, which is less than the femoral vein. The use of ultrasound guidance to aid in the placement of central venous catheters, especially in the internal jugular position, has been shown to decrease complication rates, decrease the number of attempts necessary to cannulate the vein, and decrease the amount of time necessary to perform the procedure.

Before performing central venous catheterization, obtain informed consent based on the policies of each institution. All present must agree on the patient identification, the procedure being performed, and the site of the procedure. Sterile precautions must be observed, including hand hygiene with alcohol foam/gel or antimicrobial soap, full sterile drape, sterile gloves, sterile gown, mask with face shield, and hair coverage. All persons present in the room should wear masks and hair coverage. It is helpful to have a nonsterile assistant present during the procedure.

The following guidelines are for the placement of central venous catheters using commercially available kits via Seldinger's (over guidewire) technique.

SUBCLAVIAN CENTRAL VENOUS CATHETER PLACEMENT

1. Place the patient in Trendelenburg position, and place a towel roll between the scapulae. Keep the head in neutral position or toward the side of line placement to help direction the guidewire inferiorly.

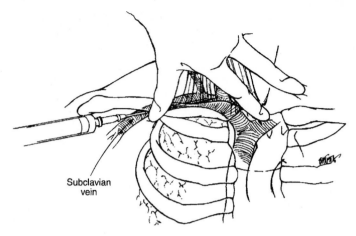

Figure 73.1. Subclavian vein anatomy and cannulation. (From Lin TL, Mohart JM, Sakurai KA. *The Washington Manual Internship Survival Guide,* 2nd ed. Philadelphia, PA: Lippincott Williams & Wilkins; 2001:195.)

2. Don sterile gown, sterile gloves, mask with face shield, and hair cover.
3. Prepare the skin with antiseptic solution (e.g., chlorhexidine or Betadine).
4. Use a sterile full-body drape and a sterile drape with a site hole or surgical towels to cover the body, head, and face, exposing only the necessary skin.
5. Flush all ports of the catheter to ensure appropriate functioning.
6. Place the index finger of the nondominant hand at the sternal notch and the thumb of the same hand on the clavicle where it bends over the first rib (approximately where the lateral third and medial two-thirds of the clavicle meet). The subclavian vein should traverse a line between the index finger and the thumb (Fig. 73.1).
7. Anesthetize the skin and subcutaneous tissue just inferior to the clavicle and lateral to the thumb.
8. With the introducer needle, bevel up, enter the skin lateral to the thumb, inferior to the clavicle (approximately 2 cm inferior and 2 cm lateral to the bend in the clavicle). Aim at the index finger (sternal notch), aspirating while advancing. It is imperative to keep the needle parallel to the floor during advancement. If the clavicle is contacted, depress the entire needle with the thumb until it passes under the clavicle, rather than changing the angle of approach. Dark blood will enter the syringe when the vein is cannulated. If there is no blood return after advancing the needle 5 cm, withdraw the needle while continuing to aspirate (frequently the vein has been pierced, and successful blood flow will be obtained during withdrawal). Redirect the needle more cephalad, and try again. Multiple repeated attempts are not recommended (Fig. 73.1). Once appropriate venous return is noted, rotate the bevel of the needle inferior.
9. Securely hold the needle, remove the syringe (placing a finger over the needle hub to reduce the risk of air embolism), and insert the guidewire. The guidewire should advance with little resistance. Leave enough of the guidewire outside the body to account for the catheter length.
10. While holding the guidewire (*always maintain control and hold of the guidewire*), remove the introducer needle. Once the introducer needle is outside the

patient's skin, hold the guidewire at the entry site and slide the needle off the guidewire.

11. Using a scalpel, make a small nick in the skin at the entry site. Ensure that the cutting edge of the scalpel is facing away from the guidewire and make a stabbing in-out motion to make the nick.

12. Pass the dilator over the guidewire, dilate the tract, and remove the dilator.

13. Ensure that the distal port of the catheter is open. Pass the catheter over the guidewire. When the catheter is near the entry site, feed the guidewire out until it emerges from the distal port on the catheter. Grasp the guidewire distally, and insert the catheter to the desired depth (15 to 16 cm for the right subclavian vein, 18 to 20 cm for the left subclavian vein, 16 to 17 cm for the right IJ vein, 17 to 18 cm for the left IJ vein).

14. Hold the catheter in place, and withdraw the guidewire.

15. Flush all ports to ensure that they are functioning properly.

16. Secure the catheter with suture or a commercially available sutureless kit.

17. Cleanse the site with antiseptic solution and place a sterile dressing.

18. Obtain a chest radiograph for placement and to evaluate for pneumothorax. The tip of the catheter should reside in the superior vena cava.

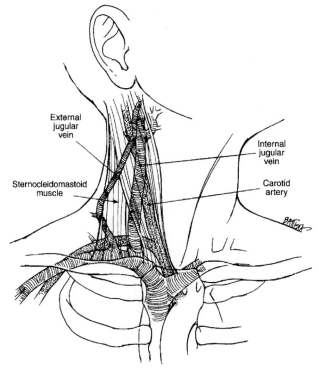

Figure 73.2. Internal jugular vein anatomy. (From Lin TL, Mohart JM, Sakurai KA. *The Washington Manual Internship Survival Guide,* 2nd ed. Philadelphia, PA: Lippincott Williams & Wilkins; 2001:191.)

INTERNAL JUGULAR CENTRAL VENOUS CATHETER PLACEMENT

(*Note:* ultrasound guidance is preferable, if available.)

1. Place the patient in Trendelenburg position, and have the patient turn his or her head 45 degrees to the direction opposite the site of catheter placement.
2. Don sterile gown, sterile gloves, mask with face shield, and hair cover.
3. Prepare the skin with antiseptic solution (e.g., chlorhexidine or Betadine).
4. Use a sterile full-body drape and a sterile drape with a site hole or surgical towels to cover the body, head, and face, exposing only the necessary skin.
5. Flush all ports of the catheter to ensure appropriate functioning.
6. Identify the triangle formed by the two heads of the sternocleidomastoid muscle and the sternum, and palpate the carotid pulse (Fig. 73.2).
7. Anesthetize the skin and subcutaneous tissue.
8. Palpate the carotid pulse. Lateral to the carotid pulse, advance the 22-gauge needle (finder needle), bevel up, at a 30- to 45-degree angle to the patient, directed at the ipsilateral nipple while aspirating. If no venous blood return is noted, withdraw the needle and change the angle to a more lateral and then more medial position. Maintain palpation of the carotid pulse. When venous blood is aspirated, make

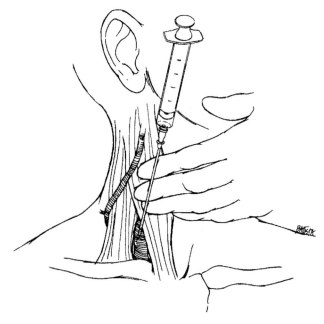

Figure 73.3. Cannulation of the internal jugular vein. (From Lin TL, Mohart JM, Sakurai KA. *The Washington Manual Internship Survival Guide,* 2nd ed. Philadelphia, PA: Lippincott Williams & Wilkins; 2001:192.).

note of the angle and depth of the finder needle, and remove the finder needle. *If the carotid artery is entered (bright red and/or pulsatile blood), remove the needle and hold pressure for 10 to 15 minutes.*

9. At the same site and angle as the internal jugular vein was entered with the finder needle, insert the introducer needle until free flow of dark venous blood is noted (Fig. 73.3).

10. Follow steps 9 through 18 for subclavian central venous catheter placement.

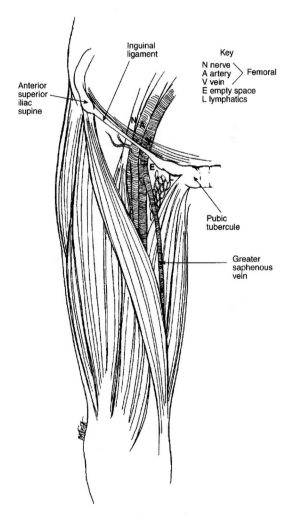

Figure 73.4. Femoral vein anatomy. (From Lin TL, Mohart JM, Sakurai KA. *The Washington Manual Internship Survival Guide,* 2nd ed. Philadelphia, PA: Lippincott Williams & Wilkins; 2001:183.)

FEMORAL CENTRAL VENOUS CATHETER PLACEMENT

1. Place the patient in the supine position, with the ipsilateral thigh slightly abducted and externally rotated.
2. Don sterile gown, sterile gloves, mask with face shield, and hair cover.
3. Prepare the skin with antiseptic solution (e.g., chlorhexidine or Betadine).
4. Use a sterile full-body drape and a sterile drape with a site hole or surgical towels to cover the body and legs, exposing only the necessary skin.
5. Flush all ports of the catheter to ensure appropriate functioning.
6. Palpate the femoral arterial pulse inferior to the inguinal ligament. The femoral vein is medial to the femoral artery (Fig. 73.4).
7. Anesthetize the skin and subcutaneous tissues, aspirating prior to injecting anesthetic.
8. Palpate the femoral pulse. With the introducer needle bevel up, enter the skin 1 cm medial to the pulse, inferior to the inguinal ligament, at a 30- to 45-degree angle (Fig. 73.5). Continue to aspirate as the needle is advanced until the return of venous blood. If the needle is advanced 5 cm with no return of venous blood, withdraw while continuing to aspirate, angle more medially, and try again. *If the femoral artery is entered (bright red and/or pulsatile blood), hold pressure for 10 to 15 minutes.*

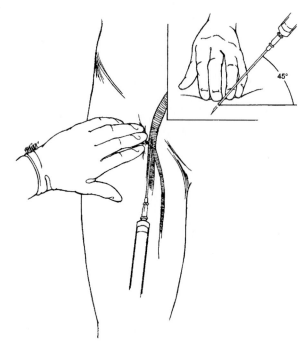

Figure 73.5. Femoral vein cannulation. (From Lin TL, Mohart JM, Sakurai KA. *The Washington Manual Internship Survival Guide,* 2nd ed. Philadelphia, PA: Lippincott Williams & Wilkins; 2001:197.)

9. Follow steps 9 through 17 for subclavian central venous catheter placement. For the femoral site, the entire length of the catheter is inserted (20 cm) and secured in place.

SUGGESTED READINGS

Hind D, Calvert N, McWilliams R, et al. Ultrasonic locating devices for central venous cannulation: meta-analysis. *BMJ.* 2003;327:361.
   Meta-analysis examining the utility and benefit of two dimensional ultrasound and doppler guidance for central venous catheter placement.
Lin TL, Mohart JM, Sakurai KA. The Washington manual internship survival guide, 2e. Philadelphia, PA: Lippincott Williams & Wilkins, 2001:157–164.
   Concise instructions on the indications, complications, and placement of central venous catheters.
McGee DC, Gould MK. Preventing complications of central venous catheterization. *N Engl J Med.* 2003;348:1123–1133.
   Review of central venous catheter placement, and the various intervention and practice techniques available to reduce and/or prevent complications of central venous catheterization.

74 Endotracheal Intubation

Michael Lippmann

Endotracheal intubation maintains airway patency, assures delivery of preset tidal volume breaths from mechanical ventilators, facilitates pulmonary toilet and helps prevent aspiration. Indications for endotracheal intubation include acute airway obstruction from trauma, infection, laryngeal edema or spasm or tumor; inability to protect the upper airway due to altered mental status from trauma, drug overdose, or cerebrovascular accident (CVA); respiratory failure and cardiopulmonary arrest (Table 74.1).

Risks include trauma to the oropharynx, hypoxemia from prolonged attempts, and unrecognized misplacement of the endotracheal tube. The incidence of complications markedly increases when intubation is attempted by inadequately trained or inexperienced providers. These providers should attempt to achieve adequate ventilation and oxygenation using bag-valve-mask devices or other advanced airway devices, which do not require visualization of the vocal cords to place.

Assessment of the upper airway anatomy facilitates recognition of potentially difficult intubations allowing practitioners formulate alternative plans and to assemble necessary equipment. An abbreviated assessment should be performed even in emergent cases. Clinicians should pay particular attention to dentition and the presence of dental appliances; the mobility of the tongue and its size relative to the oropharynx (Mallampati classification) (Fig. 74.1); range of extension and flexion of the cervical spine; mobility of the jaw; and presence of stridor. Difficult intubation may be anticipated in patients with thick or fat necks, narrow mouth openings, large tongues, and limited motion of the cervical spine.

All necessary equipment should be immediately available prior to intubation attempts. Necessary equipment includes a bag-valve-mask device, high-flow oxygen source, suction equipment, functioning laryngoscope handles and blades, appropriate-sized endotracheal tube (7.5 to 8.5 cm for most adults), stylet, syringe for endotracheal balloon inflation, medications for induction if indicated, tape or other mechanism for securing the endotracheal tube, and a device to confirm placement of the tube in the trachea.

TABLE 74.1	Indications for Endotracheal Intubation

- Acute airway obstruction
- Inability to protect the airway
- Respiratory failure
- Cardiopulmonary arrest

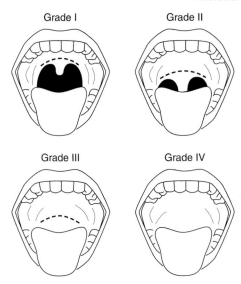

Figure 74.1. Mallampati classification. (From WK Health.)

Successful intubation requires overcoming the normal barriers to objects entering the trachea. These include reflexes arising from laryngeal stimulation, the malalignment of the major axes of the upper airway and the anatomic barriers of the tongue and epiglottis. Endotracheal intubation is extremely uncomfortable procedure and even patients with decreased mental status may cough and actively resist attempts at intubation. In addition, laryngeal stimulation increases sympathetic tone with consequent increases in blood pressure, heart rate, and intracranial pressure.

Judicious use of appropriate medications can blunt the potential adverse physiologic effects and provide sedation and amnesia. Lidocaine given as a 1.5 to 2 mg/kg bolus at least 2 minutes prior to intubation can blunt increases in intracranial pressures and is used in patients with head trauma. Agents producing sedation and anesthesia include opioids, benzodiazepines, barbiturates, etomidate, and ketamine. Decisions regarding use of specific agents are based on knowledge of their advantages and disadvantages relative to the patient's clinical status and comorbidities (Table 74.2). Paralytic agents should be used only by practitioners highly skilled in endotracheal intubation.

The "sniffing" position helps align the oral, laryngeal, and pharyngeal axes (Fig. 74.2). This position is attained by flexing the neck approximately 30 degrees and extending the head at the atlanto-occipital joint to 20 degrees. Placement of a towel under the occiput facilitates maintenance of this position.

The laryngoscope is used to displace the tongue and lift the epiglottis away from the glottic opening. Laryngoscope blades vary in size and shape. Blade sizes range from 0 to 4 with higher the number corresponding to larger blades. The curved (MacIntosh) blade has broad, flat surface, and tall flange. Straight blades include Miller, Wisconsin, and Phillips. The straight blades vary with regard to their width, presence and size of flange, and shape of distal end. Curved blades apply upward traction to the base of the tongue at the vallecula, indirectly lifting the epiglottis while straight blades lift the

TABLE 74.2 Agents Used for Intubation

Agent	Action	Advantages	Disadvantages
Lidocaine	Blunts intubation-induced increases in ICP	May also decrease arrhythmias and blunt hemodynamic response	
Fentanyl	Opioid – provides rapid onset of sedation and anesthesia	Also blocks rise in blood pressure	Increases ICP; may cause hypotension and apnea
Midazolam	Sedative-hypnotic benzodiazepine	Rapid acting with relatively short action	Negative inotrope
Thiopental	Sedative-hypnotic barbiturate	Cerebroprotective (decreases CNS metabolism)	Negative inotrope and vasodilator; bronchospasm from histamine release
Etomidate	Sedative-hypnotic carboxylated imidazole	Rapid onset of action with brief duration; cerebroprotective	Transient adrenocortical dysfunction

epiglottis directly (Figs. 74.3 and 74.4). Choice of specific equipment should be left to the individual practitioner. In general, straight blades allow visualization of a larger portion of the vocal cords as the epiglottis is removed from the field of view. It may be difficult to control a large tongue with a Miller blade, which is relatively narrow.

All equipment must be immediately available prior to intubation attempts. With the patient in the "sniff" position, the laryngoscope is held in the left hand and the blade is inserted into the right side of the mouth to the base of the tongue. The blade is then moved to the midline sweeping the tongue to the left. The laryngoscope handle and blade should align with the nasal septum. The tip of straight blades is advanced to the tip of the epiglottis while the tip of curved blades is placed in the vallecula.

The vocal cords are exposed by elevating the epiglottis through a lifting motion using the arm and shoulder in a plane 45 degrees from the horizontal. The wrist must be kept stiff to avoid a prying motion that uses the teeth as a fulcrum. When the vocal cords are visualized, the endotracheal tube is advanced from the right side of the mouth with the tip directed so that it intersects the tip of the laryngoscope blade at the level of the glottis allowing the operator to view the entry of the tube into the trachea (Fig. 74.5). The tube is advanced through the vocal cords until the cuff disappears. The cuff is then inflated with sufficient air to prevent leakage during ventilation with a bag valve. The endotracheal tube must be held firmly in place at all times to prevent displacement.

Correct tube placement is established through visualization of chest expansion and auscultation over the epigastrium and lung fields during positive pressure ventilation and confirmed using end-tidal CO_2 detection devices. Upon confirmation of placement, the endotracheal tube is secured firmly in place with either tape or a commercial device.

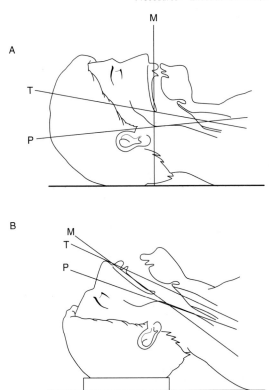

Figure 74.2. Anatomic axes for endotracheal intubation. **A:** With the head in the neutral position, the axis of the mouth (M), the axis of the trachea (T), and the axis of the pharynx (P) are not aligned with one another. **B:** If the head is extended at the atlanto-occipital joints, the axis of the mouth is correctly placed. If the back of the head is raised off the table with a pillow, thus flexing the cervical vertebral column, the axes of the trachea and pharynx are brought in line with the axis of the mouth. (From Snell RS, *Clinical Anatomy*, 7th ed. Lippincott Williams & Wilkins, 2003.)

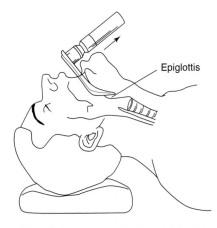

Figure 74.3. Intubation with a Macintosh blade. Blade is used anterior to the epiglottis. (From Blackbourne LH. *Advanced Surgical Recall*, 2nd ed. Baltimore, MD: Lippincott Williams & Wilkins, 2004.)

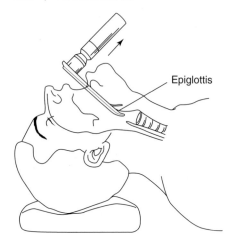

Figure 74.4. Intubation with a Miller blade. Blade is used to hold the epiglottic (posterior to the epiglottis). (From Blackbourne LH. *Advanced Surgical Recall*, 2nd ed. Baltimore, MD: Lippincott Williams & Wilkins, 2004.)

Cricoid pressure (Sellick maneuver) decreases the risk of aspiration by compressing the esophagus between the cricoid cartilage and the vertebral column. Pressure should be applied prior to intubation attempts and maintained until confirmation of correct endotracheal tube placement.

Attempts at intubation should not take longer than 1 minute. In patients where there is difficulty intubating the trachea repeated attempts increase the risk of trauma and hypoxemia. Alternate approaches to endotracheal intubation via direct laryngoscopy include laryngeal mask airways, laryngeal tube airways, flexible fiberoptic scopes, and percutaneous tracheostomy. Laryngeal mask and laryngeal tube airways are placed blindly into the upper airway and form a seal over the laryngeal inlet to ventilate and oxygenate patients while partially occluding the esophagus allowing for directed ventilation into the trachea.

Correct placement of the endotracheal tube is verified clinically visually by observing chest expansion and by auscultation over the abdomen and chest. Correct placement is further assured using an end-tidal CO_2 or esophageal detection device.

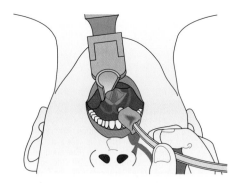

Figure 74.5. Endotracheal intubation–intubating. Illustration showing correct method for intubating victim during endotracheal intubation. (From *LifeART Image* copyright © 2007 Lippincott Williams & Wilkins. All rights reserved.)

Following confirmation the tube can be secured in place using tape or commercial device.

SUGGESTED READINGS

Blanda M, Gallo U. Emergency airway management. *Emerg Med Clin North Am.* 2003;21:1–26.
Overview of techniques for endotracheal intubation.
Butler K, Clyne B. Management of the difficult airway: alternative techniques and adjuncts.
Emerg Med Clin North Am. 2003;21:259–289.
How to recognize patients at high risk for difficult tracheal intubation and alternative techniques available to the practitioner.

75 Percutaneous Tracheostomy

Alexander C. Chen

Tracheostomy is a technique for creating an artificial airway between the neck surface and cervical trachea. There are two main tracheostomy techniques. The surgical approach uses surgical dissection to form the tract between the neck surface and the trachea. More recently, a percutaneous approach has been developed. Variations on this approach use the Seldinger technique to form the tract between the neck surface and the trachea. Although not suitable for all patients, the percutaneous approach has potential advantages over the surgical approach in appropriately selected intensive care unit (ICU) patients. A meta-analysis showed a lower rate of peristomal bleeding and postoperative infection with percutaneous tracheostomy. In addition, because percutaneous tracheostomies are commonly performed in the patient's ICU room, the risk of adverse events associated with transporting critically ill patients is reduced, and scheduling flexibility is increased. Lastly, some research supports percutaneous tracheostomies as the more cost-effective tracheostomy approach for ICU patients.

The remainder of this chapter will focus on percutaneous tracheostomies.

INDICATIONS

1. Upper airway obstruction. A surgical approach is often more appropriate for upper airway obstruction due to tumor.
2. Need for long-term mechanical ventilation.
3. Access for frequent suctioning and other airway care.
4. Treatment of severe obstructive sleep apnea when continuous positive airway pressure is ineffective or not tolerated.

CONTRAINDICATIONS

Contraindications unique to the percutaneous approach include difficult-to-palpate neck anatomy or history of prior neck surgery or radiation. Patients with high ventilatory and oxygenation requirements may be better served by a surgical approach because of the reduced ability to ventilate around the bronchoscope and likelihood of greater positive end-expiratory pressure loss during the procedure. Coagulopathies should be corrected prior to proceeding, although there are no well-validated thresholds. One center described a low rate of complications for percutaneous tracheostomy in the setting of significant thrombocytopenia as long as platelets were administered before the procedure. Hypotension can be worsened because of the significant amount of sedatives commonly needed to perform the procedure, making hypovolemia, and hypotension relative contraindications.

TIMING OF TRACHEOSTOMY PROCEDURE IN CRITICALLY ILL PATIENTS

Most patients receive tracheostomies in the ICU because of difficulty weaning from the ventilator or because they cannot protect and clear their own airways. Potential advantages of tracheostomy over prolonged endotracheal intubation include greater comfort, decreased sedation requirements, enhanced ability to participate in rehabilitation, and facilitated weaning. Optimal timing for tracheostomy in ICU patients is controversial. If prolonged intubation is predicted at admission, a tracheostomy on day 1 or 2 may be appropriate. In most patients, a tracheostomy is considered after 1 to 2 weeks of endotracheal intubation. A recent editorial argues that the preponderance of evidence supports earlier tracheostomy over prolonged endotracheal intubation, although the authors recognize that there are significant design shortcomings in the studies supporting this strategy.

PROCEDURE FOR PERCUTANEOUS TRACHEOSTOMY

Approaches differ slightly on the basis of operator preferences and the particular brand of percutaneous tracheostomy kit used. The following description describes the Ciaglia technique modified by the use of a single dilator with a hydrophilic coating.

1. Explain procedure including risks and benefits. Obtain consent.
2. A team approach makes the procedure more efficient and optimizes patient safety. The bronchoscopist is responsible for bronchoscopic guidance and maintenance of the airway. The bronchoscopist should be skilled in airway management in case of accidental extubation during the procedure. Video bronchoscopy is advantageous because it allows the operator to see the interior of the trachea continuously during the procedure. The nurse assists with intravenous anesthesia during the procedure. A respiratory therapist makes appropriate changes to the ventilator throughout the procedure. The operator performs the procedure and communicates to other members of the team to ensure coordination.
3. Increase FiO_2 to 100%.
4. Monitor blood pressure every 3 to 5 minutes; monitor other variables, including heart rate, pulse oximetry, and airway pressure, continuously.
5. A variety of anesthetic regimens can be used, although combinations of a benzodiazepine and short-acting narcotic or propofol work well. Traditionally, after deep sedation is achieved, a paralytic is administered to prevent coughing. Currently, we perform most of our procedures without a paralytic and have not had significant problems with this approach.
6. A small pad is placed under the shoulders to slightly extend the neck. The neck is prepared with chlorhexidine and a large surgical drape is used to completely cover the patient, with a small opening at the neck. The operator scrubs and dons a hat, protective eyewear, a mask, and sterile gloves and gown.
7. The operator selects the appropriate incision site by palpating the thyroid and cricoid cartilages and the sternal notch. Typically, the space between the first and second, or second and third cartilaginous rings can be approached with an incision halfway between the cricoid cartilage and the sternal notch.

8. After creating a skin wheal with lidocaine, the needle is raised to form a 90-degree angle with the trachea. The tract is anesthetized and the needle is advanced slowly while continuously aspirating. Air bubbles will appear when the needle penetrates the trachea.

9. A 1.5- to 2-cm incision through the skin and superficial subcutaneous tissue is made either horizontally or vertically.

10. A small, curved Kelley clamp is used to dissect a tract down to the trachea.

11. The bronchoscopist carefully withdraws the endotracheal tube over the bronchoscope until the tip lies just below the vocal cords and the tracheal lumen is visible. Firm pressure is applied to the trachea with the Kelly clamp to confirm placement between the appropriate cartilaginous rings.

12. Under continuous bronchoscopic visualization, the catheter-over-needle apparatus is advanced through the skin incision, between the selected tracheal rings, and into the trachea under continuous bronchoscopic surveillance. The catheter is advanced off the needle into the trachea while the needle is withdrawn.

13. The guidewire is threaded through the catheter toward the carina.

14. The catheter is removed, leaving the guidewire in place.

15. A punch dilator is advanced through the trachea and then removed.

16. Next, the curved dilator is inserted over the wire into the trachea. Remove dilator.

17. Load tracheostomy tube onto dilator and advance over guidewire. Percutaneous tracheostomy tubes have tapered ends that allow for easier tracheal insertion.

18. Next, the bronchoscopist removes the bronchoscope from the endotracheal tube and quickly inspects through the tracheostomy tube to ensure proper placement. The patient is reconnected to mechanical ventilation through the tracheostomy tube.

19. The bronchoscopist can inspect the trachea above the tracheostomy tube to rule out active bleeding and to suction blood and secretions, and then completely remove the endotracheal tube.

20. The tracheostomy tube is sewed into place, secured with tracheostomy ties, and dressed appropriately.

21. The tracheostomy tube is changed on day 10 to 14.

COMPLICATIONS

Percutaneous tracheostomy complications are typically divided into early and late categories. More common early complications include transient hypotension and minor bleeding during the procedure. Massive hemorrhage from damage to the innominate vessels has been described but is exceedingly rare. Pneumothoraces and cardiac arrests are uncommon early complications. Fractured tracheal rings occur frequently, although the clinical significance of this complication is unknown. Late complications include stomal infections, bleeding, accidental decannulation, and tracheal stenosis. Bronchoscopic visualization reduces, although does not eliminate, older described complications such as posterior tracheal perforation. Tracheal stenosis rates vary widely in the literature, with some reports finding them to be rare and others finding them to be more common in patients undergoing percutaneous tracheostomies compared with those who undergo surgical tracheostomies.

The use of different techniques and study population selection may explain some of the discrepancies in the literature. When stenosis develops in patients who have undergone percutaneous tracheostomy, they tend to be subglottic in location and may be more challenging to correct surgically.

SUGGESTED READINGS

Ahrens T, Kollef MH. Early tracheostomy. Has its time arrived? *Crit Care Med.* 2004;32:1796–1797.
Discusses controversies surrounding timing of tracheostomies.

Barba CA, Angood PB, Kauder DR, et al. Bronchoscopic guidance makes percutaneous tracheostomy a safe, cost-effective, and easy-to-tech procedure. *Surgery.* 1995;118:879–883.
Experience comparing percutaneous and surgical tracheostomies in 48 trauma patients. Percutaneous approach found to be easy to learn and perform and to be cost-effective.

Beiderlinden M, Walz MK, Sander A, et al. Complications of bronchoscopically guided percutaneous dilational tracheostomy: beyond the learning curve. *Intensive Care Med.* 2002;28:59–62.
Reviews complications in 136 percutaneous tracheostomies in a mixed surgical and medical ICU setting. Other than clinically relevant bleeding episodes in 2.9% of patients complications were rare.

Ciaglia P, Firsching R, Syniec C. Elective percutaneous dilational tracheostomy—a simple bedside procedure; a preliminary report. *Chest.* 1985;87:715–719.
Description of percutaneous technique in 134 patients.

Freeman BD, Isabella K, Lin N, et al. A meta-analysis of prospective trials comparing percutaneous and surgical tracheostomy in critically ill patents. *Chest.* 2000;118:1412–1418.
Meta-analysis reviewing studies which compared surgical to percutaneous tracheostomies. It found a lower incidence of peristomal infection, postoperative bleeding, and overall postoperative complication rate with the percutaneous compared with the surgical approach.

Raghuraman G, Rajan S, Marzouk JK, et al. Is tracheal stenosis caused by percutaneous tracheostomy different from that by surgical tracheostomy? *Chest.* 2005;127:879–885.
A small study comparing the details of tracheal stenosis in percutaneous versus surgical tracheostomies.

76 Chest Tube Insertion
Alexander C. Chen

DEFINITION

Thoracostomy refers to the insertion of a hollow, flexible tube into the pleural space.

INDICATIONS

1. Drainage of air or fluid from the pleural space.
2. Administration of therapeutic pleural agents such as sclerosants.

CONTRAINDICATIONS

1. Bleeding diatheses (prothrombin time or partial thromboplastin time greater than two times normal, platelets <50,000, or creatine level >6) should be corrected in nonemergent settings.
2. Caution is required when there is a history of thoracic surgery or pleurodesis on the side of proposed chest tube insertion. Lung tissue can adhere to the chest wall in these instances, resulting in lung injury during insertion. Image guidance or operating room placement may be required.

IMAGING

Confirmation of the suspected pleural process prior to tube placement is imperative. On standard radiographs, large bullae can mimic pneumothoraces and combinations of tumor and atelectasis can be mistaken for pleural effusions. Elevation of the hemidiaphragm in diaphragmatic paralysis or injury in the post-operative period will produce changes on routine chest radiograph that may mimic a significant pleural effusion. Attempted chest tube placement can cause significant morbidity in these situations. Lateral decubitus films may help confirm the existence of free-flowing air or fluid. In difficult cases, chest computed tomography or ultrasound imaging may be needed.

SITE SELECTION

1. Physical examination findings consistent with a pleural effusion include decreased breath sounds on auscultation, dullness to percussion, loss of tactile fremitus, and asymmetric chest wall expansion with inspiration. Physical examination findings consistent with pneumothoraces include hyperresonance and decreased

breath sounds. In tension pneumothoraces, shift of mediastinal structures may be observed.

2. For free-flowing air or fluid, chest tubes are traditionally placed in the fourth to sixth rib interspaces between the middle and anterior axillary lines. Alternatively, the second interspace in the midclavicular line can be used for drainage of pneumothoraces with small, percutaneous catheters.

3. Loculated air or fluid collections often require image guidance by ultrasound or fluoroscopy for optimal tube placement. A good understanding of the overlying anatomy is required in this situation to prevent damage to anatomic structures during tube insertion.

CHOOSING THE OPTIMAL APPROACH

The surgical and guidewire methods are the two most commonly used techniques for tube thoracostomy. Different indications dictate the appropriate approach. Loculated air or fluid collections are often more readily approached by a guidewire method. In these cases, small pockets can be safely entered with real-time visualization of a guidewire using ultrasound, fluoroscopy, or computed tomography. Small tubes ranging from 8 to 12 French have been successfully used to drain thick fluid collections, including empyemas. Recent data suggests that these smaller caliber chest tubes may be as effective as larger chest tubes for managing infected pleural spaces. Hemothoraces or large bronchopleural fistulas often require the placement of a larger tube (32 French or greater) by the surgical approach to achieve adequate drainage.

Procedure Steps

Surgical Approach

1. Explain benefits, risks, alternatives, and obtain consent.

2. Gather equipment including sterile towels, antiseptic, lidocaine, needles for local anesthesia, silk sutures, large Kelly clamps, scalpel, gauze pads, chest tube, and chest tube drainage system, as well as mask, hat, and sterile gown. Kits prepared ahead of time can simplify this process.

3. Typically, the patient is placed in a semirecumbent position with the head and shoulders about 30 degrees off the bed. The ipsilateral arm is placed above the head for exposure of the axilla and to increase the distance between ribs.

4. Clean the area with antiseptic and sterilely drape.

5. Anesthesia is primarily delivered locally, although intravenous narcotics such as fentanyl or morphine can increase patient comfort when appropriate monitoring is available. After rib identification, infiltrate subcutaneous tissue with lidocaine (Fig. 76.1). Next, inject local anesthesia down to the appropriate rib. Move needle over rib and continue to inject anesthesia. Confirm entry into air for pneumothoraces or fluid for effusions by aspirating the syringe as it is advanced. Generously anesthetize the parietal pleura. Typically, the equivalent of 25 to 40 mL of 1% lidocaine local anesthetic should achieve adequate local anesthesia.

6. Make a skin incision through the subcutaneous tissue that is wide enough to insert a finger.

7. Using medium-sized Kelly clamps, bluntly dissect to the top of the selected rib. This is done by applying forward pressure with the clamps while opening, relaxing forward pressure while closing, and repeating as necessary. Once the rib is reached,

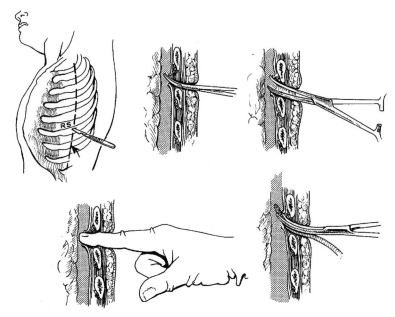

Figure 76.1. Chest tube insertion procedure (see text for details).

continue with blunt dissection over the top of the rib. A rush of air or fluid signals entry into the pleural space. As the clamps enter into the pleural space, caution is needed not to push too far, so as to prevent lung injury.

8. Place finger through tract into the pleural space. Sweep around the entry site to confirm the lack of adherent lung in the direction of chest tube placement.
9. Clamp the end of the chest tube with a Kelly clamp and guide into the pleural space. Direction is generally anteroapical for drainage of air and inferoposterior for drainage of fluid.
10. Attach external end of tube to the drainage system. Drainage of air or fluid as well as evidence of respiratory variation suggest proper placement into the pleural space.
11. Securely suture tube to prevent dislodgment. Some operators place a mattress suture at the time of the insertion, leaving the ends loose, which they use to close the incision at the time of tube removal.
12. Using occlusive gauze to seal the skin around the tube is controversial. Some authors argue that this leads to skin breakdown.
13. Dress area with a generous amount of gauze and tape.
14. Check chest x-ray for proper placement.
15. Check on chest tube output, signs of respiratory variation, and the presence of air leaks at least daily. Evaluate site for bleeding or signs of infection.
16. Remove tube when drainage is no longer indicated.

Guidewire Approach
Note: This approach may vary slightly, depending on kit used.

1. Obtain consent, position patient, and prepare area as for surgical approach.
2. Anesthetize rib and pleural space in the selected interspace.
3. Insert the introducer needle just superior to the appropriate rib. Stop just past the point where fluid or air is aspirated.
4. Remove syringe and cover needle opening with finger to prevent excessive air entry. Introduce wire into pleural space. Remove needle from pleural space leaving guidewire in pleural space.
5. Make a small skin nick at the wire entry site to allow introduction of dilators and chest tube.
6. Using sequential dilators, dilate tract into pleural space. This should be done with caution as over-insertion of dilators can lead to inadvertent lung injury. Generally, tactile feedback is present when the dilator has punctured through the parietal pleura. Dilators should be advanced a small amount beyond this point to ensure proper tract formation; further advancement beyond this point is unnecessary and potentially harmful.
7. Introduce chest tube over the wire into the pleural space. Confirm that all openings are in the pleural space. Remove wire.
8. Connect chest tube to drainage system.
9. Suture tube in place and dress with gauze and tape.
10. Check chest x-ray for proper placement.

DRAINAGE SYSTEMS

The most common drainage system for hospitalized patient is the three-bottle drainage system. The functions of the three-bottle system are most commonly incorporated into one container today. The first column serves as a drainage repository, collecting fluid that drains from the pleural space. The second column serves as a water seal, which prevents retrograde air entry into the pleural space. The third column allows for adjustment of the negative pressure applied to the pleural space.

GUIDELINES FOR CHEST TUBE REMOVAL

There is considerable practice variation involved in chest tube removal. The most important requirement is for the resolution of the initial indication for placement. For pneumothoraces, this generally means a fully expanded lung with resolution of the air leak, and for pleural fluid, this implies a maximum drainage of 100 to 150 mL/day. There are arguments for pulling at end-expiration or end-inspiration as well as arguments in favor and against tube clamping, placing on water seal, or keeping on suction prior to removal.

Our approach is to place on water seal 12 to 24 hours with a follow-up chest x-ray. If there is no significant air leak or reaccumulation of air or fluid, the tube is removed. In difficult cases, the tube can be clamped for 2 to 4 hours, with careful monitoring and a repeat chest x-ray to confirm stability. Patients can be given a small amount of narcotic prior to removal and remove sutures. Have patient make a full inspiration and pull tube out quickly while occluding the track with your other hand. Approximate the incision either by tying a previously placed mattress suture or by placing new suture. A follow-up chest x-ray should be taken 12 to 24 hours later (or sooner, if clinically indicated) to rule out recurrence of pneumothorax or pleural fluid.

COMPLICATIONS

Complications from chest tube placement are less well studied than complications associated with other common thoracic procedures. The site of placement (emergency department, intensive care unit, floor, or operating room) and circumstances of placement (emergent or elective) are undoubtedly important. One study looked at complications from chest tubes inserted by pulmonary fellows with attending supervision. Many, although not all, of the patients were in the intensive care unit. The largest number of chest tube placements in the study was for ventilator-associated or iatrogenic pneumothoraces. Problems were stratified as early (first 24 hours) or late and by size of the chest tube placed (less than or equal to 14 French or larger). Early complications included the tube not being placed in the pleural space, nonfunctional tubes, and laceration of the lung. Late complications included nonfunctional tubes, a site infection, and a leak around tube. All complications were more common with small tubes (36%) versus larger tubes (9%).

Other possible complications include hemothoraces from intercostal vessel injury or intra-abdominal placement. Infections associated with tube placement are uncommon. Prophylactic antibiotic use is supported by one meta-analysis in trauma patients, but is probably not justified in other clinical situations.

SUGGESTED READINGS

Bell RL, Ovandia P, Abdullah F, et al. Chest tube removal: end-inspiration or end-expiration? *J Trauma.* 2001;50:674–677.
  Patients randomized to end-inspiration or end-expiration removal of tube. No significant difference in outcomes found.
Collop NA, Kim S, Sahn SA. Analysis of tube thoracostomy performed by pulmonologists at a teaching hospital. *Chest.* 1997;112:709–713.
  Study of 126 tube thoracostomies performed by a pulmonary division at an academic medical center. Reviews indications and complications.
Fallon WF, Wears RL. Prophylactic antibiotics for the prevention of infectious complications including empyema following tube thoracoscopy for trauma: results of a meta-analysis. *J Trauma.* 1992;33:110–117.
  Showed a benefit for prophylactic antibiotics in trauma patients requiring chest tube placement.
Martino K, Merrit S, Boyakye K, et al. Prospective randomized trial of thoracostomy removal algorithms. *J Trauma* 1999;46:369–371.
  205 patients requiring chest tube insertion for blunt and penetrating trauma. When removal of the chest tube was indicated, patients were randomized to a water seal waiting period or to immediate removal of the chest tube. It appeared that a short period of time on water seal might allow for the detection of occult air leaks.
McVay PA, Toy PT. Lack of increased bleeding after paracentesis and thoracentesis in patients with mild coagulation abnormalities. *Transfusion.* 1991;31:164–171.
  Retrospective study of 608 patients undergoing thoracentesis or paracentesis. Argues that prophylactic plasma and platelet transfusions are unnecessary for patients with mild to moderate coagulopathies.
Rahman NM, Maskell NA, Davies CW, et al. The relationship between chest tube size and clinical outcome in pleural infection. *Chest.* 2010;137:536–543.
  405 patients with pleural infections treated with various sized chest tubes and either guide-wire or surgical technique. Showed no difference in clinical outcome between smaller caliber chest tubes and larger caliber chest tubes.
Silverman SG, Mueller PR, Saini S, et al. Thoracic empyema: management with image-guided catheter drainage. *Radiology.* 1988;169:5–9.
  43 patients treated with imaged guided catheters for empyemas. Proved successful by pre-defined criteria in 72% of patients.

Paracentesis

Chad A. Witt

Paracentesis is a procedure frequently performed in the intensive care unit for diagnostic and therapeutic purposes. Diagnostic paracentesis should be performed in patients with suspected spontaneous bacterial peritonitis (SBP) or ascites of unknown cause. In patients with significant shortness of breath and/or abdominal discomfort, therapeutic paracentesis frequently alleviates symptoms. Complications include bleeding from the paracentesis site, fluid leak, bowel or bladder perforation, and the introduction of infection.

Many patients undergoing paracentesis (especially those with underlying liver disease) are coagulopathic and/or thrombocytopenic at the time of the procedure. It has been shown in such patients that there is no need to correct the coagulopathy or transfuse platelets prior to the procedure. Paracentesis should not be performed in patients with disseminated intravascular coagulation. Additionally, in patients with small bowel obstruction, a nasogastric tube should be placed prior to the procedure. Patients with urinary retention should undergo bladder catheterization prior to paracentesis. In patients who have had multiple abdominal operations, who do not have a large amount of ascites, have pronounced organomegaly, or those who have undergone failed conventional paracentesis, performing the procedure with ultrasound guidance may be necessary.

The most common sites of paracentesis are the abdominal left lower quadrant, suprapubic, or right lower quadrant regions. Physical examination, particularly percussion and examining for shifting dullness, can help determine the ideal site. In patients with loculated ascites, ultrasound can aid in performing the procedure at the site with greatest yield. When performing a paracentesis, the catheter should not be inserted through infected/inflamed skin or tissue or hematomas.

Once the site of the procedure has been determined and all present agree on the identification of the patient, the site, and the procedure being performed, one can proceed with paracentesis.

PERFORMANCE OF PARACENTESIS

1. Sterile gloves and a mask with face shield are worn.
2. The patient should be placed supine with the head of the bed slightly elevated.
3. The site is prepared with antiseptic solution (e.g., chlorhexidine or Betadine), and a sterile draped is placed.
4. Using a 22- or 25-gauge needle, local anesthesia with 1% lidocaine is performed, starting with a subcutaneous wheel followed by deeper anesthesia. While injecting the deeper tissues, maintain continuous negative pressure on the syringe, and inject

lidocaine periodically. Maintain an angle of entry perpendicular to the abdominal wall.

5. When ascitic fluid is obtained, inject lidocaine around the peritoneum.
6. Ideally, a needle/catheter specifically designed for paracentesis (e.g., Caldwell needle) should be used, although a large-bore intravenous catheter may be used. Attach a 10-mL syringe to the catheter.
7. Using a scalpel, make a small nick in the skin at the insertion site to facilitate insertion of the paracentesis catheter.
8. Using the Z-tract technique, pull the skin 2 cm caudad before inserting the catheter (this theoretically causes the tract to close, and thus reduces the rate of leakage when the catheter is withdrawn).
9. Insert the catheter slowly, with continued negative pressure on the syringe. When ascitic fluid is obtained, stop advancing the needle/catheter system, advance the catheter over the needle, and remove the needle.

TABLE 77.1	Common Clinical Situations and Pertinent Studies for Ascitic Fluid	
Clinical situation	Studies	Comments
Concern for SBP	○ Cell count ○ Culture (blood culture bottles inoculated at bedside)	○ >250 cells/mm^3 consistent with SBP ○ Culture definitive for diagnosis. ○ Treat with third-generation cephalosporin or fluoroquinolone
Determining if ascites is secondary to portal hypertension	○ Serum albumin ○ Ascites albumin	○ SAAG ≥1.1 g/dL (portal hypertension): cirrhosis, alcohol hepatitis, cardiac ascites, portal-vein thrombosis, Budd-Chiari syndrome, liver metastases ○ SAAG <1.1 g/dL: peritoneal carcinomatosis, tuberculous peritonitis, pancreatic ascites, nephrotic syndrome, serositis
Concern for malignant ascites	○ Cytology	○ Sensitivity can be increased by sending three samples, and examining samples promptly

SBP, spontaneous bacterial peritonitis; SAAG, serum ascites albumin gradient = serum albumin − ascites albumin.

10. Obtain an adequate amount of ascitic fluid for diagnostic studies (culture bottles should be inoculated at the bedside).
11. If a therapeutic paracentesis is being performed, tubing should be connected from the catheter to the vacuum bottle.

DIAGNOSTIC CONSIDERATIONS

Diagnostic studies performed on ascitic fluid are determined by the clinical situation (Table 77.1). Other less common diagnostic studies include triglycerides (chylous ascites), amylase (pancreatic ascites), mycobacterial culture (tuberculous ascites), and carcinoembryonic antigen and/or alkaline phosphatase (hollow viscous perforation). If there is concern for SBP, fluid should be sent for cell count and culture. As previously mentioned, culture bottles should be inoculated at the bedside to improve yield. Cell count demonstrating >250 polymorphonuclear cells/mm^3 without secondary source of infection (e.g., perforated viscous) or a grossly bloody tap suggests SBP. The definitive diagnosis is based on positive culture results. In patients with findings suggestive or diagnostic of SBP, treatment should be initiated with a third-generation cephalosporin (ceftriaxone or cefotaxime) or a fluoroquinolone (ciprofloxacin or levofloxacin).

The use of albumin infusion (6 to 8 g albumin/L fluid removed) after large-volume paracentesis (5 L or more) has been shown to decrease circulatory dysfunction and the potential precipitation of hepatorenal syndrome.

SUGGESTED READINGS

Runyon BA. Management of adult patients with ascites. *Hepatology.* 2004;39:841–856.
> *An evidence based review of the diagnostic studies and their indications in patients with ascites, as well as a discussion of the treatment of several diagnoses, including refractory ascites, the hepatorenal syndrome, and SBP.*

Thomsen TW, Shaffer RW, White B, et al. Paracentesis. *N Engl J Med.* 2006;355:e21.
> *An excellent review of the indications, risks, performance of, studies to be sent, and complications of paracentesis.*

78 Lumbar Puncture
Jennifer Alexander-Brett

The lumbar puncture (LP) is commonly performed in the intensive care unit to obtain cerebrospinal fluid (CSF) for diagnostic purposes. This chapter will discuss the indications, technique, complications, and common pitfalls of performing an LP in adults.

INDICATIONS AND CONTRAINDICATIONS

It is useful to remember the old adage, "If you consider an LP, you should do it." Delay in the diagnosis of meningitis leads to inappropriate treatment and difficulty in later establishing the diagnosis when the patient fails to improve. Likewise, prompt diagnosis of subarachnoid hemorrhage results in early treatment of aneurysms and prevention of rebleeding. Table 78.1 lists common indications for LP.

There are few contraindications to LP. Coagulopathy is an important contraindication because an LP may cause an epidural hematoma leading to compression of the cauda equina. No studies have established useful cutoffs, but an international normalized ratio >1.4, partial thromboplastin time >50, and/or platelet count <100,000/mm^3 are commonly corrected with fresh-frozen plasma and/or platelet transfusions prior to an LP. In the setting of altered mental status, papilledema, focal neurologic deficit, or if there is suspicion for subarachnoid hemorrhage, a head computed tomography scan should be obtained prior to LP. Signs of herniation and large posterior fossa masses preclude an LP because the pressure drop following CSF removal can precipitate tonsillar herniation.

Other contraindications to LP include local skin infections, known spinal cord tumors, and very recent surgical instrumentation. Prior to performing an LP, informed consent must be obtained according to the policy at each institution.

TECHNIQUE

Collect the Supplies

Gather the following: sterile 20-gauge or smaller spinal needle with a stylet, a sterile 25-gauge needle and syringe for local anesthesia, topical antiseptic, sterile drape and gauze, 1% to 2% lidocaine solution, a sterile manometer, sterile surgical gloves, and tubes for collection of the fluid. With more experience, a smaller gauge spinal needle, preferably a Sprotte needle, helps reduce post-LP headaches. In morbidly obese patients, a needle longer than the standard 3.5 inches may be necessary.

Position the Patient

Lateral decubitus positioning is required to accurately measure the intracranial CSF pressure. The patient is positioned such that the hips and shoulders are squarely above

TABLE 78.1 Common Indications for Lumbar Puncture

- Diagnosis of bacterial, viral, fungal, parasitic, or mycobacterial meningitis
- Diagnosis of carcinomatosis meningitis
- Diagnosis of subarachnoid hemorrhage
- Assessing central nervous system and meningeal inflammation for diagnosis of conditions including multiple sclerosis, Devic disease, and neurosarcoidosis
- Measuring CSF protein levels for the diagnosis of Guillain–Barré syndrome
- Measuring intracranial pressure for diagnosis of pseudotumor cerebri
- Removing CSF for treatment of pseudotumor cerebri or normal-pressure hydrocephalus

CSF, cerebrospinal fluid.

one another, the back is parallel to the wall, and the patient is curled up with the knees and chin tucked deeply into the torso (Fig. 78.1). In other cases, a sitting position aids in determining the midline of the spine, increases the space between spinous processes, and may increase filling of the lumbar cistern, thus improving the chance of successful LP. In this position, the patient is positioned such that the back is straight and arched outward, with the chin tucked deeply into the chest. Ultimately, the choice of positioning should be determined by the indications for the LP, patient comfort, and operator experience.

Find the L4–5 Space

In most adults, the spinal cord ends at L1 and in a few adults it ends at L2. Therefore, the L3–4, L4–5, and L5-S1 spaces represent safe and effective locations to insert a spinal needle. In most adults, a line (Tuffier line, Fig. 78.1) drawn across the tops of both iliac crests crosses the L4 spinous process or the L4–5 space. Use the spinous space on or immediately below the Tuffier line. Attention to superficial anatomy helps ensure appropriate placement of the spinal needle.

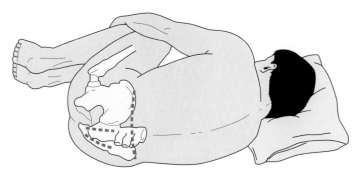

Figure 78.1. Positioning the patient. Tuffier line is indicated by the *dashed line*. (From Taylor C, Lillis CA, LeMone P. *Fundamentals of Nursing*. 2nd ed. Philadelphia, PA: JB Lippincott, 1993:543, with permission.)

Scrub and Anesthetize the Space

Scrub the location with antiseptic solution (e.g., chlorhexidine or Betadine). Using sterile gloves, place a sterile drape at the selected location with the lumbar space above it exposed. Lidocaine is injected subcutaneously and about 2 cm deep along the expected track of the spinal needle.

Insert the Spinal Needle

The spinal needle with its stylet in place should then be introduced through the skin in a tract that is angled toward the navel or about 15 degrees cephalad. The needle must be entered at midline and orthogonal to the plane of the back. The bevel should initially be perpendicular to the long axis of the body to minimize tearing of the dura and the subsequent post-LP headaches.

Advance the Spinal Needle

After penetrating the skin and subcutaneous fat, the needle should traverse the supraspinatus ligament, the interspinous ligaments, the ligamentum flavum, the epidural space, and finally the dura (Fig. 78.2). Severe pain may indicate being away from the midline. Once the needle has been inserted about 3 to 4 cm, or if a "pop" or sudden loss of resistance is experienced, remove the stylet to check for CSF. If no CSF is obtained, replace the stylet and advance the needle another 2 to 3 mm and remove

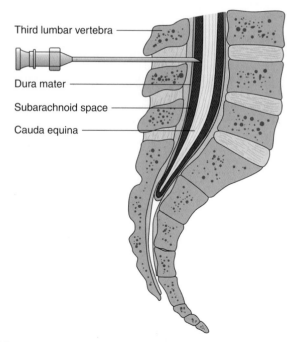

Third lumbar vertebra

Dura mater

Subarachnoid space

Cauda equina

Figure 78.2. The ideal tract of the spinal needle. (From Taylor C, Lillis CA, LeMone P. *Fundamentals of Nursing*, 2nd ed. Philadelphia, PA: JB Lippincott, 1993:543, with permission.)

the stylet again to check for CSF. Once the lumbar cistern has been entered, CSF should flow freely through the spinal needle, and the stylet can be replaced to limit CSF leakage until it can be collected or a manometer can be attached to measure CSF pressure. Hitting bone while inserting the needle indicates either incorrect angling of the needle or the skin has been entered away from the midline. When this occurs, retract the needle to the subcutaneous tissue, reposition its angle so that it is closer to being 15 degrees or less cephalad and more directed toward the midline, and then enter again. This procedure can be repeated a few times until a tract free of bone is achieved. After several attempts at the first lumbar space, using the L3–4 space (the space immediately above the Tuffier line) is permissible, but using any higher spaces risks inserting the needle into the tip of the spinal cord.

On occasion, the LP needle is inserted to the hub without obtaining CSF. This problem can be avoided by using a needle that is sufficiently long, ensuring a correct entry point and angle, and occasionally by sitting up the patient. Fluoroscopic guidance may be necessary in obese or uncooperative patients.

Measure CSF Pressure and Collect Fluid

Once the needle has entered the lumbar cistern, a manometer can be used to measure "opening" CSF pressure. This measurement is accurate only when the patient is in the lateral decubitus position and relaxed enough to allow visible respiratory excursions of the CSF in the manometer. Normal pressure is 8 to 22 cm H_2O, although it can be slightly higher in normal obese patients. The fluid in the manometer should be collected for CSF analysis. Sufficient CSF should be collected for all of the necessary tests, and additional fluid should be collected and saved in case further testing is desired. If the opening pressure is >50 cm H_2O, the minimum amount of fluid necessary should be collected. Fluid analyses are listed in Table 78.2. If the CSF appears bloody initially and later it clears, this suggests a "traumatic" tap, whereby the needle had punctured a vein en route to the lumbar cistern. Xanthochromia, or a yellowish tint to the fluid, indicates either blood products >12 to 24 hours old in

TABLE 78.2	Common Tests for Cerebrospinal Fluid (CSF) Analysis (to be Ordered Based on Clinical Concern)

- Complete cell count and differential
- CSF glucose and protein levels
- Gram stain and bacterial, fungal, and mycobacterial cultures
- Cytology and wet mount inspection
- Spectrophotometer analysis for xanthochromia
- IgG and albumin levels, serum IgG and albumin levels to determine the IgG index: (CSF–IgG/CSF–albumin)/(Serum–IgG/Serum–albumin)
- Oligoclonal bands
- PCR tests for a variety of pathogens including HSV, VZV, EBV, CMV, enteroviruses, TB, arboviruses, and toxoplasmosis
- Other tests for pathogens including syphilis (VDRL or FTA-ABS), cysticercosis, histoplasmosis, coccidioidomycosis, and malaria

IgG, immunoglobulin G; PCR, polymerase chain reaction; HSV, herpes simplex virus; VZV, varicella-zoster virus; EBV, Epstein-Barr virus; CMV, cytomegalovirus; TB, tuberculosis; VDRL, Venereal Disease Research Laboratory; FTA-ABS, fluorescent treponemal antibody-absorption.

the subarachnoid space or greatly elevated protein levels. Careful replacement of the stylet before and after collection helps avoid excessive CSF leak. After CSF collection, a closing pressure can be measured if necessary. Replace the stylet before removing the needle. Samples collected should be sent for cell count with differential, chemistry, and Gram stain/culture; additional studies may be included based on suspected underlying diagnosis (Table 78.2). Of note, samples should be analyzed as soon as possible after collection, as cell counts are prone to decline markedly over the course of hours.

COMPLICATIONS

Following the LP procedure, the patient should be placed in the supine position for 1 hour. This helps reduce post dural-puncture headaches immediately after an LP, though probably does not prevent post-LP headaches due to a dural tear and persistent CSF leakage. The latter can be reduced by appropriate spinal needle selection and proper technique. Fluids, caffeine, acetaminophen, and nonsteroidal anti-inflammatory drugs are effective in most cases of post-LP headaches. Characteristically, the headache worsens with sitting up or standing and resolves when lying down. If the headaches persist longer than 5 days, an epidural blood patch may be required.

Rarely, the patient may complain of paresthesias or pain referred to one leg. During the procedure, this indicates impingement of a nerve root, and the spinal needle should be retracted, repositioned further toward the midline, and then reinserted. Careful controlled insertion of the needle helps avoid such nerve damage. When symptoms of cord compression occur following the procedure, there is concern for an intraspinal epidermoid tumor or an epidural hematoma. In both cases, obtaining a magnetic resonance image or computed tomography is mandatory, and neurosurgical consultation is warranted if any such mass is discovered.

Other rare complications include cerebral herniation syndromes and spontaneous rupture of a subarachnoid arterial aneurysm. These can be avoided by careful physical examination and, when indicated, brain imaging prior to the LP.

SUGGESTED READINGS

Boon JM, Abrahams PH, Meiring JH, et al. Lumbar puncture: anatomical review of a clinical skill. *Clin Anat.* 2004;17:544–553.
  This comprehensive article reviews the relevant anatomy for performing a lumber puncture. It is well written and is advised particularly when one is having trouble successfully performing the procedure.
Ellenby MS, Tegtmeyer K, Lai S, et al. Lumbar puncture. *N Engl J Med.* 2006;355:e12.
  A video and accompanying article that demonstrates the proper method of performing a lumber puncture. This is highly recommended to everyone who has never performed this procedure before.

79 Thoracentesis
Alexander C. Chen

DEFINITION

Thoracentesis is a procedure in which a needle is inserted between the ribs into the pleural space for aspiration of air or fluid.

INDICATIONS

1. Evaluation of pleural effusions of unknown cause.
2. To exclude empyema or complicated parapneumonic effusions in patients with fever and pleural effusions.
3. Therapeutic removal of air or fluid from the pleural space.

RELATIVE CONTRAINDICATIONS

1. Uncooperative patient.
2. Cutaneous abnormality such as an infection at the proposed sampling site.
3. Uncorrectable bleeding diathesis that includes a prothrombin time or partial thromboplastin time >2 times normal, platelets <50,000, or a creatine level >6. The diagnostic benefits of excluding empyema or hemothorax may outweigh bleeding risks if these are diagnostic considerations.

HISTORY

1. Patients with risk factors or a history suggestive of bleeding problems should have coagulation factors measured.
2. Screen for allergies to local anesthetics.

SITE SELECTION

1. Physical examination findings consistent with pleural effusions include decreased breath sounds, dullness to percussion, loss of tactile fremitus, and asymmetric diaphragmatic excursion.
2. A lateral decubitus film, ultrasound, or computed tomography scan of the chest can exclude other entities that mimic pleural fluid on standard chest films.
3. At least 1 cm of fluid should layer out on a lateral decubitus film in order to safely sample an effusion without ultrasound guidance.

4. Using ultrasound for site selection for all thoracenteses is controversial. If readily available, potential benefit from its routine use has been found in some studies. On the other hand, experienced operators can perform thoracentesis with a low complication rate without ultrasound. If two attempts at blind thoracentesis fail to sample fluid, the use of ultrasound guidance can improve the yield for obtaining fluid. Ultrasound-guided thoracentesis can be performed safely in patients on mechanical ventilation.

PROCEDURE

1. Explain benefits, risks, answer questions, and obtain consent.
2. A number of companies offer helpful prepackaged procedure kits that simplify the gathering of needed equipment.
3. Sit patient straight up to maximize the amount of fluid in the posterior gutter. If the patient is intubated, our preference is to roll the patient on their side with the affected side up (i.e., for a right sided pleural effusion, the patient is rolled left side down and right side up).
4. The preferred site for needle insertion is generally midway between the spine and posterior axillary line. Percuss down the chest until an area of dullness is reached. Go one interspace below the area of dullness. Avoid the paraspinal area and do not go below the ninth rib interspace. If performed with ultrasound, site selection is directed by the ultrasound image.
5. Wear a mask and sterile gloves.
6. Clean area with chlorhexidine or other appropriate antiseptic.
7. Cover surrounding area with sterile drape or towels.
8. Using a 25-gauge needle filled with lidocaine, create a small skin wheal over the top of the appropriate rib.
9. Using a 22-gauge needle, go through the wheal, anesthetizing deeper levels of tissue as you go. It is important to keep the needle perpendicular to the skin surface at all times. The skin surface, top of the rib, and parietal pleura require the most anesthetic. Advance until fluid is aspirated (Fig. 79.1).
10. If using a needle without a catheter device, insert needle into previously anesthetized tract until fluid is aspirated. Collect fluid for studies.
11. If using a needle with a catheter device, first make a skin nick with a scalpel. Insert the needle and catheter device through the skin nick and advance while aspirating making certain to keep the device perpendicular to the skin surface and in line with the tract that was anesthetized. After fluid is aspirated, advance needle and catheter 2 to 3 mm further into the pleural space and then advance the catheter off the needle into the pleural space while preventing the needle from advancing further and remove the needle.
12. Using a large syringe, remove fluid for studies. Samples for chemical evaluation are typically sent in a mint green top blood tube, and cell counts in a lavender top blood tube. Cytology and microbiology samples for study can be sent in small, sterile containers. Although submission of large amounts of cytology fluid is commonly advocated, the yield for diagnosis appears to be independent of the fluid amount submitted. Fluid can be instilled in blood culture bottles in an effort to improve the yield of cultures, but this requires the submission of a separate sample to obtain a Gram stain. (See Chapter 15, "Pleural Effusion," for further guidance on fluid analysis.)

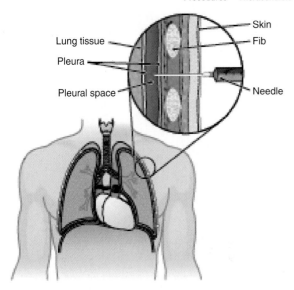

Figure 79.1. Schematic illustrating appropriate needle location for sampling and pleural effusion.

13. If performing a therapeutic procedure, connect the catheter to a syringe and collection bag system. Vacuum bottles should not be used for thoracentesis as this has been associated with an increased risk for pneumothorax. It is generally recommended that the procedure be stopped after 1200 to 1500 mL if pleural fluid is removed or if the patient develops symptoms of cough or chest discomfort to avoid re-expansion pulmonary edema. Alternatively, one can monitor pleural manometry and keep pleural pressures less than −20 cm H_2O.
14. Remove the catheter while the patient exhales to avoid entrainment of air.
15. Chest x-rays are commonly performed to exclude pneumothorax, but are probably not needed unless there are concerning symptoms or problems with the procedure that suggests that the lung may have been punctured.

COMPLICATIONS

Complications can be separated into major complications, such as pneumothorax or significant bleeding, and minor complications, such as pain or dry taps. Table 79.1 summarizes common complications.

Operator experience plays a significant role in the risk of complications, emphasizing the importance of having the proper background knowledge, and experience in the performance of the procedure.

Re-expansion pulmonary edema is a feared but uncommon complication of thoracentesis. The pathophysiology is unclear, but traditionally has been attributed to excessive negative pressure in the pleural space during pleural drainage procedures.

TABLE 79.1	Common Complications in Thoracentesis		
Complication	Overall no. (%)	Inexperienced no. (%)	Experienced no. (%)
Pain	77 (25)	64 (25)	13 (26)
Cough	37 (12)	25 (10)	12 (24)
Dry tap	33 (11)	32 (13)	1 (2)
Pneumothorax	31 (10)	29 (11)	2 (4)
Vasovagal	7 (2)	6 (2)	1 (2)
Worsened dyspnea	4 (1)	0	4 (8)

SUGGESTED READINGS

Bartter T, Mayo PD, Pratter MR, et al. Lower risk and higher yield for thoracentesis when performed by experienced operators. *Chest.* 1993;103:1873–1876.

Prospective study involving 50 consecutive thoracentesis performed by pulmonary fellows or attendings. Showed significantly lower rates of major complications compared to similar studies of procedure performed by non-pulmonary housestaff.

Collins TR, Sahn SA. Thoracentesis: clinical value, complications, technical problems, and patient experience. *Chest.* 1987;91:817–822.

Prospective study of 129 thoracenteses primarily performed by medical housestaff and students.

Jones PW, Moyers JP, Rogers JT, et al. Ultrasound-guided thoracentesis: is it a safer method? *Chest.* 2003;123:418–423.

Prospective, descriptive study of 941 thoracenteses in 605 patients. Showed a low rate of complications when thoracentesis was performed under ultrasound by experienced operators. Also showed a low incidence of re-expansion pulmonary edema regardless of the amount of fluid removed.

McVay PA, Toy PT. Lack of increased bleeding after paracentesis and thoracentesis in patients with mild coagulation abnormalities. *Transfusion.* 1991;31:164–171.

Retrospective study of 608 patients undergoing thoracentesis or paracentesis. Argues that prophylactic plasma and platelet transfusions are unnecessary for patients with mild to moderate coagulopathies.

Petersen WG, Zimmerman R. Limited utility of chest radiograph after thoracentesis. *Chest.* 2000;117:1038–1042.

Prospective, cohort involving 251 thoracenteses. Showed that clinically significant pneumothoraces were always associated with symptoms or aspiration of air.

Seneff MG, Corwin RW, Gold LH, et al. Complications associated with thoracentesis. *Chest.* 1986;90:97–100.

Prospective study of 125 procedures primarily performed by housestaff.

80 Pulmonary Artery Catheterization

Warren Isakow

Since its inception in the 1970s, the clinical use of the pulmonary artery catheter (PAC) has been controversial. The PAC provides direct pressure measurements from the right atrium (RA), right ventricle (RV), pulmonary arteries (PAs), and pulmonary capillary wedge pressure as well as a means of measuring cardiac output (CO) by thermodilution. The PAC rapidly gained favor when it was recognized how inaccurate physician assessments of these parameters were. Use of the catheter became widespread, and bedside management was often influenced by the hemodynamic parameters; however, no clinical validation of the benefit of this approach had been performed.

A number of subsequent trials in different patient populations, including surgical patients, patients with acute myocardial infarction, congestive heart failure, and acute lung injury, have shown no benefits, and possibly increased risk, from use of a PAC. A study by the acute respiratory distress syndrome clinical trials network found no differences in outcomes of patients with this syndrome who had their fluid balance guided by use of a central line with central venous pressure monitoring or use of a PAC. Routine use of the PAC should be avoided, but it still has a role in patients with pulmonary arterial hypertension and congenital heart disease, and in patients with complex fluid management issues. In addition, as new therapies emerge, information on treatment benefits may require invasive assessment of hemodynamic parameters.

Newer, noninvasive techniques to assess hemodynamic parameters are being refined and are reducing dependence on the PAC. The clinician using the PAC needs to ask how the information obtained from a PAC will change management of a specific patient, and be alert to possibly the greatest danger of the device: misinterpretation of its hemodynamic measurements. The PAC should be used for the shortest time possible and with the understanding that it is unlikely to alter the clinical course of a patient with multiple complex medical problems (Table 80.1).

PROCEDURE TECHNIQUE

The easiest insertion sites are normally the right internal jugular (RIJ) vein or the left subclavian vein; however, femoral or even brachial vein sites can be used. Prior to starting the procedure, an evaluation of any contraindications to the procedure should be made. In cases with suspected RV dysfunction, pulmonary artery hypertension, tricuspid regurgitation, or RA enlargement, consideration should be given to placing the PAC with fluoroscopic guidance, as direct visualization enhances ability to pass the PAC in difficult cases.

TABLE 80.1	Contraindications to, Indications for, and Complications of Pulmonary Artery Catheter Placement
Relative contraindications	**Complications**
Left bundle branch block	Complications related to introducer placement:
Severe coagulopathy	• Pneumothorax
	• Hemothorax
	• Hematoma at site of insertion
	• Infection at insertion site
Indications (controversial)	
Diagnosis and management of shock states	Complications related to PAC use:
Oliguric acute renal failure	• Arrhythmias
Assessment of volume status	• Right bundle branch block
Titration of therapy for cardiogenic shock	• Complete heart block (pre-existing left heart block)
Diagnosis of PAH	• Catheter thrombosis
Vasodilator testing in PAH	• Pulmonary embolism
Diagnosis of multiple cardiac disorders including pericardial constriction, VSD, RV infarction	• Pulmonary infarct
	• Line sepsis
	• Pulmonary artery rupture
	• Pulmonary artery pseudoaneurysm
Perioperative management of major procedures	• Valvular damage
	• Cardiac perforation
	• Catheter kinking

PAC, pulmonary artery catheter; PAH, pulmonary arterial hypertension; VSD, ventricular septal defect; RV, right ventricle.

The intravenous lines, pressure bags, transducers, and zeroing apparatus should all be assembled and ready prior to the sterile insertion of the PAC. It is useful to have an assistant or nurse available for the procedure. A sterile procedural field should be used, with strict attention to handwashing, mask and cap usage, sterile glove and gown use, as well as full-length drapes. The introducer catheter is inserted in a similar manner to a central venous catheter using the Seldinger technique. The introducer catheter is slightly different in that the dilator is advanced through the introducer rather than as a separate piece of equipment, as occurs with a regular central venous catheter insertion. Additionally, the guidewire and dilator are removed together at the conclusion of the introducer insertion, which leaves the introducer alone in the vessel.

The PAC (Fig. 80.1) should have all ports flushed and the balloon checked for leaks prior to insertion. In addition, the operator should check that the balloon tip does not protrude beyond the inflated balloon as this can increase the risk of vascular rupture. All ports of the PAC should be attached to the pressure transducers and flushed prior to insertion. Waving of the catheter tip prior to insertion with verification of a waveform on the monitor confirms that the catheter ports are correctly attached. Prior to starting the procedure, a final check to verify that the protective catheter sheath has been inserted over the catheter should be performed. The catheter should be oriented prior to insertion to match the natural curve in the catheter to the projected course through the vasculature.

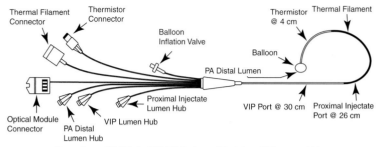

Swan-Ganz CCO/SvO₂/VIP TD Catheter (Model 746HF8 or 746F8)

Figure 80.1. Pulmonary artery catheter. (From Clark SL, Phelan JP. *Critical Care Obstetrics*, 2nd ed. Boston, MA: Blackwell Scientific, 1990:63, with permission.)

The PAC is advanced through the introducer, and when the catheter tip is in the RA, the balloon should be inflated gently. The distance from the insertion site to the RA will vary depending on site, but is usually 15 to 20 cm from the RIJ or left subclavian sites. Once the balloon is inflated and the lock on the inflating syringe has been activated, the catheter is advanced and the waveforms on the monitor are inspected. The RA waveform will increase in amplitude as the RV is entered, which normally occurs at approximately 30 cm (from a RIJ approach). The passage of the catheter through the RV is arrhythmogenic and should not be of prolonged duration. Conversion of the RV waveform to a PA waveform, as the catheter tip traverses the pulmonary valve, is identified by an increase in the diastolic pressure and the development of a dicrotic notch in the tracing (often at 40 cm). Difficulty in traversing the pulmonary valve is not uncommon in patients with pulmonary arterial hypertension from any cause and, if excessive catheter length has been advanced without this transition occurring, the most likely explanation is that the catheter is coiled in the enlarged RV. If this occurs, the balloon should be deflated and the catheter should be withdrawn until an RA tracing is obtained, after which the balloon should be inflated and the procedure attempted again. The pulmonary capillary wedge pressure tracing is identified by loss of the arterial tracing to a flatter tracing of lower amplitude than the PA diastolic pressure (often at 50 cm) (Fig. 80.2 for the pressure tracings obtained as the catheter advances).

At this point, the balloon should be deflated and the PA waveform should be observed. Gentle reinflation of the balloon while feeling for increased resistance and monitoring the waveform for overwedging is crucial. The 1.5-mL balloon should be fully inflated when a wedge tracing is obtained. If a wedge tracing is obtained and the balloon is only partially inflated, this signifies that the catheter tip is too distal and increases the risk of PA rupture by full inflation of the balloon. With this scenario, the catheter should be gently withdrawn 1 to 2 cm with the balloon deflated, and the balloon inflation procedure performed again to obtain a wedge tracing optimally at full balloon inflation. If there is no wedge tracing obtained with full inflation of the balloon, the catheter should be advanced with the balloon inflated till a wedge tracing is obtained. The catheter should never be withdrawn with the balloon inflated and should never be advanced without the balloon inflated, as this can result in perforation of the heart or a PA.

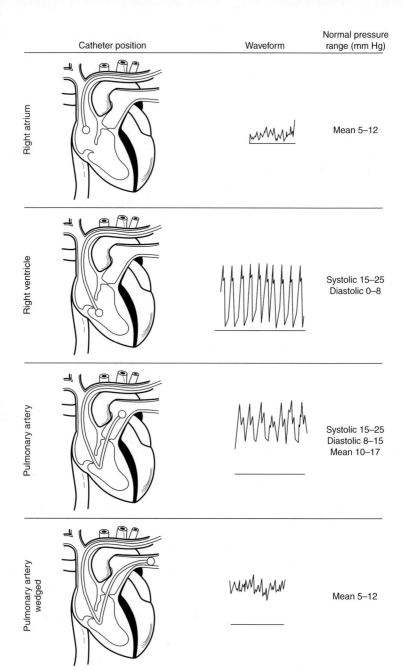

	Catheter position	Waveform	Normal pressure range (mm Hg)
Right atrium			Mean 5–12
Right ventricle			Systolic 15–25 Diastolic 0–8
Pulmonary artery			Systolic 15–25 Diastolic 8–15 Mean 10–17
Pulmonary artery wedged			Mean 5–12

Figure 80.2. Pulmonary artery catheter placement. Catheter position, corresponding waveforms, and pressures are shown. (From Clark SL, Phelan JP. *Critical Care Obstetrics*, 2nd ed. Boston, MA: Blackwell Scientific, 1990:67, with permission.)

TABLE 80.2		Examples of Hemodynamic Parameters Obtained by a Pulmonary Artery Catheter in Different Clinical Situations				
CVP (mm Hg)	RV pressures (mm Hg)	PA pressures (mm Hg)	PAOP (mm Hg)	CO (L/min)	SVR (dynes/ sec/cm^{-5})	Diagnosis
4	17–30/ 0–6	15–30/ 5–13	2–12	3–7	900–1200	Normal
10	48/12	48/30	28	2.2	3200	Cardiogenic shock
4	26/4	26/8	6	7	700	Sepsis
14	26/14	26/14	14	3.0	3000	Cardiac tamponade
16	80/30	80/40	8	3.5	1400	Pulmonary arterial hypertension
14	38/12	38/18	6	3	2800	Pulmonary embolism (acute)
2	30/2	30/12	3	2.5	2500	Hypovolemic shock

CVP, central venous pressure; RV, right ventricle; PA, pulmonary artery; PAOP, pulmonary arterial occlusion pressure; CO, cardiac output; SVR, systemic vascular resistance.

Once insertion is completed, the distance of insertion from the introducer site should be noted and recorded as a reference point. The catheter should be secured with tape and a sterile dressing and a chest x-ray should be obtained to verify catheter course, tip position, and to rule out any complications from the procedure, such as a pneumothorax. As the catheter warms up in the patient's body, it tends to soften and migrate distally, which increases the risk of overwedging, pulmonary infarction, and PA rupture with balloon inflation, so this should be re-evaluated with a daily chest x-ray as well as bedside by cautious inflation of the balloon and inspection of the waveforms (Table 80.2).

Cardiac Output Determination

Once the PAC has been verified to be correctly placed, hemodynamic data can be obtained. The catheter system must be opened to the air to set the zero point as atmospheric pressure and the catheter transducer must be referenced to the level of the heart. The CO is determined by both thermodilution and the Fick calculation. For thermodilution, a known volume (usually 5–10 mL) of cold saline is injected through the proximal port of the PAC. The distal port has a thermistor that records the change in temperature of the blood over time and displays this as the thermodilution curve. The area under the thermodilution curve is proportional to the CO (pulmonary artery flow rate) as long as there is not an intracardiac shunt (falsely elevated CO) or tricuspid regurgitation (falsely low CO). Normally, three thermodilution curves with minimal variance (<10%) are used to determine the mean CO utilizing the Stewart Hamilton equation. Figure 80.3 shows various thermodilution curves.

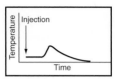

Normal thermodilution curve
With an accurate monitoring system and a patient who has adequate CO, the thermodilution curve begins with a smooth, rapid upstroke and is followed by a smooth, gradual downslope. The curve shown at left indicates that the injectant instillation time was within the recommended 4 seconds and that the temperature curve returned to baseline.

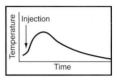

Low CO curve
A thermodilution curve representing low CO shows a rapid, smooth upstroke (from proper injection technique). However, because the heart is ejecting blood less efficiently from the ventricles, the injectant warms slowly and takes longer to be ejected from the ventricle. Consequently, the curve takes longer to return to baseline. This slow return produces a larger area under the curve, corresponding to low CO.

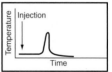

High CO curve
Again, the curve has a rapid, smooth upstroke from proper injection technique. However, because the ventricles are ejecting blood too forcefully, the injectant moves through the heart quickly and the curve returns to baseline more rapidly. The smaller area under the curve suggests higher CO.

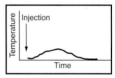

Curve reflecting poor technique
This curve results from an uneven and too slow (taking more than 4 seconds) administration of injectant. The uneven and slower than normal upstroke and the larger area under the curve erroneously indicate low CO. A kinked catheter, unsteady hands during the injection, or improper placement of the injectant lumen in the introducer sheath may also cause this type of curve.

Figure 80.3. Cardiac output measurement. Analyzing thermodilution curves.

The Fick equation can also be used to calculate the CO. The Fick principle is

$$CO = \frac{\text{Oxygen consumption}}{\text{Arteriovenous oxygen content difference} \times 10}$$

Oxygen consumption is normally assumed and is calculated by using a value for O_2 consumption at rest of 110 to 125 mL/min/m^2 depending on age and sex. The arteriovenous oxygen content calculation requires a simultaneous arterial blood gas (SaO_2) and sampling of blood from the distal port of the PAC (SvO_2) and is calculated as follows:

Arteriovenous oxygen content difference
$= 1.34 \times$ hemoglobin concentration $\times (SaO_2 - SvO_2)$.

SUGGESTED READINGS

Binanay C, Califf RM, Hasselblad V, et al. Evaluation study of congestive heart failure and pulmonary artery catheterization effectiveness: the ESCAPE trial. *JAMA.* 2005;294:1625–1633.
Randomized controlled trial in 433 patients with severe symptomatic heart failure where therapy guided by a PAC did not affect mortality or hospitalization but did increase adverse events.
Cohen MG, Kelly RV, Kong DF, et al. Pulmonary artery catheterization in acute coronary syndromes: insights from the GUSTO 2b and GUSTO 3 trials. *Am J Med.* 2005;118:482–488.

Retrospective study of 26,437 patients experiencing acute coronary syndromes. 735 patients had PAC inserted and these patients had higher mortality even after adjustments for baseline patient differences. This did not apply to patients who were in cardiogenic shock.

Connors AF Jr, Speroff T, Dawson NV, et al. The effectiveness of right heart catheterization in the initial care of critically ill patients. *JAMA.* 1996;276:889–897.

Observational study of 5735 critically ill patients, where after adjustment for treatment selection bias, PAC use was associated with increased mortality and increased resource utilization.

Eisenberg PR, Jaffe AS, Schuster DP. Clinical evaluation compared to pulmonary artery catheterization in the hemodynamic assessment of critically ill patients. *Crit Care Med.* 1984;12:549–553.

Prospective study in 103 patients which emphasized the difficulty of accurately predicting hemodynamics based on clinical evaluation. The study found that planned therapy was changed in 58% of the cases after insertion of a PAC, with unanticipated therapy added in 30% of the cases.

Harvey S, Harrison DA, Singer M, et al. Assessment of the clinical effectiveness of pulmonary artery catheters in management of patients in intensive care (PAC-Man): a randomized controlled trial. *Lancet.* 2005;366:472–477.

Large multi-center randomized controlled study in UK ICUs which noted no difference in outcomes when a PAC was used to manage critically ill patients. 46 of 486 patients had a complication from PAC insertion, none of which were fatal.

Rhodes A, Cusack RJ, Newman PJ, et al. A randomized, controlled trial of the pulmonary artery catheter in critically ill patients. *Intensive Care Med.* 2002;28:256–264.

Single center randomized trial in 201 critically ill patients did not show a mortality difference between the PAC and control groups.

Richard C, Warsjawski J, Anguel N, et al. Early use of the pulmonary artery catheter and outcomes in patients with shock and acute respiratory distress syndrome: a randomized controlled trial. *JAMA.* 2003;290:2713–2720.

Multicenter randomized study of 676 patients with septic shock, ARDS or both, where clinical management with a PAC did not affect morbidity or mortality.

Sandham JD, Hull RD, Brant RF, et al. A randomized, controlled trial of the use of pulmonary artery catheters in high-risk surgical patients. *N Engl J Med.* 2003;348:5–14.

Randomized trial in 1,994 elderly, high risk surgical patients, found no benefit to PAC directed therapy over standard care and a higher rate of pulmonary embolism in the PAC group.

Steingrub JS, Celoria G, Vickers-Lahti M, et al. Therapeutic impact of pulmonary artery catheterization in a medical/surgical ICU. *Chest.* 1991;99:1451–1455.

An expert panel rated the performance of housestaff/attending interpretation of hemodynamic data in 154 medical/surgical patients. Most housestaff/attending performance was judged appropriate and the study suggested that information derived from a PAC was instrumental in managing patients who were unresponsive to initial therapy.

Swan HJ, Ganz W, Forrester J, et al. Catheterization of the heart in man with use of a flow-directed balloon-tipped catheter. *N Engl J Med.* 1970;283:447–451.

The landmark initial description of the technique.

The National Heart, Lung, and Blood Institute Acute Respiratory Distress Syndrome (ARDS) Clinical Trials Network. Pulmonary-artery versus central venous catheter to guide treatment of acute lung injury. *N Engl J Med.* 2006;354:2213–2224.

Randomized multi-center trial in 1000 patients with acute lung injury which had an explicit fluid management algorithm. PAC use did not improve survival or organ function and was associated with more complications than therapy guided by a regular central line.

81

Alternative Hemodynamic Monitoring

Jennifer Shaffer and Warren Isakow

There are several noninvasive or minimally invasive alternatives that measure cardiac output (CO). These methods include esophageal Doppler, transpulmonary thermodilution, pulse contour analysis, partial carbon dioxide rebreathing, and thoracic electrical bioimpedance. The focus of this chapter is to describe these techniques, both their advantages, and limitations with a special focus on the esophageal Doppler.

ESOPHAGEAL DOPPLER

The esophageal Doppler has been utilized in a variety of situations including trauma patients, medical ICUs, intra-operative assessment, and for post-operative care.

Measurement of CO with the esophageal Doppler is based on measuring the velocity of blood flow through the descending aorta. The technique involves placing a transducer into the esophagus and rotating the probe to achieve an optimal signal. Blood flow velocity is measured by changes in the frequency of reflected sound waves. Stroke volume (SV) is estimated from the derivation of a time velocity integral (TVI) multiplied by aortic cross sectional area (Fig. 81.1). Once SV is calculated, the CO is determined (CO = heart rate × SV).

In addition to SV and CO, the esophageal Doppler may provide a measure of preload termed corrected flow time (FTc). FTc is systolic flow time corrected for heart rate; it is represented on the monitor display as the waveform's base. Normal values range between 330 and 360 msec. Achieving the longest possible FTc for a patient correlates well with finding the optimal level of left ventricular filling or preload. The maximum or peak velocity is the waveform's height and can serve as a measure of contractility. The normal range for peak flow velocity declines with age.

Preload	$\Longrightarrow$ Flow time	Peak velocity by age	
Contractility	$\Longrightarrow$ Peak velocity	20 years	90–120 cm/sec
Afterload	$\Longrightarrow$ Velocity and flow time	50 years	70–100 cm/sec
		70 years	50–80 cm/sec

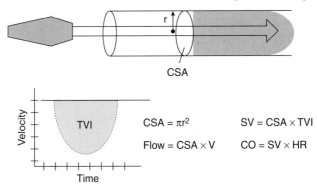

Figure 81.1. Schematic representation of the method for determining volumetric flow. This method is applicable for any laminar flow for which the cross-sectional area (*CSA*) of the flow chamber can be determined. The product of cross-sectional area and the time velocity integral (*TVI*) is stroke volume (*SV*). Cardiac output (*CO*) can be calculated as the product of SV and heart rate. See text for further details.

Following both the FTc and peak velocity helps to optimize resuscitation efforts in a wide spectrum of patients and clinical situations. For example, in hypovolemic shock the monitor displays a narrow waveform base with a corresponding decrease in FTc (<330 msec) and relatively normal peak velocity. The administration of fluid would increase the waveform base, or lengthen the FTc. If the underlying condition is myocardial depression, the initial waveform shows a low peak velocity and normal FTc. Inotropic therapy improves the peak velocity or contractility in such a situation (Fig. 81.2).

The device is easy to interpret and easy to setup. The probe is placed orally and advanced until approximately the mid-thoracic area, 35 to 40 cm. It is possible to leave the esophageal Doppler in place as long as two weeks, but it is important to test the position of the probe to ensure the optimal signal. The device is safe to use in most patients including patients with coagulopathies. Probe placement in patients with known varices is a relative contraindication.

One drawback to this technique is the limitation to sedated, mechanically venti-lated patients. There are also several assumptions in the calculation of SV and CO that affect its ability to give precise measurements. The SV is estimated from the proportion of blood flow that reaches the descending aorta. It is assumed that there is a constant 70/30 division of flow between the descending aorta (70%) and the brachiocephalic and coronary arteries (30%). The cross sectional area of the aorta is estimated based on a nomogram utilizing characteristics of the patient (age, gender, weight). Therefore if significant aortic pathology (aneurysm or dilation) is present, the absolute derived values may not be accurate. The mathematical model also assumes that the aorta is cylindrical with constant laminar flow running parallel to the esophagus. In reality, flow may be turbulent due to arrhythmia, anemia, or aortic valve disease. The presence of any of these factors makes it difficult to obtain a consistent signal and the presence of severe atherosclerosis or kyphoscoliosis may alter the fixed angle of the probe.

Esophageal Doppler monitoring is most useful when the device is used to obtain serial measurements to detect trends and response to therapy. Absolute values are not

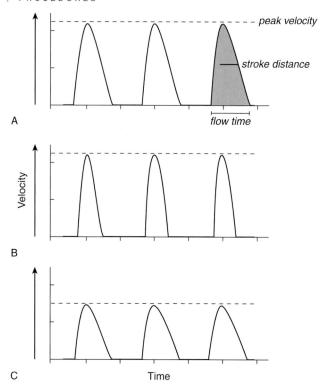

Figure 81.2. Schematic diagram of esophageal Doppler waveforms obtained during normovolemia (**A**), hypovolemia (**B**), and left ventricular failure (**C**). The primary measurements obtained during esophageal Doppler monitoring are stroke distance (the area under the waveform during systole), the peak velocity, and the ejection time during systole ("flow time"). Note that during hypovolemia and heart failure, stroke distance is decreased. In addition, ideally, during hypovolemia, flow time is decreased but peak velocity is maintained, whereas during heart failure, flow time is normal but peak velocity is reduced. (From Isakow W, Schuster DP. Extravascular lung water measurements and hemodynamic monitoring in the critically ill: bedside alternatives to the pulmonary artery catheter. *Am J Physiol Lung Cell Mol Physiol.* 2006;291:1118–1131, used with permission.)

as important as trend analysis and this concept is explained in Chapter 82 (Functional Hemodynamic Monitoring). Improved outcomes utilizing esophageal Doppler guided management have been shown in surgical patients undergoing orthopedic procedures.

TRANSPULMONARY THERMODILUTION

In contrast to the pulmonary artery (PA) thermodilution technique, transpulmonary thermodilution measures CO by detecting a cold bolus within the peripheral arterial system. The cold injectate is administered through a central venous catheter and detected by a thermistor-tipped arterial catheter placed into the radial, axillary, or femoral artery. CO is calculated by the Stewart–Hamilton equation similar to PA thermodilution (Chapter 85). The benefit with the transpulmonary technique is the ability to obtain CO readings as well as other markers of preload (global end diastolic volume [GEDV], intrathoracic blood volume [ITBV]) and extra-vascular lung water (EVLW), without a PA catheter.

Transpulmonary CO values are generally greater than the PA thermodilution values. It has been proposed that there is an unaccounted loss of cold indicator in the lung which would explain the difference as well as overcorrection for recirculation artifact.

Thermodilution measurements can be used not only to measure flow, but also to measure the volume through which flow is measured (i.e., from the point of injection to the point of detection). Figure 81.3 depicts a typical thermodilution curve utilizing transpulmonary thermodilution and explains the concept of mean transit time and downslope time. The derived volumes can be seen graphically in Figure 81.4:

• Intrathoracic thermal volume (ITTV) = CO × Mean transit time of the thermal indicator
• Pulmonary thermal volume (PTV) = CO × Downslope time of the thermal indicator
• Global end-diastolic volume (GEDV) = ITTV-PTV and provides a preload marker of moderate strength.
• ITBV = 1.25 × GEDV −28.4 (mL)

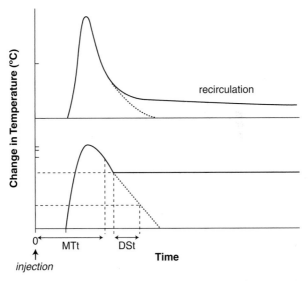

Figure 81.3. Diagrammatic representation of temperature-time curve during a thermodilution measurement, plotted on linear-linear (*top*) and log-linear scales (*bottom*). The dotted lines in each case represent what the curve would have looked like in the absence of recirculation of the thermal indicator. Note that the decay of the thermal curve becomes linear when graphed on the semi-log scale (*bottom*). Also shown are typical points used to measure the mean transit time (MTt) and the downslope time (DSt). (From Isakow W, Schuster DP. Extravascular lung water measurements and hemodynamic monitoring in the critically ill: bedside alternatives to the pulmonary artery catheter. *Am J Physiol Lung Cell Mol Physiol.* 2006;291:1118–1131, used with permission.)

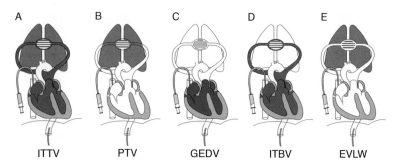

A   B   C   D   E

ITTV   PTV   GEDV   ITBV   EVLW

Figure 81.4. Schematic diagrams of different volumes that can be measured (dark-shaded areas) with the transpulmonary thermodilution technique. **A:** ITTV, intrathoracic thermal volume; **B:** PTV, pulmonary thermal volume; **C:** GEDV, global end-diastolic volume; **D:** ITBV, intrathoracic blood volume; **E:** EVLW, extravascular lung water. (From Isakow W, Schuster DP. Extravascular lung water measurements and hemodynamic monitoring in the critically ill: bedside alternatives to the pulmonary artery catheter. *Am J Physiol Lung Cell Mol Physiol.* 2006;291:1118–1131, used with permission).

- Extravascular lung water (EVLW) = ITTV-ITBV and may be used to help guide fluid administration or distinguish between hydrostatic pulmonary edema and acute lung injury.

The clinical utility of EVLW is not clear. Increases in EVLW may be used as an indication of early pulmonary edema. It has been found that mortality is greater when EVLW rises above 15 mL/kg. However, currently there is no established protocol using EVLW in patients with sepsis or ALI/ARDS. The value for EVLW is subject to error in certain situations. It is found to be overestimated in cases of severe lung injury. It is underestimated in patients with acute pulmonary embolism where the loss of perfusion affects the ability of the thermal indicator to detect all areas of lung water.

PULSE CONTOUR ANALYSIS

Pulse contour methods use the arterial pressure waveform to predict vascular flow and calculate SV. Most devices require calibration to provide a correction factor for differences in the arterial system. Indeed there are several assumptions necessary to derive the aortic pressure waveform from the shape of the peripheral pulse. Therefore, most models use either transpulmonary thermodilution or lithium dilution techniques as a reference point to derive CO. Current systems available include: PiCCO (Pulsion Medical Systems, Munich, Germany), PulseCO (LiDCO Ltd, Cambridge, UK), and Flo Trac/Vigileo (Edwards LifeSciences, Irvine, CA, USA). Thermodilution is used in the PiCCO device, lithium is the indicator for PulseCO, while the Flo Trac/Vigileo device does not require any dilution technique.

Pulse contour analysis requires arterial line placement, and for the PiCCO or PulseCO devices a central venous catheter must be placed for calibration. Each device uses a different mathematical model of pressure and flow that must account for the changes in aortic impedance, arterial compliance, and systemic resistance. Calibration is generally needed to derive the correction factors for these mathematical algorithms. The Flo Trac/Vigileo uses demographic data to extrapolate its correction factor.

Pulse contour analysis provides continuous CO monitoring in contrast to the PAC thermodilution technique that is intermittent.

The CO provided by the pulse contour analysis is subject to error as well. These devices are limited by dynamic changes in vascular resistance, which would require re-calibration. It is generally recommended to re-calibrate the PiCCO and PulseCO devices every eight hours. The Flo Trac/Vigileo does not require calibration, but may not be reliable in patients with reduced peripheral resistance such as in sepsis. Performance is also affected by the presence of aortic regurgitation, aortic aneurysm, and dampened waveforms. The PulseCO system cannot be used in patients taking lithium therapy or paralytics because this alters the sensors ability to detect the indicator. Such limitations should be taken into account when deciding which hemodynamic monitoring device to use. These devices can provide extremely useful information like pulse pressure variation and SV variation in patients who are totally mechanically ventilated (no spontaneous respiratory effort), in normal sinus rhythm and on a ventilator with adequate tidal volumes. This concept is explained in Chapter 82, Functional Hemodynamic Monitoring.

PARTIAL CARBON DIOXIDE REBREATHING

This technique relies on the Fick principle to calculate CO. The Fick equation is based on the belief that oxygen uptake from the lung is completely transferred into the bloodstream. CO therefore is calculated as a ratio between oxygen consumption and the arteriovenous difference in oxygen content. In the partial carbon dioxide (CO_2) rebreathing technique, the Fick principle is applied to carbon dioxide instead of oxygen. Several devices are necessary to obtain the appropriate measurements. These consist of a CO_2 infrared sensor, an airflow or pressure pneumotachometer, a pulse oximeter, and a disposable rebreathing loop. No central lines are required to measure CO_2 content. The value for venous CO_2 is eliminated from the equation by measuring CO_2 under normal and rebreathing conditions.

The modified Fick equation requires an estimate of venous CO_2, arterial CO_2 content, and an adjustment for the slope of the CO_2 dissociation curve. The venous content is represented by the change in CO_2 during normal (N) minute ventilation versus rebreathing (R) conditions. Arterial CO_2 is estimated from end-tidal CO_2 at the end of both maneuvers multiplied by the slope (S) of the CO_2 dissociation curve.

$$CO = \frac{vCO_2(N) - vCO_2(R)}{S \times \Delta etCO_2}$$

Intrapulmonary shunt can affect this equation by changing the blood flow participating in gas exchange. The degree of shunting in severe lung injury may not be easily estimated and adjusted by the system. Some devices incorporate peripheral oxygen saturation and PaO_2 on blood gases to account for shunting. Nonetheless, underlying lung disease, varying tidal volumes, and hemodynamic instability can alter the precision of this technique.

THORACIC BIOIMPEDANCE

In thoracic bioimpedance, SV is estimated from changes in the electrical resistance over time as a low magnitude current is applied. The patient does not detect the low level of current, and this technique is considered the least invasive of the available devices. It requires placement of six electrodes: two on the upper chest wall or neck, and four in the lower. The electrical current follows the path of least resistance, which is aortic blood flow. As the left heart contracts, there is a change in aortic blood volume and therefore a decrease in impedance. For the calculation of SV, the amount of electrically participating tissue is estimated from gender, height, and weight of the patient. The surrounding tissue fluid volume becomes important in the precision of impedance measurements.

The change in surrounding tissue fluid volume and the effect of respiration on pulmonary blood volume must be accounted for in the calculation of aortic blood flow. This technique is sensitive to acute changes in tissue water content such as pulmonary edema, effusions, and anasarca. The electrodes cannot be moved during the measurement because it is a calculation of change over time. The calculation also depends on a constant R-R interval, therefore arrhythmias will cause error in measurement of SV and CO. These are reasons for the limited use of thoracic impedance in the ICU population.

CONCLUSION

The decision to use one form of hemodynamic monitoring over the other depends on the understanding of the limitations of each device. At Washington University, the esophageal Doppler is often used for its easy placement, ease of interpretation, and quick results. It provides continuous CO monitoring as well as components of cardiac preload, contractility, and afterload. Regardless of the method chosen, the clinical picture and physical exam are crucial in interpreting the hemodynamic parameters provided by these devices.

SUGGESTED READINGS

Brown LM, Liu KD, Matthay MA. Measurement of extravascular lung water using the single indicator method in patients: research and potential clinical value. *Am J Physiol Lung Cell Mol Physiol.* 2009;297:547–558.
 Reviews the accuracy of single indicator methods, limitations of measuring EVLW, and clinical trials using EVLW as a predictor of response to therapy or disease progression.
Funk DJ, Moretti EW, Gan TJ. Minimally invasive cardiac output monitoring in the perioperative setting. *Anesth Analg.* 2009;108(3):887–897.
 Provides more in depth review of the evidence to support the use of esophageal Doppler, thoracic electrical bioimpedance, pulse contour, and transpulmonary thermodilution techniques. This article also gives more detail to the theory of thoracic bioimpedance.
Isakow W, Schuster D. Extravascular lung water measurements and hemodynamic monitoring in the critically ill: bedside alternatives to the pulmonary artery catheter. *Am J Physiol Lung Cell Mol Physiol.* 2006;291(6):1118–1131.
 A comprehensive review of the theoretical, validation, and empirical databases for transpulmonary thermodilution and esophageal Doppler measurements.
Morgan P, Al-Subaie N, Rhodes A. Minimally invasive cardiac output monitoring. *Curr Opin Crit Care.* 2008;14(3):322–326.
 Reports the evidence to support using pulse contour techniques and a closer look at the different commercially available devices.
Young BP, Low LL. Noninvasive monitoring cardiac output using partial CO_2 rebreathing. *Crit Care Clin.* 2010;26(2):383–392.
 This article reviews the use of partial carbon dioxide rebreathing devices to determine cardiac output and their application for hemodynamic monitoring in the ICU and operating room.

82 Functional Hemodynamic Monitoring

Jennifer Shaffer and Warren Isakow

Hemodynamic instability is very common in the intensive care unit (ICU). Clinical impressions regarding a patient's hemodynamic profile can often be erroneous resulting in potentially harmful interventions. The need for accurate hemodynamic information to guide patient care resulted in the widespread use of the pulmonary artery catheter (PAC). The lack of benefit observed in prospective randomized controlled trials and the inherent invasiveness of the PAC has renewed interest in alternative modes of hemodynamic monitoring and the assessment of volume responsiveness.

Basic principles of hemodynamic optimization focus on improving oxygen delivery to the tissues by restoring adequate circulating volume, restoring perfusion by optimizing cardiac output (CO) and mean arterial pressure (MAP) and ensuring an adequate oxygen carrying capacity (optimal hemoglobin and hemoglobin saturation with oxygen).

Volume responsiveness refers to the increase in CO or stroke volume (SV) that occurs in response to a fluid challenge.

STATIC MARKERS OF VOLUME RESPONSIVENESS

Figures 82.1 and 82.2 explain the concept of volume responsiveness by depicting the Frank Starling curve of a normal heart. Clinicians have generally utilized static hemodynamic values, most commonly intravascular pressures, to predict which patients will benefit from fluid challenges. Table 82.1 summarizes the static markers commonly used in ICUs to help predict volume responsiveness.

CENTRAL VENOUS PRESSURE

Figure 82.3 shows a normal central venous pressure (CVP) tracing. CVP tracings in disease states are often characteristic:

- In atrial fibrillation, the a wave is lost
- In states of atrioventricular dissociation, large cannon a waves may occur as the atrium contracts against a closed tricuspid valve.
- In patients with tricuspid regurgitation, a large fused cv wave is seen.
- Tricuspid stenosis results in giant a waves and a reduced y descent.

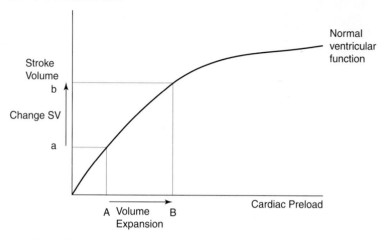

Figure 82.1. Volume responsive: Increase in stroke volume in response to a fluid challenge in a patient with normal biventricular function and on the steep portion (low preload) of the Frank Starling curve.

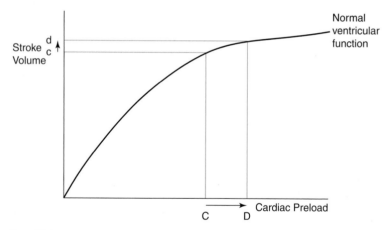

Figure 82.2. Volume unresponsive: Minimal augmentation of stroke volume despite volume expansion in a patient with normal biventricular function on the flat portion (high preload) of the Frank Starling curve.

- In constrictive pericarditis, the y descent is prominent and becomes steeper during inspiration.
- In cardiac tamponade, the x descent is preserved and the y descent is attenuated.

CVP is used extensively in ICUs to make clinical decisions regarding volume status due to the high prevalence of central lines and the ease of acquisition from an existing catheter. However, there is no association between CVP and circulating blood volume. The CVP is the intravascular pressure in the major thoracic veins, measured

TABLE 82.1 Static Markers of Volume Responsiveness

Parameter	Required elements	Invasiveness	Values	Comments
CVP	Central venous line	+	Normal: 1–8 cm H_2O Target: 8–12 cm H_2O during sepsis	Most frequently used parameter due to ease of attainment. Predictive power of a single CVP value to predict volume responsiveness is in the 50% range.
PAOP	Central access with a 8.5 French introducer catheter to insert the PAC	++++	Normal: 4–12 cm H_2O	Approximates LAP and LVEDP. Used as a surrogate for LVEDV assuming a linear pressure/volume relationship in the left ventricle. Single PAOP reading has a positive predictive value in the 50% range for assessing volume responsiveness. May be useful diagnostically when all parameters obtained from the PAC are evaluated.
GEDVI	Central venous catheter and thermistor-tipped femoral arterial line to perform transpulmonary thermodilution. (PiCCO® system)	+++	Normal: 680–800 mL/m²	GEDVI is a moderate predictor of volume responsiveness. When utilized with SVV obtained from the PiCCO® system, may improve ability to detect volume responsiveness.
LVEDA	Transesophageal echocardiography	++	LVED diameter: 49 ± 4 mm LVED volume: 102 ± 20 mL	Requires expertise and not available routinely in most ICUs. LVEDV is approximated using LVEDA by assuming ventricular geometry. Overall, LVEDA alone is a poor predictor of volume responsiveness

CVP, central venous pressure; PAOP, pulmonary artery occlusion pressure; GEDVI, global end-diastolic volume index; LVEDA, left ventricular end-diastolic area; PAC, pulmonary artery catheter.

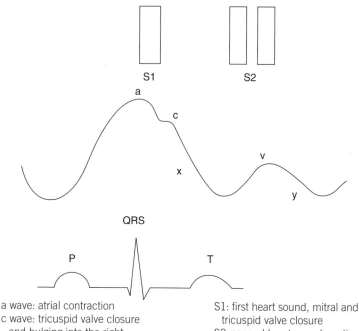

a wave: atrial contraction
c wave: tricuspid valve closure
   and bulging into the right
   atrium or transmitted pulsation
   from the carotid artery
x descent: atrial relaxation
v wave: atrial filling
y wave: atrial emptying

S1: first heart sound, mitral and
   tricuspid valve closure
S2: second heart sound, aortic
   and pulmonary valve closure
P wave: atrial depolarization
QRS complex: ventricular
   depolarization
T wave: ventricular repolarization

Figure 82.3. Normal CVP tracing.

relative to atmospheric pressure. It provides an estimate of right atrial pressure as it is ideally measured at the junction of the superior vena cava and the right atrium. There are many factors that affect the CVP including blood volume, vascular tone, right ventricular function and compliance, tricuspid valve disease, cardiac rhythm, intrathoracic pressure (respiratory efforts and PEEP) as well as patient position. The ability of any CVP value to accurately predict volume responsiveness is in the 56% range. A decrease in CVP is a relatively late sign of intravascular volume depletion particularly in patients with intact vascular tone. For all these reasons, CVP alone should not be utilized to guide fluid management decisions, but should be combined with knowledge of the patients underlying pathophysiology and additional hemodynamic parameters.

DYNAMIC MARKERS OF VOLUME RESPONSIVENESS

A dynamic assessment of volume responsiveness is possible at the bedside and essentially consists of challenging the patient's Frank Starling curve. The principle is to induce a change in preload and monitor the response by documenting changes in the SV, CO, or other surrogates.

Commonly used techniques of inducing a change in preload are as follows:

- Infusing a fluid bolus
- Passive leg raising which auto-transfuses about 200–300 mL of blood in the lower extremities back into the central circulation
- Utilizing the natural cyclic changes that occur in right ventricular SV, left ventricular preload, and ultimately left ventricular SV due to mechanical ventilation induced changes in right ventricular preload. Large mechanical ventilation induced changes in left ventricular SV will occur in patients with biventricular preload reserve with no change occurring if one or both of the ventricles is preload independent. To utilize this technique, that patient needs to be in normal sinus rhythm, totally mechanically ventilated with no spontaneous breathing attempts and the tidal volume needs to be adequate (normally 8–10 mL/kg)

Commonly used techniques of detecting a change in preload induced by one of the challenges above are as follows:

- Dynamic real-time monitoring of SV or CO utilizing esophageal or suprasternal Doppler. If the SV or CO increases by more than 15% with a fluid challenge or in response to a passive leg raise maneuver, the patient is volume responsive. If the response is in the 10% to 15% range, the patient is likely volume responsive and if associated with evidence of end-organ hypoperfusion, the patient may benefit from fluid loading. If the change in SV or CO is <10%, the patient is likely not volume responsive and is functioning on the flatter portion of their Frank Starling curve.
- Dynamic changes in descending aortic blood flow velocity utilizing esophageal Doppler. A similar cutoff of 10% to 15% is used for volume responsiveness if this technique is used.
- Measuring arterial pulse contour analysis and pulse pressure or SV variation. A pulse pressure variation (PPV) or stroke volume variation (SVV) of >10% to 12% predict volume responsiveness with high sensitivity and specificity (Fig. 82.4).

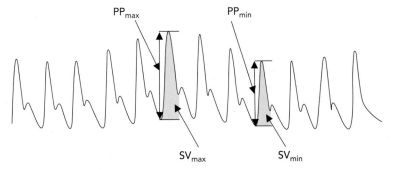

Figure 82.4. Arterial pressure tracing showing the presence of pulse pressure variation (PPV) and stroke volume variation (SVV).

Pulse pressure variation $= 100 \times (PP_{max} - PP_{min})/(PP_{max} + PP_{min})/2$
Stroke volume variation $= 100 \times (SV_{max} - SV_{min})/(SV_{max} + SV_{min})/2$

Functional hemodynamic monitoring and the assessment of volume responsiveness should only be used if a patient has

- hemodynamic instability (MAP <65 mm Hg)
- evidence of tissue hypoperfusion (urine output <20 mL/hr, anxiety, confusion, lethargy, HR >100 b/min, lactate >2.2 mmol/L)

These criteria should be met before embarking on fluid challenges as many individuals in an ICU may be fluid responsive, but may not be in need of fluid administration. It is the clinical scenario that determines the need for utilizing any hemodynamic monitoring and intervention strategy.

Once the patient is deemed to be hemodynamically unstable, the next step in the evaluation is determination of preload responsiveness using one of the dynamic markers noted above with adequate fluid boluses. If the patient is preload responsive, serial fluid boluses and serial evaluations of continuing preload responsiveness should be performed until the patient is no longer hemodynamically unstable or no longer preload responsive. The septic patient who is persistently hypotensive and no longer preload responsive will require vasopressors titrated. In addition, further diagnostic workup with bedside echocardiography should be performed to identify cardiogenic dysfunction, which would benefit from inotropic support or to identify another cause (pericardial tamponade, right ventricular dysfunction in acute pulmonary embolism, etc.).

ScvO₂ MONITORING

ScvO$_2$ is often used in the ICU as a surrogate of the true SvO$_2$ and reflects the balance between oxygen delivery and demand. A normal SvO$_2$ is between 65% and 75% and studies in critically ill patients which simultaneously measured the variables, show that the ScvO$_2$ is about 5% to 7% higher than the SvO$_2$ but that the variables track in the same direction with changes in a patient's condition. The ScvO$_2$ is, therefore, useful for trend analysis. The determinants of the ScvO$_2$ are shown in Figure 82.5.

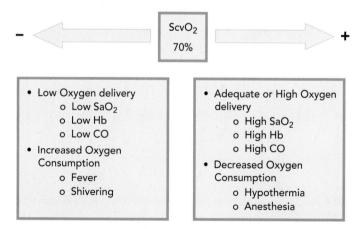

Figure 82.5. Variables affecting the ScvO$_2$.

SUGGESTED READINGS

Durairaj L, Schmidt G. Fluid therapy in resuscitated sepsis. *Chest.* 2008;133:252–263.

An excellent review of fluid therapy as well as the static and dynamic predictors of volume responsiveness in the ICU.

Marik PE, Baram M, Vahid B. Does central venous pressure predict fluid responsiveness? A systematic review of the literature and the tale of the seven mares. *Chest.* 2008;134:172–178.

A literature review of the utility of the CVP as a marker of volume responsiveness.

Monnet X, Teboul JL. Volume responsiveness. *Curr Opin Crit Care.* 2007;13:549–553.

A review of volume responsiveness focusing on the effect of respiratory variation on hemodynamic signals.

Monnet X, Rienzo M, Osman D. Passive leg raising predicts fluid responsiveness in the critically ill. *Crit Care Med.* 2006;34:1402–1407.

A study utilizing esophageal Doppler monitoring of aortic blood flow together with passive leg raising to predict volume responsiveness. A leg raise induced increase of aortic blood flow > or = 10% predicted fluid responsiveness with a sensitivity of 97% and a specificity of 94%.

Osman D, Ridel C, Ray P, et al. Cardiac filling pressures are not appropriate to predict hemodynamic response to volume challenge. *Crit Care Med.* 2007;35:64–68.

A retrospective study in a medical ICU showing that a CVP of < 8 mm Hg and a PAOP of < 12 mm Hg predicted volume responsiveness with a positive predictive value of only 47% and 54% respectively.

Rivers EP, Ander DS, Powell D. Central venous oxygen saturation monitoring in the critically ill patient. *Curr Opin Crit Care.* 2001;7:204–211.

Excellent review article on ScvO$_2$ monitoring, including pathophysiologic aspects, clinical use and comparison to SvO$_2$.

Thiel SW, Kollef MH, Isakow W. Noninvasive stroke volume measurement and passive leg raising predict volume responsiveness in medical ICU patients: an observational cohort study. *Crit Care.* 2009;13(4):R111.

A prospective study in medical ICU patients which revealed that a totally noninvasive suprasternal Doppler probe and passive leg raising was able to predict volume responsiveness with a sensitivity of 80% and specificity of 92%. The CVP in this study was not able to differentiate between volume responders and non-responders.

83 Pericardiocentesis

Jennifer Shaffer and Warren Isakow

Pericardiocentesis is indicated in the emergent setting to treat cardiac tamponade or as a diagnostic procedure for pericardial effusions. It is the insertion of a needle to remove fluid from the pericardial sac. This fluid may be bloody, purulent, or transudative. The procedure is often performed by a cardiologist with echocardiography or fluoroscopy. If the reason for pericardiocentesis is tamponade, then it may be done at the bedside urgently as a lifesaving procedure. This chapter will discuss the indications for immediate pericardiocentesis and the key steps necessary to aspirate fluid at the bedside.

Pericardiocentesis is performed in the critical care setting to relieve tamponade. Tamponade is a condition in which fluid accumulates in the pericardial space and compresses the heart. It is a clinical diagnosis classically marked by hypotension, jugular venous distension, and muffled heart sounds. These clinical signs known as Beck's Triad are a result of decreased stroke volume and impaired venous return from the cushion of fluid surrounding the heart. The presence of pulsus paradoxus (a decrease in systolic pressure >10 mm Hg during inspiration) is a more specific physical exam finding of tamponade when an effusion is present. Additional signs of tamponade include electrical alternans and low voltage on electrocardiogram.

It is generally recommended to perform a transthoracic echocardiogram to confirm the presence of an effusion before proceeding to pericardiocentesis. In the post cardiac surgery patient, a transesophageal echocardiogram is preferred because of the high likelihood of a loculated, posterior effusion. Nonetheless, if tamponade develops into obstructive shock there may not be sufficient time to obtain the echocardiogram and a bedside pericardiocentesis must be immediately performed.

The amount of fluid necessary to cause tamponade varies and depends on the rapidity of accumulation. In cases of malignant effusions, the fluid may collect gradually and stretch the pericardial sac to the point that it contains over 1 L of fluid before creating tamponade. In contrast, trauma may quickly lead to tamponade with only 100 mL of fluid or blood. A list of possible causes of cardiac tamponade in the ICU is found in Table 83.1. The most common cause of tamponade is malignancy.

The safety of the procedure is improved with the use of echocardiography to guide needle placement. It is recommended by the American College of Cardiology, American Heart Association (ACC/AHA) to perform pericardiocentesis with echocardiography to lower the risk of complications. Minor complications include coronary laceration, pneumothorax, arrhythmias, and puncture of the ventricle or peritoneal cavity. The incidence of such complications approximates 5% with transthoracic echocardiography, but as high as 17% without imaging guidance. Major complications such as ventricular rupture and death are less frequent. In a series published by the Mayo

TABLE 83.1	Causes of Cardiac Tamponade in the ICU

Neoplasm

Infectious pericarditis (viral, bacterial, tubercular, parasitic)

Uremia

Postmyocardial infarction with ventricular rupture

Complication of a catheter-based procedure (pacemaker lead insertion, central line placement, or coronary catheterization)

Compressive hematoma after cardiothoracic surgery

Traumatic hemopericardium

Systemic autoimmune diseases (systemic lupus erythematosus, rheumatoid arthritis)

Aortic dissection

Drugs (hydralazine, procainamide, isoniazid, minoxidil, anticoagulation treatment)

Idiopathic

Institute, the major complication rate was 1.2% over a 21-year period (Tsang et al., *Mayo Clin Proc.* 2002;77:429–436).

There are only a few relative contraindications for pericardiocentesis. These include coagulopathy (INR >1.4), thrombocytopenia (platelets <50,000), and small effusions located in a posterior, loculated space. Aortic dissection is an absolute contraindication. A surgical procedure such as subxiphoid pericardiostomy is preferred in cases where effusions are likely malignant. The surgical approach allows for a pericardial window, which reduces the rate of recurrence. Leaving a catheter in place for prolonged drainage after pericardiocentesis has a similar rate of recurrence as placing a pericardial window. Catheter drainage is typically left in place for 24 to 48 hours as the rate of fluid output diminishes. Catheter pericardiocentesis is the treatment of choice and given a class I recommendation by the 2004 European Society of Cardiology guidelines on pericardial disease.

The decision to perform a bedside pericardiocentesis is based on hemodynamic instability and the development of obstructive shock. Intubation should be avoided because it will worsen shock caused by tamponade. Vasopressors have limited capacity to improve organ perfusion. The following steps outline the procedure.

STEPS FOR BEDSIDE PERICARDIOCENTESIS

1. *Gather the necessary equipment,* which is available at most centers in a prepackaged pericardiocentesis kit. Equipment includes, but is not limited to:
   a. Antiseptic (Betadine or chlorhexidine gluconate)
   b. Local anesthetic (lidocaine 1%)
   c. Sterile drapes, gown, cap, and face mask
   d. Syringes, 20 mL and 60 mL
   e. Scalpel, No. 11
   f. Needles, 18 ga, 1.5 in; 25 ga, 5/8 in
   g. Spinal needle, 18 ga, 7.5 to 12 cm

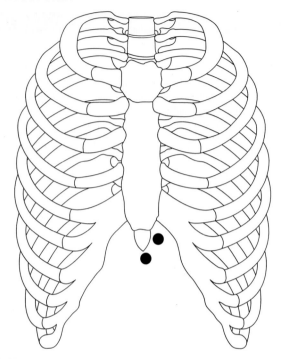

Figure 83.1. Most common sites for needle insertion.

2. *Patient positioning:* Ensure the patient is on cardiac monitoring with supplemental oxygen. If time permits, decompress the stomach with a nasogastric tube. Place the head of the bed at a 45-degree angle to cause fluid to collect inferiorly and to bring the heart closer to the anterior chest wall.

3. *Identify insertion site:* Locate the patient's xiphoid process and left costal margin by palpation. The most common sites of needle insertion are marked in Figure 83.1 by black dots.

4. *Prep site:* Use sterile technique with antiseptic solution, drapes, and anesthetize the skin with lidocaine if time allows.

5. *Needle insertion:* First make a small incision at the insertion site with the scalpel. Fill the 20-mL syringe with 10 mL of sterile saline, evacuate the air, and attach to the 18-gauge needle. As the needle is advanced, place constant suction on the syringe. Stop to inject saline (0.5 to 1 mL) intermittently to prevent tissue from clogging the needle.

6. *Needle angle:* The needle should be advanced toward the left shoulder at a 45-degree angle to the abdominal wall. The needle is slowly advanced past the posterior rib border, then flattened to a 15-degree angle.

7. *Needle advancement:* Continue advancing the needle until pericardial fluid is returned. ST segment elevation or abrupt ECG changes indicate myocardial injury. In this case, the needle should be slowly withdrawn back.

8. *Aspiration:* Remove the 20 mL syringe and replace with the larger available syringe to continue to aspirate as much fluid as possible. In obstructive shock, removal of 50 mL of fluid can cause rapid improvement in cardiac output.

9. *Pericardial drain placement:* Pericardial drains help prevent reaccumulation of fluid in the next 1 to 2 days. First, insert the guidewire found in the pericardiocentesis kit into the needle. Remove the needle over the wire, and keep the wire in hand to avoid losing its place. Slide a 6 to 8 French dilator over the wire to form a tract. A larger skin incision may be needed to advance the dilator. Remove the dilator, and then advance the drainage catheter over the guidewire into the pericardial space. The guidewire is removed and discarded leaving the catheter available for draining the effusion. Suture in place and cover with sterile dressing. Fluid can be removed through a three-way stopcock until the patient is hemodynamically improved.

10. *Continued catheter drainage:* There are two options for continued drainage of the pericardial fluid. The catheter may be directly connected to tubing and placed on a suction bulb; or the tubing can be left to gravity drainage. To maintain patency, the tubing should be flushed with saline every 1 to 2 hours. Another alternative is to fill the tubing and catheter with urokinase. In this case, the tubing must then be opened every 2 to 4 hours to drain for 1 hour.

11. *Diagnostic studies:* There are several possible studies to obtain depending on the clinical situation. The fluid may be sent for cell count with differential, glucose, protein, Gram stain, culture (aerobic, anaerobic, AFB), hematocrit, lactate dehydrogenase, cytology, tumor markers, hematocrit, rheumatoid factor (RF), and antinuclear antibody (ANA).

SUGGESTED READINGS

Cheitlin MD, Armstrong WF, Aurigemma GP, et al. ACC/AHA/ASE 2003 guideline update for the clinical application of echocardiography. *J Am Coll Cardiol.* 2003;42:954–970. American College of Cardiology Web Site. Available at: www.acc.org/clinical/guidelines/echo/index.pdf.
Clinical guidelines for the use of echocardiography.

Imazio M, Brucato A, Trinchero R, et al. Diagnosis and management of pericardial diseases. *Nat Rev Cardiol.* 2009;6:743–751.
Review of pericardial disease with focus on management of acute and chronic pericarditis.

Maisch B, Seferovic PM, Ristic AD, et al. Guidelines on the diagnosis and management of pericardial diseases executive summary; The Task force on the diagnosis and management of pericardial diseases of the European society of cardiology. *Eur Heart J.* 2004;25:587.
Provides a review of the evidence used to create the current guidelines on managing constrictive pericarditis, tamponade, and acute pericarditis.

Spodick DH. Acute cardiac tamponade. *N Engl J Med.* 2003;349:684–690.
In depth review of causes, diagnosis, and management of cardiac tamponade.

84

End-of-Life Care in the Intensive Care Unit

Jonathan M. Green

Despite individuals' stated preference to die at home, the majority of persons die in institutions. In 2001, only 20% to 25% of U.S. deaths were at home, with the remaining in hospitals (approximately 50% to 60%) and nursing homes (20% to 25%). Of hospital deaths, almost half occurred in the intensive care units (ICUs). In 1995, the SUPPORT trial documented a number of deficiencies in end-of-life care in ICUs, including poor communication between physician and patient about preferences for cardiopulmonary resuscitation, failure to write do not resuscitate orders for patients who desire them, and inadequately treated pain and discomfort during the final days of life. Thus, it is critical that the ICU physician develop the skills and techniques appropriate to managing the dying patient. In this chapter, I will discuss issues common to providing good end-of-life care to all patients, as well as those issues unique to the ICU patient population.

ESTABLISHING GOALS OF CARE

Patients admitted to ICUs are at an increased risk of death and also face the prospect of being subjected to invasive procedures and treatments. Studies have demonstrated that as the potential for good outcome declines, so does willingness to undergo highly burdensome treatment regimens. However, in one study, 26% of those surveyed stated they strongly agreed with receiving ICU care despite an outcome predicted to be a persistent vegetative state or terminal illness. Conversely, between 1% and 2% of patients did not wish to undergo ICU care, even if they were to be returned to a fully functional health status. Given these disparities in individual patient preferences, it is essential to establish appropriate goals of care either prior to admission or early in the course of an ICU stay.

On admission to the ICU, the staff should ascertain whether a patient has previously appointed a durable power of attorney for health care and/or completed an advance directive. If so, these documents should be obtained and, if possible, the contents of them should be discussed with the patient. However, the majority of patients have neither document, and despite the presence of life-limiting illness, many will have not discussed end-of-life care with either their personal physician or family members. Thus, it may be that these discussions are occurring in the ICU setting for the first time. If the patient is capable of participating, discussions to establish goals of care should be held directly with him or her. The outcome of these discussions should then be shared by the patient and physician together with the patient's family and loved ones, as directed by the patient. If the patient is not decisional either because of the acute condition or previous underlying disease, the discussion should be held with an appropriate surrogate (see "Surrogate Decision-making").

The purpose of the goals of care discussion is to ascertain what the patient and family's expectations are for the hospitalization. In addition, the physician should elicit the values, preferences, and wishes of the patient with respect to what the patient views as an acceptable outcome for the ICU stay. This may range from hope for cure to a desire for a pain-free death, or anywhere in between. Patients often have multiple seemingly contradictory goals, in which case the physician should help in clarification and prioritization. It is equally important for the physician to provide prognostic information and advise the patient and family as to what can reasonably be expected during the hospitalization. Disparities between the patient's and physician's goals are frequent sources of conflict in the ICU. If significant differences are identified, ongoing discussions to identify reasons for the disagreement and reach a consensus are crucial. Possible reasons may include misunderstandings on the part of the patient or family as to nature of the disease or treatment options, or failure of the physician to appreciate cultural differences or other values inherent to the individual patient. It is also important to recognize that the goals may shift during the course of an acute illness. Therefore, as the clinical scenario changes, ongoing discussions to re-evaluate the goals of care are necessary.

SURROGATE DECISION MAKING

Patients in the ICU are often unable to participate in decision-making because of either their acute illness or underlying disease process. In these instances, appropriate surrogates must be identified. Many, but not all, states have a legal order of surrogacy established. It is important to be familiar with the relevant laws in the state in which you practice. For the purposes of this discussion, a valid surrogate can be defined as an individual who can faithfully represent the goals, values, and wishes of the patient, and act accordingly and in the patient's best interest. Typically, it is presumed that family members are best able to fill this role; however, persons not related to the patient may also be able to serve as a valid surrogate. As implied by the definition, the role of the surrogate is to represent the patient's wishes. However, this is often a difficult task, and is almost always colored by the surrogate's own values and preferences. Studies of surrogate decision-making have shown that surrogates accurately represent the patient only 50% to 70% of the time.

There are often multiple individuals who could be considered a valid surrogate. The family may choose to appoint one person as spokesperson, or may prefer to decide as a group. Not infrequently, there is disagreement among them as to what the patient's wishes would be. If the patient has appointed a specific individual as durable power of attorney for health care, then in the absence of specific evidence that he or she is not acting in good faith, that individual should serve as primary decision-maker. Most often, there is no one individual specified. It is important that the critical care physician work to guide the family and help them reach consensus. Typically, a series of family meetings in which the disputed issues are explored will lead to consensus and resolution. It is often helpful to include nurses, social workers, chaplains, and other team members in these discussions.

The standards for surrogate decision-making are (a) substituted judgment and (b) best interest. The substituted judgment standard asks the surrogate to guide the team as to what decision the patient would make in this circumstance, essentially asking if the patient could speak for himself or herself, what he or she would say. If the patient and surrogate have had specific discussions that inform this decision, then this approach may be reasonable. Often, however, no such discussion has taken place, leaving the surrogate to speculate. The best interest standard asks the surrogate to help the physician determine whether the proposed treatment is in the best interest of the patient, weighing the potential benefits and burdens of the treatment with what is known about the goals and values of the patient. This standard can also be problematic because in the absence of specific information, it is difficult to determine what an acceptable outcome is and what level of treatment burden the patient would tolerate for that outcome. Typically, both surrogates and caregivers underestimate the willingness of patients to undergo aggressive interventions and the quality of life that patients deem to be acceptable.

WITHDRAWING AND WITHHOLDING LIFE-SUSTAINING TREATMENTS

Critical care physicians are often faced with decisions to limit life-sustaining treatment. In one large study of 851 patients admitted to a medical ICU requiring mechanical ventilation, almost 20% had ventilatory support withdrawn. These decisions can be a source of distress and conflict for health care providers as well as patients and families. The ethical basis for withdrawal of life-sustaining treatment stems directly from the principle of respect for autonomy. It is well accepted by the medical profession and society at large that a patient, and therefore by extension the surrogate, may make an informed decision to refuse any proposed treatment, even if the physician believes that such a decision is not in their best interest. From this, it follows directly that patients may opt to discontinue any treatment once initiated. If this were not the case, many patients might be reluctant to initiate potentially beneficial therapies for fear they would not be permitted to stop at a later time. Conflicts may arise when the health care provider believes that discontinuation of life-sustaining interventions violates the principles of beneficence and nonmaleficence, or because they think such actions are in opposition to their own conscience. Alternatively, surrogates may wish to continue aggressive care despite the recommendation of the team that such treatments are only prolonging an inevitable death (see "Futility").

Most commonly, withdrawal of life-sustaining treatments is equated with discontinuation of mechanical ventilation. However, discontinuation of hemodynamic support, hemodialysis, transfusions, or other interventions also may be considered in this context. The decision to withdraw life-sustaining treatments should be approached in a manner similar to all other treatment decisions. Although ultimate responsibility lies with the attending physician, it is particularly important in this circumstance that opinions of other health care providers are given voice and considered. The goal of withdrawal of life-sustaining interventions is to remove treatments that are no longer congruent with the patient's goals and are therefore no longer appropriate. If the patient is not decisional, it is essential that there has been prior discussion with the surrogate(s) and that they are in agreement with the proposed plan. This should be documented in the medical record.

Attention to the patient's comfort is paramount throughout the patient's ICU stay, but assumes particular importance during the process of withdrawal of life-sustaining treatments. Reluctance to administer adequate doses of analgesics and sedatives can result in undue and unacceptable levels of suffering to both the patient and surviving family members. There is ethical and legal consensus that although respiratory

TABLE 84.1	**The Rule of Double Effect**

An action with two possible consequences, one good and one bad, is morally permissible if the action:
1. Is not in itself immoral.
2. Is undertaken only with the intention of achieving the possible good effect, without intending the possible bad effect, even though the bad effect may be foreseen.
3. The action does not bring about the good effect solely by means of the bad effect.
4. Is undertaken for a proportionately grave reason.

depression or hypotension may be a foreseeable consequence of these medications, if the intent is to relieve specific symptoms such as pain or dyspnea, it is essential to treat in adequate doses despite the possibility that death may be hastened. Ethically, the justification for this has been termed *the rule of double effect* (Table 84.1). Doses of medication vary considerably depending on the patient. Most commonly, narcotics such as morphine or fentanyl are given in combination with a benzodiazepine, typically either midazolam or lorazepam. The medications should be administered initially as a bolus followed by continuous infusion. Each increase in infusion rate should be preceded by an appropriate bolus to allow for a rapid achievement of steady-state levels. Individual patients may have greatly differing medication requirements, depending on their illness and previous exposure to the drugs. Therefore, the dosage needs to be titrated to individual patient needs. Neuromuscular blocking agents should not be used as they do not provide any palliative effect to the patient and make assessment of comfort impossible.

If mechanical ventilation is to be discontinued, paralytic agents should be discontinued and their effect allowed to wear off. The patient is first placed on continuous positive airway pressure/peak systolic velocity settings of 5/5 mm Hg, adequate sedation is administered to minimize dyspnea and the patient is then extubated. There should be frequent assessment by the nursing and medical staff for comfort. Family members are given the option of being present during the extubation, depending solely on their personal preferences. If possible, the monitor screen in the patient's room should be turned off to allow the family to focus on the patient without distraction.

FUTILITY

The issue of medical futility has been a subject of prolonged and intense controversy. Typically, futility debates arise in the ICU when the health care team believes that continued aggressive interventions are highly unlikely to lead to patient survival, yet the patient's surrogate insists that all measures continue. Frustration on the part of the physicians and other team members results in the declaration that further treatment is futile, in an attempt to rationalize discontinuation of treatment without the consent of the surrogate. However, this is ethically problematic, and there remains no clear consensus on an approach to futility. Moreover, most clinical situations in which these conflicts arise can be favorably resolved by improved communication between the physician and family.

Bernard Lo provides three specific conditions that define interventions that are futile in the strict sense. (a) The intervention has no pathophysiologic rationale. An example of this would be the treatment of a Gram-negative infection with an antibiotic such as vancomycin. (b) Cardiac arrest occurs as a result of refractory hypotension or hypoxemia despite maximal supportive therapy. Performance of cardiopulmonary resuscitation in such a circumstance will be ineffective in restoring circulation. (c) The intervention has been tried and already failed in the patient. Treatments that meet these strict criteria do not need to be provided. However, these are clearly the minority of clinical situations in which futility is discussed. Many other looser futility criteria have been proposed, but these are problematic. Most of these rely on subjective determinations of what is an acceptable probability of a favorable outcome, or on determinations of quality of life.

Some groups have developed policies on futility that focus on process and conflict resolution rather than on absolute definitions. The advantage of these is that a defined series of steps are taken that result in enhanced communication. Ultimately, it is the process of increased communication between the health care providers and family members that leads to the satisfactory resolution of these difficult situations. Unilateral decision-making with regard to limiting life-sustaining care for critically ill patients using futility as a rationale is highly discouraged for several reasons. First, the criteria are often incorrectly and inconsistently applied, and perhaps most importantly, such action can lead to extreme distress and anger among the surviving family members. This is not to imply that physicians need to be held hostage to unreasonable demands of unrealistic families, but that the focus should be on continued communication to reach a plan of care that is acceptable to all involved parties.

DETERMINATION OF DEATH BY WHOLE-BRAIN CRITERIA

In 1981, the President's Commission for the Study of Ethical Problems in Medicine and Biomedical and Behavioral Research recommended a uniform standard for the determination of death. This stated that "An individual who has sustained either (1) irreversible cessation of circulatory and respiratory functions or (2) irreversible cessation of all functions of the entire brain, including the brainstem, is dead. A determination of death must be made in accordance with accepted medical standards." Although death by cardiopulmonary criteria is understood and well accepted by physicians and lay people alike, declaration of death by whole-brain criteria can be more problematic. Many families and religious groups are reluctant to accept this determination.

Determination of death by whole-brain criteria requires examination by an experienced physician. Essential elements include that the patient is in deep coma, that brainstem function is documented to be absent, the cause of coma is established and sufficient to account for the loss of brainstem function, that the possibility of recovery of any brain function is excluded, and that cessation of all brain function persists for an appropriate period of observation and/or trial of therapy (Table 84.2). Implicit in this is that reversible causes such as drug intoxications, severe metabolic disturbances, and hypothermia have been excluded as causes for the coma. The definition does not require the use of specialized testing, but in some instances cerebral perfusion scanning or electroencephalography testing may be helpful to document the absence of cerebral blood flow or electrical activity.

After the determination of death, the family should not be told the patient is "brain-dead," as this terminology is confusing to many. Instead, they should be

TABLE 84.2	Whole-Brain Criteria for Death

An individual with irreversible cessation of all functions of the entire brain, including the brainstem is dead.
1. Cerebral functions are absent.
   Presence of deep coma, cerebral unreceptivity and unresponsiveness.
2. Brainstem functions are absent.
   Absence of pupillary, corneal, oculocephalic, oculovestibular, oropharyngeal, and respiratory reflexes.
3. Irreversibility is recognized by:
   The cause of coma is established and is sufficient to account for the loss of brain function.
   The possibility of recovery of any brain function is excluded.
   The cessation of all brain functions persists for an appropriate period of observation and/or trial of therapy.

informed that the patient has been pronounced dead by neurologic or whole-brain criteria. All previously initiated life-sustaining treatments, such as mechanical ventilation and pressor support, should be withdrawn. In some circumstances, the clinician may elect to continue these for a limited time to allow family members to come to the bedside or for arrangements to be made for organ donation. It is not necessary to provide sedation or analgesia to the patient at this time.

CONCLUSION

Physicians caring for the critically ill will continue to face challenges in providing appropriate care for the dying patient. Many factors, including increases in technology and an aging population, will almost certainly lead to greater numbers of patients dying in ICUs. Enhanced communication between care providers, patients, and families at all stages of the illness is a key to assuring that a satisfactory outcome is achieved.

SUGGESTED READINGS

Angus DC, Barnato AE, Linde-Zwirble WT, et al. Use of intensive care at the end of life in the United States: an epidemiologic study. *Crit Care Med.* 2004;32:638–643.

Cook D, Rocker G, Marshall J, et al. Withdrawal of mechanical ventilation in anticipation of death in the intensive care unit. *N Engl J Med.* 2003;349:1123–1132.

Elpern EH, Patterson PA, Gloskey D, et al. Patients' preferences for intensive care. *Crit Care Med.* 1992;20:43–47.
   This study interviewed patients that had been in an ICU, and determined whether they would undergo ICU level care again given four specific outcome scenarios.

Fried TR, Bradley EH, Towle VR, et al. Understanding the treatment preferences of seriously ill patients. *N Engl J Med.* 2002;346:1061–1066.
   This study documents how patients modify their preferences in response to specific treatment strategies, weighing treatment burden against possible outcomes.

Halevy A, Brody BA. A multi-institution collaborative policy on medical futility. *JAMA.* 1996;276:571–574.

Lo B. Resolving ethical dilemmas: a guide for clinicians. Philadelphia, PA: Lippincott Williams & Wilkins, 2005.

This is an outstanding text examining contemporary medical ethical issues in a practical way.

Murphy DJ, Barbour E. GUIDe (Guidelines for the Use of Intensive Care in Denver): a community effort to define futile and inappropriate care. *New Horiz.* 1994;2:326–331.

The Presidents Commission for the Study of Ethical Problems in Medicine and Biomedical and Behavioral Research. Defining death: medical, legal, and ethical issues in the definition of death. Washington, DC: US Government Printing Office, 1981:159–166.

Shalowitz DI, Garrett-Mayer E, Wendler D. The accuracy of surrogate decision makers: a systematic review. *Arch Intern Med.* 2006;166:493–497.

This study is a meta-analysis demonstrating the difficulty in relying on surrogate decision makers to guide treatment plans.

Support Principal Investigators. A controlled trial to improve care for seriously ill hospitalized patients. The study to understand prognoses and preferences for outcomes and risks of treatments (SUPPORT). *JAMA.* 1995;274:1591–1598.

This large multicenter trial demonstrated significant gaps in communication about critical end-of-life issues in intensive care units. However, in a second, intervention phase, implementation of enhanced communication strategies failed to improve outcomes.

Teno J. Facts on Dying, March 19, 2004. Center for Gerontology and Health Care Research, Brown University. Available at: http://www.chcr.brown.edu/dying/2001DATA.HTM. Accessed October 2, 2006.

85

Common Equations and Rules of Thumb in the Intensive Care Unit

Warren Isakow

PULMONARY EQUATIONS

Alveolar Gas Equation

$$PAO_2 = FiO_2(PB - PH_2O) - \frac{PaCO_2}{R}$$

Where PAO_2 = alveolar partial pressure of oxygen,
   FiO_2 = fraction of inspired oxygen,
   PB = barometric pressure (760 mm Hg at sea level),
   PH_2O = water vapor pressure,
   $PaCO_2$= partial pressure of carbon dioxide in the blood,
   R = respiratory quotient, assumed to be 0.8.

Alveolar-arterial Oxygen Gradient

$$PAO_2 - PaO_2$$

Normal value is between 3 and 15 mm Hg, and is influenced by age. In a healthy 60-year-old person, it may be as high as 28 mm Hg.
   For FiO_2 = 21%, should be 5 to 25 mm Hg
   For FiO_2 = 100%, should be <150 mm Hg

Partial Pressure of Arterial Carbon Dioxide

$$PaCO_2 = K \times \frac{VCO_2}{(1 - Vd/Vt) \times VA}$$

Where $PaCO_2$= the partial pressure of carbon dioxide in the blood,
   K = constant,
   VCO_2 = carbon dioxide production,
   Vd/Vt = dead space ratio of each tidal volume breath,
   VA = minute ventilation.

Lung Compliance

$$\text{Compliance}_{static} = \frac{\text{Tidal volume}}{\text{Plateau pressure} - \text{PEEP (positive end-expiratory pressure)}}$$

Normal compliance in an intubated patient $= 0.05$ to 0.07 L/cm H_2O

Airway Resistance

$$\text{Airway resistance} = \frac{\text{(Peak inspiratory pressure} - \text{Plateau pressure)}}{\text{(Peak inspiratory flow)}}$$

Normal resistance in an intubated patient is 4 to 6 cm $H_2O \cdot L^{-1} \cdot sec^{-2}$.

ACID–BASE EQUATIONS

Acute Respiratory Acidosis or Respiratory Alkalosis

$$\Delta pH = 0.008 \times \Delta PaCO_2 \text{ (from 40)}$$

Chronic Respiratory Acidosis or Respiratory Alkalosis

$$\Delta pH = 0.003 \times \Delta PaCO_2 \text{ (from 40)}$$

Metabolic Acidosis

$$\text{Predicted } PaCO_2 = 1.5 \times [HCO_3^-] + 8 \ (\pm 2)$$
$$\text{Bicarbonate deficit (mEq/L)} = [0.5 \times \text{body weight (kg)} \times (24 - [HCO_3^-])]$$

Metabolic Alkalosis

$$\text{Predicted } PaCO_2 = 0.7 \times [HCO_3^-] + 21(\pm 1.5) \text{ (when } [HCO_3^-] \text{ is } <40 \text{ mEq/L)}$$
$$\text{Predicted } PaCO_2 = 0.75 \times [HCO_3^-] + 19(\pm 7.5) \text{ (when } [HCO_3^-] \text{ is } >40 \text{ mEq/L)}$$
$$\text{Bicarbonate excess} = [0.4 \times \text{body weight (kg)} \times ([HCO_3^-] - 24)]$$

Validity of the Data, Henderson's Equation for Concentration of H^+

$$[H^+] = 24 \times \frac{PaCO_2}{HCO_3^-}$$

pH	[H$^+$] (mmol/L)
7.60	25
7.55	28
7.50	32
7.45	35
7.40	40
7.35	45
7.30	50
7.25	56
7.20	63
7.15	71

Anion Gap

$$\text{Anion Gap} = [Na^+] - ([CL^-] + [HCO_3^-]) = 10 \pm 4$$

The anion gap should be corrected for albumin, and for every decrease of 1 g/dL in albumin, a decrease of 2.5 mmol in the anion gap will occur.

Delta Gap

$$\Delta\text{gap} = (AG - 12) - (24 - [HCO_3^-]) = 0 \pm 6$$

Positive delta gap signifies a concomitant metabolic alkalosis or respiratory acidosis. Negative delta gap signifies a concomitant normal anion gap metabolic acidosis or chronic respiratory alkalosis.

RENAL EQUATIONS

Calculated Osmolarity

$$\text{Osmolarity (mM)} = 2 \times [Na^+] + \frac{BUN\ (mg/dL)}{2.8} + \frac{Glucose\ (mg/dL)}{18} + \frac{ETOH}{4.8}$$

Where ETOH = alcohol.

Osmolar Gap

Osmolar gap = Measured osmolarity – calculated osmolarity. (Normal is <10 mOsm.)

Estimated Creatinine Clearance

$$\text{Creatinine Clearance} = \frac{140 - Age\ (years)}{Serum\ creatinine\ (mg/dL) \times 72} \times \text{weight (kg)} (\times 0.85 \text{ in females})$$

Creatinine Clearance

$$\text{Creatinine clearance} = \frac{[Urine\ creatinine\ (mg/dL)] \times [Urine\ volume\ (mL/day)]}{[Plasma\ creatinine\ (mg/dL)] \times (1{,}440\ min/day)}$$

Fractional Excretion of Sodium (FENa$^+$)

$$\text{FENa}^+ = \frac{[\text{Urine Na}^+] \times [\text{Plasma creatinine}]}{[\text{Urine creatinine}] \times [\text{Plasma Na}^+]}$$

Fractional Excretion of Urea (FE urea)

$$\text{FE Urea} = \frac{[\text{Urine urea}] \times [\text{Plasma creatinine}]}{[\text{BUN}] \times [\text{Urine creatinine}]}$$

Correcting Sodium for Hyperglycemia

$$\text{Corrected Na}^+ = 0.016\,(\text{Measured Glucose} - 100) + \text{Measured Na}$$

Free Water Deficit

$$\text{Free Water Deficit} = 0.4 \times \text{Lean Body Weight} \times \left[\frac{\text{Plasma }[\text{Na}^+]}{140} - 1\right]$$

Formula for Correcting Hyponatremia

$$\text{Sodium deficit} = (\text{desired }[\text{Na}^+] - \text{current }[\text{Na}^+]) \times 0.6 \times \text{body weight (kg)}$$

HEMODYNAMIC EQUATIONS

Mean Arterial Pressure (MAP) (70–100 mm Hg)

$$\text{MAP} = 1/3\,(\text{Pulse Pressure}) + \text{Diastolic BP (blood pressure)}$$

Where pulse pressure = systolic BP – diastolic BP

Arterial Oxygen Content (CaO$_2$) (18 to 21 mL O$_2$/dL)

$$\text{CaO}_2 = \{1.39 \times [\text{Hb (g/dL)}] \times \text{SaO}_2\} + 0.003 \times \text{PaO}_2$$

Mixed Venous Oxygen Content (CvO$_2$) (14.5 to 15.5 mL O$_2$/dL)

$$\text{CvO}_2 = \{1.39 \times [\text{Hb (g/dL)}] \times \text{SvO}_2\} + 0.003 \times \text{MvO}_2$$

Arterial-Mixed Venous Oxygen Content Difference (3.5 to 5.5 mL O$_2$/dL)

$$\text{avDO}_2 = \text{CaO}_2 - \text{CvO}_2$$

Cardiac Output (CO) (4 to 7 L/min)

1.
$$\text{CO} = \text{heart rate} \times \text{stroke volume}$$

2.
$$\text{CO (Fick principle)} = \frac{\text{Oxygen consumption} \times 10}{\text{CaO}_2 - \text{CvO}_2}$$

Cardiac Index (CI) (2.5 to 4 L/min/m²)

$$CI = CO/BSA$$

Where Body Surface Area (BSA, in m²) $= [\text{height (cm)}]^{0.718} \times [\text{weight (kg)}]^{0.427} \times 0.007449$.

Stroke Volume (SV) (50 to 120 mL per contraction)
Stroke Volume Index (SVI) (35 to 50 mL/m²)

$$SVI = SV/BSA$$

Oxygen Delivery (mL/min) (1000 mL/min)

$$O_2 \text{ delivery} = CO \times CaO_2 \times 10$$

Systemic Vascular Resistance (SVR) (800 to 1200 dyne·s·cm⁻⁵)

$$SVR \text{ (dyne} \cdot s \cdot cm^{-5}) = 80 \times \frac{MAP - CVP}{CO}$$

Pulmonary Vascular Resistance (PVR) (120 to 220 dyne·s·cm⁻⁵)

$$PVR \text{ (dyne} \cdot s \cdot cm^{-5}) = 80 \times \frac{\text{Mean PAP} - PAOP}{CO}$$

Drug–Drug Interactions
Jamie M. Rosini and Scott T. Micek

TABLE 86.1	Cytochrome P450 Enzyme Family Substrates, Inhibitors, and Inducers			
Substrates				
1A2	2C9	2C19	2D6	3A4
Acetaminophen	Celecoxib	Amitriptyline	Amitriptyline	Alprazolam
Cyclobenzaprine	Ibuprofen	Citalopram	Carvedilol	Aripiprazole
Imipramine	Irbesartan	Clopidogrel	Codeine	Buspirone
Haloperidol	Losartan	Cyclophos-	Dextromethor-	Calcium
Mexiletine	Phenytoin	phamide	phan	Channel
Olanzapine	Sulfonylureas	Diazepam	Haloperidol	Blockers
Ondansetron	Torsemide	Imipramine	Imipramine	Carbama-
Theophylline	(S) Warfarin	Phenytoin	Lidocaine	zepine
(R) Warfarin		Proton pump	Metoprolol	Conivaptan
		inhibitors	Metoclopra-	Cyclosporine
			mide	Diazepam
			Mexiletine	Fentanyl
			Ondansetron	Hydrocortisone
			Paroxetine	Lidocaine
			Propafenone	Midazolam
			Propranolol	Protease
			Risperidone	Inhibitors
			Tramadol	Sildenafil
			Venlafaxine	Sirolimus
				Statins (except
				pravastatin)
				Tacrolimus
Inhibitors				
(Increase the serum and tissue concentration of substrates)				
Amiodarone	Amiodarone	Cimetidine	Amiodarone	Amiodarone
Cimetidine	Fluconazole	Fluoxetine	Bupropion	Cimetidine
Ciprofloxacin	Isoniazid	Ketoconazole	Cimetidine	Clarithromycin

(continued)

TABLE 86.1	Cytochrome P450 Enzyme Family Substrates, Inhibitors, and Inducers (*Continued*)

Inhibitors

1A2	2C9	2C19	2D6	3A4
Clarithromycin	Metronidazole Sulfametho- xazole Voriconazole	Lansoprazole Omeprazole Voriconazole	Duloxetine Fluoxetine Haloperidol Paroxetine Methadone Quinidine Ritonavir Sertraline	Conivaptan Diltiazem Erythromycin Itraconazole Ketoconazole Protease Inhibitors Quinupristin- dalfopristin Verapamil Voriconazole

Inducers

(Decrease the serum and tissue concentration of substrates)

Carbamazepine Rifampin Tobacco	Bosentan Phenobar- bital Rifampin	Bosentan Carbamaze- pine Rifampin	Dexametha- sone Rifampin	Bosentan Carbamazepine Glucocorticoids Phenobarbital Phenytoin Rifabutin Rifampin St. John's wort

TABLE 86.2 Frequent Drug–Drug Interactions in Critically Ill Patients

Medication	Interacting drug	Effect[a]
Cardiac		
Amiodarone	2C9, 2D6, 3A4 Substrates (Table 86.1)	↑ Substrate
		↑ Digoxin
	Digoxin	
Beta-blockers (2D6 substrates)	2D6 Inhibitors (Table 86.1)	↑ Beta-blocker
Carvedilol	Carbamazepine	↓ Beta-blocker
Metoprolol	Phenytoin	↓ Beta-blocker
Propranolol	Rifampin	↓ Beta-blocker
Digoxin	Amiodarone	↑ Digoxin
	Clarithromycin	↑ Digoxin
	Erythromycin	↑ Digoxin
	Esomeprazole	↓ Digoxin
	Quinidine	↑ Digoxin
	Verapamil	↑ Digoxin
Diltiazem/verapamil (3A4 inhibitors)	3A4 Substrates (Table 86.1)	↑ Substrate
Lidocaine	Amiodarone	↑ Lidocaine
Antiepileptics		
Carbamazepine (enzyme inducer, 3A4 substrate)	1A2, 2C19, 3A4 Substrates (Table 86.1)	↓ Substrate
		↑ Carbamazepine
	Clarithromycin	↑ Carbamazepine
	Diltiazem	↑ Carbamazepine
	Erythromycin	↑ Carbamazepine
	Quinupristin-dalfopristin	↑ Carbamazepine
	Verapamil	
Oxcarbamazepine	Phenytoin	↑ Phenytoin
	Verapamil	↓ Oxcarbamazepine
Phenytoin (enzyme inducer)	3A4 Substrates (Table 86.1)	↓ Substrate
Antimicrobials		
Azithromycin	Antacids	↓ Azithromycin
	Cyclosporine	↑ Cyclosporine
	Digoxin	↑ Digoxin
	Tacrolimus	↑ Tacrolimus
Carbapenems	Valproic acid	↓ Valproic acid
Clindamycin	Aminoglycosides	↑ Nephrotoxicity
	Erythromycin	↓ Erythromycin
	Neuromuscular blocking agents	↑ Neuromuscular blockade
Ciprofloxacin (1A2 inhibitor)	1A2 Substrates (Table 86.1)	↑ Substrate
	Cyclosporine	↓ Ciprofloxacin
	Sucralfate	↓ Ciprofloxacin
	Calcium, iron, antacids	↓ Oral Ciprofloxacin

(continued)

TABLE 86.2	Frequent Drug–Drug Interactions in Critically Ill Patients (*Continued*)	
Medication	Interacting drug	Effect[a]
Antimicrobials		
Clarithromycin (1A2, 3A4 inhibitor)	1A2, 3A4 Substrates (Table 86.1)	↑ Substrate
	Digoxin	↑ Digoxin
Colistin	Neuromuscular blocking agents	↑ Neuromuscular blockade
Linezolid	SSRIs	↑ Serotonin concentrations
	Tramadol	↑ Linezolid
	Tricyclic antidepressants	↑ Linezolid
Piperacillin-tazobactam	Methotrexate	↑ Methotrexate
Quinupristin-dalfopristin (3A4 inhibitor)	3A4 Substrates (Table 86.1)	↑ Substrate
Vancomycin	NSAIDs	↑ Vancomycin
Antifungals		
Caspofungin	Carbamazepine	↓ Caspofungin
	Cyclosporine	↑ Caspofungin
	Dexamethasone	↓ Caspofungin
	Phenytoin	↓ Caspofungin
	Rifampin	↓ Caspofungin
	Tacrolimus	↓ Tacrolimus
Fluconazole, voriconazole (2C9, 3A4 inhibitor)	2C9, 3A4 Substrates (Table 86.1)	↑ Substrate
Itraconazole	3A4 Substrates (Table 86.1)	↑ Substrate
Ketoconazole (3A4 inhibitor)	Acid suppressants	↓ Oral capsule form itra/ketoconazole
Posaconazole	3A4 Substrates (Table 86.1)	↑ Substrate
	Cimetidine	↓ Posaconazole (avoid concomitant use)
	Phenytoin	↓ Posaconazole (avoid concomitant use)
	Rifabutin	↓ Posaconazole (avoid concomitant use)
Antivirals		
Foscarnet	Ciprofloxacin	↑ Seizures

[a] ↑, increase serum/tissue concentration; ↓, decrease serum/tissue concentration.
SSRIs, selective serotonin reuptake inhibitors; NSAIDs, nonsteroidal anti-inflammatory drugs.

TABLE 86.3 | Drugs Associated with QT-Interval Prolongation[a]

Antiarrhythmic agents
Amiodarone
Disopyramide
Dofetilide
Flecainide
Ibutilide
Procainamide
Propafenone
Quinidine
Sotalol

Antimicrobials
Azithromycin
Clarithromycin
Erythromycin
Telithromycin
Foscarnet
Ciprofloxacin
Levofloxacin
Moxifloxacin
Pentamidine
Azole antifungals

Antidepressants
Amitriptyline
Desipramine
Imipramine
Doxepin
Fluoxetine
Fluoxetine
Sertraline
Venlafaxine

Antipsychotics
Droperidol
Haloperidol
Quetiapine
Risperidone
Thioridazine
Chlorpromazine
Ziprasidone

Other Agents
Dolasetron
Indapamide
Methadone
Octreotide
Tacrolimus
Tizanidine
Tyrosine kinase inhibitors

[a]The combination of these agents may increase the risk for adverse arrhythmic event including torsades de pointes.
From Li EC, Esterly JS, Pohl S, et al. Drug-induced QT-interval prolongation: considerations for clinicians. *Pharmacotherapy.* 2010;30:684–701.

TABLE 86.4	Drugs with Serotonergic Properties[a]

Increased release of serotonin
Amphetamines and derivatives	MAOIs
Cocaine	Mirtazapine
Levodopa	

Inhibition of serotonin metabolism
| Linezolid | Selegiline |
| MAOIs | St. John's wort |

Impaired presynaptic reuptake
Amphetamines and derivatives	SSRIs
Bupropion	St. John's wort
Cocaine	Tramadol
Dextromethorphan	Trazodone
Fentanyl	Tricyclic antidepressants
Meperidine	Venlafaxine
Propoxyphene	

Direct serotonin receptor agonism
| 5-HT1 receptor agonists (i.e., sumatriptan) | Buspirone |
| Lithium | Carbamazepine |

[a]The combination of these agents may increase the risk for serotonin toxicity manifested by a triad of symptoms including: (1) cognitive changes, (2) autonomic instability, and (3) neuromuscular excitability.

MAOIs, monoamine oxidase inhibitors; SSRIs, selective serotonin reuptake inhibitors.

From Taylor JJ, Wilson JW, Estes LL. Linezolid and serotonergic drug interactions: a retrospective survey. *Clin Infect Dis.* 2006;43:180–187, with permission.

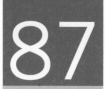

Common Drug Dosages and Side Effects

Lee P. Skrupky and Scott T. Micek

TABLE 87.1	Shock		
Drug class/ prototypes	Dosing	Rare toxicities	Common toxicities
Norepinephrine	0.02–3 μg/kg/min	Tissue hypoxia, tachycardia, arrhythmias, myocardial ischemia, extravasation-associated tissue necrosis	Hyperglycemia
Epinephrine	0.01–0.1 μg/kg/min	Tachycardia, arrhythmias, myocardial ischemia, splanchnic and renal hypoxia, extravasation-associated tissue necrosis	Tachycardia, hyperglycemia
Phenylephrine	0.5–10 μg/kg/min	Bradycardia, reduced cardiac output, myocardial ischemia, extravasation-associated tissue necrosis	—
Dopamine	5–20 μg/kg/min	myocardial ischemia, tissue hypoxia, extravasation-associated tissue necrosis	Tachycardia, arrhythmias

(continued)

Drug class/prototypes	Dosing	Rare toxicities	Common toxicities
TABLE 87.1	**Shock (*Continued*)**		
Vasopressin	0.01–0.04 U/min	Reduced cardiac output, myocardial ischemia, hepatosplanchnic hypoperfusion, thrombocytopenia, hyponatremia, ischemic skin lesions	—
Dobutamine	2.5–20 μg/kg/min	Arrhythmias	Tachycardia
Milrinone	50 μg/kg bolus, then 0.25–0.75 μg/kg/min	Thrombocytopenia, arrhythmias	Hypotension
Corticosteroids Hydrocortisone	Septic Shock: 200–300 mg/day in 3–4 divided doses	—	Short-term: hyperglycemia, mood changes, insomnia, gastrointestinal irritation, increased appetite Long-term: osteoporosis, acne, thin skin, fat redistribution, muscle wasting, cataracts HPA axis suppression, increased blood pressure, infection
Mineralocorticoids Fludrocortisone	Septic shock: 50–100 μg PO q24h	—	Increased blood pressure, edema, hypernatremia, hypokalemia
Drotrecogin alfa	24 μg/kg/hr × 96 hr	—	Bleeding

[a]Toxicities were classified as "rare" and "common" in a relative fashion for each agent. This table does not include an exhaustive list of possible adverse effects.
HPA, hypothalamic-pituitary-adrenal; PO, by mouth; IV, intravenous.

TABLE 87.2	Respiratory Disorders		
Drug class/ prototypes	Dosing	Rare toxicities	Common toxicities
ARDS, status asthmaticus, COPD exacerbation			
Corticosteroids Methylpred-nisolone	1–2 mg/kg/day in 3–4 divided doses, tapering schedule dependant on disease process	—	Short term: hyperglycemia, mood changes, insomnia, gastrointestinal irritation, increased appetite. Long term: osteoporosis, acne, thin skin, fat redistribution, muscle wasting, cataracts, HPA axis suppression, increased blood pressure, infection
Beta-agonists Albuterol Levalbuterol	2–4 puffs BID to QID 0.63–0.125 mg TID	Tachycardia, insomnia, irritability/nervousness, tremor, hyperglycemia, hypokalemia	—
Anticholinergics Ipratropium	2–4 puffs BID to QID	Dry mucous membranes, tachycardia	—
Pulmonary hypertension			
Calcium channel blockers Diltiazem Nifedipine[a]	up to 720 mg/day up to 240 mg/day both in divided doses	Gingival hyperplasia, increased cardiovascular events	Peripheral edema flushing, headache, dizziness, hypotension
Warfarin	Target goal INR	Skin necrosis, purple-toe syndrome	Bleeding
Prostacyclins Epoprostenol	2–50 ng/kg/min IV 5000–20,000 ng/mL continuous nebulization	—	Jaw pain, nausea, headache, flushing, hypotension, infusion-site pain*

(continued)

TABLE 87.2	Respiratory Disorders (*Continued*)		
Drug class/ prototypes	Dosing	Rare toxicities	Common toxicities
Treprostinil*	10–150 ng/kg/min SC		
Iloprost	2.5–5 μg inhaled 6–9 times daily		
Endothelin antagonists		Hepatotoxicity, anemia	Headache, hypotension,
Bosentan	62.5 mg PO bid × 1 month, then 125 mg PO BID, as tolerated	Hepatotoxicity, anemia	flushing Peripheral edema
Ambrisen-tan	5–10 mg PO daily		
PDE-5 inhibitors		Vision changes	Headache, hypotension,
Sildenafil	20–40 mg PO TID		flushing, dyspepsia
Nitric oxide	5–40 parts per million	Methemoglo-binemia, elevated nitrogen dioxide	Hypotension
Pulmonary embolism			
Unfractionated heparin	80 U/kg bolus, then 18 U/kg/hr, adjust to aPTT 1.5–2.5 × control	Type II heparin-induced thrombocy-topenia, hyperkalemia	Bleeding, type I heparin-induced thrombocytopenia bleeding
Alteplase	100 mg IV over 2 hr	—	Bleeding

*a*Immediate-release form.

HPA, hypothalamic-pituitary-adrenal; BID, twice daily; QID, four times a day; INR, international normalized ratio; IV, intravenous; SC, subcutaneously; PO, by mouth.

TABLE 87.3	Cardiac Disorders		
Drug class/ prototypes	Dosing	Rare toxicities	Common toxicities
	Acute myocardial infarction		
Aspirin	160–325 mg PO daily	Tinnitus, anaphylaxis, gastritis	Bleeding, dyspepsia
Beta-blockers		Heart block, bronchospasm, depression, nightmares, altered glucose metabolism, dyslipidemia, sexual dysfunction	Bradycardia, hypotension, fatigue, malaise, cold extremities
Metoprolol	5 mg IV q5min × 3 dose 50–200 mg PO q12h		
Esmolol	500 μg/kg bolus, then 50–300 μg/kg/min		
Nitrates		—	Headache, flushing, dizziness, hypotension, tachycardia
Nitroglycerin	10–200 μg/min		
Isosorbide dinitrate	5–40 mg PO TID		
Isosorbide mononitrate	30–120 mg PO daily		
Morphine	1–4 mg IV q5min	Respiratory depression, hypotension, pruritus	Constipation, dyspepsia, nausea, drowsiness, dizziness
Fibrinolytics	STEMI	—	Bleeding
Alteplase	15 mg bolus, then 0.75 mg/kg (up to 50 mg) × 30 min, then 0.5 mg/kg (up to 35 mg) × 60 min (max, 100 mg over 90 min		
Reteplase	10 mg IV, then 10 mg IV 30 min after first dose		
Tenecteplase	One time bolus: $\leq$60 kg = 30 mg 61–70 kg = 35 mg 71–80 kg = 40 mg 81–90 kg = 45 mg $\geq$90 kg = 50 mg		
Streptokinase	1.5 million units over 2 hr		

(continued)

| TABLE 87.3 | Cardiac Disorders (*Continued*) |

Drug class/ prototypes	Dosing	Rare toxicities	Common toxicities
Unfractionated heparin	60 U/kg bolus, then 12 U/kg/hr, adjust to aPTT 1.5–2.5 × control	Type II heparin-induced thrombocytopenia, hyperkalemia	Bleeding, type I heparininduced thrombocytopenia bleeding
Low-molecular-weight Heparins		—	
Enoxaparin	1 mg/kg SC q12h		
Dalteparin	120 U/kg SC q12h		
Direct thrombin inhibitors	PCI	Hypersensitivity reactions*	Bleeding
Argatroban	350 μg/kg bolus, then 25 μg/kg/min		
Bivalirudin	1 mg/kg bolus, then 2.5 mg/kg/hr		
GPIIb/IIIa inhibitors	PCI:	Thrombocytopenia	Bleeding
Abciximab	0.25 mg/kg bolus, then 0.125 μg/kg/min		
Eptifibatide	180 μg/kg bolus, then 2 μg/kg/min		
Tirofiban	0.4 μg/kg/min × 30 min, then 0.1 μg/kg/min		
Clopidogrel	75 mg PO daily	Thrombotic thrombocytopenic purpura	Nausea, vomiting, diarrhea, bleeding
Arrhythmias and conduction abnormalities			
Atropine	1 mg IV q3–5min	—	Dry eyes, dry mouth, urinary retention, tachycardia
Epinephrine	1 mg IV q3–5min	—	Tachycardia, hypertension
Vasopressin	40 units IV		
Procainamide	15–18 mg/kg bolus then 1–6 mg/min	Torsade de pointes	Diarrhea, nausea, vomiting
Lidocaine	1–1.5 mg/kg bolus (may repeat doses 0.5–0.75 mg/kg in 5–10 min up to max 3 mg/kg), then 1–4 mg/min	Confusion, drowsiness, slurred speech, psychosis, paresthesias, muscle twitching, seizures, bradycardia	—

(*continued*)

TABLE 87.3 | Cardiac Disorders (*Continued*)

Drug class/ prototypes	Dosing	Rare toxicities	Common toxicities
Amiodarone	300 mg bolus, then 1 mg/min for 6 hr, then 0.5 mg/min for ≥18 hr	Heart block, pulmonary fibrosis, hypo/hyperthyroidism, blue-gray skin discoloration, torsade de pointes, corneal microdeposits, optic neuropathy	Bradycardia, hypotension, nausea
Calcium channel blockers Diltiazem	0.25 mg/kg bolus (may repeat 0.35 mg/kg bolus after 15 min), then 5–15 mg/hr	Heart block, heart failure, exacerbation	Bradycardia, hypotension, constipation (verapamil > diltiazem) headache, flushing, edema
Verapamil	5 mg bolus (may repeat up to total 20 mg), then 5–15 mg/hr		
Adenosine	6 mg IV, if not effective in 1–2 min can give 12 mg, may repeat 12 mg	—	Flushing, lightheadedness, headache, nervousness/ anxiety
Congestive heart failure			
Nesiritide	2 μg/kg bolus, then 0.01–0.03 μg/kg/min	—	Hypotension, increased serum creatinine
Digoxin	Load: 10–15 μg/kg; give 50% of load in initial dose, then 25% at 6–12 hr intervals × 2 Maintenance: 0.125–0.5 mg/day (Dose should be reduced by 20%–25% when changing from oral to IV)	Arrhythmias, heart block, visual disturbances (blurred or yellow vision), mental disturbances	Bradycardia
ACE inhibitors Captopril Lisinopril Enalapril Ramipril	6.25–50 mg PO TID 2.5–40 mg PO BID 2.5–10 mg PO BID 1.25–5 mg PO BID	Anaphylaxis, angioedema	Cough, hyperkalemia, hypotension, renal insufficiency

(continued)

TABLE 87.3	Cardiac Disorders (*Continued*)		
Drug class/ prototypes	Dosing	Rare toxicities	Common toxicities
Aldosterone receptor Antagonists		Gynecomastia (spironolactone > eplerenone), hyponatremia	Hyperkalemia
Spironolac- tone	12.5–50 mg PO daily		
Eplerenone	25–50 mg PO daily		
Loop diuretics*a*		Ototoxicity	Hypokalemia, hypomagnesemia, hypocalcemia, orthostatic hypotension, azotemia
Furosemide	20–80 mg/day IV/PO in 2–3 divided doses		
Torsemide	10–20 mg IV/PO daily		
Bumetanide	0.5–2 mg/day in 1–2 doses		
Hypertensive emergencies			
Nitroprusside	Usual, 0.25–3 μg/kg/min Max, 10 μg/kg/min	Muscle spasm	Nausea, vomiting, hypotension, tachycardia, thiocyanate and cyanide toxicity
Nicardipine	3–15 mg/hr	—	Hypotension, tachycardia, headache, flushing, peripheral edema
Labetalol	20–40 mg (max, 80 mg) as IV bolus at 10–20 min intervals, then 0.5–2 mg/min if needed	Heart block, bron- choconstriction	Hypotension, bradycardia, nausea, vomiting
Clonidine	0.1–0.3 mg PO BID–TID	—	Drowsiness, dizziness, hypotension, bradycardia, dry mouth
Hydralazine	10–40 mg IV q4–6h or 10–75 mg PO TID-QID	Drug-induced lupuslike syndrome, rash peripheral neuropathy	Hypotension, tachycardia, flushing, headache
Enalaprilat	1.25–5 mg IV q6h	Anaphylaxis, angioedema	Hypotension, hyperkalemia, renal insufficiency

*a*Usual starting doses are listed for furosemide and torsemide; dosing is highly variable and much larger doses are often used.
PO, by mouth; IV, intravenous; TID, three times a day; STEMI, ST-segment elevation myocardial infarction; aPTT, activated partial thromboplastin time; PCI, percutaneous coronary intervention; BID, twice daily.

TABLE 87.4 | **Electrolyte Abnormalities**

Drug class/ prototypes	Dosing	Rare toxicities	Common toxicities
		Hyponatremia	
Conivaptan	20 mg IV bolus, then 0.8–1.6 mg/hr IV continuous infusion	—	Diarrhea, hypokalemia
		Hyperkalemia	
Regular Humulin insulin	10–20 units IV (given with dextrose, every ~1 unit for 4–5 g dextrose)	Local skin reactions	Hypoglycemia, hypokalemia, weight gain
Sodium bicarbonate	1 mEq/kg IV	Extravasation-associated tissue necrosis	Metabolic alkalosis, hypernatremia, hypokalemia
Albuterol	10–20 mg nebulized over 30–60 min	Tachycardia, insomnia, irritability/ nervousness tremor, hyperglycemia, hypokalemia	—
Calcium gluconate	1 g IV over 2 min	Arrhythmias, phlebitis (chloride > gluconate)	Hypercalcemia, constipation (oral)
		Hypercalcemia	
Bisphosphonates Pamidronate	60–90 mg IV bolus	Thrombophlebitis; bone, joint, muscle pain	Fever, fatigue
Zoledronic acid	4 mg IV bolus		
Calcitonin	Initial 4 U/kg IM q12h, up to 8 U/kg IM q6h	Allergic reaction	Facial flushing, nausea, vomiting
		Hypophosphatemia	
Phosphate salts Potassium phosphate* Sodium phosphate†	0.08–0.16 mmol/kg IV over 6 hr	—	Hyperphosphatemia Hypocalcemia Hypomagnesemia, Hyperkalemia,* hypernatremia,† diarrhea (oral)

IV, intravenously; IM, intramuscularly.

TABLE 87.5	Endocrine Disorders		
Drug class/ prototypes	Dosing	Rare toxicities	Common toxicities
	Hypothyroid		
Thyroid hormones Levothyroxine	Myxedema coma: 50–100 μg IV q6–8h × 24 hr, then 100 μg IV q24h	Signs and symptoms of hyperthyroidism with excessive doses (tachycardia, angina pectoris, arrhythmias, myocardial infarction, heat intolerance, diaphoresis, hyperactivity)	—
	Hyperthyroid		
Thiourea drugs Propylthio-uracil*	Initial 300–600 mg/day in 3 divided doses q8h, main-tenance 50–300 mg per day	Agranulocytosis, aplastic anemia, hepatotoxicity, lupuslike syndrome, hypoprothrombine-mia, polymyositis*	Rash, arthralgias, fever, leukopenia, nausea, vomiting
Methimazole	Initial 30–60 mg/day in 3 divided doses q8h, Maintenance 5–30 mg per day		
Beta-blockers Propranolol	10–40 mg PO q6h	Heart block, bronchospasm, depression, nightmares, altered glucose metabolism, dyslipidemia, sexual dysfunction	Bradycardia, hypotension, fatigue, malaise, cold extremities
SS potassium iodide	1–2 drops PO q12h	Hypersensitivity reactions	Metallic taste, nausea, stomach upset, diarrhea, salivary gland swelling

(continued)

TABLE 87.5	Endocrine Disorders (*Continued*)		
Drug class/ prototypes	Dosing	Rare toxicities	Common toxicities
Adrenal insufficiency			
Corticosteroids Hydrocortisone Dexamethasone	100 mg IV q8h 10 mg IV prior to ACTH stimulation test	—	Short term: hyperglycemia, mood changes, insomnia, gastrointestinal irritation, increased appetite Long term: osteoporosis, acne, thin skin, fat redistribution, muscle wasting, cataracts HPA axis suppression, increased blood pressure, infection
Mineralocorticoids Fludrocortisone	50–200 μg PO q24h	—	Increased blood pressure, edema, hypernatremia, hypokalemia
Insulin	—	Local skin reactions	Hypoglycemia, hypokalemia, weight gain

IV, intravenous; PO, by mouth; ACTH, adrenocorticotropin hormone; HPA, hypothalamic-pituitary-adrenal; PRN, as needed; NSAIDs, nonsteroidal anti-inflammatory drugs; TID, three times a day.

TABLE 87.6	Oncologic Emergencies		
Drug class/ prototypes	Dosing	Rare toxicities	Common toxicities
Allopurinol	600–800 mg/day in 2–3 divided doses	Nausea, vomiting	Rash
Rasburicase	0.2 mg/kg/day	Hypersensitivity reactions, methemoglobinemia, hemolysis	Nausea, vomiting, fever, headache, rash, diarrhea, constipation

IV, intravenous; PO, by mouth; ACTH, adrenocorticotropin hormone; HPA, hypothalamic-pituitary-adrenal; PRN, as needed; NSAIDs, nonsteroidal anti-inflammatory drugs; TID, three times a day.

TABLE 87.7	Temperature Regulation		
Drug class/ prototypes	Dosing	Rare toxicities	Common toxicities
Acetaminophen	325–1000 mg PO q4–6h PRN	Hepatotoxicity	—
NSAIDs		Gastric ulceration, bleeding, acute renal failure, increased risk of cardiovascular events	Gastric irritation, nausea
Ibuprofen	200–800 mg PO q3–6h PRN		
Ketorolac	15–30 mg IM or 10 mg PO PRN		
Dantrolene	1–2.5 mg/kg IV; may repeat q5–10 min to max cumulative dose 10 mg/kg	Hepatotoxicity, muscle weakness	Drowsiness, dizziness, diarrhea, nausea, vomiting
Bromocriptine	2.5–5 mg PO TID	—	Headache, dizziness, nausea, diarrhea, hypotension, nasal congestion

IV, intravenous; PO, by mouth; ACTH, adrenocorticotropin hormone; HPA, hypothalamic-pituitary-adrenal; PRN, as needed; NSAIDs, nonsteroidal anti-inflammatory drugs; TID, three times a day.

TABLE 87.8	Toxicology		
Drug class/ prototypes	Dosing	Rare toxicities	Common toxicities
Activated charcoal	25–100 g	Bowel obstruction	Vomiting, constipation, fecal discoloration (black)
Naloxone	0.4–2 mg IV q2min, up to 10 mg	Abrupt reversal may cause withdrawal symptoms (sweating, agitation, hypertension, tachycardia, nausea, vomiting, cardiovascular events, seizures) pulmonary edema	—
Flumazenil	0.2–0.5 mg IV q1min, up to 5 mg	Abrupt reversal may cause withdrawal symptoms (sweating, agitation, hypertension, tachycardia, nausea, vomiting, cardiovascular events, seizures)	—
N-Acetylcysteine	Oral 140 mg/kg loading dose, then 70 mg/kg q4h × 17 doses IV 150 mg/kg bolus, then 12.5 mg/kg/hr × 4 hr, then 6.25 mg/kg/hr × 16 hr	Anaphylactic reactions	Nausea, vomiting (oral), unpleasant odor (oral)

(continued)

TABLE 87.8	Toxicology (*Continued*)		
Drug class/ prototypes	Dosing	Rare toxicities	Common toxicities
Deferoxamine	1 g IV bolus, then 500 mg IV q4h × 2 doses	Infusion-related reactions (hypotension, tachycardia, erythema, urticaria) anaphylactic reactions acute respiratory distress syndrome	Urine discoloration (orange-red)
Fomepizole	15 mg/kg IV bolus, then 10 mg/kg IV q12h × 4 doses, then 15 mg/kg IV q12h until ethylene glycol or methanol level <20	—	—

IV, intravenous.

TABLE 87.9	Infectious Diseases		
Drug class/ prototypes	Dosing	Rare toxicities	Common toxicities
Antibacterial agents			
Penicillins Ampicillin Aqueous penicillin G	2–3 g IV q4–6h 2–4 million U IV q4h	Anaphylaxis, seizures, hemolytic anemia, neutropenia, thrombocytope- nia, drug fever	Diarrhea, nausea, vomiting, rash
Antistaphylococcal Penicillins Nafcillin Oxacillin	2 g IV q4–6h 2 g IV q4–6h	Anaphylaxis, neutropenia, thrombocytope- nia, acute interstitial nephritis, hepatotoxicity	Diarrhea, nausea, vomiting, rash
B-lactam/ B-lactamase Inhibitors Amoxicillin/ clavulanate Ampicillin/ sulbactam	875 mg PO BID 1.5–3 g IV q6h	Anaphylaxis, seizures, hemolytic anemia, neutropenia, thrombocytope- nia, *Clostridium difficile* colitis, cholestatic jaundice,* drug fever	Diarrhea, nausea, vomiting, rash
Piperacillin/ Tazobactam* Ticarcillin/ clavulanate	3.375–4.5 g IV q6h 3.1 g IV q4–6h		
Cephalosporins Cefazolin Cefoxitin Ceftriaxone Cefepime	1–2 g IV q8h 1–2 g IV q4–8h 1–2 g IV q12–24h 500 mg–2 g IV q8–12h	Anaphylaxis, seizures, neutropenia, thrombocytope- nia, drug fever	Diarrhea, nausea, vomiting, rash
Carbapenems Imipenem Meropenem Ertapenem Doripenem	500 mg–1 g IV q6–8h 1 g IV q8h 1 g IV q24h 500 mg IV q8h	Anaphylaxis, seizures (imipenem> meropenem> ertapenem), *C. difficile* colitis, drug fever	Diarrhea, nausea, vomiting

(continued)

TABLE 87.9	Infectious Diseases (*Continued*)		
Drug class/ prototypes	Dosing	Rare toxicities	Common toxicities
Glycopeptides Vancomycin	15 mg/kg IV q12h	Ototoxicity, nephrotoxicity, Red-man syndrome (unlikely without concomitant nephrotoxins), thrombocytopenia	
Telavancin	7.5 mg/kg IV q24h	Nephrotoxicity, QTc prolongation, nausea, vomiting, taste sense altered	
Oxazolidinones Linezolid	600 mg IV/PO q12h	More common with long-term use: peripheral and optic neuropathy, myelosuppression Possible with short-term use: lactic acidosis	Diarrhea
Lipopeptides Daptomycin	4–6 mg/kg IV q24h	Myopathy, anemia	Diarrhea, constipation, vomiting
Streptogramin Quinupristin/ dalfopristin	7.5 mg/kg IV q8h	—	Arthralgia, myalgia, inflammation, pain, edema at infusion site, hyperbiliru-binemia
Aminoglycosides Amikacin	— 8 mg/kg IV q12h or 15 mg/kg extended interval	— —	Nephrotoxicity Ototoxicity
Gentamicin	3 mg/kg bolus, then 2 mg/kg IV q8h or 5–7 mg/kg extended interval		
Tobramycin	See gentamicin		

(*continued*)

TABLE 87.9	Infectious Diseases (*Continued*)		
Drug class/ prototypes	Dosing	Rare toxicities	Common toxicities
Fluoroquinolones Ciprofloxacin	500–750 mg PO BID or 400 mg IV q8–12h	Anaphylaxis, QTc prolongation, joint toxicity in children, tendon rupture	Nausea, vomiting, diarrhea, photosensitivity, rash
Levofloxacin	500–750 mg IV/PO q24h		CNS stimulation, dizziness, somnolence
Moxifloxacin	400 mg IV/PO q24h		
Macrolides Erythromycin*	250–500 mg PO qid or 0.5–1 g IV q6h	QTc prolongation (erythromycin > clarithromycin > azithromycin), cholestasis*	Nausea, vomiting, diarrhea, abnormal taste
Azithromycin	250–500 mg IV/PO daily		
Clarithromycin	250–500 mg PO BID		
Ketolides Telithromycin	800 mg PO q24h	Acute hepatic failure, QTc prolongation, Exacerbations of myasthenia gravis	Nausea, vomiting, diarrhea
Clindamycin	600–900 mg IV q8h	*C. difficile* colitis	Nausea, vomiting, diarrhea, abdominal pain, rash
Tetracyclines Tetracycline*	250–500 mg PO q6h	Tooth discoloration and retardation of bone growth (in children), renal tubular necrosis,* dizziness,† vertigo,† pseudotumor cerebri	Photosensitivity, diarrhea
Doxycycline	100 mg IV/PO q12h		
Minocycline†	200 mg PO, then 100 mg PO q12h		
Glycylcyclines Tigecycline	100 mg bolus, then 50 mg IV q12h	—	Nausea, vomiting, diarrhea

(*continued*)

TABLE 87.9 | Infectious Diseases (*Continued*)

Drug class/ prototypes	Dosing	Rare toxicities	Common toxicities
Trimethoprim/ sulfamethoxazole	5 mg/kg IV q8h (based on the trimethoprim component)	Myelosuppression, Stevens–Johnson syndrome, hyperkalemia, aseptic meningitis, hepatic necrosis	Rash, nausea, vomiting, diarrhea
Metronidazole	500 mg IV/PO q8h	Seizures, peripheral neuropathy	Nausea, vomiting, metallic taste, disulfiram-like reaction
Antifungal agents			
Azoles		Hepatic failure, increased AST/ALT, cardiovascular toxicity,* hypertension,* edema,* QTc prolongation	Nausea, vomiting, diarrhea rash, visual disturbances,[†] phototoxicity[†]
Fluconazole	100–800 mg PO/IV daily		
Itraconazole*	200 mg IV/PO q24h		
Voriconazole[†]	4 mg/kg IV q12h or 200 mg PO BID		
Posaconazole	200–400 mg PO TID-BID		
Amphotericin B products		Nephrotoxicity (less common with lipid formulations), acute liver failure, myelosuppression	Acute infusion-related reactions, hypokalemia, hypomagne-semia
Amphotericin B deoxycholate	0.3–1.5 mg/kg q24h		
ABLC	5 mg/kg IV q24h		
ABCD	3–4 mg/kg IV q24h		
Liposomal amphotericin B	3–5 mg/kg IV q24h		
Echinocandins		Hepatotoxicity, infusion-related rash, flushing, itching	—
Caspofungin	70 mg IV bolus, then 50 mg IV q24h		
Micafungin	50–150 mg IV q24h		
Anidulafungin	200 mg IV bolus, then 100 mg IV q24h		
Flucytosine	25–37.5 mg/kg PO q6h	Myelosuppression, hepatotoxicity, confusion, hallucinations, sedation	Nausea, vomiting, diarrhea, rash

(*continued*)

TABLE 87.9	Infectious Diseases (*Continued*)		
Drug class/ prototypes	Dosing	Rare toxicities	Common toxicities
Antiviral agents			
Nucleoside analogs		Nephrotoxicity, rash, encephalopathy, inflammation at injection site phlebitis	Bone marrow suppression,[†] headache, nausea, vomiting, diarrhea (with oral forms)
Acyclovir	400 mg PO TID or 5 mg/kg IV q8h		
Valacyclovir[†]	1000 mg PO q8h		
Ganciclovir[†]	5 mg/kg IV q12h		
Valganci- clovir	900 mg PO daily–BID		
Amantadine	100 mg PO BID	CNS disturbances (amantadine > rimantadine)	Nausea, vomiting, anorexia, xerostomia
Rimantadine	100 mg PO BID		
Neuraminidase inhibitors		Anaphylaxis,* bronchospasm,[†]	Nausea, vomiting,* cough,[†] local discomfort[†]
Oseltamivir*	75 mg PO BID		
Zanamivir[†]	10 mg inhaled q12h		
Cidofovir	5 mg/kg IV weekly plus probenecid 2 g PO 3 hr before the infusion and then 1 g at 2 and 8 hr after the infusion	Anemia, neutropenia, fever, rash	Nephrotoxicity, uveitis/iritis, nausea, vomiting
Foscarnet	60 mg/kg IV q8h or 90 mg/kg IV q12h	Seizures, anemia, fever	Nephrotoxicity, electrolyte abnormalities (hypocalcemia, hypomagne- semia, hypokalemia, hypophos- phatemia), nausea, vomiting, diarrhea, headache

IV, intravenous; PO, by mouth; BID, two times a day; AST/ALT, alanine aminotransferase/aspartate aminotransferase; TID, three times a day.

TABLE 87.10	Hepatic Disorders		
Drug class/ prototypes	Dosing	Rare toxicities	Common toxicities
Lactulose	20–30 g (30–45 mL) PO q2h until initial stool, then adjust to maintain 2–3 soft stools/day	—	Diarrhea, flatulence, nausea
Neomycin	500–2000 mg PO q6–12h	Nephrotoxicity, neurotoxicity	Nausea, vomiting, diarrhea, irritation or soreness of mouth or rectal area
Rifaximin	400 mg PO TID		Headache
Nonspecific Beta-Blockers		Heart block, bronchospasm, depression, nightmares, altered glucose metabolism, dyslipidemia, sexual dysfunction	Bradycardia, hypotension, fatigue, malaise, cold extremities
Propranolol	20–80 mg PO q12h		
Nadolol	20–80 mg PO q24h		
Spironolactone	12.5–100 mg PO q24h	Gynecomastia, hyponatremia	Hyperkalemia

PO, by mouth.

TABLE 87.11 Gastrointestinal Disorders

Drug class/ prototypes	Dosing	Rare toxicities	Common toxicities
Proton pump inhibitors Pantoprazole	20–40 mg PO q12–24h 80 mg IV bolus, then 8 mg/hr × 72 hr	Headache, dizziness, somnolence, diarrhea, constipation, nausea	—
Omeprazole	20–40 mg PO q12–24h		
Lansoprazole	30–60 mg PO q12–24h		
Esomeprazole	20–40 mg PO q24h		
Octreotide	25–50 μg IV bolus, then 25–50 μg/hr infusion	Arrhythmias, conduction abnormalities, hypothyroidism, cholelithiasis (long-term use)	Diarrhea, flatulence, nausea, abdominal cramps, bradycardia, dysglycemia

PO, by mouth; IV, intravenous.

TABLE 87.12	Neurologic Disorders		
Drug class/ prototypes	Dosing	Rare toxicities	Common toxicities
Status epilepticus			
Benzodiazepines		Paradoxical excitation, hypotension, respiratory depression (high doses)	CNS depression
Lorazepam	0.1 mg/kg at 2 mg/min up to 8 mg		
Midazolam	0.2 mg/kg bolus, then 0.75–10 μg/kg/min		
Phenytoin	20 mg/kg IV bolus, then 5–7 mg/kg day	Idiosyncratic: rash, fever, bone marrow suppression, Steven-Johnson syndrome, hepatitis	Concentration-dependent: nystagmus, diplopia, ataxia, sedation, lethargy, mood/behavior changes, coma, seizures
Fosphenytoin	20 mg phenytoin equivalents/kg IV/IM bolus	Associated with chronic use: gingival hyperplasia, folic acid deficiency, hirsutism, acne, vitamin D deficiency, osteomalacia	IV form: hypotension, bradycardia, phlebitis
Phenobarbital	20 mg/kg IV bolus	Rash, bone marrow suppression	Sedation, nystagmus, ataxia, nausea, vomiting IV form: hypotension, bradycardia, respiratory depression
Propofol	30–250 μg/kg/min	Pancreatitis, propofol infusion syndrome	Hypotension, bradycardia, CNS depression, hyper-triglyceridemia
Levetiracetam	500–1000 mg IV/PO q12h	Behavioral disturbances	Somnolence, nausea, vomiting

(continued)

TABLE 87.12	Neurologic Disorders (*Continued*)		
Drug class/ prototypes	Dosing	Rare toxicities	Common toxicities
Valproate	1000–2500 mg/day IV/PO in 2–4 divided doses	Hepatotoxicity, pancreatitis, thrombocy-topenia, hyper-ammonemia, rash	Somnolence, diplopia nausea, vomiting, diarrhea
Intracranial pressure elevation			
Hypertonic saline (23.4% NaCl)	For mannitol-refractory patients: 30–50 mL q3–6h as needed (central line only) 0.686 mL of 23.4% saline is equiosmolar to 1 g of mannitol	—	Hypernatremia, hyperchloremia
Mannitol	1–1.5 g/kg IV bolus, then 0.25–1 g/kg q3–6h as needed	—	Hypotension, acute renal failure, fluid and electrolyte imbalances
Stroke			
Alteplase	Ischemic stroke: 0.9 mg/kg IV (NOT to exceed 90 mg), infused over 60 min with 10% of the dose given as an initial bolus over 1 min	—	Bleeding
Factor VII	Hemorrhagic stroke: 1.2–4.8 mg IV	Thrombosis	Hypertension

(*continued*)

TABLE 87.12	Neurologic Disorders (*Continued*)		
Drug class/ prototypes	Dosing	Rare toxicities	Common toxicities
ICU delirium			
Haloperidol	2–80 mg IV/PO q6h	QTc prolongation, extrapyramidal side effects (dystonia, akathisia, pseudoparkin-sonism, tardive dyskinesia), neuroleptic malignant syndrome	CNS depression, orthostatic hypotension
ICU sedation			
Benzodiazepines Lorazepam	2–4 mg bolus, 0.5–4 mg/hr	Paradoxical excitation, hypotension, respiratory depression (high doses)	CNS depression
Midazolam	1–5 mg bolus, 1–10 mg/hr		
Propofol	25–100 μg/kg/min	Pancreatitis, propofol infusion syndrome	Hypotension, bradycardia, CNS depression, hyper-triglyceridemia
Dexmedeto-midine	0.2–1.5 μg/kg/hr	—	Hypotension, bradycardia

IV, intravenous; IM, intramuscular; PO, by mouth; ICU, intensive care unit.

TABLE 87.13	Hematopoietic Disorders		
Drug class/ prototypes	Dosing	Rare toxicities	Common toxicities
Direct thrombin inhibitors Lepirudin*	Initial 0.1–0.15 mg/kg/hr infusion, adjust based on aPTT measurements	Allergic reactions*	Bleeding
Argatroban	Initial 2 μg/kg/min, adjust based on aPTT measurements		
DDAVP	0.3 μg/kg slow IV	Hyponatremia, hypotension, tachycardia, thrombosis	Facial flushing
Phytonadione (vitamin K)	1–10 mg q24h Can be given PO, SQ, or IV	IV form: anaphylaxis, hypotension	—
Warfarin	Initial 1–5 mg/day, adjust based on INR measurements	Skin necrosis, purple-toe syndrome	Bleeding

aPTT, activated partial thromboplastin time; IV, intravenous; PO, by mouth; SQ, subcutaneous; INR, international normalized ratio.

TABLE 87.14	Pregnancy[a]		
Drug class/ prototypes	Dosing	Rare toxicities	Common toxicities
Magnesium	4–6 g IV over 15–20 min, then 2 g/hr infusion	—	
Phenytoin	20 mg/kg IV bolus, then 5–7 mg/kg day	Idiosyncratic: rash, fever, bone marrow suppression, Steven-Johnson syndrome, hepatitis Associated with chronic use: gingival hyperplasia, folic acid deficiency, hirsutism, acne, vitamin D deficiency, osteomalacia	
Labetalol	100–800 mg PO q8–12h, max 2.4 g/day	Heart block, bronchoconstriction drug-induced lupuslike syndrome, rash, peripheral neuropathy	Hypotension, bradycardia, nausea, vomiting,
Hydralazine	10–40 mg IV q4–6h or 10–75 mg PO TID–QID		hypotension, tachycardia, flushing, headache

IV, intravenous; PO, by mouth; TID, three times a day; QID, four times a day.

Index

Note: Page numbers followed by *f* indicate figures; page numbers followed by *t* indicate tables; page numbers followed by *a* indicate algorithms; page numbers followed by *b* indicate boxes.